Medical Terminology

FOR HEALTH CARE PROFESSIONALS

NINTH EDITION

Jane Rice, RN, CMA-C

Medical Assisting Program Director, Retired
Georgia Northwestern Technical College
Rome, Georgia

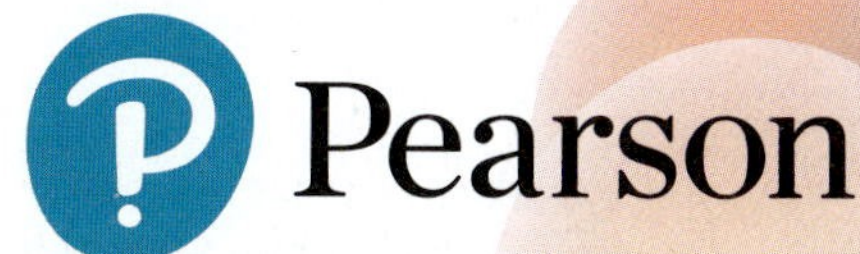

330 Hudson Street, NY NY 10013

DEDICATION

In special memory of my parents, Warren Galileo and Elizabeth Styles Justice, and my sister, Betty Sue Nelson

Publisher: Julie Levin Alexander
Assistant to Publisher: Sarah Henrich
Director, Portfolio Management: Marlene McHugh Pratt
Executive Portfolio Manager: John Goucher
Managing Content Producer: Nicole Ragonese
Portfolio Management Assistant: Erica Viviani
Development Editor: Lynda Hatch
Director of Marketing: David Gesell
Executive Marketing Manager: Brittany Hammond
Media Program Manager: Amy Peltier
Media Project Manager: William Johnson
Production Editor: Patty Donovan, SPi Global
Operations Specialist: Mary Ann Gloriande
Senior Art Director: Mary Siener
Cover Designer: Laurie Entringer
Composition: SPi Global
Printer/Binder: LSC Communications/Kendallville
Cover Printer: Lehigh-Phoenix Color/Hagerstown
Cover Image: Pasieka/Science Photo Library/Getty Images

Credits and acknowledgments borrowed from other sources and reproduced, with permission, in this textbook appear on the appropriate page within text.

Library of Congress Cataloging-in-Publication Data

Names: Rice, Jane, author.
Title: Medical terminology for health care professionals / Jane Rice.
Description: 9th edition. | Hoboken, New Jersey : Pearson Education, Inc., 2016.
Identifiers: LCCN 2016042119 | ISBN 9780134495347 | ISBN 0134495349
ISubjects: | MESH: Medicine | Anatomy | Terminology as Topic | Terminology
Classification: LCC R123 | NLM W 15 | DDC 610.1/4—dc23 LC record available at https://lccn.loc.gov/2016042119

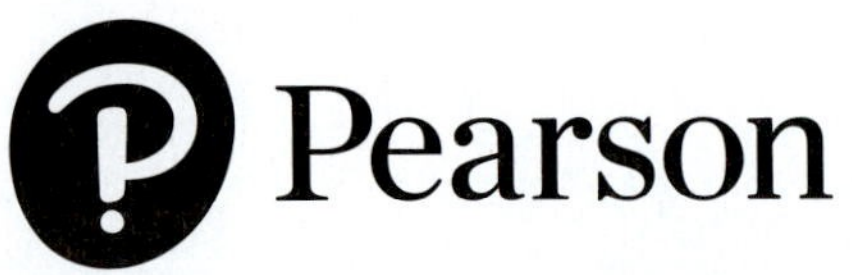

4 17
ISBN-13: 978-0-13-449534-7
ISBN-10: 0-13-449534-9

CONTENTS IN BRIEF

PREFACE

The ease with which students learn component parts directly associated with a body system or specialty area is the key to the time-proven approach found in *Medical Terminology for Health Care Professionals*, now in its ninth edition. Suffixes and prefixes are presented in Chapters 2 and 3, and reinforced throughout the text as they become integrated with combining forms and roots to form the medical words of the featured body system or specialty area.

The text's strengths include:

1. **A word-building approach.** Learn medical terminology by building medical terms from commonly used word parts. **Combining Forms Tables** with meanings are included in the **Building Your Medical Vocabulary** sections in each body system chapter. This makes it easier and faster for students to learn the foundations of key terms pertaining to each system.
2. **The Rice Method.** The Building Your Medical Vocabulary sections present all words in alphabetical order. This format shows those terms with the same prefix, word root, and/or combining form together, thereby reinforcing the ease of learning medical terminology using the Rice approach.
3. **Accurate and complete coverage of human anatomy.** Presents concise coverage of all major body structures and functions, organized by body system.
4. **Study and Review** sections include the following:
   - ***Study and Review I*** covers all questions relating to the anatomy and physiology of the chapter and includes an anatomy labeling exercise.
   - ***Study and Review II*** covers word parts, identifying medical terms, and matching exercises. It includes exercises for **Medical Case Snapshots**, case study vignettes that provide an opportunity to relate the medical terminology to a precise patient care presentation.
   - ***Study and Review III*** consists of an array of learning exercises, such as *Building Medical Terms*, *Combining Form Challenge*, and *Select the Right Term*. Also included in this section are the questions relating to *Diagnostic and Laboratory Tests*, *Abbreviations*, and the *Practical Application* exercise.
   - ***Practical Application*** exercises include a variety of medical record analyses and ICD-10-CM terminology questions.
5. **Visually appealing with new art and photos.**

The ninth edition builds upon this framework and presents an exciting blend of fresh ideas merged with proven methods.

A Special Feature New to this Edition: Insights

A Note from the Author

Insights is a new feature that brings to light some of the latest medical coding terminology being used in *The Complete Official Codebook ICD-10-CM, 2016*. When planning the revision of this text many peer reviewers and instructors gave valuable input. One subject kept coming up, the ICD-10-CM, which had recently been revised and is now being used in all United States healthcare treatment settings. I found the concept of updating the terminology of my book to correspond with the ICD-10-CM compelling. The addition of coding information and terminology from the ICD-10-CM in the **Insights** feature will be extraordinarily helpful to many of the students who desire a career in healthcare. I believe that this new feature is so distinctive and helpful that it sets apart this terminology book from others. —*Jane Rice*

Features At A Glance

Here is a sneak peek at what makes *Medical Terminology for Health Care Professionals* so dynamic and trusted as a learning resource.

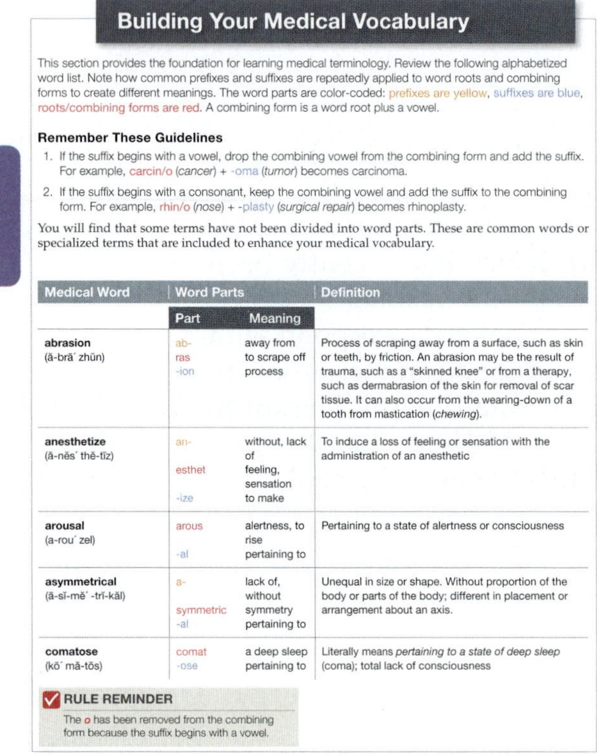

Building Your Medical Vocabulary

This section provides the foundation for learning medical terminology. Review the following alphabetized word list. Note how common prefixes and suffixes are repeatedly applied to word roots and combining forms to create different meanings. The word parts are color-coded: prefixes are yellow, suffixes are blue, roots/combining forms are red. A combining form is a word root plus a vowel.

Remember These Guidelines

1. If the suffix begins with a vowel, drop the combining vowel from the combining form and add the suffix. For example, carcin/o (*cancer*) + -oma (*tumor*) becomes carcinoma.
2. If the suffix begins with a consonant, keep the combining vowel and add the suffix to the combining form. For example, rhin/o (*nose*) + -plasty (*surgical repair*) becomes rhinoplasty.

You will find that some terms have not been divided into word parts. These are common words or specialized terms that are included to enhance your medical vocabulary.

Medical Word	Word Parts		Definition
	Part	Meaning	
abrasion (ă-brā´ zhŭn)	ab- ras -ion	away from to scrape off process	Process of scraping away from a surface, such as skin or teeth, by friction. An abrasion may be the result of trauma, such as a "skinned knee" or from a therapy, such as dermabrasion of the skin for removal of scar tissue. It can also occur from the wearing-down of a tooth from mastication (*chewing*).
anesthetize (ă-nĕs´ thĕ-tīz)	an- esthet -ize	without, lack of feeling, sensation to make	To induce a loss of feeling or sensation with the administration of an anesthetic
arousal (a-rou´ zel)	arous -al	alertness, to rise pertaining to	Pertaining to a state of alertness or consciousness
asymmetrical (ā-sĭ-mĕ´ -trĭ-kăl)	a- symmetric -al	lack of, without symmetry pertaining to	Unequal in size or shape. Without proportion of the body or parts of the body; different in placement or arrangement about an axis.
comatose (kō´ mă-tōs)	comat -ose	a deep sleep pertaining to	Literally means *pertaining to a state of deep sleep* (coma); total lack of consciousness

RULE REMINDER

The *o* has been removed from the combining form because the suffix begins with a vowel.

- **Building Your Medical Vocabulary—**The heart of every chapter, this section is an alphabetized word list that shows how word parts are built, pronounced, and defined. The word parts are color-coded with prefixes in yellow, roots and combining forms in red, and suffixes in blue. Also included is a table of combining forms with definitions.

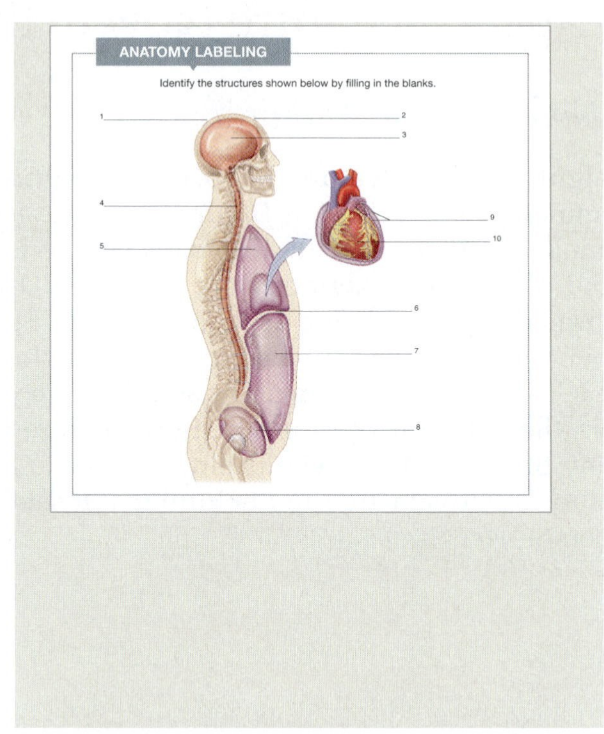

- **Designed for Visual Learners—**Most pages are highlighted by a vibrant and instructive image. Examples include anatomically precise diagrams, authentic medical photographs, and engaging labeling activities.

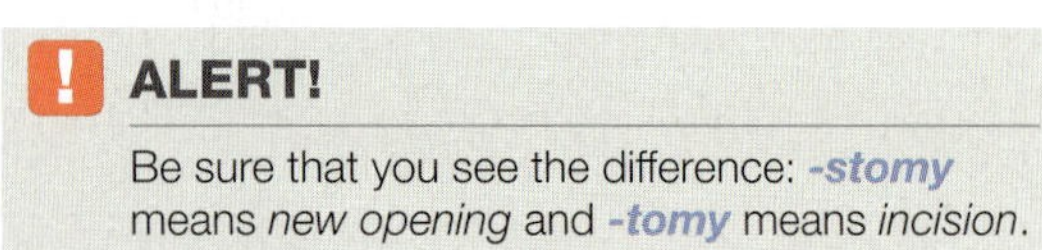

ALERT!

Be sure that you see the difference: ***-stomy*** means *new opening* and ***-tomy*** means *incision*.

- **ALERT!—**Offers singular to plural spelling and other tips.

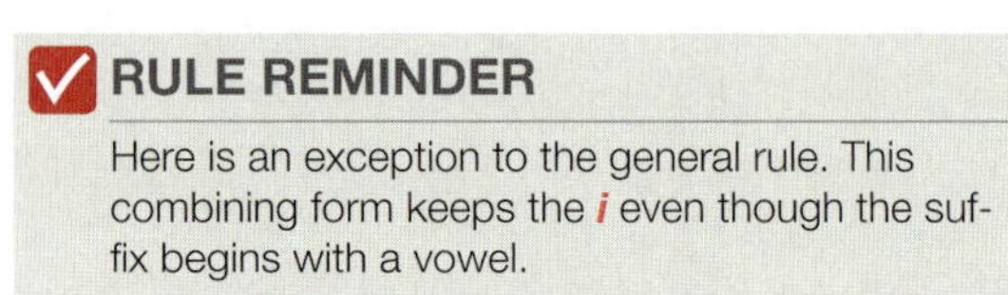

RULE REMINDER

Here is an exception to the general rule. This combining form keeps the ***i*** even though the suffix begins with a vowel.

- **Rule Reminder—**Reinforces the rules that govern medical terminology.

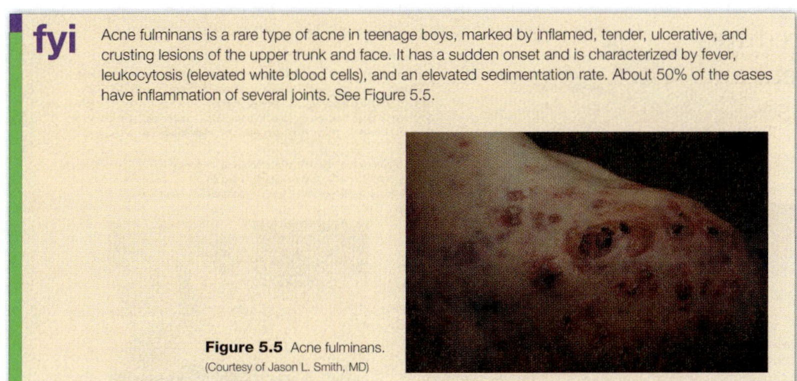

fyi Acne fulminans is a rare type of acne in teenage boys, marked by inflamed, tender, ulcerative, and crusting lesions of the upper trunk and face. It has a sudden onset and is characterized by fever, leukocytosis (elevated white blood cells), and an elevated sedimentation rate. About 50% of the cases have inflammation of several joints. See Figure 5.5.

Figure 5.5 Acne fulminans.
(Courtesy of Jason L. Smith, MD)

- **FYI—**Contains interesting medical information to broaden knowledge and pique interest.

- **INSIGHTS—**Familiarizes the reader with some of the latest coding terminology being used in *The Complete Official Codebook ICD-10-CM, 2016.*

insights *Laterality* (side of the body affected) is a new coding convention added to relevant ICD-10-CM codes to increase specificity. Designated codes for conditions such as fractures, burns, ulcers, and certain neoplasms will require documentation of the side/region of the body where the condition occurs. In ICD-10-CM, laterality code descriptions include right, left, bilateral, or unspecified designations. Over one-third of the expansion of ICD-10-CM codes is due to the addition of laterality.

Example:

Physician office documentation: "patient complains of hearing loss (right); large right cerumen impaction"
ICD-10-CM code: H61.21—impacted cerumen, right ear

Drug Highlights

Type of Drug	Description and Examples
emollients	Substances that are generally oily in nature. These substances are used for dry skin caused by aging, excessive bathing, and psoriasis. EXAMPLE: Desitin
keratolytics	Agents that cause or promote loosening of horny (keratin) layers of the skin. These agents may be used for acne, warts, psoriasis, corns, calluses (hardened skin), and fungal infections. EXAMPLES: Duofilm, Keralyt, and Compound W
local anesthetic agents	Agents that inhibit the conduction of nerve impulses from sensory nerves and thereby reduce pain and discomfort. These agents may be used topically to reduce discomfort associated with insect bites, burns, and poison ivy. EXAMPLES: Solarcaine and Xylocaine
antihistamine agents	Agents that act to prevent the action of histamine. Used to help relieve symptoms, such as itching, in allergic responses and contact dermatitis. EXAMPLE: Benadryl (diphenhydramine)
antipruritic agents	Agents that prevent or relieve itching EXAMPLES: Topical—tripelennamine HCl; Oral—Benadryl (diphenhydramine HCl) and hydroxyzine HCl
antibiotic agents	Agents that destroy or stop the growth of microorganisms. These agents are used to prevent infection associated with minor skin abrasions and to treat superficial skin infections and acne. Several antibiotic agents are combined in a single product to take advantage of the different antimicrobial spectrum of each drug. EXAMPLES: Neosporin, Polysporin, and Mycitracin
antifungal agents	Agents that destroy or inhibit the growth of fungi and yeast. These agents are used to treat fungus and/or yeast infection of the skin, nails, and scalp. EXAMPLES: Equate antifungal cream (clotrimazole) and Lamisil (terbinafine)
antiviral agents	Agents that combat specific viral diseases. EXAMPLE: Zovirax (acyclovir) is used in the treatment of herpes simplex virus types 1 and 2, varicella zoster, Epstein–Barr, and cytomegalovirus
anti-inflammatory agents	Agents used to relieve the swelling, tenderness, redness, and pain of inflammation. Topically applied corticosteroids are used in the treatment of dermatitis and psoriasis. EXAMPLES: Carmol HC (hydrocortisone acetate; urea) and Temovate (clobetasol propionate) Oral corticosteroids are used in the treatment of contact dermatitis, such as in poison ivy, when the symptoms are severe. EXAMPLE: prednisone 12-day unipak

- **Drug Highlights—**Presents essential pharmacology information that relates to the subject of the chapter. The trade names of drugs and their availability were verified at the time of this text's publication, in order to provide the most up-to-date information possible.

- **Diagnostic and Laboratory Tests—**Provides an overview of current tests and procedures that are used in the physical assessment and diagnosis of certain conditions/diseases.

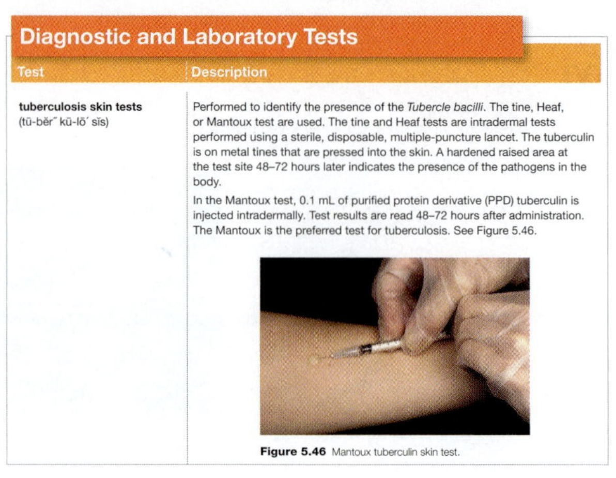

Diagnostic and Laboratory Tests

Test	Description
tuberculosis skin tests (tū-bĕr″ kū-lō′ sĭs)	Performed to identify the presence of the *Tubercle bacilli*. The tine, Heaf, or Mantoux test are used. The tine and Heaf tests are intradermal tests performed using a sterile, disposable, multiple-puncture lancet. The tuberculin is on metal tines that are pressed into the skin. A hardened raised area at the test site 48–72 hours later indicates the presence of the pathogens in the body. In the Mantoux test, 0.1 mL of purified protein derivative (PPD) tuberculin is injected intradermally. Test results are read 48–72 hours after administration. The Mantoux is the preferred test for tuberculosis. See Figure 5.46.

Figure 5.46 Mantoux tuberculin skin test.

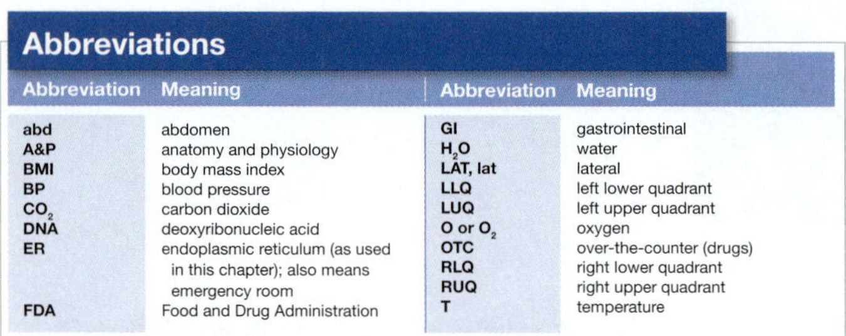

Abbreviations

Abbreviation	Meaning	Abbreviation	Meaning
abd	abdomen	GI	gastrointestinal
A&P	anatomy and physiology	H_2O	water
BMI	body mass index	LAT, lat	lateral
BP	blood pressure	LLQ	left lower quadrant
CO_2	carbon dioxide	LUQ	left upper quadrant
DNA	deoxyribonucleic acid	O or O_2	oxygen
ER	endoplasmic reticulum (as used in this chapter); also means emergency room	OTC	over-the-counter (drugs)
		RLQ	right lower quadrant
		RUQ	right upper quadrant
FDA	Food and Drug Administration	T	temperature

- **Abbreviations—**Provides commonly used abbreviations with their meanings in an at-a-glance table format. These abbreviations are specific to each chapter's content.

- **Practical Application—**Real-world medical practice sections that challenge readers to apply their understanding of each chapter while interacting with medical records.

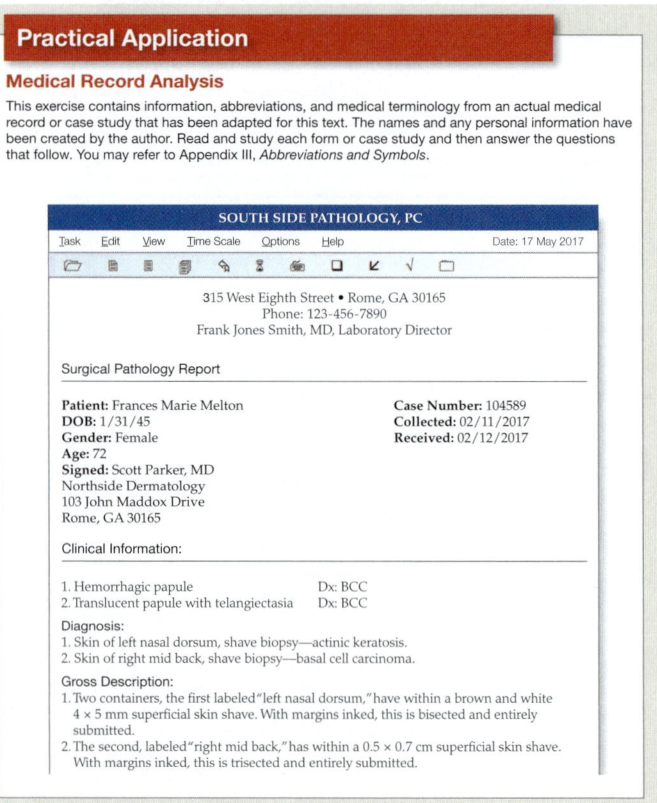

Practical Application

Medical Record Analysis

This exercise contains information, abbreviations, and medical terminology from an actual medical record or case study that has been adapted for this text. The names and any personal information have been created by the author. Read and study each form or case study and then answer the questions that follow. You may refer to Appendix III, *Abbreviations and Symbols*.

SOUTH SIDE PATHOLOGY, PC

Task Edit View Time Scale Options Help Date: 17 May 2017

315 West Eighth Street • Rome, GA 30165
Phone: 123-456-7890
Frank Jones Smith, MD, Laboratory Director

Surgical Pathology Report

Patient: Frances Marie Melton
DOB: 1/31/45
Gender: Female
Age: 72
Signed: Scott Parker, MD
Northside Dermatology
103 John Maddox Drive
Rome, GA 30165

Case Number: 104589
Collected: 02/11/2017
Received: 02/12/2017

Clinical Information:

1. Hemorrhagic papule Dx: BCC
2. Translucent papule with telangiectasia Dx: BCC

Diagnosis:
1. Skin of left nasal dorsum, shave biopsy—actinic keratosis.
2. Skin of right mid back, shave biopsy—basal cell carcinoma.

Gross Description:
1. Two containers, the first labeled "left nasal dorsum," have within a brown and white 4 × 5 mm superficial skin shave. With margins inked, this is bisected and entirely submitted.
2. The second, labeled "right mid back," has within a 0.5 × 0.7 cm superficial skin shave. With margins inked, this is trisected and entirely submitted.

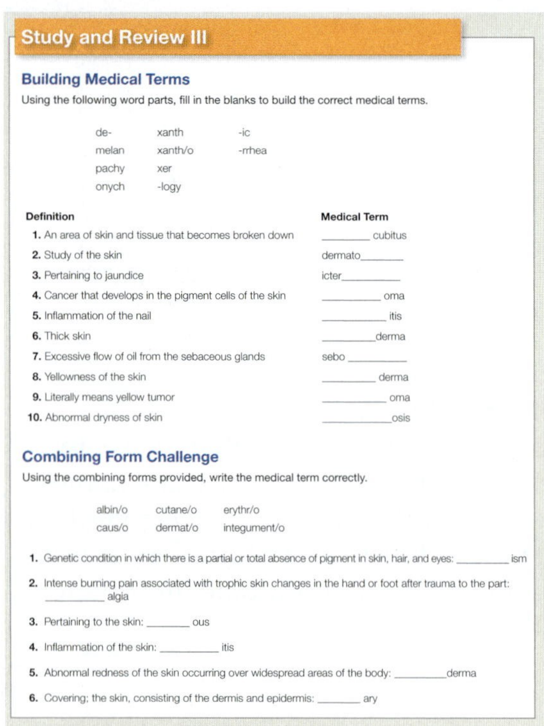

Study and Review III

Building Medical Terms

Using the following word parts, fill in the blanks to build the correct medical terms.

de-	xanth	-ic
melan	xanth/o	-rrhea
pachy	xer	
onych	-logy	

Definition	Medical Term
1. An area of skin and tissue that becomes broken down	_______ cubitus
2. Study of the skin	dermato_______
3. Pertaining to jaundice	icter_______
4. Cancer that develops in the pigment cells of the skin	_______ oma
5. Inflammation of the nail	_______ itis
6. Thick skin	_______derma
7. Excessive flow of oil from the sebaceous glands	sebo _______
8. Yellowness of the skin	_______ derma
9. Literally means yellow tumor	_______ oma
10. Abnormal dryness of skin	_______osis

Combining Form Challenge

Using the combining forms provided, write the medical term correctly.

albin/o	cutane/o	erythr/o
caus/o	dermat/o	integument/o

1. Genetic condition in which there is a partial or total absence of pigment in skin, hair, and eyes: _______ ism
2. Intense burning pain associated with trophic skin changes in the hand or foot after trauma to the part: _______ algia
3. Pertaining to the skin: _______ ous
4. Inflammation of the skin: _______ itis
5. Abnormal redness of the skin occurring over widespread areas of the body: _______derma
6. Covering; the skin, consisting of the dermis and epidermis: _______ ary

- **Study and Review I, II, and III—**Self-paced study guide sections featuring a wide variety of exercises, including Case Studies.

MyMedicalTerminologyLab™

The ultimate personalized learning tool is available at **www.mymedicalterminologylab.com**. This online course correlates with the textbook and is available for purchase separately or for a discount when packaged with the book. MyMedicalTerminologyLab is an immersive study experience that contains fun quizzes, word games, videos, and other self-study challenges. The system allows learners to track their own progress through the course and use a personalized study plan to achieve success.

MyMedicalTerminologyLab saves instructors time by providing quality feedback, ongoing individualized assessments for students, and instructor resources all in one place. It offers instructors the flexibility to make technology an integral part of their courses, or a supplementary resource for students.

Visit **www.mymedicalterminologylab.com** to log in to the course or purchase access. Instructors seeking more information about discount bundle options or for a demonstration, please contact your Pearson sales representative.

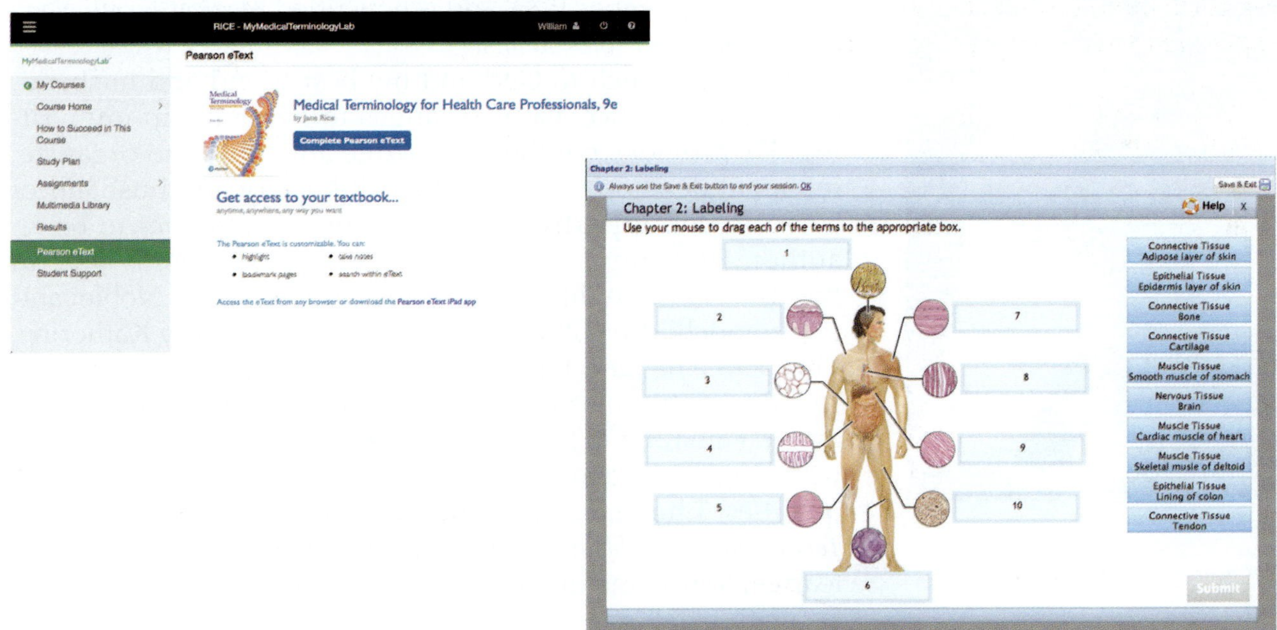

COMPREHENSIVE INSTRUCTIONAL PACKAGE

Perhaps the most gratifying part of an educator's work is the "aha" learning moment when the light bulb goes off and a student truly understands a concept—when a connection is made. Along these lines, Pearson is pleased to help instructors foster more of these educational connections by providing a complete battery of resources to support teaching and learning. Qualified adopters are eligible to receive a wealth of materials designed to help instructors prepare, present, and assess. For more information, please contact your Pearson sales representative or visit **www.pearsonhighered.com/educator**.

ABOUT THE AUTHOR

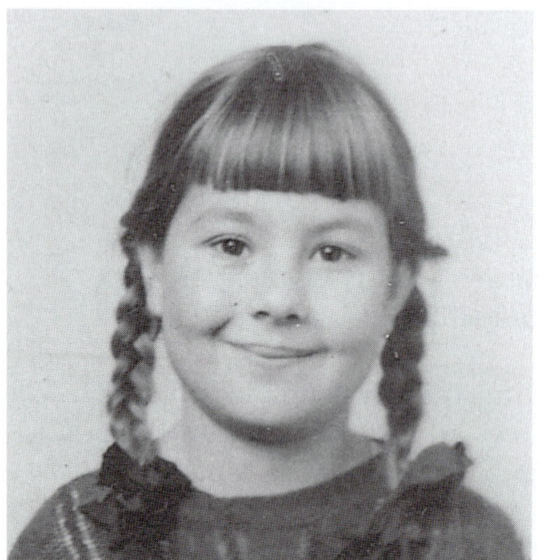

Source: Jane Rice

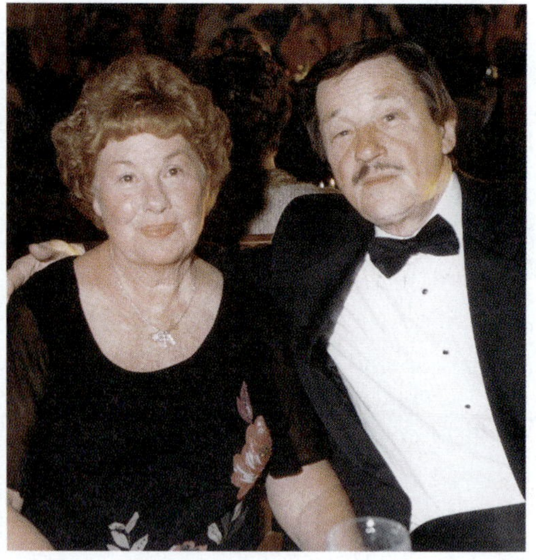

Source: Jane Rice

The year is 1947 and I am a little girl with brown hair that is braided into pigtails. I am very shy and afraid, for, you see, I am in the second grade and I cannot read. Not one little word. The teacher discovered this and made me sit on a tall metal stool in front of the classroom with a dunce cap on my head. Still to this day, I get very nervous when I have to get up in front of a crowd of people.

My mother taught me to read because back then, there were no special classes for children with learning disabilities. I did not learn "phonetics" but memorized everything. I still have trouble pronouncing words, but I can tell you all you want to know about a medical word.

After the death of two brothers, my father, and the impending death of my mother, I prayed for something else to do, something that would help take away the pain and the hurt. In 1982, my prayers were answered with a most precious gift: *Medical Terminology with Human Anatomy*, which was first published in September 1985, and is now titled *Medical Terminology for Health Care Professionals*.

I owe so much to God and my best friend and husband, Charles Larry Rice. God continues to guide me in my writing. He provides me the knowledge and ability to organize, research, develop, and then to write. Larry, my husband of 50 years, is supportive and gives me the freedom to be an author. He is my love and hero. Also, I express my love to the flowers in my life: Melissa Rice-Noble, Doug Noble, and our grandchildren: Zachary, Benjamin, Jacob, Mary Katherine, Elizabeth Ann, and Emily Sarah.

Although I am now retired, I had a wonderful teaching career. I am forever beholden to the many wonderful students who taught me so much and touched my life with their unique qualities. I hope and pray that this ninth edition of *Medical Terminology for Health Care Professionals* will enable you, the learner, to become the professional that you choose to be.

Jane Rice, RN, CMA-C

ACKNOWLEDGMENTS

First, I would like to offer my warmest thanks to all of the individuals who have accepted my medical terminology text as their book of choice. Over the past 31 years, I have been blessed with the gift of writing. It is my desire for this edition to make learning a wonderful experience for you, the learner and educator.

I want to express my gratitude to each person who worked so hard on this project and provided his or her unique talents to create and develop this edition. A sincere thank you to all the exceptional people at Pearson, especially John Goucher, Portfolio Manager—Health Professions. To Lynda Hatch—you were with me all the way. Through your guidance and excellent work, this ninth edition of my "dream" has reached a new dimension. To Jason Smith, MD, and Kristi Ware, CMA, Northwest Georgia Dermatology, Rome, Georgia—A special thank you for providing me with much of the art used for this text.

Editorial Development Team

The content and format of *Medical Terminology for Health Care Professionals* are the result of an incredible collaboration of expert educators from all around. This book represents the collective insights, experience, and thousands of hours of work performed by members of this development team. Their influence will continue to have an impact for decades to come. Let us introduce the members of our team.

Nicole Claussen, MS, CST, FAST
Kirtland Community College
Roscommon, MI

Dianne Finkelstein, DC
Molloy College
Rockville Centre, NY

Judith Hurtt, MEd
East Central Community College
Decatur, MS

Jennifer C. Hutchinson, PhD(c), RN
Liberty University
Lynchburg, VA

Nikki Marhefka, EdM, MT(ASCP), CMA(AAMA)
Central Penn College
Summerdale, PA

Alyssa Pliml, RN
Southwestern Michigan College
Dowagiac, Michigan

Nehal Rangnekar, MS, CPC
Dallas County Community College
District, TX

Lisa Smith, CST, FA
Quinsigamond Community College
Worcester, MA

J. Ryan Walther, MHA, ARRT(RT)
El Centro College School of Allied Health and Nursing
Dallas, TX

Gary Williams Jr., BS, NRP
University of Maryland Baltimore County
Baltimore, MD

A COMMITMENT TO ACCURACY

As a learner embarking on a career in health care you probably already know how critically important it is to be precise in your work. Patients and coworkers will be counting on you to avoid errors on a daily basis. Likewise, we owe it to you—the reader—to ensure accuracy in this book. We have gone to great lengths to verify that the information provided in *Medical Terminology for Health Care Professionals* is complete and correct. To this end, here are the steps we have taken:

1. **Editorial review.** We have assembled a large team of developmental consultants to critique every word and every image in this book. No fewer than 12 content experts have read each chapter for accuracy. In addition, some members of our developmental team were specifically assigned to focus on the precision of each illustration that appears in the book.
2. **Medical illustrations.** A team of medically trained illustrators was hired to prepare each piece of art that graces the pages of this book. These illustrators have a higher level of scientific education than the artists for most textbooks, and they worked directly with the author and members of our development team to make sure that their work was clear, correct, and consistent with what is described in the text.
3. **Accurate ancillaries.** The teaching and learning ancillaries are often as important to instruction as the textbook itself. Therefore we took steps to ensure accuracy and consistency of these components by reviewing every ancillary component.

While our intent and actions have been directed at creating an error-free text, we have established a process for correcting any mistakes that may have slipped past our editors. Pearson takes this issue seriously and therefore welcomes any and all feedback that you can provide along the lines of helping us enhance the accuracy of this text. If you identify any errors that need to be corrected in a subsequent printing, please send them to:

Pearson Health Science Editorial
Medical Terminology Corrections
221 River Street
Hoboken, NJ 07030

Thank you for helping Pearson reach its goal of providing the most accurate medical terminology textbooks available.

DETAILED CONTENTS

Chapter 1

Introduction to Medical Terminology

plural suffix combining form abbreviation root spelling pronunciation prefix

Learning Outcomes

On completion of this chapter, you will be able to:

1. Describe the fundamental elements that are used to build medical words.
2. List three guidelines that will assist you with the building and spelling of medical words.
3. State the importance of correct spelling in medical terminology.
4. Explain the use of abbreviations when writing and documenting data.
5. Analyze, build, spell, and pronounce medical words.
6. Describe the purpose of medical coding and the ICD-10-CM, and identify the terminology related to it.
7. Understand the general components of a patient's medical record.
8. List and describe the four parts of the SOAP chart note record.
9. Identify and define selected abbreviations.
10. Apply your acquired knowledge of medical coding terminology by successfully completing the *Practical Application* exercise.

Comprehension of Fundamental Word Structure

Medical terminology is the study of terms that are used in the art and science of medicine. It is a specialized language with its origin arising from the Greek influence on medicine. Hippocrates was a Greek physician who lived from 460 to 377 BC and whose vital role in medicine is still recognized today. He is called the "Father of Medicine" and is credited with establishing early ethical standards for physicians. Because of advances in scientific computerized technology, many new terms are coined daily; however, most of these terms are composed of word parts that have their origins in ancient Greek or Latin. Because of this foreign origin, it is necessary to learn the English translation of terms when learning the fundamentals of word structure.

Fundamentals of Word Structure

The fundamental elements in medical terminology are the component parts used to build medical words. The abbreviations used for component parts in this text are **P (prefix)**, **R (root)**, **CF (combining form)**, and **S (suffix)**. (The word parts are color-coded to make identification easier.) The key to learning medical terminology is through the word-building technique used in this text. Combining forms and word roots are integrated into each chapter of the text, according to body system or specialty area. Suffixes and prefixes are presented in Chapters 2 and 3 and then will continue to be repeated throughout the text. To build your medical vocabulary, all you have to do is recall the word parts that you have learned and then link them with the new component parts presented in each chapter.

Presented throughout the Building Your Medical Vocabulary sections, which are the heart of every chapter, is a feature called **Alert!** It is designed to help you in the identification, building, and spelling of medical words. You will be assisted in the formation of plural endings and in the recall of word parts. These short tidbits of information will draw your attention to interesting learning concepts. A new feature, **Insights**, brings to light some of the terminology of the ICD-10-CM and is included in the vocabulary sections and throughout the text. The purpose and use of the ICD-10-CM is explained later in the chapter in the section titled "Medical Coding."

Prefix

The term *prefix* means *to fix before* or *to fix to the beginning* of a word. A prefix can be a syllable or a group of syllables. Prefixes are united with or placed at the beginning of words to alter or modify their meanings or to create entirely new words. For example, the word ***ex / cis / ion*** means *the process of cutting out; surgical removal*. Note its component parts:

ex-	**P** (prefix) meaning *out*
cis	**R** (root) meaning *to cut*
-ion	**S** (suffix) meaning *process*

Word Root

A *root* is a word or word element from which other words are formed. It is the foundation of the word. The root conveys the central meaning of the word and forms the base to which prefixes and suffixes are attached for word modification.

For example, the word ***mal / format / ion*** means *the process of being badly shaped; deformed*. Note its component parts:

mal-	**P** (prefix) meaning *bad*
format	**R** (root) meaning *a shaping*
-ion	**S** (suffix) meaning *process*

Combining Form

A *combining form* is a word root to which a vowel has been added. A combining vowel (*a, e, i, o, u*, and sometimes *y*) links the root to the suffix or the word root to another root. The combining vowel does not have a meaning of its own. The vowel *o* is used more often than any other to make combining forms. Combining forms can be found at the beginning of a word or within the word.

For example, the word ***chem / o / therapy*** means *treatment of disease by using chemical agents*. Note the relationship of its component parts:

chem/o	**CF** (combining form) meaning *chemical*
-therapy	**S** (suffix) meaning *treatment*

Suffix

The term *suffix* means *to fasten on, beneath, or under*. A suffix can be a syllable or group of syllables united with or placed at the end of a word to alter or modify the meaning of the word or to create a new word. When you break down a word to understand it or when you give the meaning of the word or read its definition, you usually begin with the meaning of the suffix.

For example, the word ***centi / grade*** means *having 100 steps or degrees; unit of temperature measurement* (Celsius scale) and the word ***centi / meter*** means *unit of measurement in the metric system; one hundredth of a meter*:

centi-	**P** (prefix) meaning *one hundred, one hundredth*
-grade	**S** (suffix) meaning *a step*
centi-	**P** (prefix) meaning *one hundred, one hundredth*
-meter	**S** (suffix) meaning *measure*

Word roots and combining forms, together with their definitions, are included in each chapter according to the cell, tissue, organ, system, or element they describe. This arrangement makes it possible for you to form associations between medical terms and the various body systems. To reinforce the learning process, the text provides you a general anatomy and physiology overview for each of the body systems.

This text presents an alphabetical listing of the medical words within the Building Your Medical Vocabulary sections. The alphabetical format groups together those terms with the same prefix, word root, and/or combining form, thereby reinforcing the ease of learning medical terminology using the Rice approach.

Principles of Component Parts

As you learn definitions for prefixes, roots, combining forms, and suffixes, you will discover that some component parts have the same meanings as others. This occurs most often with words that relate to the organs of the body and the diseases that affect them. The existence of more than one component part for a particular meaning can be traced to differences in the Greek or Latin words from which they originated. Most of the terms for the body's organs originated from Latin words, whereas terms describing diseases that affect these organs have their origins in Greek. For example:

- **Uterus.** Latin word for one of the organs of the female reproductive system, the womb
- **Metr/i.** Greek **CF** (combining form) for uterus (womb)
- **Endometriosis.** Pathological condition in which endometrial tissue has been displaced to various sites in the abdominal or pelvic cavity: **endo- (P)**, meaning *within*; **metr/i (CF)**, meaning *uterus*; and **-osis (S)**, meaning *condition*

In this text, definitions are worded in an attempt to establish a relationship with the meanings given for each word part. For example, the medical term **adhesion** is divided into two word parts: **adhes (R)**, meaning *stuck to*, and **-ion (S)**, meaning *process*. The definition given is *process of being stuck together*.

Identification of Medical Words

When identifying medical words, you will learn to distinguish among and select the appropriate component parts for the meaning of the word. For example, the word **microscope** means an instrument for examining small objects. Note the following: *micro- + -scope*; not *-scope + micro*. With the proper placement of component parts (**P** + **S**) the definition translates micro- (small) and -scope (instrument for examining).

Vocabulary Words

You will find that some terms have not been divided into word parts. These are common words or specialized terms that are included to enhance your medical vocabulary. These terms were selected because of their usage in medical records/reports, case studies, and in various medical and surgical specialty areas. For example, **abate**, which means *to lessen, decrease, or cease*. This term is used to note the lessening of pain or the decrease in severity of symptoms. *The patient's arthritic pain did not **abate** , even though she followed the prescribed treatment plan.*

Spelling

Medical words of Greek origin are often difficult to spell because many of them begin with a silent letter or have a silent letter within the word. The following are examples of words that begin with silent letters:

Silent Beginning	Pronounced	Medical Term	Pronunciation Guide
gn	n	**g**nathic	(năth´ ĭk)
kn	n	**k**nuckle	(nŭk´ ĕl)
mn	n	**m**nemonic	(nĭ-mŏn´ ĭk)
pn	n	**p**neumonia	(nū´ -mō´ nĭ-ă)
ps	s	**p**sychiatrist	(sī-kī´ ă-trĭst)
pt	t	**p**tosis	(tō´ sĭs)

The following example is a medical term that contains a silent letter within the word:

Silent Letter	Medical Term	Pronunciation Guide
g	phle**g**m	(flĕm)

Correct spelling is extremely important in medical terminology because the addition or omission of a single letter can change the meaning of a word to something entirely different. The following examples illustrate this point:

Term/Letter Change	Meaning of Term	Term/Letter Change	Meaning of Term
a**b**duct	To lead **away** from the middle	ar**te**ritis	Inflammation of an **artery**
a**d**duct	To lead **toward** the middle	ar**th**ritis	Inflammation of a **joint**

Prefixes and Suffixes That Are Frequently Misspelled

Following are some of the prefixes and suffixes that often contribute to spelling errors:

Prefix	Meaning	Suffix	Meaning
ante-	before, forward	**-poiesis**	formation
anti-	against	**-ptosis**	prolapse, drooping, sagging, falling down
ecto-	out, outside, outer	**-ptysis**	spitting
endo-	within, inner	**-rrhage**	to burst forth, bursting forth
hyper-	above, beyond, excessive	**-rrhagia**	to burst forth, bursting forth
hypo-	below, under, deficient	**-rrhaphy**	suture
inter-	between	**-rrhea**	flow, discharge
intra-	within	**-rrhexis**	rupture
para-	beside, alongside, abnormal	**-scope**	instrument for examining
per-	through	**-scopy**	visual examination, to view, examine
peri-	around	**-tome**	instrument to cut
pre-	before, in front of	**-tomy**	incision
pro-	before	**-tripsy**	crushing
super-	above, beyond	**-trophy**	nourishment, development
supra-	above, beyond		

Building and Spelling Medical Words

Follow these guidelines for building and spelling medical words.

1. If the suffix begins with a vowel, drop the combining vowel from the combining form and add the suffix. For example, necr/*o* (*death*) + -osis (*condition*) becomes necrosis when we drop the *o* from necr*o*.

2. If the suffix begins with a consonant, keep the combining vowel and add the suffix to the combining form. For example, cardi/*o* (*heart*) + -logy (*study of*) becomes cardiology; we keep the *o* on the combining form.
3. Keep the combining vowel between two or more roots in a term. For example, gastr/*o* (*stomach*) + enter/*o* (*intestine*) + -logy (*study of*) becomes gastroenterology and we keep the two combining vowels.

As a way to help you remember "how to" build and spell medical words, **Rule Reminder** is a feature designed to draw your attention to terms in the Building Your Medical Vocabulary sections that follow specific rules. We hope you find this feature to be beneficial to your learning process!

Formation of Plural Endings

To change the following singular endings to plural endings, substitute the plural endings as illustrated:

Singular Ending	Plural Ending	Singular Ending	Plural Ending
a as in burs**a**	to **ae** as in burs**ae**	**ix** as in appendi**x**	to **ices** as in appendi**ces**
ax as in thor**ax**	to **aces** as in thor**aces** or **es** as in thorax**es**	**nx** as in phala**nx**	to **ges** as in phalan**ges**
en as in foram**en**	to **ina** as in foram**ina**	**on** as in spermatozo**on**	to **a** as in spermatozo**a**
is as in cris**is**	to **es** as in cris**es**	**um** as in ov**um**	to **a** as in ov**a**
is as in ir**is**	to **ides** as in ir**ides**	**us** as in nucle**us**	to **i** as in nucle**i**
is as in femor**is**	to **a** as in femor**a**	**y** as in arter**y**	to **i** and add **es** as in arter**ies**

Use of Abbreviations

An **abbreviation** is a process of shortening a word or phrase into appropriate letters. It is used as a form of communication in writing and documenting data. The Institute for Safe Medication Practices (ISMP) and The Joint Commission (TJC) developed a list of abbreviations considered to be dangerous because of the potential for misinterpretation. It is recommended that facilities using abbreviations for documentation keep a list of approved and unapproved abbreviations on hand and readily accessible.

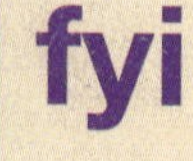

To view the list of unapproved abbreviations from the ISMP and TJC, go to *www.ismp.org/Tools/errorproneabbreviations.pdf* or *www.jointcommission.org/facts_about_do_not_use_list*.

When using abbreviations, caution must be exercised. Many have more than one meaning, such as ***ER***, which means *emergency room* and *endoplasmic reticulum*, and ***PA***, which means *physician assistant*, *posteroanterior*, and *pernicious anemia*. It is essential that you use or translate the correct meaning for the abbreviation being used. If there is any question about which abbreviation to use, it is best to spell out the word or phrase and not use an abbreviation.

An **acronym** is a word formed by the combining of initial letters, or syllables and letters, of a series of words or a compound term. Any shortened form of a word is an abbreviation, but an acronym is a special type of abbreviation that can be pronounced as a word. For example: HIPAA is an acronym for Health Insurance Portability and Accountability Act.

An **initialism** is another type of abbreviation. It is formed by the initial letters of a series of words or a compound term, but is not pronounced as a word. Example: DOB (date of birth), each letter is pronounced.

In each chapter of this text, you will find selected abbreviations with their meanings. These abbreviations are in current use and are directly associated with the subject of the chapter. In the appendices, you will find an expanded alphabetical list of commonly used abbreviations and symbols. The abbreviations are presented using capital letters without periods except in those cases where lowercase letters and periods represent the norm or preferred method.

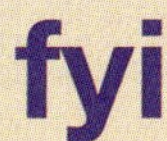

An **eponym** is a disease, structure, operation, or procedure named for the person who discovered or described it first. For example: Alzheimer disease is named for Alois Alzheimer, a neuropathologist who in 1906 identified an unusual disease of the cerebral cortex and described the amyloid plaques and neurofibrillary tangles that are its characteristics.

Pronunciation

Pronunciation of medical words may seem difficult; however, it is very important to correctly pronounce medical words with the same or very similar sounds in order to convey their correct meanings. As in spelling, one mispronounced syllable can change the meaning of a medical word. The following guide will help you to pronounce each medical word in this text correctly.

PRONUNCIATION GUIDE

This text uses a *phonetic* type of pronunciation guide adapted from *Taber's Cyclopedic Medical Dictionary*. This system uses symbols called *diacritics* (shown in the table below) to help you pronounce the word correctly. You should practice speaking each term aloud when working with the various lists of medical terms or vocabulary words.

ACCENT MARKS	Marks used to indicate stress on certain syllables. *Example:* an″ tə -sep´ tik (antiseptic)
Single ´	Used to indicate stress on certain syllables; a single accent mark is called a *primary accent* and is used with the syllable that has the strongest stress (primary syllable).
Double ″	Used to indicate syllables that are stressed less than primary syllables; a double accent mark is called a *secondary accent*.
DIACRITICS	Marks placed over or under vowels to indicate the long or short sound of the vowel.
Macron ¯	Indicates the long sound of the vowel. *Example:* mī´ krō-skōp (microscope)
Breve ˘	Indicates the short sound of the vowel. *Example:* măks´ ĭ-măl (maximal)
Schwa ə	Indicates the central vowel sound of most unstressed syllables. *Example:* bou´əl (bowel)

Building Your Medical Vocabulary

This section provides the foundation for learning medical terminology. Review the following alphabetized word list. Note how common prefixes and suffixes are repeatedly applied to word roots and combining forms to create different meanings. The word parts are color-coded: prefixes are yellow, suffixes are blue, roots/combining forms are red.

Remember These Guidelines

1. If the suffix begins with a vowel, drop the combining vowel from the combining form and add the suffix. For example, necr/o (*death*) + -osis (*condition*) becomes necrosis.
2. If the suffix begins with a consonant, keep the combining vowel and add the suffix to the combining form. For example, chem/o (*chemical*) + -therapy (*treatment*) becomes chemotherapy.

You will find that some terms have not been divided into word parts. These are common words or specialized terms that are included to enhance your medical vocabulary.

Medical Word	Word Parts		Definition
	Part	Meaning	
abate (ă-bāt′)			To lessen, ease, decrease, or cease. Used to note the lessening of pain or the decrease in severity of symptoms.
abnormal (ăb-nōr′ măl)	ab- norm -al	away from rule pertaining to	Pertaining to away from the norm or rule. A condition that is considered to be not normal.
abscess (ăb′ sĕs)			Localized collection of pus, which may occur in any part of the body
acute (ă-cūt′)			Sudden, sharp, severe; used to describe a disease that has a sudden onset, severe symptoms, and a short course
adhesion (ăd′ hē-zhŭn)	adhes -ion	stuck to process	Literally means *a process of being stuck together*. An abdominal adhesion usually involves the intestines and is caused by inflammation or trauma. This type of adhesion may cause an intestinal obstruction and require surgery.
afferent (ăf′ ĕ rĕnt)			Carrying impulses toward a center
ambulatory (ăm′ bū-lăh-tōr″ ē)			Condition of being able to walk, not confined to bed
antidote (ăn′ tĭ-dōt)			Substance given to counteract poisons and their effects

Medical Word	Word Parts: Part	Word Parts: Meaning	Definition
antipyretic (ăn″ tĭ-pī-rĕt′ ĭk)	anti- pyret -ic	against fever pertaining to	Pertaining to an agent that is used to lower an elevated body temperature (fever)
antiseptic (ăn″ tə-sĕp′ tĭk)	anti- sept -ic	against putrefaction pertaining to	Pertaining to an agent that works against sepsis (*putrefaction*); a technique or product used to prevent or limit infections
antitussive (ăn″ tĭ-tŭs′ ĭv)	anti- tuss -ive	against cough nature of, quality of	Pertaining to an agent that works against coughing
apathy (ăp′ ă-thē)			Condition in which one lacks feelings and emotions and is indifferent
asepsis (ā-sĕp′ sĭs)	a- -sepsis	without decay	Without decay; *sterile*, free from all living microorganisms
axillary (ax) (ăks′ ĭ-lār-ē)	axill -ary	armpit pertaining to	Pertaining to the armpit
biopsy (Bx) (bī′ ŏp-sē)	bi(o) -opsy	life to view	Surgical removal of a small piece of tissue for microscopic examination; used to determine a diagnosis of cancer or other disease processes in the body

! ALERT!

To change biops**y** to its plural form, you change the ***y*** to ***i*** and add ***es*** to make *biopsies*.

Medical Word	Word Parts: Part	Word Parts: Meaning	Definition
cachexia (kă-kĕks′ ē-ă)	cac- -hexia	bad condition	Condition of ill health, malnutrition, and wasting. It may occur in chronic diseases such as cancer and pulmonary tuberculosis.
centigrade (C) (sĕn′ tĭ-grād)	centi- -grade	one hundred, one hundredth a step	Literally means *having 100 steps* or *degrees*; unit of temperature measurement (Celsius scale) with a boiling point at 100° and a freezing point at 0°. Each degree of temperature change is 0.01 (1/100) of the scale.
centimeter (cm) (sĕn′ tĭ-mē-tĕr)	centi- -meter	one hundred, one hundredth measure	Unit of measurement in the metric system; one hundredth of a meter

Medical Word	Word Parts		Definition
	Part	**Meaning**	
chemotherapy (kē″ mō-thĕr′ ă-pē)	chem/o -therapy	chemical treatment	The use of chemical agents in the treatment of disease, specifically drugs used in cancer therapy
chronic (krŏn′ ĭk)			Pertaining to time; denotes a disease with little change or of slow progression; the opposite of acute
diagnosis (Dx) (di″ ăg-nō′ sĭs)	dia- -gnosis	through knowledge	The process of identifying a disease or disorder, which is generally determined through the use of scientific and skillful methods of knowledge. Several types of information are used for diagnosis, including signs and symptoms. *Example:* chest pain that radiates to the neck, jaw, or left arm is diagnosis code I20.9 *angina pectoris, unspecified,* in the ICD-10-CM.

ALERT!

To change diagnos***is*** to its plural form, you change ***is*** to ***es*** to create *diagnoses*.

Medical Word	Part	Meaning	Definition
diaphoresis (dī″ ă-fō-rē′ sĭs)	dia- -phoresis	through to carry	To carry through sweat glands; *profuse sweating*
disease (dĭ-zēz′)			Literally means *lack of ease*; a pathological condition of the body that presents with a series of symptoms, signs, and laboratory findings peculiar to it and sets it apart from normal or other abnormal body states; a disruption of normal functioning of the body by a process that can be congenital or infectious, or the failure of normal activity to maintain and sustain health
disinfectant (dĭs″ ĭn-fĕk′ tănt)	dis- infect -ant	apart to infect forming	Chemical substance that can be applied to objects to destroy pathogenic microorganisms, such as bacteria
efferent (ĕf″ ĕrĕnt)			Carrying impulses away from a center
empathy (ĕm′ pă-thē)			The ability to sense intellectually and emotionally the feelings of another person
epidemic (ĕp″ i-dĕm′ ik)	epi- dem -ic	upon people pertaining to	Pertaining to upon the people; the rapid, widespread occurrence of an infectious disease that can be spread by any pathological organism transmitted by and to humans, birds, insects, etc.

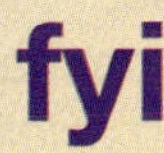

fyi The H1N1 (swine flu) reached an *epidemic* level in 2009, and in the same year the World Health Organization (WHO) declared it a worldwide pandemic, with more than 207 countries and overseas territories or communities being affected.

Medical Word	Word Parts: Part	Word Parts: Meaning	Definition
etiology (ē″ tē-ŏl′ ō-jē)	eti/o -logy	cause study of	Study of the cause(s) of disease
excision (ĕk-si′ zhŭn)	ex- cis -ion	out to cut process	Process of cutting out, surgical removal
febrile (fē′ brĭl)			Pertaining to fever, a sustained body temperature (T) above 98.6°F
gram (g) (grăm)			Unit of weight in the metric system; a cubic centimeter or a milliliter of water is equal to the weight of a gram
heterogeneous (hĕt″ ĕr-ō-jē′ nĭ-ŭs)	hetero- gene -ous	different formation, produce pertaining to	Literally means *pertaining to a different formation*; composed of unlike substances; the opposite of homogeneous
illness (ĭl′ nĭs)			State of being sick
incision (ĭn-sĭzh′ ŭn)	in- cis -ion	in, into to cut process	Process of cutting into
kilogram (kg) (kĭl′ ō-grăm)	kil/o -gram	a thousand a weight	Unit of weight in the metric system; 1000 g; a kilogram is equal to 2.2 lb

RULE REMINDER

This term keeps the combining vowel ***o*** because the suffix begins with a consonant.

Medical Word	Word Parts: Part	Word Parts: Meaning	Definition
liter (L) (lē′ tĕr)			Unit of volume in the metric system; 1000 mL; a liter is equal to 33.8 fl oz or 1.0567 qt
macroscopic (măk″ rō-skŏp′ ĭk)	macr/o scop -ic	large to examine pertaining to	Pertaining to objects large enough to be examined by the naked eye
malaise (mă-lāz′)			A general feeling of discomfort, uneasiness; often felt by a patient who has a chronic disease

Medical Word	Word Parts		Definition
	Part	Meaning	
malformation (măl″ fōr-mā′ shŭn)	mal- format -ion	bad a shaping process	Literally means *a process of being badly shaped, deformed*; a structural defect that fails to form normal shape and therefore can affect the function (e.g., *cleft palate*)

RULE REMINDER

The ***o*** has been removed from the combining form because the suffix begins with a vowel.

Medical Word	Part	Meaning	Definition
malignant (mă-lĭg′ nănt)	malign -ant	bad kind forming	Literally means *formation of a bad kind*; growing worse, harmful, cancerous
maximal (măks′ ĭ-măl)	maxim -al	greatest pertaining to	Pertaining to the greatest possible quantity, number, or degree
microgram (mcg) (mī′ krō-grăm)	micro- -gram	small a weight	Unit of weight in the metric system; one-millionth of a gram or one-thousandth of a milligram (0.001 mg)
microorganism (mī″ krō-ōr′ găn-ĭzm)	micro- organ -ism	small organ condition	Small living organisms that are not visible to the naked eye
microscope (mī′ krō-skōp)	micro- -scope	small instrument for examining	Scientific instrument designed to view small objects
milligram (mg) (mĭl′ ĭ-grăm)	milli- -gram	one-thousandth a weight	Unit of weight in the metric system; 0.001 g
milliliter (mL) (mĭl′ ĭ-lē″ tĕr)	milli- -liter	one-thousandth liter	Unit of volume in the metric system; 0.001 L
minimal (mĭn′ ĭ-măl)	minim -al	least pertaining to	Pertaining to the least possible quantity, number, or degree
morbidity (morbĭd' ĭty)	morbid -ity	sick condition	State of being diseased; ill, sick; refers to the disease rate or number of cases of a particular disease in a given age range, gender, occupation, or other relevant population-based grouping
mortality (mŏr-tăl′ ĭ-tē)	mortal -ity	human being condition	Being human, subject to death; refers to the death rate reflected by the population in a given region, age range, or other relevant statistical grouping

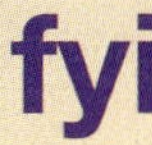

Top 10 Leading Causes of Death in the United States

1. Heart disease
2. Cancer (CA)
3. Chronic lower respiratory disease (infectious diseases)
4. Accidents (unintentional injuries)
5. Stroke (cerebrovascular accident [CVA])
6. Alzheimer disease (AD)
7. Diabetes (diabetes mellitus [DM])
8. Influenza and pneumonia
9. Kidney disease (nephritis, nephrotic syndrome, nephrosis)
10. Suicide (intentional self-harm)

Medical Word	Word Parts: Part	Word Parts: Meaning	Definition
multiform (mŭl′ tĭ-form)	multi- -form	many, much shape	Occurring in or having many shapes; an object that has more than one defined shape
necrosis (nĕ-krō′ sis)	necr -osis	death condition	Abnormal condition of tissue death
oncology (ŏng-kŏl′ ō-jē)	onc/o -logy	tumor study of	Literally means *the study of tumors*; the study of the etiology, the characteristics, treatments, etc., of cancer
pallor (păl′ or)			Paleness, a lack of color
palmar (păl′ mar)	palm -ar	palm pertaining to	Pertaining to the palm of the hand
paracentesis (păr″ ă-sĕn-tē′ sĭs)	para- -centesis	beside surgical puncture	Surgical puncture of a body cavity for fluid removal
prognosis (prŏg-nō′ sĭs)	pro- -gnosis	before knowledge	Literally means *a state of foreknowledge*; prediction of the course of a disease and the recovery rate of the affected person
prophylactic (prō-fi-lăk′ tĭk)	prophylact -ic	guarding pertaining to	Pertaining to preventing or protecting against disease or pregnancy
pyrogenic (pī″ rō-jĕn′ ĭk)	pyr/o -genic	heat, fire formation, produce	Pertaining to the production of heat; *a fever*
radiology (rā″ dē-ŏl′ ō-jē)	radi/o -logy	ray, x-ray study of	Study of x-rays and other imaging modalities that use x-rays
rapport (ră-pōr′)			Relationship of understanding between two individuals, especially between the patient and the physician

Medical Word	Word Parts		Definition
	Part	**Meaning**	
sequela (sē-kwē´ lă)			Abnormal condition that follows and is the result of a disease, treatment, or injury, such as deafness after treatment with an *ototoxic* drug (ot/o, *ear*; tox, *poison*; -ic, *pertaining to*)

ALERT!

To change sequel***a*** to its plural form, you add an ***e*** to create *sequelae*.

insights In ICD-10-CM, *sequelae* is defined as a late effect, the residual effect (condition produced) after the acute phase of an illness or injury has ended. There is no time limit on when a late effect code can be used. The residual effect may be apparent early, such as in cerebral infarction, or it may occur months or years later, such as joint damage due to the previous injury.

Medical Word	Part	Meaning	Definition
syndrome (sĭn´ drōm)	syn- -drome	together, with that which runs together	A group of signs and symptoms occurring together that characterize a specific disease or pathological condition
thermometer (thĕr-mŏm´ ĕ-tĕr)	therm/o -meter	hot, heat instrument to measure	An instrument used to measure degree of heat, especially the temperature of a person

RULE REMINDER

This term keeps the combining vowel ***o*** because the suffix begins with a consonant.

Medical Word	Part	Meaning	Definition
triage (trē-ahzh´)			A system of prioritizing and classifying patient injuries to determine priority of need and treatment

Medical Coding

Medical coding is the process of assigning alphanumeric characters that represent the diagnoses patients have been given and the services they are to receive. **Alphanumeric** refers to a character set with alphabetic characters (A–Z) and numerals (0–9). For example: A69.21 is the code for meningitis due to Lyme disease in the ***International Classification of Diseases, 10th Revision, Clinical Modification*** **(ICD-10-CM)**, which is used throughout the United States.

Diagnosis codes identify the reasons that healthcare services were provided. **Procedure codes** describe the types of services, such as laboratory or radiology, and types of procedures, such as surgery, ordered for patients. The combination of diagnosis codes and related procedure codes provides the basis for financial reimbursement to healthcare professionals and facilities from third-party payers for services rendered.

The Health Insurance Portability and Accountability Act (HIPAA) mandates the approved code-sets for all covered entities, such as medical offices and hospitals, which handle claims related to healthcare services. On a broader scale, medical codes are used to compile and report statistics, within the United States and worldwide, regarding mortality, morbidity, and health trends. Within the coding system, medical terminology is the language used for identifying the diseases and conditions that are coded.

Worldwide, the present coding system, developed by the World Health Organization (WHO), is the ***International Classification of Diseases, 10th Revision*** **(ICD-10)**, which was implemented for mortality coding and classification for death certificates. The United States developed a Clinical Modification (ICD-10-CM) for medical diagnoses based on the WHO ICD-10. The Centers for Medicare & Medicaid Services (CMS) developed a new Procedure Coding System (ICD-10-PCS) for inpatient procedures. Thus, the ICD-10-CM/PCS consists of two parts:

1. **ICD-10-CM** The clinical modification (diagnosis classification system) was developed by the Centers for Disease Control and Prevention (CDC) for use in all United States healthcare treatment settings. Diagnosis coding under this system uses three to seven alpha and numeric digits and full code titles.
2. **ICD-10-PCS** The procedure classification system was developed by the CMS for use in the United States for inpatient hospital settings only. The new procedure coding system uses seven alpha or numeric digits.

This classification system, which went into effect on October 1, 2015, provides significant improvements over the previous code (ICD-9-CM) by offering more detailed information and the ability to expand to capture additional advancements in clinical medicine. The greater level of detail in the new code-sets includes laterality, severity, and complexity of disease conditions, which will enable more precise identification and tracking of specific conditions. Terminology and disease classification are now consistent with new technology and current clinical practice. Injuries, poisonings, and other external causes are much more detailed in ICD-10-CM, including the severity of injuries and how and where they occurred. Pregnancy trimester is now designated for ICD-10-CM codes in the pregnancy, delivery, and puerperium chapter. Postoperative codes are expanded and now distinguish between intraoperative and postprocedural complications. There are new concepts that did not exist in the previous code, such as underdosing, blood type, the Glasgow Coma Scale, and alcohol level.

The ICD-10-CM is divided into the Alphabetic Index, an alphabetical list of terms and their corresponding code, and the Tabular List, a chronological list of codes divided into chapters based on body system or condition. The Alphabetic Index consists of the following parts: the Index of Diseases and Injury, the Index of External Causes of Injury, the Table of Neoplasms, and the Table of Drugs and Chemicals.

Current Procedural Terminology (CPT) is a medical code set that is used to report medical, surgical, and diagnostic procedures and services to entities such as physicians, health insurance companies, and accreditation organizations. CPT codes are used in conjunction with the ICD-10-CM diagnostic coding during the electronic medical billing process. Physicians, medical offices, and hospital outpatient and other outpatient facilities will continue to use CPT for procedure coding when sending patients for outpatient (OP) testing (they will not use ICD-10-PCS for procedure coding, which pertains to inpatient hospital settings only). The narrative reason/symptoms for the test should be used on the outpatient testing order form, not the ICD-10 code.

The tabular list of the ICD-10-CM is an alphanumerically sequenced list of all diagnosis codes, divided into 21 chapters based on cause, etiology, and body system. See *Insights: ICD-10-CM Tabular List with Associated Medical/Surgical Specialty*.

INSIGHTS

ICD-10-CM Tabular List with Associated Medical/Surgical Specialty

Chapter	Title	Code Range	Associated Specialty Area
1	Certain Infectious and Parasitic Diseases	A00–B99	Infectious diseases
2	Neoplasms	C00–D49	Oncology
3	Diseases of the Blood and Blood-forming Organs and Certain Disorders Involving the Immune Mechanism	D50–D89	Allergy/Immunology/ Hematology
4	Endocrine, Nutritional, and Metabolic Diseases	E00–E89	Endocrinology
5	Mental, Behavioral and Neurodevelop-mental Disorders	F01–F99	Psychiatry (Psych)
6	Diseases of the Nervous System	G00–G99	Neurology (Neuro)
7	Diseases of the Eye and Adnexa	H00–H59	Ophthalmology
8	Diseases of the Ear and Mastoid Process	H60–H95	Otorhinolaryngology (commonly called ear, nose, and throat [ENT])
9	Diseases of the Circulatory System	I00–I99	Cardiology
10	Diseases of the Respiratory System	J00–J99	Pulmonology
11	Diseases of the Digestive System	K00–K95	Gastroenterology
12	Diseases of the Skin and Subcutane-ous Tissue	L00–L99	Dermatology (Derm)
13	Diseases of the Musculoskeletal Sys-tem and Connective Tissue	M00–M99	Orthopedics (Orth)
14	Diseases of the Genitourinary System	N00–N99	Gynecology (GYN)/ Nephrology/Urology
15	Pregnancy, Childbirth and the Puerperium	O00–O9A	Obstetrics (OB)
16	Certain Conditions Originating in the Perinatal Period	P00–P96	Neonatology

Chapter	Title	Code Range	Associated Specialty Area
17	Congenital Malformations, Deformations and Chromosomal Abnormalities	Q00–Q99	Genetics/Obstetrics/Pediatrics/Perinatology/other specialties associated with affected body systems
18	Symptoms, Signs and Abnormal Clinical and Laboratory Findings, Not Elsewhere Classified	R00–R99	Pathology/Radiology/Internal Medicine/various other specialties
19	Injury, Poisoning and Certain Other Consequences	S00–T88	Trauma/Toxicology/various other specialties depending on injury
20	External Causes of Morbidity	V00–Y99	
21	Factors Influencing Health Status and Contact with Health Services	Z00–Z99	

Medical Records

Electronic Health Record

The **electronic health record (EHR)** is an electronic record of health-related information for an individual that is created, gathered, managed, and consulted by authorized healthcare clinicians and staff. Included in this information are patient demographics, progress notes, problems, medications, vital signs, past medical history, immunizations, laboratory data, radiology images, and personal data such as age, weight, and billing information. The EHR automates and streamlines the clinician's workflow. The EHR has the ability to generate a complete record of a clinical patient encounter, as well as supporting other care-related activities directly or indirectly via interface, including evidence-based decision support, quality management, and outcomes reporting.

An EHR is generated and maintained within an institution, such as a hospital, clinic, or physician's office. Its purpose is to give patients, physicians, and other healthcare providers, employers, or insurers access to a patient's medical records across facilities.

Sections contained within the medical record will vary according to the physician's preference, type of practice, cost, and regulatory requirements. Many of the EHR software programs have a prescription component that can be accessed by clicking on the prescription tab. This program can store thousands of drug names with their usual dosages. With just a few clicks, an entire prescription can be created.

A patient's medical record, electronic or paper, is often referred to as a *chart* or *file*. The general components of a patient's medical record include the following:

- **Patient Data.** Information that is provided by the patient and then updated as necessary. It is data that relates directly to the patient, including last name, first name, gender, date of birth (DOB), marital status, street address, city, state, zip code, telephone number, insurance information, employment status, address and phone number of employer, name and contact information for the person who is responsible for the patient's bill, and vital information concerning who should be contacted in case of an emergency.

- **Medical History (Hx).** Document describing past and current history of all medical conditions experienced by the patient.
- **Physical Examination (PE).** Record that includes a current head-to-toe assessment of the patient's physical condition.
- **Consent Form.** Signed document by the patient or legal guardian giving permission for treatment.
- **Informed Consent Form.** Signed document by the patient or legal guardian that explains the purpose, risks, and benefits of a procedure and serves as proof that the patient was properly informed before undergoing a procedure.
- **Physician's Orders.** Record of the prescribed care, medications, tests, and treatments for a given patient.
- **Nurse's Notes.** Record of a patient's care that includes vital signs, particularly temperature (T), pulse (P), respiration (R) [TPR], and blood pressure (BP). The nurse's notes can also include treatments, procedures, and patient's responses to such care. See Figure 1.1.
- **Physician's Progress Notes.** Documentation given by the physician regarding the patient's condition, results of the physician's examination, summary of test results, plan of treatment, and updating of data as appropriate (assessment and diagnosis [Dx]).
- **Consultation Reports.** Documentation given by specialists whom the physician has asked to evaluate the patient.
- **Ancillary/Miscellaneous Reports.** Documentation of procedures or therapies provided during a patient's care, such as physical therapy, respiratory therapy, or chemotherapy.
- **Diagnostic Tests/Laboratory Reports.** Documents providing the results of all diagnostic and laboratory tests performed on the patient.
- **Operative Report.** Documentation from the surgeon detailing the operation, including the preoperative and postoperative diagnosis, specific details of the surgical procedure, how well the patient tolerated the procedure, and any complications that occurred.
- **Anesthesiology Report.** Documentation from the attending anesthesiologist or nurse anesthetist that includes a detailed account of anesthesia during surgery, which drugs were used, dose and time given, patient response, monitoring of vital signs, how well the patient tolerated the anesthesia, and any complications that occurred.

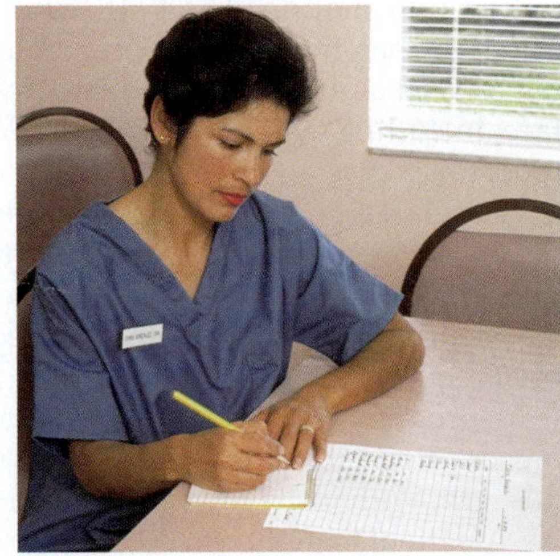

Figure 1.1 The healthcare professional is making notes before entering patient information into the electronic health record.

Source: Pearson Education, Inc.

- **Pathology Report.** Documentation from the pathologist regarding the findings or results of samples taken from the patient, such as bone marrow, blood, or tissue.
- **Discharge Summary (also called Clinical Resumé, Clinical Summary, or Discharge Abstract).** Outline summary of the patient's hospital care, including date of admission, diagnosis, course of treatment and patient's response(s), results of tests, final diagnosis, follow-up plans, and date of discharge.

SOAP: Chart Note

The **SOAP**—subjective, objective, assessment, plan—chart note is a method of documentation employed by healthcare providers to write out notes in a patient's chart, along with other common formats, such as the admission note. Documenting patient encounters in the medical record is an integral part of medical/surgical practice workflow, starting with patient appointment scheduling, to writing out notes, to medical billing. The SOAP note is a method of displaying patient data in a concise, organized format and is written to improve communication among those caring for the patient. The length and focus of each component of a SOAP note varies depending on the specialty area. The four parts of a SOAP chart note follow.

1. **Subjective**. This describes the patient's current condition in narrative form and is information provided by the patient. It includes symptoms that the subject (patient) feels and describes to the healthcare professional. These symptoms arise within the individual and are not perceptible to an observer. Examples include pain, nausea, dizziness, tightness in the chest, lump in the throat, weakness of the legs, and "butterflies" in the stomach. The healthcare professional can see the physical reaction of the patient to the symptom but not the actual symptom. Subjective symptoms can be verbally expressed by a parent or a significant other. Also included in the subjective section is the patient's chief complaint (CC), presenting symptom, or presenting complaint stated by the patient and described in the patient's own words. This includes the concern that brings a patient to a doctor.
2. **Objective**. Symptoms that can be observed, such as those that are seen, felt, smelled, heard, or measured by the healthcare provider. Included in the objective analysis are the vital signs (TPR and BP) and data relating to the physical examination (PE) such as height (Ht); weight (Wt); general appearance; and condition of the lungs, heart, abdomen, musculoskeletal and nervous systems, and the skin. The results of laboratory and diagnostic tests may also be included. *Please note that it may be common practice for the nurse or other medical professional assisting the physician to record the patient's vital signs, allergies, and chief complaint at the top of the chart, instead of within the SOAP chart note.*
3. **Assessment**. Interpretation of the subjective and objective findings. Generally includes a diagnosis, including a differential diagnosis, or in some cases will rule out a disease/condition.
4. **Plan**. Includes the management and treatment regimen for the patient; may include laboratory tests, radiological tests, physical therapy, diet therapy, medications, medical and surgical interventions, patient referrals such as counseling and finding a support group, patient teaching, and follow-up directions.

A SOAP chart note should express current patient data, including the date of the visit, patient's name, date of birth, age, and gender.

Abbreviations

Abbreviation	Meaning
ax	axillary
BP	blood pressure
Bx	biopsy
C	centigrade, Celsius
CC	chief complaint
CDC	Centers for Disease Control and Prevention
cm	centimeter
CMS	Centers for Medicare & Medicaid Services
Derm	dermatology
DOB	date of birth
Dx	diagnosis
EHR	electronic health record
ENT	ear, nose, throat (larynx) (otorhinolaryngology)
g	gram
GYN	gynecology
HIPAA	Health Insurance Portability and Accountability Act
Ht	height
ICD	International Classification of Diseases
kg	kilogram
L	liter
mcg	microgram
mg	milligram
mL	milliliter
Neuro	neurology
OB	obstetrics
OP	outpatient
Orth	orthopedics
P	pulse
Path	pathology
PE	physical examination
PCS	procedure coding system
Psych	psychiatry, psychology
R	respiration
SOAP	subjective, objective, assessment, plan
T	temperature
TPR	temperature, pulse, respiration
WHO	World Health Organization
Wt	weight

Study and Review

Word Parts

Prefixes

Give the definitions of the following prefixes.

1. a- ____________________

2. ab- ____________________

3. anti- ____________________

4. cac- ____________________

5. centi- ____________________

6. dia- ____________________

7. hetero- ____________________

8. mal- ____________________

9. micro- ____________________

10. mill- ____________________

11. multi- ____________________

12. para- ____________________

13. pro- ____________________
14. syn- ____________________
15. dis- ____________________
16. epi- ____________________
17. ex- ____________________
18. in- ____________________

Roots and Combining Forms

Give the definitions of the following roots and combining forms.

1. adhes ____________________
2. axill ____________________
3. centr/i ____________________
4. chem/o ____________________
5. format ____________________
6. gene ____________________
7. kil/o ____________________
8. macr/o ____________________
9. necr ____________________
10. norm ____________________
11. onc/o ____________________
12. organ ____________________
13. pyr ____________________
14. pyr/o ____________________
15. radi/o ____________________
16. scop ____________________
17. sept ____________________
18. therm/o ____________________
19. tuss ____________________
20. infect ____________________
21. dem ____________________
22. eti/o ____________________
23. cis ____________________
24. malign ____________________
25. maxim ____________________
26. minim ____________________
27. palm ____________________
28. prophylact ____________________

Suffixes

Give the definitions of the following suffixes.

1. -al ____________________
2. -ary ____________________
3. -centesis ____________________
4. -drome ____________________
5. -form ____________________
6. -genic ____________________
7. -gnosis ____________________
8. -grade ____________________
9. -gram ____________________
10. -hexia ____________________

11. -ic ______________________

12. -ion ______________________

13. -ism ______________________

14. -ive ______________________

15. -liter ______________________

16. -logy ______________________

17. -meter ______________________

18. -osis ______________________

19. -ous ______________________

20. -phoresis ______________________

21. -scope ______________________

22. -sepsis ______________________

23. -therapy ______________________

24. -ar ______________________

Identifying Medical Terms

In the spaces provided, write the medical terms for the following meanings.

1. ______________________ Process of being stuck together

2. ______________________ Without decay

3. ______________________ Pertaining to the armpit

4. ______________________ Use of chemical agents in the treatment of disease

5. ______________________ Pertaining to a different formation

6. ______________________ Process of being badly shaped, deformed

7. ______________________ Scientific instrument designed to view small objects

8. ______________________ Occurring in or having many shapes

9. ______________________ Study of tumors

Matching

Select the appropriate lettered meaning for each of the following words.

________	**1.** abate	**a.**	Literally means *lack of ease*
________	**2.** antipyretic	**b.**	State of being sick
________	**3.** cachexia	**c.**	Pertaining to protecting against disease or pregnancy
________	**4.** diagnosis	**d.**	Pertaining to an agent that is used to lower an elevated body temperature (fever)
________	**5.** disease	**e.**	A system of prioritizing and classifying patient injuries to determine priority of need and treatment
________	**6.** etiology	**f.**	To lessen, ease, decrease, or cease
________	**7.** illness	**g.**	Determination of the cause and nature of a disease
________	**8.** prognosis	**h.**	New disease
________	**9.** prophylactic	**i.**	Literally means *a state of foreknowledge*
________	**10.** triage	**j.**	Condition of ill health, malnutrition, and wasting
		k.	Study of the cause(s) of disease

Abbreviations

Place the correct word, phrase, or abbreviation in the space provided.

1. CC ________________________________

2. ax ________________________________

3. biopsy ________________________________

4. weight ________________________________

5. Neuro ________________________________

6. ear, nose, throat (otorhinolaryngology) ________________________________

7. dermatology ________________________________

8. gram ________________________________

9. GYN ________________________________

10. Orth ________________________________

Practical Application

Medical Coding

Write your answer to the following questions about terms and abbreviations used in medical coding.

1. Medical coding is the process of assigning __________ characters that represent the diagnoses patients have been given and the services they are to receive.
2. __________ codes identify the reasons that healthcare services were provided.
3. Within the coding system, __________ ____________ is the language used for identifying the diseases and conditions that are coded.
4. The procedure coding system was developed by the ______________________ (CMS) for use in the United States for inpatient hospital settings only.
5. Physicians will continue to use _________________ (CPT) when sending patients for outpatient (OP) testing.

Matching

Select the appropriate lettered meaning for each of the following.

___________	**1.** HIPAA	**a.** clinical modification
___________	**2.** WHO	**b.** Procedure Coding System
___________	**3.** CM	**c.** Health Insurance Portability and Accountability Act
___________	**4.** PCS	**d.** Centers for Medicare & Medicaid Services
___________	**5.** ICD	**e.** World Health Organization
___________	**6.** CMS	**f.** alphabetic characters
___________	**7.** CPT	**g.** Centers for Disease Control and Prevention
___________	**8.** A–Z	**h.** outpatient
___________	**9.** OP	**i.** International Classification of Diseases
___________	**10.** CDC	**j.** Current Procedural Terminology

MyMedicalTerminologyLab™

MyMedicalTerminologyLab is a premium online homework management system that includes a host of features to help you study. Registered users will find:

- A multitude of activities and assignments built within the MyLab platform
- Powerful tools that track and analyze your results—allowing you to create a personalized learning experience
- Videos and audio pronunciations to help enrich your progress
- Streaming lesson presentations (Guided Lectures) and self-paced learning modules
- A space where you and your instructor can check your progress and manage your assignments

Chapter 2

Suffixes

-rrhea
-stasis -oma
-logy -genesis
-pathy -itis
-uria
-trophy

Learning Outcomes

On completion of this chapter, you will be able to:

1. Understand how suffixes are used when building medical words.
2. Name adjective, noun, and diminutive suffixes.
3. Identify suffixes that have more than one meaning.
4. Recognize suffixes that pertain to pathological conditions.
5. Identify selected suffixes common to surgical and diagnostic procedures.
6. Recognize terminology included in the ICD-10-CM.
7. Analyze, build, spell, and pronounce medical words.
8. Apply your acquired knowledge of ICD-10-CM terminology by successfully completing the *Practical Application* exercise.

Overview of Suffixes

The term **suffix** means *to fasten on, beneath, or under*. A suffix can be a syllable or group of syllables united with or placed at the end of a word to alter or modify the meaning of the word or to create a new word. A suffix can be connected to a prefix, a root, or to a combining form to make new words. For example, the suffix *-ic* (which means *pertaining to*) can be combined with the root *gastr* (which means *stomach*) to make the medical word *gastr/ic* (*pertaining to the stomach*) or the suffix *-itis* (which means *inflammation*) can be combined with the root *gastr* to make another medical word, *gastr/itis* (*inflammation of the stomach*).

A compound suffix is made up of more than one word component. It too is added to a root or a combining form to modify its meaning. For example, look at the suffix *-ectomy* (which means *surgical excision*). It is a combination of three word elements: *ec*, a prefix meaning *out*; *tom*, a root meaning *to cut*; and *-y*, a suffix meaning *process*. When the resulting suffix *-ectomy* is added to the root *gastr*, it forms the medical word *gastr/ectomy*, which means *surgical excision of the stomach* or literally *the process to cut out the stomach*.

Whenever you change the suffix, you alter the meaning of the word to which it is attached. For example, adding the suffix *-tomy* (*incision*) to the combining form *gastr/o* forms the medical word *gastr/o/tomy* (*incision into the stomach*). Notice that in the definition, the meaning associated with the suffix (*incision*) precedes the meaning associated with the combining form (*stomach*) to which it is attached. The term *gastr/o/tomy* means or can be read as *incision into* (the suffix) *the stomach* (the combining form).

Review the following guidelines, which were presented in Chapter 1. These will help you with the building and spelling of medical words.

1. If the suffix begins with a vowel, drop the combining vowel from the combining form and add the suffix. For example: gynec/*o* (*female*) + -oid (*resemble*) becomes gynecoid when we drop the *o* from gyneco.
2. If the suffix begins with a consonant, keep the combining vowel and add the suffix to the combining form. For example, lip/*o* (*fat*) + -lysis (*destruction*) becomes lipolysis, and we keep the *o* on the combining form lipo.
3. Keep the combining vowel between two or more roots in a term. For example, electro (*electricity*) + cardio (*heart*) + -gram (*record*) becomes electrocardiogram, and we keep the combining vowels.

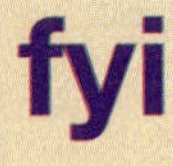

When giving the meaning of the word or reading its definition, you usually begin with the meaning of the suffix. Examples: gynec/*oid* means to *resemble* a female; sperm/i/*cide* is an agent that *kills* sperm; poly/*dipsia* means *thirst* that is excessive.

General Use Suffixes

A collection of suffixes common to medical terminology is listed in Table 2.1. Note that all are preceded by a hyphen (-) to signify that they are to be linked to the end of a root, combining form, or, in some cases, a prefix. Example words are included for each suffix along with their definition. As you progress through this text, the understanding of word parts and the process of building medical words will become easier and easier for you. You do not need to learn all the word parts at one time or the definition of each example word. Start with 10 and then add 10 more and soon you will be surprised at how much you have learned.

Table 2.1 Selected Suffixes for General Use

Suffix	Meaning	Example Word	Word Definition
-algesia	condition of pain	an/*algesia*	Condition in which there is a lack of the sense of pain
-ant	forming	malign/*ant*	Literally means formation of a bad kind; growing worse, harmful, cancerous
-ase	enzyme	amyl/*ase*	Enzyme that breaks down starch
-ate	use, action	exud/*ate*	An oozing of pus or serum
-blast	immature cell, germ cell	oste/o/*blast*	Bone-forming cell
-cide	to kill	sperm/i/*cide*	Agent that kills sperm
-crit	to separate	hemat/o/*crit*	Blood test that separates solids from plasma in the blood by centrifuging the blood sample
-cuspid	point	bi/*cuspid*	Having two points or cusps
-cyst	bladder, sac	blast/o/*cyst*	A structure formed in the early embryogenesis of mammals, after the formation of the morula, but before implantation
-cyte	cell	neur/o/*cyte*	Nerve cell, neuron
-dipsia	thirst	poly/*dipsia*	Excessive thirst
-drome	that which runs together	syn/*drome*	A group of signs and symptoms occurring together that characterize a specific disease or pathological condition
-er	relating to, one who	radi/o/graph/*er*	Person skilled in making x-ray records
-gen	formation, produce	muta/*gen*	Agent that causes a change in the genetic structure of an organism
-genesis	formation, produce	spermat/o/*genesis*	Formation of spermatozoa
-ide	having a particular quality	radi/o/nucl/*ide*	A radioactive atom identified by its atomic number, mass, and energy state
-ive	nature of, quality of	connect/*ive*	Having the nature of connecting or binding together
-liter	liter	milli/*liter*	Unit of volume in the metric system; 0.001 L
-logy	study of	gynec/o/*logy*	Study of the female, especially the diseases of the female reproductive organs and the breasts
-lymph	clear fluid, serum, pale fluid	peri/*lymph*	Serous fluid of the inner ear
-or	one who, a doer	doct/*or*	Literally means to teach; one who is a recipient of an advanced degree, such as doctor of medicine (MD)
-phil	attraction	bas/o/*phil*	White blood cell that has an attraction for a base dye
-stasis	control, stop, stand still	meta/*stasis*	Spreading process (out of control) of cancer from a primary site to a secondary site
-therapy	treatment	hydro/*therapy*	Treatment using scientific application of water
-thermy	heat	dia/*thermy*	Treatment using high-frequency current to produce heat within a part of the body
-um	tissue, structure	epi/thel/i/*um*	Structure that covers the internal and external organs of the body and the lining of vessels, body cavities, glands, and organs
-uria	urination, condition of urine	hemat/*uria*	Presence of blood in the urine

Grammatical Suffixes

Grammatical suffixes are those that can be attached to a word root to form a part of speech, especially a noun or an adjective, or to make a medical word singular or plural in its form. They are also used to indicate a diminutive form of a word that specifies a smaller version of the object indicated by the word root. You will find that many of these suffixes are the same as those used in the English language. See Tables 2.2–2.4.

Table 2.2 Adjective Suffixes That Mean *Pertaining To*

Suffix	Word Analysis	Word Definition
-ac	cardi/*ac*	Pertaining to the heart
-ad	cephal/*ad*	Pertaining to the head
-al	con/genit/*al*	Pertaining to presence at birth
-ar	muscul/*ar*	Pertaining to the muscles
-ary	integument/*ary*	Pertaining to the skin (a covering)
-ic	norm/o/cephal/*ic*	Pertaining to a normal appearance of the head as used in the objective description during a physical examination
-ile	pen/*ile*	Pertaining to the penis
-ior	anter/*ior*	Pertaining to a surface or part situated toward the front of the body
-ose	grandi/*ose*	Pertaining to a feeling of greatness
-ous	edemat/*ous*	Pertaining to an abnormal condition in which the body tissues contain an accumulation of fluid
-tic	cyan/o/*tic*	Pertaining to an abnormal condition of the skin and mucous membranes caused by oxygen deficiency in the blood
-us	de/cubit/*us*	Pertaining to a bedsore
-y	a/ton/*y*	Pertaining to a lack of normal tone or tension

Table 2.3 Noun Suffixes That Mean *Condition*, *Treatment*, or *Specialist*

Suffix	Word Analysis	Word Definition
-esis	enur/*esis*	Condition of involuntary emission of urine; bedwetting
-ia	a/lopec/*ia*	Condition of loss of hair; baldness
-iatry	pod/*iatry*	Treatment of diseases and disorders of the foot
-ician	obstetr/*ician*	Physician who specializes in treating the female during pregnancy, childbirth, and postpartum
-ism	embol/*ism*	Condition in which a blood clot obstructs a blood vessel
-ist	cardi/o/log/*ist*	Physician who specializes in the study of the heart
-osis	hyper/hidr/*osis*	Condition of excessive sweating
-y	an/encephal/*y*	Congenital condition in which there is a lack of development of the brain

Table 2.4 Diminutive Suffixes That Mean *Small* or *Minute*

Suffix	Word Analysis	Word Definition
-icle	ventr/*icle*	Literally means *little belly*; a small cavity or chamber within a body or organ
-ole	bronchi/*ole*	One of the smaller subdivisions of the bronchial tubes
-ula	mac/*ula*	Small spot or discolored area of the skin
-ule	pust/*ule*	Small, elevated, circumscribed lesion of the skin that is filled with pus

Suffixes That Have More Than One Meaning

Some suffixes can have more than a single meaning, thereby making it a little more difficult when defining the medical terms to which they are attached. An alphabetical listing of some of these suffixes is included in Table 2.5.

Table 2.5 Selected Suffixes That Have More Than One Meaning

Suffix	Meanings
-ate	use, action, having the form of, possessing
-blast	immature cell, germ cell, embryonic cell
-ectasis	dilation, distention, stretching, expansion
-gen	formation, produce
-genesis	formation, produce
-genic	formation, produce
-gram	a weight, mark, record
-ive	nature of, quality of
-lymph	serum, clear fluid, pale fluid
-lysis	destruction, separation, breakdown, loosening, dissolution
-penia	lack of, deficiency, abnormal reduction
-plasm	a thing formed, plasma
-plegia	stroke, paralysis, palsy
-ptosis	prolapse, drooping, falling down, sagging
-rrhea	flow, discharge
-scopy	to view, examine, visual examination
-spasm	tension, spasm, contraction
-staxis	dripping, trickling
-trophy	nourishment, development
-y	process, condition, pertaining to

Suffixes That Pertain to Pathological Conditions

Suffixes that carry meanings such as pain, weakness, swelling, softening, inflammation, and tumor are often combined with roots or combining forms to describe pathological conditions. Table 2.6 is an alphabetical listing of some of the more frequently used suffixes associated with disease conditions and disorders.

Table 2.6 Selected Suffixes That Pertain to Pathological Conditions

Suffix	Meaning	Pathological Condition	Definition of Condition
-algia	pain, ache	dent/*algia*	Pain in a tooth; toothache
-asthenia	weakness	my/*asthenia*	Muscular weakness and abnormal fatigue
-betes	to go	dia/*betes*	General term used to describe diseases characterized by excessive discharge of urine
-cele	hernia, tumor, swelling	cyst/o/*cele*	Hernia of the bladder that protrudes into the vagina
-cusis	hearing	presby/*cusis*	Impairment of hearing that occurs with aging
-derma	skin	xer/o/*derma*	Dry skin
-dynia	pain, ache	ot/o/*dynia*	Pain in the ear, earache
-ectasis	dilation, distention	bronch/i/*ectasis*	Chronic dilation of a bronchus or bronchi, with a secondary infection that usually involves the lower portion of a lung
-edema	swelling	papill/*edema*	Swelling of the optic disk, usually caused by increased intracranial pressure (ICP)
-emesis	vomiting	hyper/*emesis*	Excessive vomiting
-ion	process	in/fect/*ion*	Process whereby a pathogenic (*disease-producing*) microorganism invades the body, reproduces, multiplies, and causes disease
-itis	inflammation	burs/*itis*	Inflammation of a bursa (*padlike sac between muscles, tendons, and bones*)
-kinesis	motion	hyper/*kinesis*	Excessive muscular movement and motion; inability to be still; also known as hyperactivity
-lepsy	seizure	narc/o/*lepsy*	Chronic condition with recurrent attacks of uncontrollable drowsiness and sleep
-lexia	diction, word, phrase	dys/*lexia*	Condition in which an individual has difficulty in reading and comprehending written language
-malacia	softening	oste/o/*malacia*	Softening of the bones
-mania	madness	pyro/*mania*	Impulse-control disorder consisting of a compulsion to set fires or to watch fires
-megaly	enlargement, large	acr/o/*megaly*	Characterized (in the adult) by marked enlargement and elongation of the bones of the face, jaw, and extremities
-mnesia	memory	a/*mnesia*	Condition in which there is a loss or lack of memory

(*continued*)

Table 2.6 Selected Suffixes That Pertain to Pathological Conditions *(continued)*

Suffix	Meaning	Pathological Condition	Definition of Condition
-noia	mind	para/*noia*	Mental disorder characterized by highly exaggerated or unwarranted mistrust or suspiciousness
-oid	resemble	carcin/*oid*	Slow growing type of cancer that typically begins in the lining of the digestive tract
-oma	tumor	carcin/*oma*	Malignant tumor arising in epithelial tissue
-opia	sight, vision	presby/*opia*	Vision defect in which parallel rays come to a focus beyond the retina; occurs normally with aging; farsightedness
-oxia	oxygen	hyp/*oxia*	Deficient amount of oxygen in the blood cells and tissues
-pathy	disease, emotion	retin/o/*pathy*	Any disease of the retina
-penia	deficiency	oste/o/*penia*	Deficiency of bone tissue, regardless of the cause
-pepsia	to digest	dys/*pepsia*	Difficulty in digestion; indigestion
-phagia	to eat, to swallow	a/*phagia*	Loss or lack of the ability to eat or swallow
-phasia	to speak, speech	dys/*phasia*	Impairment of speech caused by a brain lesion
-phobia	fear	acr/o/*phobia*	Fear of heights
-plasia	formation, produce	hyper/*plasia*	Excessive formation and growth of normal cells
-plasm	a thing formed, plasma	neo/*plasm*	New thing formed, such as an abnormal growth or tumor
-plegia	paralysis, stroke	hemi/*plegia*	Slight paralysis that affects one side of the body
-pnea	breathing	sleep a/*pnea*	Temporary cessation of breathing during sleep
-ptosis	drooping, prolapse, sagging	blephar/o/*ptosis*	Drooping of the upper eyelid(s)
-ptysis	spitting	hem/o/*ptysis*	Spitting up blood
-rrhage	bursting forth	hem/o/*rrhage*	Excessive bleeding; bursting forth of blood
-rrhea	flow, discharge	rhin/o/*rrhea*	Discharge from the nose
-rrhexis	rupture	my/o/*rrhexis*	Rupture of a muscle
-spasm	tension, spasm, contraction	my/o/*spasm*	Spasmodic contraction of a muscle
-trophy	nourishment, development	hyper/*trophy*	Literally means *excessive nourishment*

ALERT!

Memorize these suffixes that begin with **rrh**: ***-rrhage*** (*bursting forth*), ***-rrhea*** (*flow, discharge*), ***-rrhexis*** (*rupture*). Also recall the surgical procedure suffix ***-rrhaphy*** (*suture*).

Suffixes Associated with Surgical and Diagnostic Procedures

Suffixes with meanings such as puncture, surgical excision, instrument to measure, and new opening are often combined with roots or combining forms to describe surgical and/or diagnostic procedures. See Table 2.7 for an alphabetical listing of some of the more frequently used suffixes associated with surgery and diagnosis.

Table 2.7 Selected Suffixes Used in Surgical and Diagnostic Procedures

Suffix	Meaning	Example Word	Word Definition
-centesis	surgical puncture	amni/o/*centesis*	Surgical puncture of the amniotic sac to obtain a sample of amniotic fluid containing fetal cells that are examined
-clasis	a break	oste/o/*clasis*	The intentional surgical fracture of a bone to correct a deformity
-desis	binding	arthr/o/*desis*	Surgical binding of a joint; surgical fixation of a joint
-ectomy	surgical excision, surgical removal, resection	vas/*ectomy*	Surgical procedure in which the vas deferens are clamped, cut, or otherwise sealed providing permanent sterility by preventing transport of sperm out of the testes
-gram	a weight, mark, record	dactyl/o/*gram*	Fingerprint
-graph	instrument for recording	electr/o/cardi/o/*graph*	Medical diagnostic device used for recording the electrical impulses of the heart muscle
-graphy	recording	mamm/o/*graphy*	Process of obtaining x-ray pictures of the breast using a low-dose x-ray system
-ize	to make, to treat, or combine with	an/esthet/*ize*	To induce a loss of feeling or sensation with the administration of an anesthetic
-lysis	destruction, separation, breakdown, loosening	lip/o/*lysis*	Destruction of fat
-meter	instrument to measure, measure	audi/o/*meter*	Medical instrument used to measure hearing
-metry	measurement	pelvi/*metry*	Measurement of the expectant mother's pelvic dimensions to determine whether it will be possible to deliver a fetus through the normal vaginal route
-opsy	to view	bi/*opsy*	Surgical removal of a small piece of tissue for microscopic examination
-pexy	surgical fixation	gastr/o/*pexy*	Surgical fixation of the stomach to the abdominal wall for correction of displacement
-pheresis	remove	plasma/*pheresis*	Removal of blood from the body and centrifuging it to separate the plasma from the blood and reinfusing the cellular elements back into the patient
-plasty	surgical repair	rhin/o/*plasty*	Surgical repair of the nose

(*continued*)

Table 2.7 Selected Suffixes Used in Surgical and Diagnostic Procedures *(continued)*

Suffix	Meaning	Example Word	Word Definition
-rrhaphy	suture	my/o/*rrhaphy*	Suture of a muscle wound
-scope	instrument for examining	ophthalm/o/*scope*	Medical instrument used to examine the interior of the eye
-scopy	visual examination, to view, examine	lapar/o/*scopy*	Visual examination of the abdominal cavity
-stomy	new opening	ile/o/*stomy*	Creation of a new opening through the abdominal wall into the ileum
-tome	instrument to cut	derma/*tome*	Instrument used to cut the skin for grafting
-tomy	incision	myring/o/*tomy*	Surgical incision of the tympanic membrane to remove unwanted fluids from the ear
-tripsy	crushing	lith/o/*tripsy*	Crushing of a kidney stone

ALERT!

Be sure that you see the difference: ***-stomy*** means *new opening* and ***-tomy*** means *incision*.

Building Your Medical Vocabulary

This section provides the foundation for learning medical terminology. Review the following alphabetized word list. Note how common prefixes and suffixes are repeatedly applied to word roots and combining forms to create different meanings. The word parts are color-coded: prefixes are yellow, suffixes are blue, roots/combining forms are red. A combining form is a word root plus a vowel.

Remember These Guidelines

1. If the suffix begins with a vowel, drop the combining vowel from the combining form and add the suffix. For example, carcin/o (*cancer*) + -oma (*tumor*) becomes carcinoma.
2. If the suffix begins with a consonant, keep the combining vowel and add the suffix to the combining form. For example, rhin/o (*nose*) + -plasty (*surgical repair*) becomes rhinoplasty.

You will find that some terms have not been divided into word parts. These are common words or specialized terms that are included to enhance your medical vocabulary.

Medical Word	Word Parts		Definition
	Part	Meaning	
abrasion (ă-brā´ zhŭn)	ab- ras -ion	away from to scrape off process	Process of scraping away from a surface, such as skin or teeth, by friction. An abrasion may be the result of trauma, such as a "skinned knee" or from a therapy, such as dermabrasion of the skin for removal of scar tissue. It can also occur from the wearing-down of a tooth from mastication (*chewing*).
anesthetize (ă-nĕs´ thĕ-tīz)	an- esthet -ize	without, lack of feeling, sensation to make	To induce a loss of feeling or sensation with the administration of an anesthetic
arousal (a-rou´ zel)	arous -al	alertness, to rise pertaining to	Pertaining to a state of alertness or consciousness
asymmetrical (ā-sĭ-mĕ´ -trĭ-kăl)	a- symmetric -al	lack of, without symmetry pertaining to	Unequal in size or shape. Without proportion of the body or parts of the body; different in placement or arrangement about an axis.
comatose (kō´ mă-tōs)	comat -ose	a deep sleep pertaining to	Literally means *pertaining to a state of deep sleep* (coma); total lack of consciousness

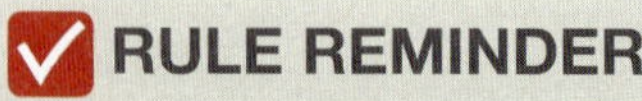

RULE REMINDER

The ***o*** has been removed from the combining form because the suffix begins with a vowel.

Medical Word	Word Parts		Definition
	Part	**Meaning**	
epithelium (ĕp″ ĭ-thē′ lē-ŭm)	epi- thel/i -um	upon, above nipple tissue, structure	Structure that covers the internal and external organs of the body and the lining of vessels, body cavities, glands, and organs. It is the layer of cells forming the outermost layer of the skin and the surface layer of mucous and serous membranes.

ALERT!

To change epitheli***um*** to its plural form, you change the ***um*** to ***a*** to create *epithelia*.

Medical Word	Part	Meaning	Definition
exogenous (ĕks-ŏj′ ĕ-nŭs)	ex(o)- gen -ous	out formation, produce pertaining to	Pertaining to originating outside the body or an organ of the body or produced from external causes, such as a disease caused by a bacterial or viral agent foreign to the body
grandiose (grăn′ dē-ōs)	grand/i -ose	great pertaining to	Pertaining to a feeling of *greatness*. In psychiatry, it refers to a person's unrealistic and exaggerated concept of self-worth, importance, wealth, and ability.

RULE REMINDER

Here is an exception to the general rule. This combining form keeps the ***i*** even though the suffix begins with a vowel.

Medical Word	Part	Meaning	Definition
gynecoid (jĭn′ ĕ-koyd)	gynec -oid	female resemble	Literally means *to resemble a female*; gynecoid pelvis is the normal shape of the birth canal that allows for the exit of the average fetus
infection (ĭn-fĕk′ shŭn)	infect -ion	to infect process	Process whereby a pathogenic (*disease-producing*) microorganism invades the body, reproduces, multiplies, and causes disease. Examples of disease-producing microorganisms are bacteria, viruses, mycoses (fungi), helminths (worms), and protozoa. See Figure 2.1.

(*continued*)

Medical Word	Word Parts		Definition
	Part	Meaning	

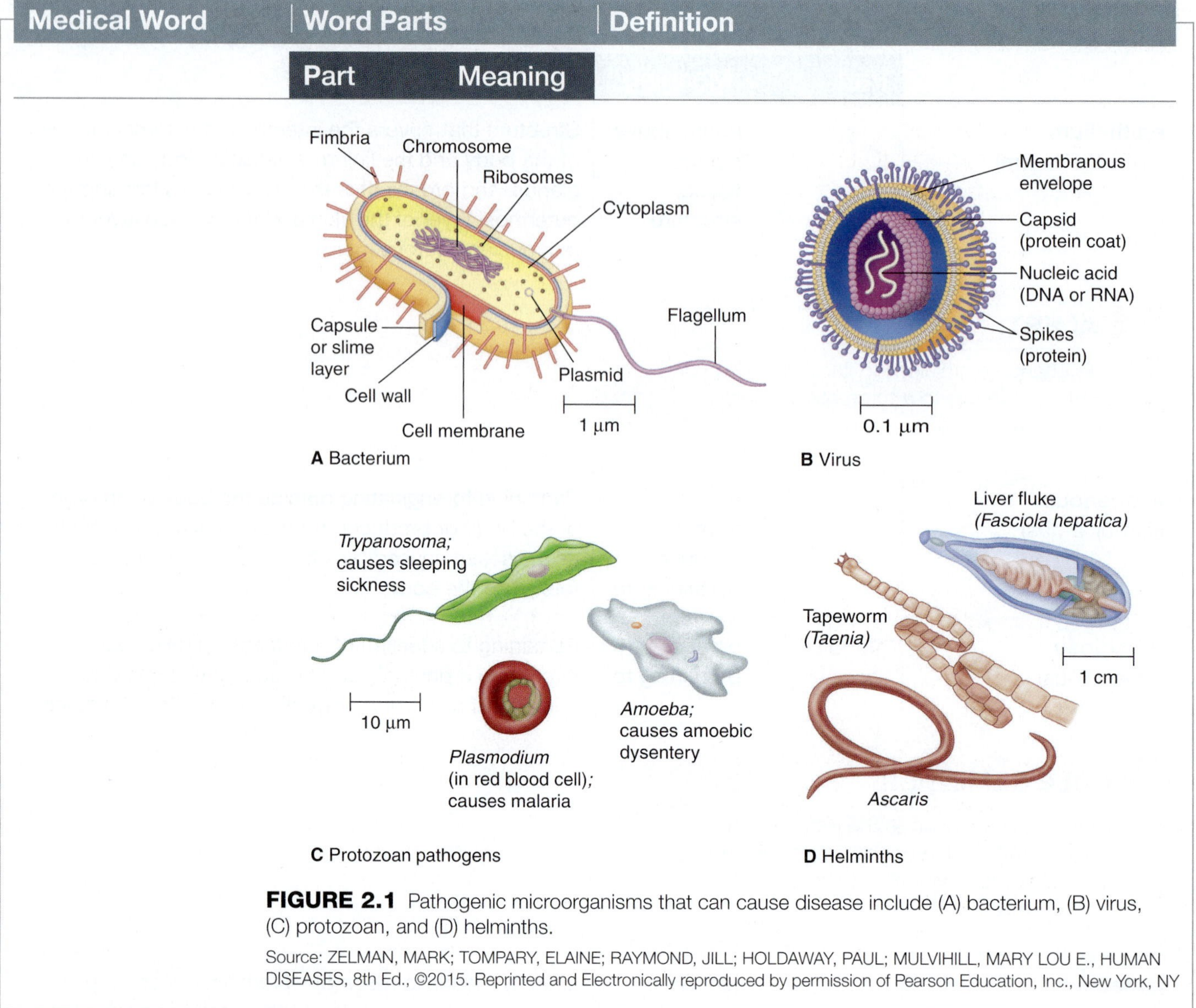

FIGURE 2.1 Pathogenic microorganisms that can cause disease include (A) bacterium, (B) virus, (C) protozoan, and (D) helminths.

Source: ZELMAN, MARK; TOMPARY, ELAINE; RAYMOND, JILL; HOLDAWAY, PAUL; MULVIHILL, MARY LOU E., HUMAN DISEASES, 8th Ed., ©2015. Reprinted and Electronically reproduced by permission of Pearson Education, Inc., New York, NY

(*continued*)

Medical Word	Word Parts		Definition
	Part	Meaning	

insights The following terms, used in ICD-10-CM, Chapter 1, *Certain Infectious and Parasitic Diseases* (A00–B99), are associated with the causative agents or signs of some infections and diseases.

arthropods	Invertebrate animals (mosquitoes, ticks, mites, fleas, sand fleas, lice) that can transmit diseases to humans and animals. They function as hematophagous (hemat/o [blood], phag [to eat], -ous [pertaining to]) **vectors** (carriers) that transmit disease through their bite. Only female mosquitos bite to get a blood meal for their growing eggs. Arthropods are the largest animal *phylum* (scientific way of grouping together related organisms), comprising about 85% of all known animals in the world. See Figure 2.2.

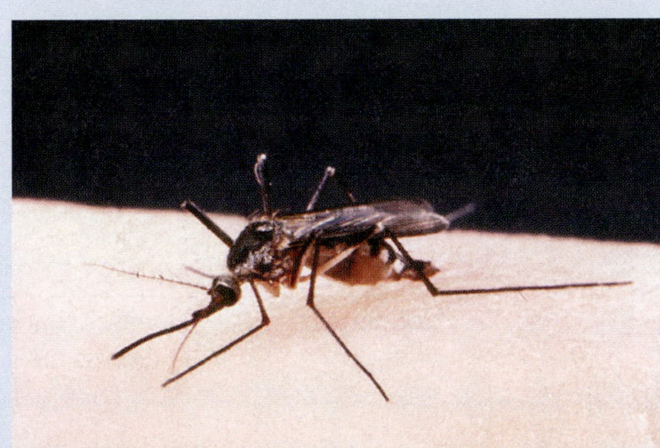

FIGURE 2.2 The *Aedes* mosquito, one of the vectors responsible for causing West Nile virus encephalitis.
Courtesy Centers for Disease Control and Prevention (CDC)/Robert S. Craig.

helminths	Wormlike animals (vermiform parasites). Broadly classified into tapeworms, flukes, and roundworms, these parasites often live in the gastrointestinal tract of their hosts, but may also burrow into other organs, where they induce physiological damage. ***Helminthiasis*** is the term used for the patient having intestinal parasites or worms.
mycoses	Fungal infections
nonsuppurative	Pertaining to inflammation without the production of pus
prion infections	Disease caused by a protein-like infectious particle (prion). Prions cause a number of diseases in animals and humans known as spongiform encephalopathies (brain diseases), in which the brain becomes damaged with holes. Mad cow disease in cattle is a prion infection.
protozoal	Pertaining to single-celled parasitic organisms (protozoa) with flexible membranes and the ability to move. They can cause amebic dysentery, sleeping sickness, and malaria.

(*continued*)

Medical Word	Word Parts		Definition
	Part	**Meaning**	

rickettsiosis Infection with rickettsiae, the most common being Rocky Mountain spotted fever and epidemic typhus. See Figure 2.3.

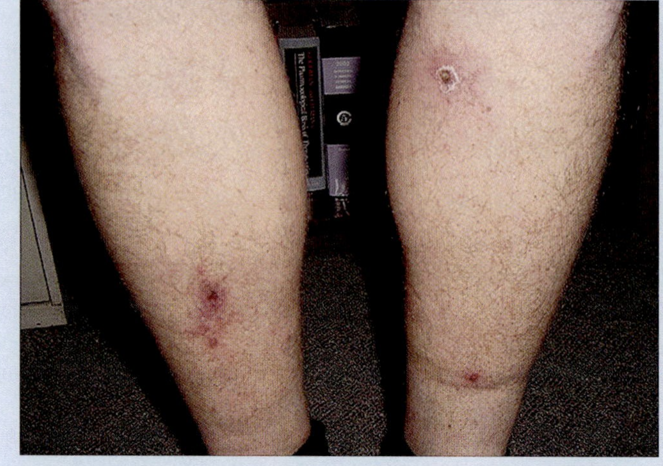

Figure 2.3 Inoculation eschars associated with the site of tick attachment in a patient infected with rickettsial infection *R. parkeri*.
Courtesy Centers for Disease Control and Prevention (CDC).

spirochetal Pertaining to spirochetes, especially infections caused by them, such as syphilis.

zoonoses Diseases that are communicable (transmissible) from animals to humans. Examples are viruses, bacteria, parasites, and mycoses.

Medical Word	Part	Meaning	Definition
irregular (ĭr-rĕg´ ū-lăr)	ir- regul -ar	not rule pertaining to	Pertaining to not being regular
nasolabial (nā´´ zō-lā´ bĭ-ăl)	nas/o labi -al	nose lip pertaining to	Pertaining to the nose and lip
palpate (păl´ pāt)	palp -ate	touch use, action	To use the hands or fingers to examine by touch; to feel
sanguineous (sang-gwin´ ē-ŭs)			Pertaining to or containing blood
sanguinopurulent (sang´´ gwĭ-no-pu´ ru-lent)			Containing blood and pus
sepsis (sēp´ sĭs)	sep -sis	putrefaction condition	Pathological condition in which bacteria are present in the blood; the spread of infection from its initial site to the bloodstream. *Note:* In the ICD-10-CM, the term *sepsis* replaced *septicemia*.

Medical Word	Word Parts		Definition
	Part	Meaning	
steroid (stĕr´ oyd)	ster -oid	solid resemble	Literally means *resembling a solid substance*; applies to any one of a large group of substances chemically related to sterols; natural steroid hormones include androgens, estrogens, and adrenal cortex secretions
trauma (traw´ mă)			Physical injury or wound caused by external force, violence, or a toxic substance; also refers to psychological injury resulting from a severe emotional shock, which can cause disordered feelings and/or behavior
turgor (tur´ jor)	turg -or	swelling one who	Generally refers to the expected resiliency of the skin caused by the outward pressure of the cells and interstitial fluid. An evaluation of the skin turgor is an essential part of physical assessment.

Study and Review

Identifying Suffixes

Underline the suffixes in the following medical words.

1. cardiac
2. cephalad
3. enuresis
4. obstetrician
5. bronchiole
6. pustule
7. dentalgia
8. diabetes
9. hyperemesis
10. hemoptysis

Defining Suffixes

Give the meaning of the following suffixes.

1. -asthenia ______________________
2. -ion ______________________
3. -itis ______________________
4. -malacia ______________________
5. -megaly ______________________
6. -pathy ______________________
7. -penia ______________________
8. -pepsia ______________________
9. -phobia ______________________
10. -rrhexis ______________________
11. -al ______________________
12. -ar ______________________

13. -ate ____________________

14. -ia ____________________

15. -ize ____________________

16. -oid ____________________

17. -or ____________________

18. -ose ____________________

19. -ous ____________________

20. -um ____________________

Using Suffixes to Build Medical Words

Using a suffix from the following list, build the appropriate medical word.

-al	*-ior*	*-ar*	*-ile*
-ary	*-osis*	*-ia*	*-ula*
-icle	*-us*		

1. Condition of excessive sweating — hyper/hidr/__________
2. Pertaining to muscles — muscul/__________
3. Small spot or discolored area of the skin — mac/__________
4. Condition of loss of hair — a/lopec/__________
5. Literally means *little belly* — ventr/__________
6. Pertaining to a bedsore — de/cubit/__________
7. Pertaining to the skin — integument/__________
8. Pertaining to the penis — pen/__________
9. Pertaining to present at birth — con/genit/__________
10. Pertaining to toward the front of the body — anter/__________

Identifying Medical Terms

In the spaces provided, write the medical terms for the following meanings.

1. ______________________ Process of scraping away from a surface
2. ______________________ To induce a loss of feeling or sensation
3. ______________________ Pertaining to a state of alertness or consciousness
4. ______________________ Unequal in size or shape
5. ______________________ The process whereby a pathogenic organism invades the body and causes disease
6. ______________________ Pertaining to a state of deep sleep
7. ______________________ Refers to the expected resiliency of the skin
8. ______________________ Pertaining to a feeling of greatness
9. ______________________ To resemble a female
10. ______________________ To use the hands or fingers to examine by touch

Practical Application

ICD-10-CM Terminology

Write your answers in the spaces provided.

1. The largest animal phylum that makes up about 85% of all known animals in the world is known as ____________.
2. A ____________ is the scientific way of grouping together related organisms.
3. The term used for the patient having intestinal parasites or worms is ____________
4. A ____________ is a protein-like infectious particle.
5. What is the term that means pertaining to single-celled parasitic organisms with flexible membranes and the ability to move? ____________
6. A ____________ is an organism, such as fleas, mosquitoes, ticks, that transmits a pathogen from one source to another.
7. The term that means pertaining to or containing blood is ____________.
8. The term that is used to describe fungal infections is ____________.
9. The term ____________ means pertaining to spirochetes, especially infections caused by them, such as syphilis.
10. What is the term that means pertaining to inflammation without the production of pus? ____________

Chapter 3

Prefixes

sub- intra- hydro- bi- mono- anti- poly- dys- endo- ex- hyper-

Learning Outcomes

On completion of this chapter, you will be able to:

1. Understand how prefixes are used when building medical words.
2. Name prefixes that are commonly used in medical terminology.
3. Identify prefixes that have more than one meaning.
4. Recognize prefixes that pertain to position or placement.
5. Identify selected prefixes that pertain to numbers and amounts.
6. Analyze, build, spell, and pronounce medical words.

Overview of Prefixes

The term **prefix** means *to fix before* or *to fix to the beginning* of a word. A prefix can be a syllable or a group of syllables. Prefixes are united with or placed at the beginning of words to alter or modify their meanings or to create entirely new words. For example, by adding the prefix *ab-* to the root *norm*, and the suffix *-al*, the word **ab/norm/al** is created. As you know, there is a big difference between normal and abnormal. Ab/norm/al means *pertaining to away from the norm*. Remember that when giving the meaning of the word or reading its definition, you usually begin with the meaning of the suffix. Note the component parts of the word *abnormal*:

ab-	P or prefix meaning	*away from*
norm	R or root meaning	*norm*
-al	S or suffix meaning	*pertaining to*

Not all medical words have a prefix, but when they do, the prefix will alter or modify the meaning of the word. For example, see the following list of medical words that were formed by uniting various prefixes with a single suffix (*-pnea*).

Prefix	Suffix	Medical Word	Word Definition
a- (lack of)	-pnea (breathing)	apnea	Temporary absence of (lack of) breathing
brady- (slow)	-pnea (breathing)	*brady*pnea	Slow breathing
dys- (difficult)	-pnea (breathing)	*dys*pnea	Difficult breathing
eu- (good, normal)	-pnea (breathing)	*eu*pnea	Good, normal breathing
hyper- (excessive)	-pnea (breathing)	*hyper*pnea	Excessive breathing
hypo- (deficient)	-pnea (breathing)	*hypo*pnea	Deficient breathing
tachy- (rapid)	-pnea (breathing)	*tachy*pnea	Rapid breathing

General Use Prefixes

See Table 3.1 for a collection of prefixes that are commonly used in medical terminology. These prefixes can be linked with a word root or a suffix.

Table 3.1 Selected Prefixes for General Use

Prefix	Meanings	Example Words	Word Definitions
a, an-	no, without, lack of, apart	*a*/mnes/ia	Condition in which there is a loss or lack of memory
		an/emia	Literally *a lack of red blood cells*
anti-, contra-	against	*anti*/gen	Invading foreign substance that induces the formation of antibodies
		contra/cept/ion	Process of preventing conception
auto-	self	*auto*/trans/fus/ion	Process of infusing a patient's own blood
brachy-	short	*brachy*/therapy	Radiation therapy in which the radioactive substance is inserted into a body cavity or organ. The source of radiation is located a short distance from the body area being treated.

(*continued*)

Table 3.1 Selected Prefixes for General Use *(continued)*

Prefix	Meanings	Example Words	Word Definitions
brady-	slow	*brady*/card/ia	Abnormally slow heartbeat defined as less than 60 beats per minute
cac-, mal-	bad	*cac*/hexia	Condition of ill health, malnutrition, and wasting; may occur in chronic diseases such as cancer and pulmonary tuberculosis
		mal/format/ion	The process of being badly shaped, deformed
dia-	through, between	*dia*/gnosis	Determination of the cause and nature of a disease
dys-	bad, difficult, painful, abnormal	*dys*/meno/rrhea	Difficulty or painful monthly flow (menses or menstruation)
eu-	good, normal	*eu*/pnea	Good or normal breathing
ex-, exo-	out, away from	*ex*/cis/ion	Process of cutting out, surgical removal
		exo/crine	Pertains to a type of gland that secretes into ducts (duct glands); examples include sweat glands, salivary glands, mammary glands, stomach, liver, and pancreas
hetero-	different	*hetero*/sexu/al	Pertaining to the opposite sex; refers to an individual who has a sexual preference and relationship with the opposite sex
homeo-	similar, same, likeness, constant	*homeo*/stasis	State of equilibrium maintained in the body's internal environment; an important fundamental principle of physiology that permits a body to maintain a constant internal environment despite changes in the external environment
hydro-	water	*hydro*/cele	Accumulation of fluid in a saclike cavity
micro-	small	*micro*/cephal/us	Abnormally small head
oligo-	scanty, little	*oligo*/meno/rrhea	Scanty monthly flow (menses, menstruation)
pan-	all	*pan*/cyto/penia	Lack of the cellular elements of the blood
pseudo-	false	*pseudo*/cyesis	False pregnancy
sym-, syn-	together, with	*sym*/physis	State of growing together
		syn/erget/ic	Pertaining to certain muscles that work together

Prefixes That Have More Than One Meaning

Just like suffixes, many prefixes have more than one meaning. See Table 3.2. To be able to identify the correct meaning of the prefix, you will need to analyze the definition of the medical word. For example, in the medical word **dyspnea** (difficult breathing), *dys-* means *difficult*. Note that *dys-* also means *bad*, *painful*, or *abnormal*, but in dyspnea these meanings do not apply. As you learn the various component parts that are used to build medical words, you will acquire the knowledge to select and use the correct meaning for each word.

Table 3.2 Selected Prefixes That Have More Than One Meaning

Prefix	Meanings	Prefix	Meanings
a-, an-	no, not, without, lack of, apart	**extra-**	outside, beyond
ad-	toward, near	**hyper-**	above, beyond, excessive
bi-	two, double	**hypo-**	below, under, deficient
de-	down, away from	**in-**	in, into, not
di-	two, double	**mega-**	large, great
dia-	through, between, complete	**meta-**	beyond, over, between, change
dif-, dis-	apart, free from, separate	**para-**	beside, alongside, abnormal
dys-	bad, difficult, painful, abnormal	**poly-**	many, much, excessive
ec-, ecto-	out, outside, outer	**post-**	after, behind
end-, endo-	within, inner	**pre-**	before, in front of
ep-, epi-	upon, over, above	**pro-**	before, in front of
eu-	good, normal	**super-**	upper, above
ex-, exo-	out, away from	**supra-**	above, beyond

Prefixes That Pertain to Position or Placement

Prefixes that carry meanings such as *away from, toward, before, above,* and *below* are often combined with roots and suffixes to describe a position or placement. See Table 3.3 for an alphabetical listing of some of the more frequently used prefixes associated with position or placements.

TABLE 3.3 Prefixes That Pertain to Position or Placement

Prefix	Meanings	Example Words	Word Definitions
ab-	away from	*ab*/duct/ion	Process of moving a body part away from the middle
ad-	toward, near, to	*ad*/duct/or	Muscle that draws a part toward the middle
ana-	up, apart, backward	*ana*/trop/ia	Tendency of eyeballs to turn upward
ante-	before, forward	*ante*/flex/ion	The process of bending forward of an organ or part
cata-	down	*cata*/bol/ism	Literally *a casting down*; a breaking of complex substances into more basic elements
circum-, peri-	around	*circum*/cis/ion	Surgical process of removing (a cutting around) the foreskin of the penis
		peri/cardi/al	Pertaining to the pericardium, the sac surrounding the heart
endo-	within, inner	*endo*/card/itis	Inflammation of the endocardium (inner lining of the heart)
epi-	upon, above, over	*epi*/gastr/ic	Pertaining to the region above the stomach

(*continued*)

TABLE 3.3 Prefixes That Pertain to Position or Placement *(continued)*			
Prefix	Meanings	Example Words	Word Definitions
ex-	out, away from	*ex*/cis/ion	Process of cutting out; surgical removal
extra-	outside, beyond	*extra*/corpor/eal (circulation)	Pertaining to the circulation of the blood outside the body via a heart-lung machine or hemodialyzer
hyper-	above, beyond, excessive	*hyper*/tens/ion	High blood pressure
hypo-	below, under, deficient	*hypo*/tens/ion	Low blood pressure
inter-	between	*inter*/cost/al	Pertaining to between the ribs
intra-	within, into	*intra*/uter/ine	Pertaining to within the uterus
meso-	middle	*meso*/derm	A middle layer of the embryo lying between the ectoderm and endoderm
para-	beside, alongside	*para*/plegia	Paralysis of the lower part of the body and of both legs
retro-	backward	*retro*/vers/ion	Process of being turned backward, such as the displacement of the uterus with the cervix pointed forward
sub-	below, under, beneath	*sub*/lingu/al	Pertaining to below the tongue
supra-	above, beyond, superior	*supra*/ren/al	Two small glands located on top (above) of each kidney, also called adrenal glands

Prefixes That Pertain to Numbers and Amounts

Prefixes with meanings such as *both, ten, double, many, half,* and *none* are often combined with roots or suffixes to describe numbers or amounts. See Table 3.4 for an alphabetical list of some of the more frequently used prefixes associated with numbers and amounts.

Table 3.4 Prefixes That Pertain to Numbers and Amounts			
Prefix	Meanings	Example Word	Word Definitions
ambi-	both	*ambi*/later/al	Pertaining to both sides
bi-	two, double	*bi*/later/al	Pertaining to two sides
bin-	twice, two	*bin*/aur/al	Pertaining to both ears
centi-	one hundredth	*centi*/meter	Unit of measurement in the metric system; one hundredth of a meter
deca-	ten	*deca*/gram	A weight of 10 grams
di(s)-	two, apart	*dis*/locat/ion	Displacement of a bone from a joint
milli-	one thousandth	*milli*/liter	Unit of volume in the metric system; 0.001 L
mono-	one	*mono*/nucle/osis	Condition of excessive amounts of mononuclear leukocytes in the blood
multi-	many, much	*multi*/para	Refers to a woman who has given birth to two or more children and is written as para 2 (3, 4, 5, etc.)

(continued)

Table 3.4 Prefixes That Pertain to Numbers and Amounts *(continued)*

Prefix	Meanings	Example Word	Word Definitions
nulli-	none	*nulli*/para	Refers to a woman who has never delivered a viable offspring and is written as para 0
poly-	many	*poly*/uria	Excessive urination
primi-	first	*primi*/para	Refers to a woman who has had one birth at more than 20 weeks' gestation, regardless of whether the infant is born alive or dead and is written as para 1
quadri-	four	*quadri*/plegia	Paralysis of all four extremities and usually the trunk due to injury to the spinal cord in the cervical spine
semi-, hemi-	half	*semi*/lun/ar	Valves of the aorta and pulmonary artery; shaped like a crescent (half-moon)
		hemi/plegia	Paralysis of one half of the body when it is divided along the median sagittal plane
tri-	three	*tri*/som/y	Genetic condition of having three chromosomes instead of two that causes birth defects, such as Down syndrome
uni-	one	*uni*/later/al	Pertaining to one side

Building Your Medical Vocabulary

This section provides the foundation for learning medical terminology. Review the following alphabetized word list. Note how common prefixes and suffixes are repeatedly applied to word roots and combining forms to create different meanings. The word parts are color-coded: prefixes are yellow, suffixes are blue, roots/combining forms are red.

You will find that some terms have not been divided into word parts. These are common words or specialized terms that are included to enhance your medical vocabulary.

Medical Word	Word Parts		Definition
	Part	Meaning	
afebrile (ă-fĕb´ rĭl)	a- febr -ile	without fever pertaining to	Literally means *pertaining to without fever*; the patient's temperature would be within a normal range of 98.6°F
anicteric (ăn″ ĭk-tĕr´ ĭk)	an- icter -ic	without jaundice pertaining to	Term used to describe a condition that is without signs of jaundice (yellowish discoloration of the skin, whites of the eyes, mucous membranes, and body fluids), such as anicteric hepatitis (a mild form of hepatitis in which there is no jaundice)
arrest (ă-rĕst´)			To stop, inhibit, restrain. A condition of being stopped, such as occurs in cardiac arrest when cardiac output and effective circulation stop.
bifurcation (bī´ fŭr-kā´ shŭn)	bi- furcat -ion	two fork process	The process of having two forks or two branches or two divisions; the point of forking.

insights In ICD-10-CM, *bifurcation (congenital)* is coded as Q44.1 for the gallbladder, Q63.8 for the kidney pelvis, and Q63.8 for the renal pelvis; there are six other codes included under this subcategory.

Medical Word	Part	Meaning	Definition
concentration (kŏn-sĕn-trā´ shŭn)	con- centrat -ion	with, together center process	In psychology, the process of being able to bring to the center one thought and focus on it, while excluding other thoughts
decompensation (dē-kŏm-pen-sā´ shŭn)	de- compensat -ion	down, away from to make good again process	Failure of a system. In cardiology—failure of the heart to maintain adequate circulation; in psychology—failure of the defense mechanism system that may occur during a relapsing of a mental condition.

Medical Word	Word Parts: Part	Word Parts: Meaning	Definition
enucleate (ē-nū´ klē-āt)			Literally means *to remove the kernel of*. It is used to describe the removal of the eyeball surgically or to remove a cataract surgically. It also means to remove a part or a mass in its entirety.
extraocular (ěks˝ tră-ŏk´ ū-lăr)	extra- ocul -ar	outside eye pertaining to	Pertaining to outside the eye, as used in describing the extraocular eye muscles. These are the muscles that control eye movement and eye coordination.

RULE REMINDER

The ***o*** has been removed from the combining form because the suffix begins with a vowel.

Medical Word	Word Parts: Part	Word Parts: Meaning	Definition
hyperactive (hī˝ pěr-ăk´ tĭv)	hyper- act -ive	excessive act nature of, quality of	Nature or quality of excessive activity; this can refer to the entire organism or to a particular entity such as the thyroid, heart, or muscles. It may also describe an individual who exhibits constant overactivity.
hypoplasia (hī˝ pō-plā´ zē-ă)	hypo- -plasia	under formation	Underdevelopment of a tissue, organ, or body
insomnia (ĭn-sŏm´ nē-ah)	in- somn -ia	not sleep condition	Condition of not being able to sleep. People with insomnia can have difficulty falling asleep, wake up often during the night and have trouble going back to sleep, wake up too early in the morning, or experience unrefreshing sleep.
intercellular junctions (ĭn˝ ter-sěl-ū-lăr)	inter- cell(ul) -ar	between cell pertaining to	Pertaining to the microscopic space between cells that are important in assisting the transfer of small molecules across capillary walls
intraoperative (in˝ trah-op´er-a˝ tiv)	intra- operat -ive	within to work quality of	Occurring during a surgical operation or procedure
latent (lā´ tent)			Lying hidden; quiet, not active; for example, tuberculosis (TB) may be latent for extended periods of time and become active under certain conditions
lumen (lū´ měn)			Space within an artery, vein, intestine, or tube. It is also the hollow core of a hypodermic needle, which forms an oval-shaped opening when exposed at the beveled (flat, slanted surface) point.

Medical Word	Word Parts		Definition
	Part	Meaning	
multifocal (mŭl″ tĭ-fō′ kăl)	multi- foc -al	many focus pertaining to	Pertaining to or arising from many locations
occlusion (ŏ-kloo′ zhŭn)			Process of closing or state of being closed such as of a passage or lumen
parasternal (păr-ă-stĕrn′ ăl)	para- stern -al	beside sternum, breastbone pertaining to	Pertaining to either side of the sternum (breastbone)
patent (pă′ tĕnt)			Wide open; freely open; for example, a lumen would be patent (opposite of occlusion)
pericardial (pĕr-ĭ-kăr′ dē-ăl)	peri- cardi -al	around heart pertaining to	Pertaining to the pericardium (a fibrous sac surrounding the heart)
polydactyly (pŏl″ ē-dăk′ tĭ-lē)	poly- dactyl -y	many finger or toe pertaining to	Pertaining to having more than the normal number of fingers and toes; for example, a person having six fingers or toes

RULE REMINDER

The ***o*** has been removed from the combining form because the suffix ***-y*** is a vowel.

Medical Word	Part	Meaning	Definition
postprocedural (pōst-prō-sē′ jūr-al)	post- procedur -al	after to proceed pertaining to	Pertaining to the period of time after surgery
premenstrual (prē-mĕn′ stroo-ăl)	pre- menstru -al	before to discharge the menses pertaining to	Pertaining to the number of days before the discharge of the menses (the monthly flow of bloody fluid from the endometrium via the vagina)
react (rē-ăkt′)	re- -act	again to act	Literally means *to act again*; to respond to a stimulus; to participate in a chemical reaction
regurgitation (rē-gŭr″ jĭ-tā′ shŭn)	re- gurgitat -ion	backward to flood process	Process of a backward flow of solids or foods from the stomach to the mouth or the backflow of blood through a defective heart valve

Medical Word	Word Parts		Definition
	Part	**Meaning**	
sign (sīn)			Any objective clinical evidence of an illness or disordered function of the body. A sign can be seen, heard, measured, or felt by the examiner.
subacute (sŭb″ ă-kūt′)	sub- acute	below sharp	Literally means *below sharp*. It is used to describe the course of a disease process or the healing process following tissue injury; designated as the midground between acute and chronic.
superinfection (soo″ pĕr-ĭn-fĕk′ shŭn)	super- infect -ion	upper, above to infect process	An infection following a previous infection produced by an overgrowth of a resistant strain of bacteria, fungi, or yeast. It can occur as an adverse effect of antibiotic usage or overusage.
symptom (sĭm′ tŭm)			Any perceptible change in the function of the body that indicates disease; symptoms may be acute, chronic, relapsing, remitting, and can have a systemic or local effect; they can be classified as objective (can be observed and measured), subjective (felt and described by the patient), and cardinal (the vital signs: temperature [T], pulse [P], respiration [R], and blood pressure [BP]).
unconscious (ŭn-kŏn′ shŭs)	un- consci -ous	not aware pertaining to	An abnormal state in which the person is not aware of his or her environment. In this state the person experiences no sensory impressions and is unresponsive neurologically.

Study and Review

Identifying Prefixes

Underline the prefixes in the following medical words.

1. apnea
2. bradypnea
3. dyspnea
4. eupnea
5. hyperpnea
6. hypopnea
7. tachypnea
8. binary
9. concentration
10. extraocular

Defining Prefixes

Give the meaning of the following prefixes.

1. anti- ______________________
2. brachy- ______________________
3. dia- ______________________
4. hetero- ______________________
5. homeo- ______________________
6. hydro- ______________________
7. micro- ______________________
8. oligo- ______________________
9. pan- ______________________
10. pseudo- ______________________
11. a- ______________________
12. an- ______________________
13. bi- ______________________
14. bin- ______________________
15. con- ______________________
16. de- ______________________
17. extra- ______________________
18. hyper- ______________________
19. hypo- ______________________
20. in- ______________________
21. inter- ______________________
22. multi- ______________________
23. para- ______________________
24. peri- ______________________
25. poly- ______________________
26. pre- ______________________
27. re- ______________________
28. sub- ______________________
29. super- ______________________
30. un- ______________________

Using Prefixes to Build Medical Words

Using a prefix from the following list, build the appropriate medical word.

an-	*hypo-*	*poly-*
bi-	*inter-*	*sub-*
de-	*multi-*	*un-*
hyper-		

1. Pertaining to without jaundice ________________ icteric
2. Nature or quality of excessive activity ________________ active
3. Pertaining to arising from many locations ________________ focal
4. Failure of a system ________________ compensation
5. Pertaining to the microscopic space between cells ________________ cellular
6. The process of having two forks ________________ furcation
7. Pertaining to having more than the normal number of fingers and toes ________________ dactyly
8. Underdevelopment of a tissue, organ, or body ________________ plasia
9. Below sharp ________________ acute
10. Pertaining to not being aware ________________ conscious

Identifying Medical Terms

In the spaces provided, write the medical terms for the following meanings.

1. ______________________ Pertaining to without fever
2. ______________________ Pertaining to outside the eye
3. ______________________ Condition of not being able to sleep
4. ______________________ To stop, inhibit, restrain
5. ______________________ To remove the kernel of
6. ______________________ Space within an artery, vein, intestine, or tube
7. ______________________ Wide open
8. ______________________ To act again
9. ______________________ Any objective evidence of an illness
10. ______________________ Any perceptible change in the function of the body that indicates disease

Chapter

4 Organization of the Body

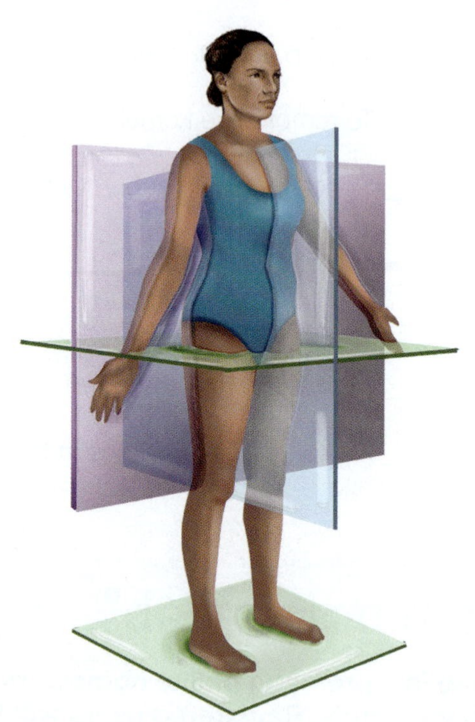

Learning Outcomes

On completion of this chapter, you will be able to:

1. Define terms that describe the body and its structural units.
2. List the systems of the body and the organs in each system.
3. Define terms that are used to describe direction, planes, and cavities of the body.
4. Understand word analysis as it relates to head-to-toe assessment.
5. Recognize terminology included in the ICD-10-CM.
6. Analyze, build, spell, and pronounce medical words.
7. Comprehend the drugs highlighted in this chapter.
8. Identify and define selected abbreviations.
9. Apply your acquired knowledge of ICD-10-CM terminology by successfully completing the *Practical Application* exercise.

Anatomy and Physiology

This chapter introduces you to terms describing the body and its structural units. To aid you, these terms have been grouped into two major sections: The first offers an overview of the units that make up the human body, and the second covers terms used to describe anatomical positions and locations.

The human body is made up of atoms, molecules, organelles, cells, tissues, organs, and systems. See Figure 4.1. All of these parts normally function together in a unified and complex process known as **homeostasis** (a state of equilibrium that is maintained within the body's internal environment). This means that the body's fluid composition, its volume and characteristics, and its temperature (T), blood pressure (BP), and the exchange of oxygen (O_2) and carbon dioxide (CO_2) remain within normal limits. By maintaining homeostasis, the cells of the body are in an environment that meets their needs and permits them to function optimally under changing conditions.

Human Body: Levels of Organization

Atoms

An **atom** is the smallest, most basic chemical unit of an element. It consists of a nucleus that contains protons and neutrons and is surrounded by electrons. A **proton** is a positively charged particle; a **neutron** is without any electrical charge. An **electron** is a negatively charged particle that revolves around the nucleus of an atom.

Chemical elements are made up of atoms, which can be classified on the basis of their atomic number into groups called elements. An **element** is a substance that cannot be broken down by chemical means into any other substance. There are 118 elements listed on the Periodic Table from atomic numbers 1 (hydrogen) to 118 (ununoctium).

Elements found in the human body include aluminum, carbon, calcium, chlorine, cobalt, copper, fluorine, hydrogen, iodine, iron, manganese, magnesium, nitrogen, oxygen, phosphorus, potassium, sodium, sulfur, and zinc. The mass of the human body is made up of just six elements: oxygen, carbon, hydrogen, nitrogen, calcium, and phosphorus. See Table 4.1.

Molecules

A **molecule** is a chemical combination of two or more atoms that form a specific chemical compound. In a water molecule (H_2O), oxygen forms polar covalent (sharing of electrons) bonds with two hydrogen atoms. **Water** is a tasteless, clear, odorless liquid that makes up 65% of a male's body weight and 55% of a female's body weight. Water is the most important constituent of all body fluids, secretions, and excretions. It is an ideal transportation medium for inorganic and organic compounds.

Cells

The body consists of millions of cells working individually and with each other to sustain life. For the purposes of this text, **cells** are considered the basic building blocks for the various structures that together make up a human being. There are several types of cells, with each specialized to perform specific functions. The size and shape of a cell are generally related directly to its function. See Figure 4.2.

For example, cells forming the skin overlap each other to form a protective barrier, whereas nerve cells are usually elongated with branches connecting to other cells for the transmission of sensory impulses. Despite these differences, however, cells can

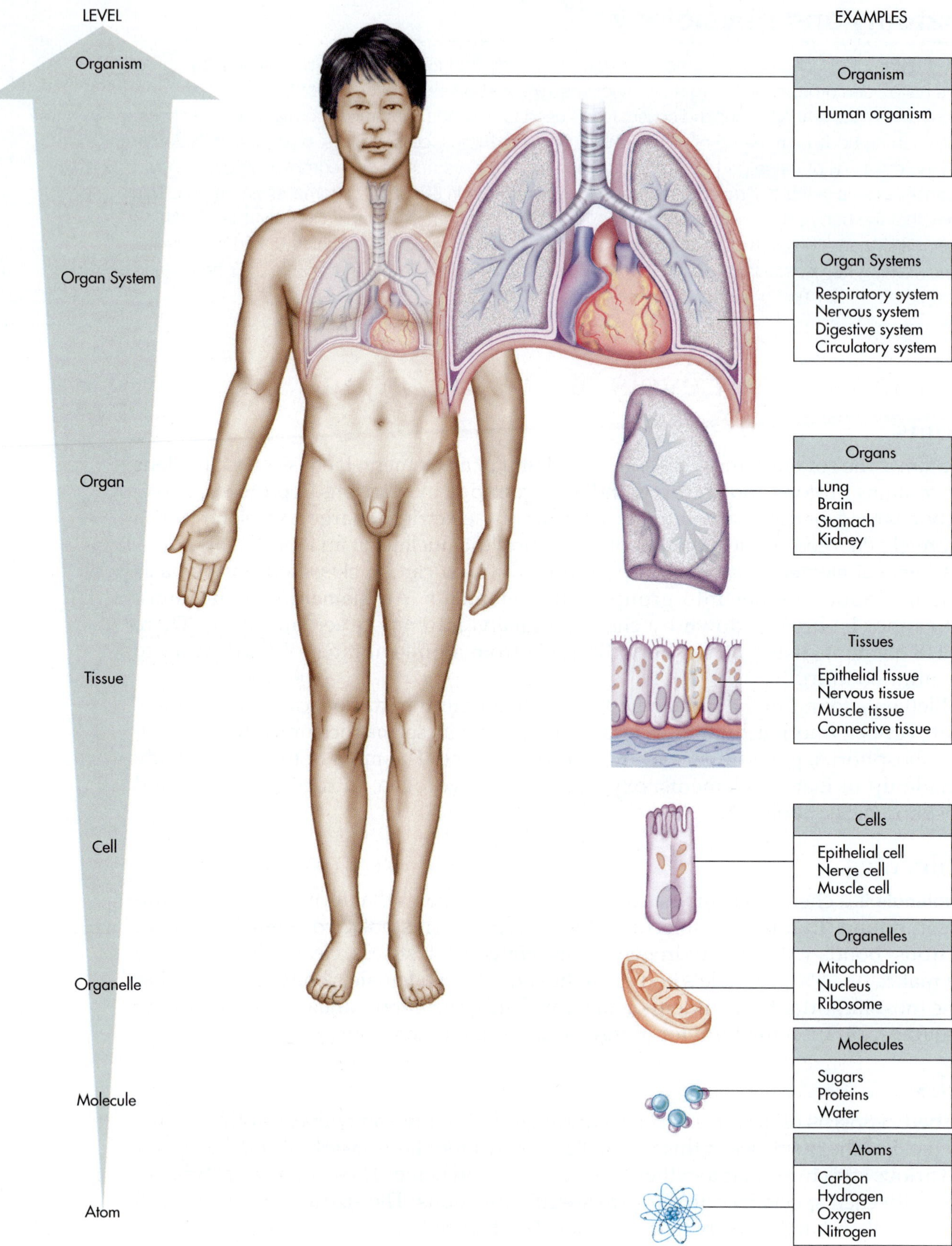

Figure 4.1 Human body: levels of organization.

Table 4.1 Elements Found in the Human Body

Symbol	Element	Symbol	Element
Al	Aluminum	Mn	Manganese
C	Carbon	Mg	Magnesium
Ca	Calcium	N	Nitrogen
Cl	Chlorine	O or O_2	Oxygen
Co	Cobalt	P	Phosphorus
Cu	Copper	K	Potassium
F	Fluorine	Na	Sodium
H	Hydrogen	S	Sulfur
I	Iodine	Zn	Zinc
Fe	Iron		

generally be said to have a number of common components. The major parts of the cell are the cell membrane, cytoplasm, and nucleus. See Figure 4.3 and Table 4.2.

CELL MEMBRANE

The outer covering of the cell is called the **cell membrane**. Cell membranes have the capability of allowing some substances to pass into and out of the cell while denying passage to other substances. This selectivity allows cells to receive nutrition and dispose of waste just as a human being eats food and disposes of waste.

CYTOPLASM

Cytoplasm is the substance between the cell membrane and the nuclear membrane. It is a jellylike material that is mostly water. The cytoplasm provides storage and work areas for the cell. The work and storage elements of the cell, called *organelles* (little organs), are the endoplasmic reticulum (ER), ribosomes, Golgi apparatus, mitochondria, lysosomes, and centrioles.

NUCLEUS

The **nucleus** is responsible for the cell's metabolism, growth, and reproduction. It is the central portion of the cell that contains the **chromosomes** (microscopic bodies that carry the genes that determine hereditary characteristics). A single gene makes up each segment of deoxyribonucleic acid (DNA) and is located in a specific site on the chromosome. The human body has 23 pairs of chromosomes. A **genome** is the complete set of genes and chromosomes tucked inside each of the body's trillions of cells. Genes determine an individual's physical traits such as hair, skin, and eye color, body structure, and metabolic activity. See Figure 4.4.

Stem Cells

Stem cells are the precursors of all body cells. Stem cells have three general properties: They are capable of dividing and renewing themselves for long periods, they are unspecialized, and they can give rise to specialized cell types. Some primary sources of stem cells include embryos, adult tissues, and umbilical cord blood. An embryonic cell

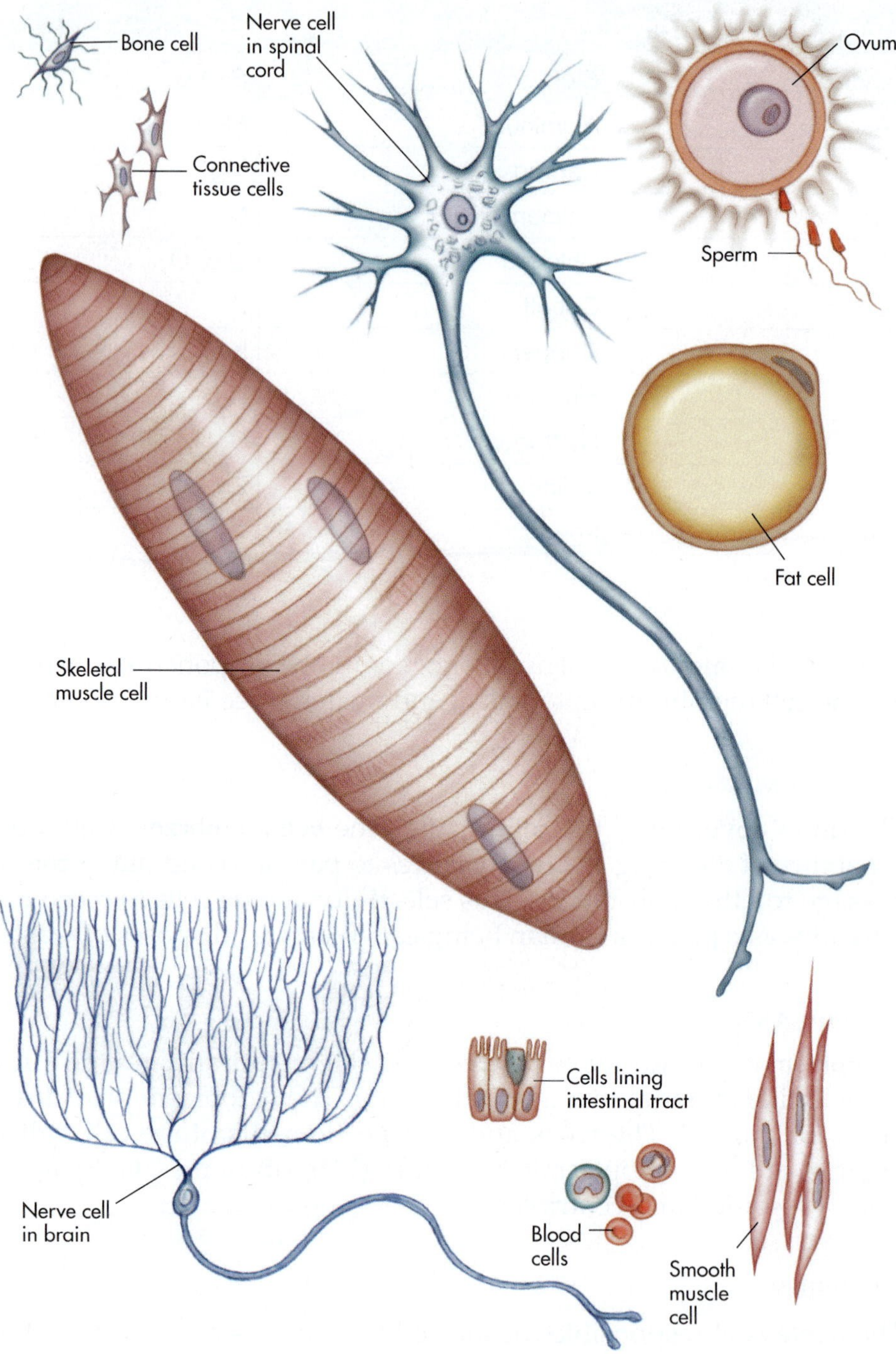

Figure 4.2 Cells are the basic building blocks of the human body. They have many different shapes and vary in size and function. These examples show the range of forms and sizes with the dimensions they would have if magnified approximately 500 times.

is an unspecialized cell that can turn itself into any type of tissue. Embryonic stem cells are derived primarily from frozen **in vitro** (in glass, as in a test tube) fertilized embryos. An adult stem cell is a more specialized cell found in many kinds of tissue, such as bone marrow, skin, and the liver. An umbilical cord cell is a rich source of precursors of mature blood cells. It is obtained from cord blood at the time of birth.

Stem cells can now be grown and transformed into specialized cells with characteristics consistent with cells of various tissues such as muscles or nerves through cell culture. Highly plastic adult stem cells from a variety of sources, including umbilical cord blood and bone marrow, are used in medical therapies, which are often referred to as **regenerative** or **reparative medicine**.

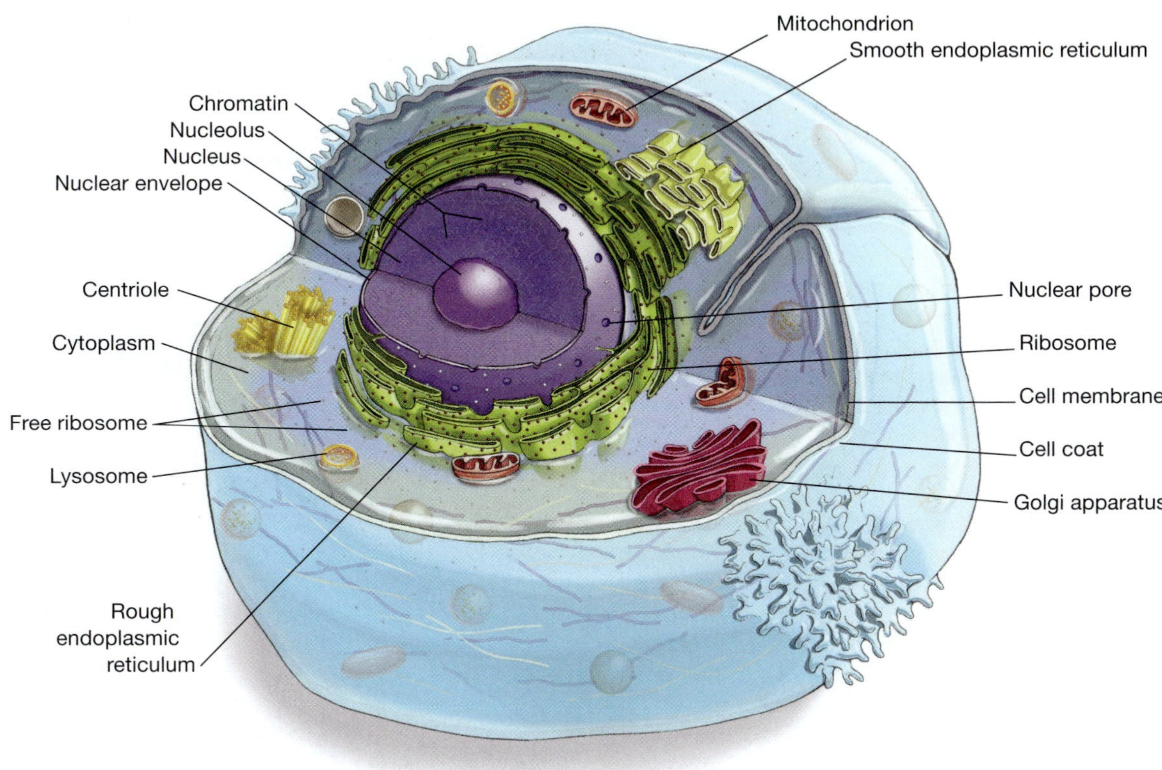

Figure 4.3 Major parts of a cell.

Table 4.2 Major Cell Structures and Primary Functions

Cell Structures	Primary Functions
Cell membrane	Protects the cell; provides for communication via receptor proteins; surface proteins serve as positive identification tags; allows some substances to pass into and out of the cell while denying passage to other substances; this selectivity allows cells to receive nutrition and dispose of waste
Cytoplasm	Provides storage and work areas for the cell; the work and storage elements of the cell, called *organelles*, are the ribosomes, endoplasmic reticulum, Golgi apparatus, mitochondria, lysosomes, and centrioles
Ribosomes	Make enzymes and other proteins; nicknamed “protein factories”
Endoplasmic reticulum (ER)	Carries proteins and other substances through the cytoplasm
Golgi apparatus	Chemically processes the molecules from the endoplasmic reticulum and then packages them into vesicles; nicknamed “chemical processing and packaging center”
Mitochondria	Involved in cellular metabolism and respiration; provides the principal source of cellular energy and is the place where complex, energy-releasing chemical reactions occur continuously; nicknamed “power plants”
Lysosomes	Contain enzymes that can digest food compounds; nicknamed “digestive bags”
Centrioles	Play an important role in cell reproduction
Cilia	Hairlike processes that project from epithelial cells; help propel mucus, dust particles, and other foreign substances from the respiratory tract
Flagellum	“Tail” of the sperm that enables the sperm to “swim” or move toward the ovum
Nucleus	Controls every *organelle* (little organ) in the cytoplasm; contains the genetic matter necessary for cell reproduction as well as control over activity within the cell’s cytoplasm; responsible for the cell’s metabolism, growth, and reproduction

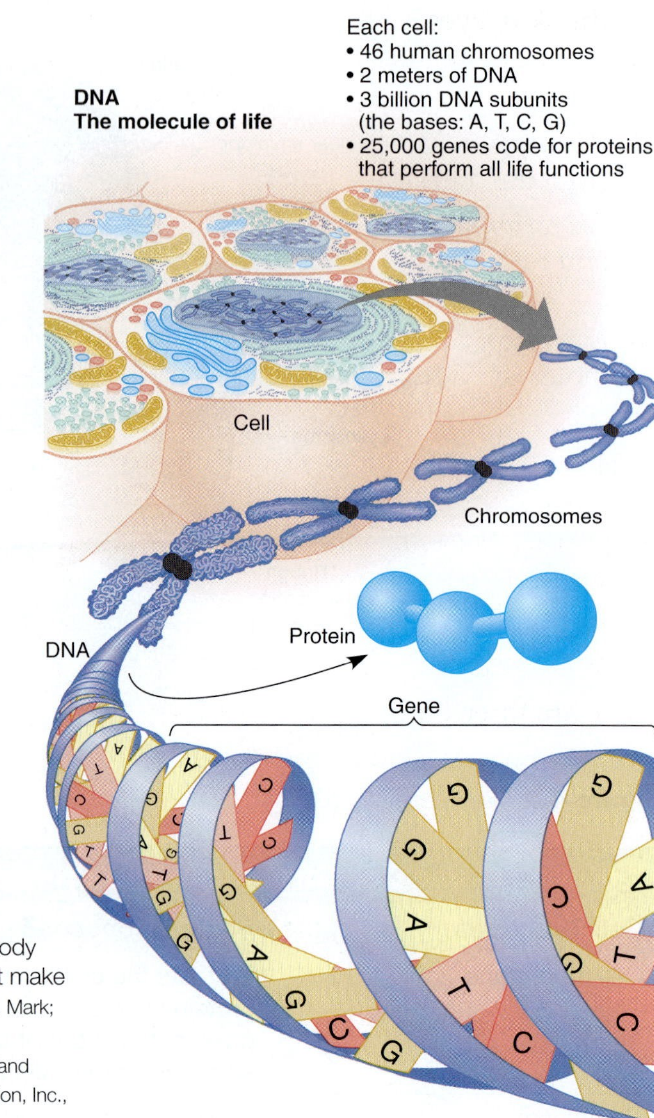

Figure 4.4 Each cell nucleus throughout the body contains the genes, DNA, and chromosomes that make up the majority of an individual's genome. (Zelman, Mark; Tompary, Elaine; Raymond, Jill; Holdaway, Paul; Mulvihill, Mary Lou E., Human Diseases, 8th Ed., ©2015. Reprinted and Electronically reproduced by permission of Pearson Education, Inc., New York, NY.)

Tissues

A **tissue** is a grouping of similar cells that together perform specialized functions. There are four basic types of tissue in the body: *epithelial*, *connective*, *muscle*, and *nerve*. Each of the four basic tissues has several subtypes named for their shape, appearance, arrangement, or function. The following sections describe the four basic types of tissue.

EPITHELIAL TISSUE

Epithelial tissue appears as sheetlike arrangements of cells, sometimes several layers thick, that form the outer surfaces of the body and line the body cavities and the principal tubes and passageways leading to the exterior. These cells form the secreting portions of glands and their ducts and are important parts of certain sense organs. There are six main functions of epithelial tissue:

1. ***Protection.*** Protects underlying tissue from mechanical injury, harmful chemicals and pathogens, and excessive water loss.

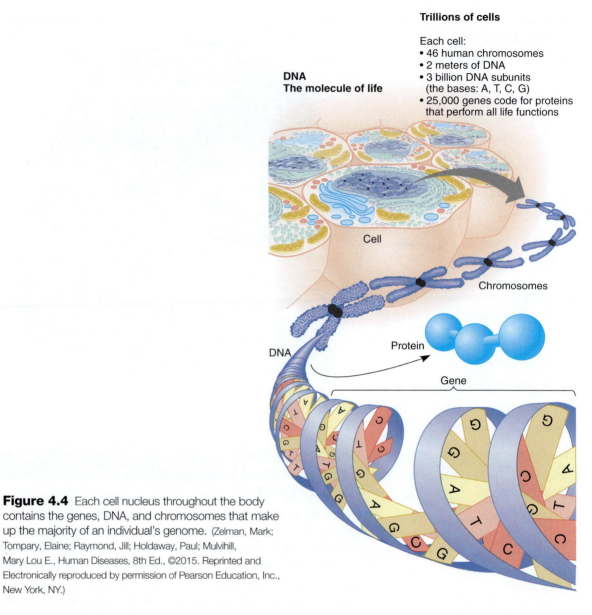

2. ***Sensation.*** Sensory stimuli are detected by specialized epithelial cells found in the skin, eyes, ears, and nose and on the tongue.
3. ***Secretion.*** In glands, epithelial tissue is specialized to secrete specific chemical substances such as enzymes, hormones, and lubricating fluids.
4. ***Absorption.*** Certain epithelial cells lining the small intestine absorb nutrients from the digestion of food.
5. ***Excretion.*** Epithelial tissues in the kidney excrete waste products from the body and reabsorb needed materials from the urine. Sweat is also excreted from the body by epithelial cells in the sweat glands.
6. ***Diffusion.*** Simple epithelium (found in the walls of capillaries and lungs) promotes the diffusion of gases, liquids, and nutrients.

CONNECTIVE TISSUE

The most widespread and abundant of the body tissues, **connective tissue** forms the supporting network for the organs of the body, sheaths the muscles, and connects muscles to bones and bones to joints. Bone is a dense form of connective tissue.

MUSCLE TISSUE

There are three types of **muscle tissue**:

1. **Skeletal muscle** or *voluntary muscle* is striated in appearance and is anchored by tendons to bone. They are used to effect skeletal movement such as locomotion and in maintaining posture. An average adult male is made up of 42% skeletal muscle and an average adult female is made up of 36% (as a percentage of body mass).
2. **Smooth muscle** or *involuntary muscle* is found within the walls of organs and structures such as the esophagus, stomach, intestines, bronchi, uterus, urethra, bladder, blood vessels, and the arrector pili in the skin. Unlike skeletal muscle, smooth muscle is not under conscious control and is under the control of the autonomic nervous system.
3. **Cardiac muscle** is also an involuntary muscle and is a specialized form of striated tissue found only in the heart. Cardiac muscle is under the control of the autonomic nervous system.

NERVE TISSUE

Nerve tissue consists of nerve cells (neurons) and supporting cells called *neuroglia*. It has the properties of excitability and conductivity and functions to control and coordinate the activities of the body.

Organs

Multiple different tissues serving a common purpose or function make up structures called **organs**. Examples are the brain, skin, or heart.

Systems

A group of different organs functioning together for a common purpose is called a **system**. The various body systems function in support of the body as a whole. Figure 4.5 shows the organ systems of the body. Each body system is discussed in the following chapters.

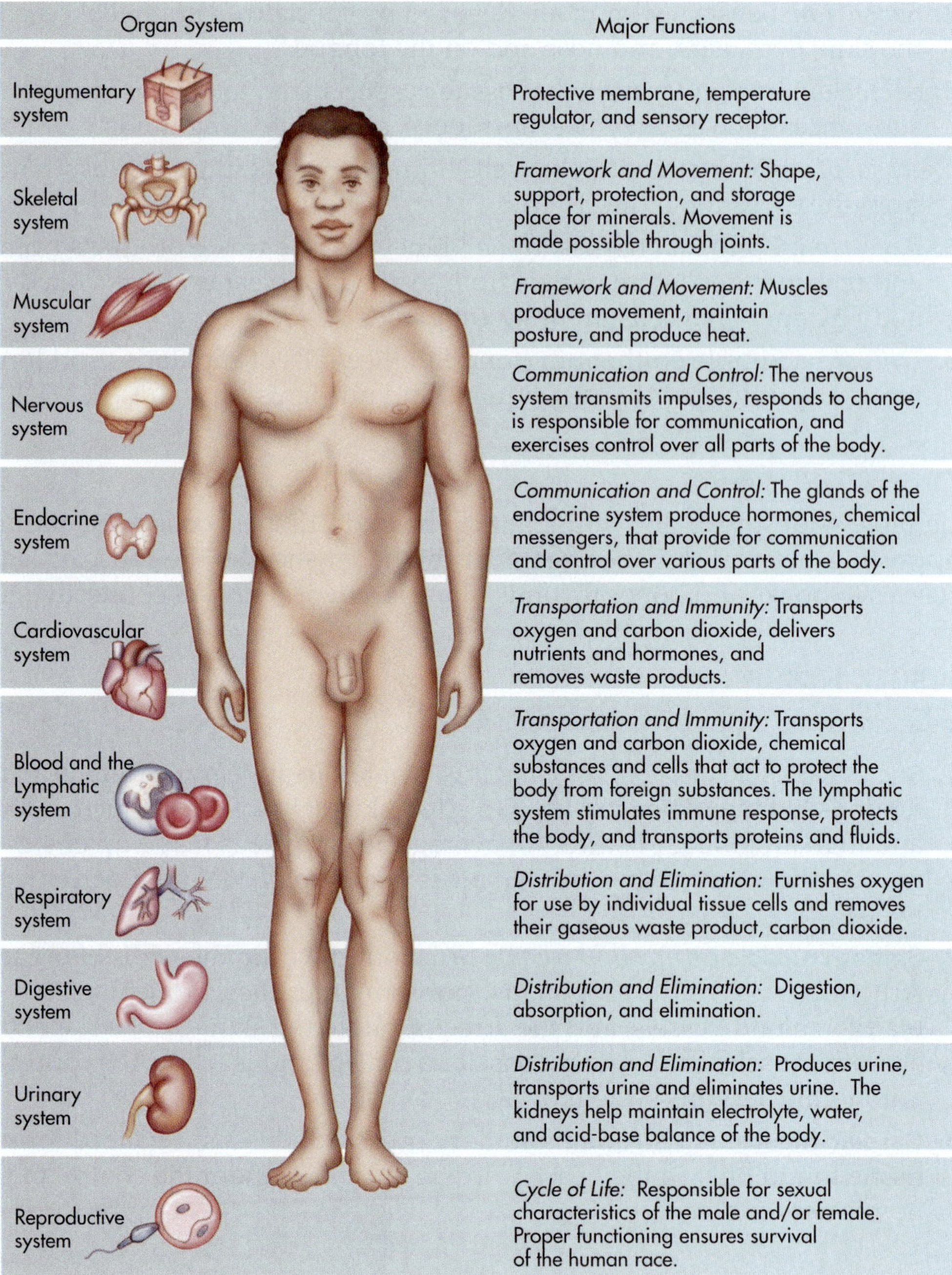

Organ System
Major Functions
Integumentary system
Protective membrane, temperature regulator, and sensory receptor.
Skeletal system
Framework and Movement: Shape, support, protection, and storage place for minerals. Movement is made possible through joints.
Muscular system
Framework and Movement: Muscles produce movement, maintain posture, and produce heat.
Nervous system
Communication and Control: The nervous system transmits impulses, responds to change, is responsible for communication, and exercises control over all parts of the body.
Endocrine system
Communication and Control: The glands of the endocrine system produce hormones, chemical messengers, that provide for communication and control over various parts of the body.
Cardiovascular system
Transportation and Immunity: Transports oxygen and carbon dioxide, delivers nutrients and hormones, and removes waste products.
Blood and the Lymphatic system
Transportation and Immunity: Transports oxygen and carbon dioxide, chemical substances and cells that act to protect the body from foreign substances. The lymphatic system stimulates immune response, protects the body, and transports proteins and fluids.
Respiratory system
Distribution and Elimination: Furnishes oxygen for use by individual tissue cells and removes their gaseous waste product, carbon dioxide.
Digestive system
Distribution and Elimination: Digestion, absorption, and elimination.
Urinary system
Distribution and Elimination: Produces urine, transports urine and eliminates urine. The kidneys help maintain electrolyte, water, and acid-base balance of the body.
Reproductive system
Cycle of Life: Responsible for sexual characteristics of the male and/or female. Proper functioning ensures survival of the human race.

Figure 4.5 Organ systems of the body with major functions.

Anatomical Locations and Positions

Four primary reference systems have been adopted to provide uniformity to the anatomical description of the body. These reference systems are **direction**, **planes**, **cavities**, and **structural unit**. The standard **anatomical position** for the body is erect, head facing forward, arms by the sides with palms to the front. Left and right are from the subject's point of view, not from the point of view of the person doing the examination. See Figure 4.6.

Direction

Directional and positional terms describe the location of organs or body parts in relationship to one another. They are used in describing physical assessment of a patient's presenting complaints and in pinpointing the location of a given sign or symptom. Table 4.3 lists the terms used to describe direction and position, including their combining forms (CFs).

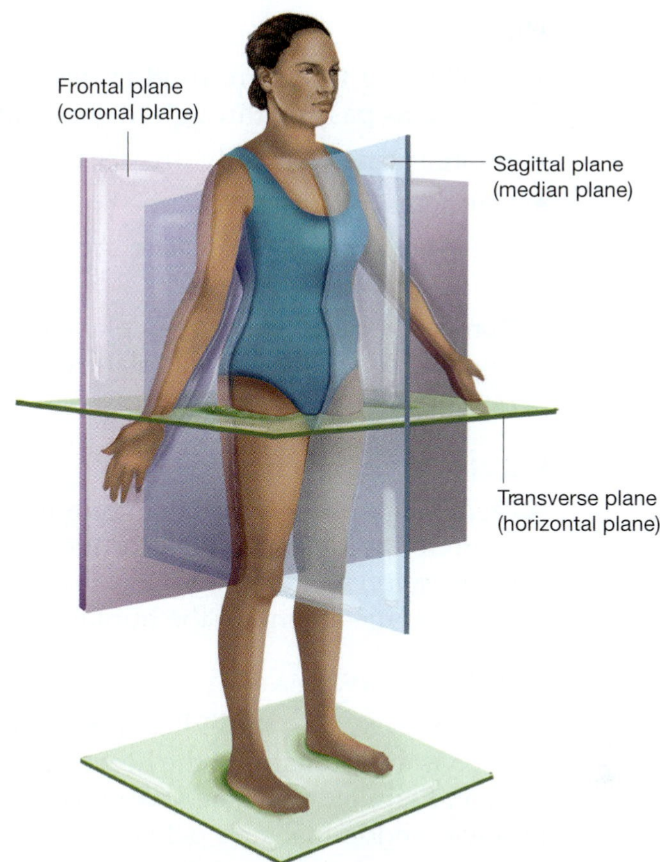

Figure 4.6 Standard anatomical position and planes of the body.

TABLE 4.3 Directional and Positional Terms

Term	Combining Form (CF)	Description	Example
superior		Above, in an upward direction, toward the head. *Note: super-* is a prefix (P) that means *upper, above*.	The head is superior to the neck of the body.
inferior	(infer/o)	Below or in a downward direction; more toward the feet or tail	The feet are inferior to the head of the body.
anterior	(anter/o)	In front of or before, the front side of the body	The breasts are located on the anterior side of the body.
posterior	(poster/o)	Toward the back, back side of the body	The nape is the back of the neck and is located on the posterior side of the body.
cephalic	(cephal/o)	Pertaining to the head; superior in position	A cephalic presentation is one in which any part of the head of the fetus is presented during delivery.
caudal	(caud/o)	Pertaining to the tail; inferior in position	The cauda equina (horse's tail) is a bundle of spinal nerves below the end of the spinal cord.
medial	(medi/o)	Nearest the midline or middle	The umbilicus is a depressed point in the medial area of the abdomen.
lateral	(later/o)	To the side, away from the middle	In the anatomical position, the arm is located on the lateral side of the body.
proximal	(proxim/o)	Nearest the point of attachment or near the point of origin	The proximal end of the humerus (upper bone of the arm) joins with part of the shoulder bone.
distal	(dist/o)	Away from the point of attachment or far from the point of origin	The distal end of the humerus joins with part of the elbow.

Planes

The following terms are used to describe the imaginary planes that are depicted in Figure 4.6 as passing through the body and dividing it into various sections.

- **Sagittal plane**. Vertically divides the body or structure into *right* and *left sides*.
- **Midsagittal plane**. Divides the body or structure into *right* and *left halves*.
- **Transverse** or **horizontal plane**. Any plane that divides the body into *superior* and *inferior* portions.
- **Coronal** or **frontal plane**. Any plane that divides the body at right angles to the midsagittal plane. The coronal plane divides the body into *anterior* (ventral) and *posterior* (dorsal) portions.

Cavities

A *cavity* is a hollow space containing body organs. Body cavities are classified into two groups according to their location. On the front is the **ventral cavity** (also called the *anterior cavity*) and on the back is the **dorsal cavity** (also called the *posterior cavity*). The various cavities found in the human body are depicted in Figure 4.7.

VENTRAL CAVITY

The ventral cavity is the hollow portion of the human torso extending from the neck to the pelvis and containing the heart and the organs of respiration, digestion, reproduction, and elimination. The ventral cavity can be subdivided into three distinct areas: thoracic, abdominal, and pelvic.

- **Thoracic cavity**. The area of the chest containing the heart and the lungs. Within this cavity, the space containing the **heart** is called the **pericardial cavity** and the spaces surrounding each **lung** are known as the **pleural cavities**. Other organs located in the thoracic cavity are the esophagus, trachea, thymus, and certain large blood and lymph vessels.
- **Abdominal cavity**. The space below the diaphragm, commonly referred to as the *belly*; contains the stomach, intestines, and other organs of digestion.
- **Pelvic cavity**. The space formed by the bones of the pelvic area; contains the organs of reproduction and elimination.

DORSAL CAVITY

The dorsal cavity contains the structures of the nervous system and is subdivided into the cranial cavity and the spinal cavity.

- **Cranial cavity**. The space in the skull containing the brain.
- **Spinal cavity**. The space within the bony spinal column that contains the spinal cord and spinal fluid.

ABDOMINOPELVIC CAVITY

The **abdominopelvic cavity** is the combination of the abdominal and pelvic cavities. It is divided into nine regions.

Nine Regions of the Abdominopelvic Cavity. As a ready reference for locating visceral organs, anatomists divided the abdominopelvic cavity into nine regions (see Figure 4.8A). A grid pattern drawn across the abdominopelvic cavity delineates these regions:

- **Right hypochondriac**. Upper right region at the level of the ninth rib cartilage
- **Left hypochondriac**. Upper left region at the level of the ninth rib cartilage
- **Epigastric**. Region over the stomach

- **Right lumbar**. Right middle lateral region
- **Left lumbar**. Left middle lateral region
- **Umbilical**. In the center, between the right and left lumbar regions; at the navel
- **Right iliac (inguinal)**. Right lower lateral region
- **Left iliac (inguinal)**. Left lower lateral region
- **Hypogastric**. Lower middle region below the navel

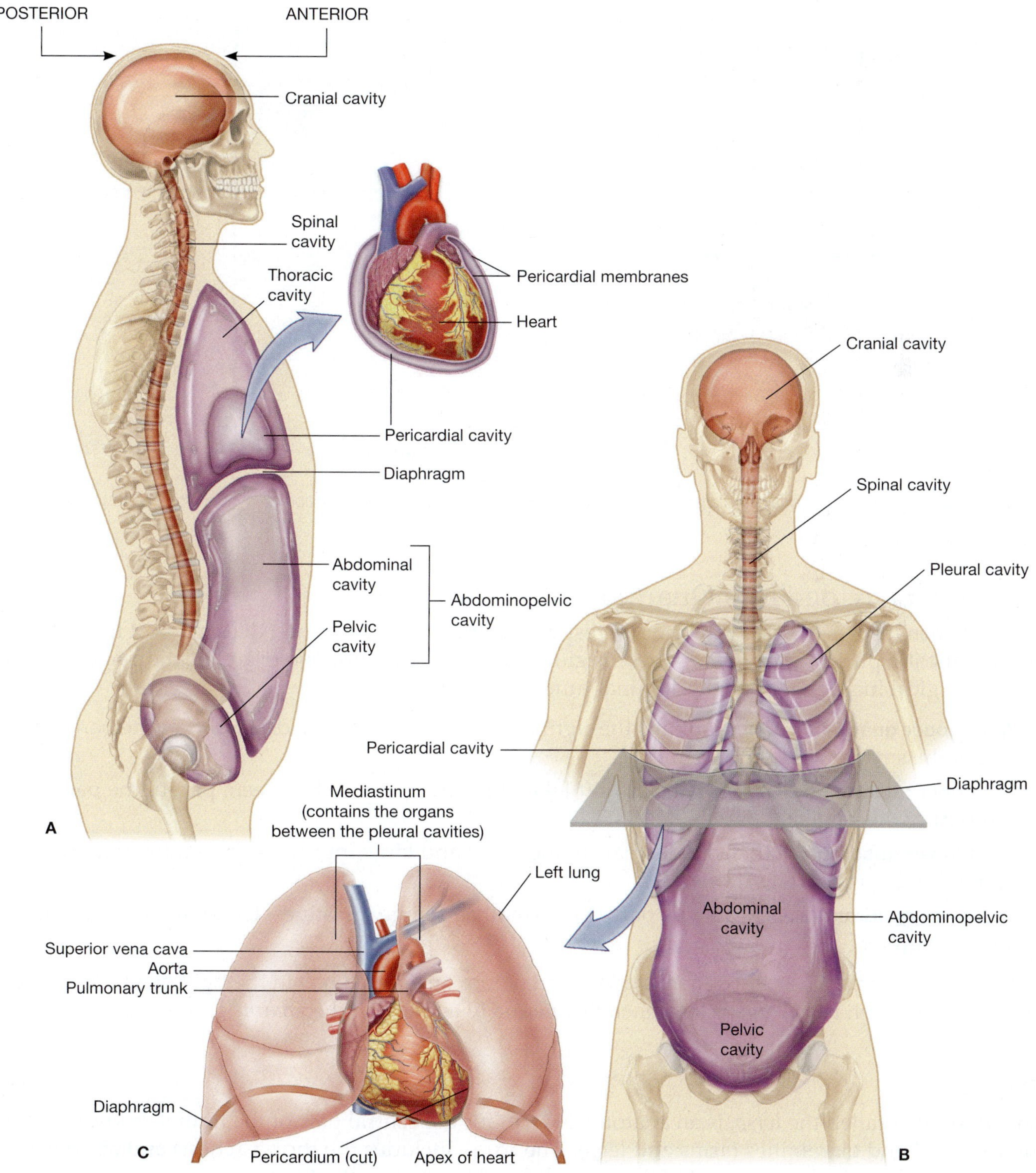

Figure 4.7 Body cavities. (A) Lateral view of a sagittal section through the body. (B) Anterior view of a frontal section through the body. (C) Location of the heart within the mediastinum of the thoracic cavity.

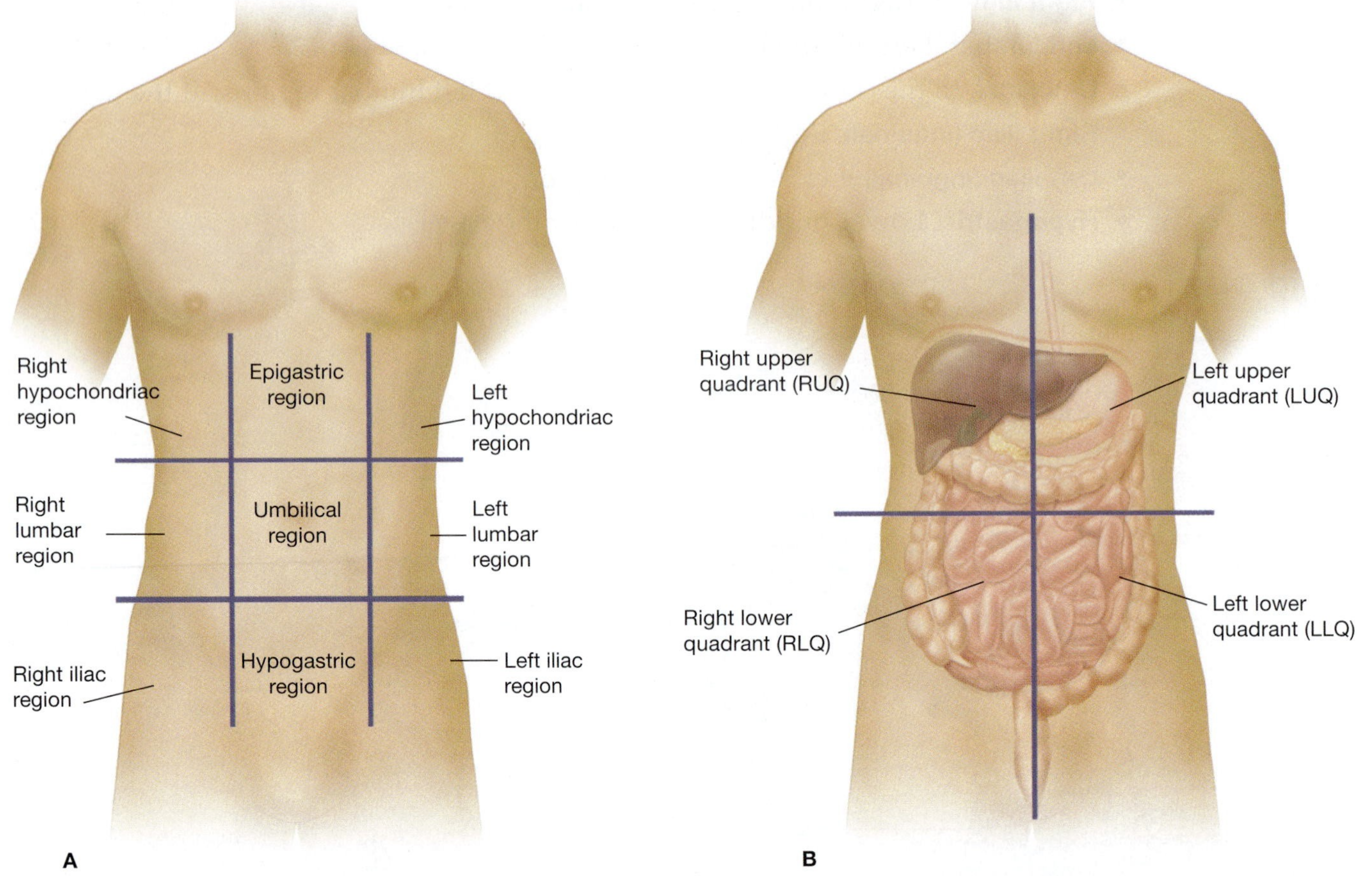

Figure 4.8 (A) The nine regions of the abdominopelvic cavity. (B) The four regions of the abdomen, which are referred to as *quadrants*.

Abdomen Divided into Quadrants

The **abdomen (abd)** is divided into four corresponding regions (quadrants) that are used for descriptive and diagnostic purposes. By using these regions, one may describe the exact location of pain, a skin lesion, surgical incision, and/or abdominal tumor. See Figure 4.8B.

- **Right upper quadrant (RUQ)**. Contains the right lobe of the liver, gallbladder, part of the pancreas, and part of the small and large intestines
- **Left upper quadrant (LUQ)**. Contains the left lobe of the liver, stomach, spleen, part of the pancreas, and part of the small and large intestines
- **Right lower quadrant (RLQ)**. Contains part of the small and large intestines, appendix, right ovary, right fallopian tube, right ureter
- **Left lower quadrant (LLQ)**. Contains part of the small and large intestines, left ovary, left fallopian tube, left ureter

Note: Some organs, such as the urinary bladder and uterus, are located half in the right quadrant and half in the left quadrant. These organs are generally referred to as being in the *midline* of the body.

Trunk

The **trunk**, also called the *torso*, is an anatomical term for the central part of the human body, not including the head and extremities (arms and legs). The trunk includes the thorax (chest) and abdomen. The trunk is also described as that part of the body defined by the length of the vertebral column with reference to the posterior or back of the body. The trunk also contains many of the main groups of muscles in the body, including the pectoral, abdominal, and lateral groups. The muscles and organs mainly originating from thoracic vertebral segments are innervated by various peripheral nerves.

Most vital organs are located within the trunk. In the upper chest, the heart and lungs are protected by the rib cage. The abdomen contains the majority of organs responsible for digestion. The liver plays an essential role in the normal metabolism of carbohydrates, fats, and proteins. It produces bile necessary for the breakdown of large fat globules into smaller particles. Digestion and absorption take place chiefly in the small intestine where digested nutrients pass into the villi through diffusion and in the large intestine digestion and absorption are completed. The gallbladder stores and concentrates bile. Other organs found in the trunk are the kidneys, which produce urine; the ureters, which pass it to the bladder for storage; and the urethra, which excretes urine and in the male, passes sperm through the seminal vesicles. The pelvic region contains the reproductive organs.

Head-to-Toe Assessment

The terminology associated with head-to-toe assessment can be useful when studying the organization of the body and in understanding information contained in a patient's medical record. Body areas, along with their word parts, are provided in Table 4.4.

Table 4.4 Body Area Terminology

Body Area	Word Part(s)	Body Area	Word Part(s)
abdomen (belly)	abdomin/o	liver	hepat/o
ankle (tarsus)	tars/o	lungs	pulm/o; pulmon/o; pneum/o; pneumon/o
arm	brach/i; brachi/o	mouth	or/o
back	poster/o	muscles	muscul/o; my/o
bones	oste/o	navel	umbilic/o; omphal/o
breast	mast/o; mamm/o	neck	cervic/o
cheek	bucc/o	nerves	neur/o
chest	thorac/o	nose	rhin/o; nas/o
ear	aur/i; ot/o	ribs	cost/o
elbow	cubit/o; olecran/o	side	later/o
eye	ophthalm/o; ocul/o; opt/o	skin	derm/a; dermat/o; derm/o; cutane/o
finger	dactyl/o	skull	crani/o
foot	pod/o	stomach	gastr/o
gums	gingiv/o	teeth	dent/i
hand	manus; chir/o	temples	tempor/o
head	cephal/o	thigh bone	femor/o
heart	cardi/o	throat	pharyng/o
hip or hip joint	coxa	tongue	lingu/o; gloss/o
leg	crur/o	wrist (carpus)	carp/o

Study and Review I

Anatomy and Physiology

Write your answers to the following questions.

1. The ________________ consist of millions of ________________ working individually and with each other to ________________ life.

2. The outer covering of the cell is known as the ________________, which has the capability of allowing some substances to pass into and out of the cell.

3. The common parts of the cell are the ________________, ________________, and ________________.

4. Three functions of the cell's nucleus are ________________, ________________, and ________________.

5. An ________________ is an unspecialized cell that can turn itself into any type of tissue.

6. List the six functions of epithelial tissue.

a. ________________ **b.** ________________

c. ________________ **d.** ________________

e. ________________ **f.** ________________

7. ________________ tissue is the most widespread and abundant of the four body tissues.

8. Name the three types of muscle tissue.

a. ________________ **b.** ________________

c. ________________

9. Two properties of nerve tissue are ________________ and ________________.

10. Define *organ*. ________________.

11. Define *body system*. ________________.

12. Name the organ systems listed in this text.

a. ________________ **b.** ________________

c. ________________ **d.** ________________

e. ________________ **f.** ________________

g. ______________________ h. ______________________

i. ______________________ j. ______________________

k. ______________________

13. Define the following directional terms.

a. superior ________________ **b.** anterior ________________

c. posterior ________________ **d.** cephalic ________________

e. medial ________________ **f.** lateral ________________

g. proximal ________________ **h.** distal ________________

14. The ________________________________ vertically divides the body. It passes through the midline to form a right and left half.

15. The ______________ plane is any plane that divides the body into superior and inferior portions.

16. The ______________ plane is any plane that divides the body at right angles to the plane described in Question 14.

17. List the three distinct cavities that are located in the ventral cavity.

a. ______________________ **b.** ______________________

c. ______________________

18. Name the two distinct cavities located in the dorsal cavity.

a. ______________________ **b.** ______________________

ANATOMY LABELING

Identify the structures shown below by filling in the blanks.

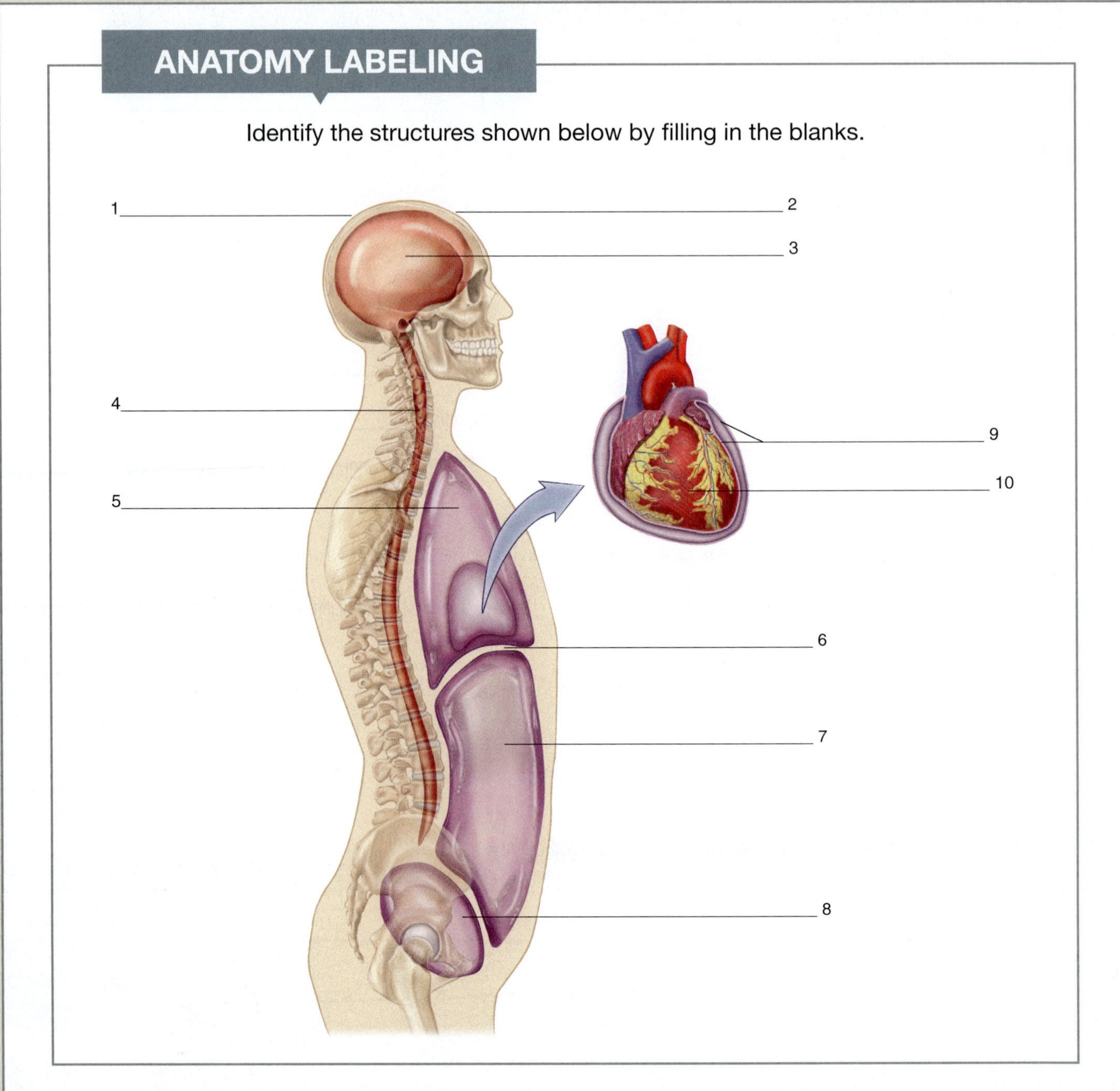

Building Your Medical Vocabulary

This section provides the foundation for learning medical terminology. Review the following alphabetized word list. Note how common prefixes and suffixes are repeatedly applied to word roots and combining forms to create different meanings. The word parts are color-coded: prefixes are yellow, suffixes are blue, roots/combining forms are red. A combining form is a word root plus a vowel. The chart below lists the combining forms for the word roots in this chapter and can help to strengthen your understanding of how medical words are built and spelled.

Remember These Guidelines:

1. If the suffix begins with a vowel, drop the combining vowel from the combining form and add the suffix. For example, adip/o (*fat*) + -ose (*pertaining to*) becomes adipose.
2. If the suffix begins with a consonant, keep the combining vowel and add the suffix to the combining form. For example, hist/o (*tissue*) + -logy (*study of*) becomes histology.

You will find that some terms have not been divided into word parts. These are common words or specialized terms that are included to enhance your medical vocabulary.

Combining Forms of the Organization of the Body

adip/o	fat	**kary/o**	cell's nucleus
andr/o	man	**later/o**	side
anter/o	toward the front	**medi/o**	toward the middle
bi/o	life	**organ/o**	organ
caud/o	tail	**path/o**	disease
cyt/o	cell	**phen/o**	to show
dist/o	away from the point of origin	**physi/o**	nature
dors/o	backward	**poster/o**	behind, toward the back, back
hist/o	tissue	**proxim/o**	near the point of origin
hydr/o	water	**somat/o**	body
infer/o	below	**ventr/o**	near or on the belly side of the body
inguin/o	groin		
		viscer/o	body organs

Medical Word	Word Parts: Part	Word Parts: Meaning	Definition
adipose (ăd′′ ĭ-pōs)	adip -ose	fat pertaining to	Pertaining to fatty tissue throughout the body

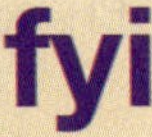

fyi *Adiposity* is the condition of being obese. The recommended measurement of **obesity** is the body mass index (BMI), a key index for relating weight to height. To determine a person's BMI, weight in kilograms (kg) is divided by height in meters squared. The National Institutes of Health (NIH) now defines normal weight, overweight, and obesity according to BMI rather than the traditional height/weight charts. Overweight is a BMI of 27.3 or more for women and 27.8 or more for men. Obesity is a BMI of 30 or more for both males and females (about 30 pounds overweight).

insights In ICD-10-CM, *morbid (severe) obesity* (E66.01) is due to excess calories. The term *overweight* is not recognized as a clinical term for high adiposity obesity.

Medical Word	Word Parts: Part	Word Parts: Meaning	Definition
ambilateral (ăm′′ bĭ-lăt′ ĕr-ăl)	ambi- later -al	both side pertaining to	Pertaining to both sides
anatomy (ăn-ăt′ ō-mē)	ana- -tomy	up; apart incision	Literally means *to cut up* or *to cut apart*; the study of the structure of an organism such as humans.

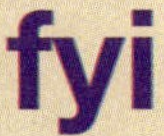

fyi A method that can be used to learn about the anatomy of the body of a once-living thing is termed *dissection*. To *dissect* means to separate tissues and parts of a cadaver for anatomical study.

Medical Word	Word Parts: Part	Word Parts: Meaning	Definition
android (ăn′ droyd)	andr -oid	man resemble	To resemble man
apex (ā′ pĕks)			Pointed end of a cone-shaped structure
base (bās)			Lower part or foundation of a structure
bilateral (bī-lăt′ ĕr-ăl)	bi- later -al	two side pertaining to	Pertaining to two sides
biology (bī-ŏl′ ō-jē)	bi/o -logy	life study of	Study of life
center (sĕn′ tĕr)			Middle or midpoint of a body

Medical Word	Word Parts		Definition
	Part	Meaning	
chromosome (krō-mō-sōm)	chromo- -some	color body	Microscopic bodies in the nucleus that carry the genes that determine hereditary characteristics
cytology (sī-tŏl′ ō-jē)	cyt/o -logy	cell study of	Study of cells
dehydrate (dē-hī′ drāt)	de- hydr -ate	down, away from water use, action	To remove water; to lose or be deprived of water from the body; to become dry
diffusion (dĭ-fū′ zhŭn)	dif- fus -ion	apart to pour process	The process whereby particles in a fluid move from an area of high concentration to an area of lower concentration, resulting in an even distribution of the particles in the fluid
ectomorph (ĕk′ tō-morf)	ecto- -morph	outside form, shape	Slender physical body form; linear physique

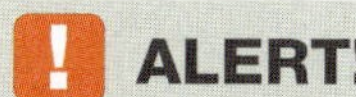

ALERT!

Note that ***ecto-*** means *outside*, while ***endo-*** means *within.*

Medical Word	Part	Meaning	Definition
endomorph (ĕn′ dō-morf)	endo- -morph	within form, shape	Round and soft physical body form
filtration (fĭl-trā′ shŭn)	filtrat -ion	to strain through process	Process of filtering or straining particles from a solution
gene (jēn)			Hereditary unit that transmits and determines one's characteristics or hereditary traits
histology (hĭs-tŏl′ ō-jē)	hist/o -logy	tissue study of	Study of tissue

! RULE REMINDER

This term keeps the combining vowel ***o*** because the suffix begins with a consonant.

Medical Word	Part	Meaning	Definition
homeostasis (hō″ mē-ō-stā′ sĭs)	homeo- -stasis	similar, same control, stop, stand still	State of equilibrium maintained in the body's internal environment; an important fundamental principle of physiology that permits a body to maintain a constant internal environment despite changes in the external environment

Medical Word	Word Parts: Part	Word Parts: Meaning	Definition
horizontal (hŏr′ ă-zŏn′ tăl)	horizont -al	horizon pertaining to	Pertaining to the horizon, of or near the horizon, lying flat, even, level
human genome (hŭ′ măn jē′ nōm)			Complete set of genes and chromosomes tucked inside each of the body's trillions of cells
inguinal (ĭng′ gwĭ-năl)	inguin -al	groin pertaining to	Pertaining to the groin, of or near the groin
internal (ĭn-tĕr′ nal)	intern -al	within pertaining to	Pertaining to within or the inside
karyogenesis (kăr″ ē-ō-jĕn′ ĕ-sĭs)	kary/o -genesis	cell's nucleus formation, produce	Formation of a cell's nucleus
lateral (Lat, lat) (lăt′ ĕr-ăl)	later -al	side pertaining to	Pertaining to the side

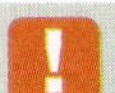

RULE REMINDER

The *o* has been removed from the combining form because the suffix begins with a vowel.

insights *Laterality* (side of the body affected) is a new coding convention added to relevant ICD-10-CM codes to increase specificity. Designated codes for conditions such as fractures, burns, ulcers, and certain neoplasms will require documentation of the side/region of the body where the condition occurs. In ICD-10-CM, laterality code descriptions include right, left, bilateral, or unspecified designations. Over one-third of the expansion of ICD-10-CM codes is due to the addition of laterality.

Example:

Physician office documentation: "patient complains of hearing loss (right); large right cerumen impaction"
ICD-10-CM code: H61.21—impacted cerumen, right ear

Medical Word	Word Parts: Part	Word Parts: Meaning	Definition
medial (mē′ dē-al)	medi -al	toward the middle pertaining to	Pertaining to the middle or midline
mesomorph (mĕs′ ō-morf)	meso- -morph	middle form, shape	Well-proportioned body form marked by predominance of tissue derived from the mesoderm (the middle layer of cells in the developing embryo)

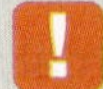

ALERT!

Meso- means *middle*. Using the suffix ***-morph*** and the prefixes ***ecto-***, ***endo-***, and ***meso-***, build three medical terms that describe body forms.

Medical Word	Word Parts		Definition
	Part	**Meaning**	
organic (or-găn´ ĭk)	organ -ic	organ pertaining to	Pertaining to an organ or organs; pertaining to or derived from vegetable or animal forms of life
pathology (pă-thŏl´ ō-jē)	path/o -logy	disease study of	Study of disease
perfusion (pur-fŭ´ zhŭn)	per- fus -ion	through to pour process	Literally means *a process of pouring through*; as passing of a fluid through spaces; to supply the body with nutritive fluid via the bloodstream
phenotype (fē´ nō-tīp)	phen/o -type	to show type	Physical appearance or type of makeup of an individual
physiology (fĭz″ ē-ŏl´ ō-jē)	physi/o -logy	nature study of	Study of the function (nature) of living organisms; anatomy and physiology (A&P) is the combination of the study of the anatomy and physiology of the human body
protoplasm (prō-tō-plăzm)	proto- -plasm	first a thing formed, plasma	Essential matter inside of a living cell
somatotrophic (sō″ mă-tō-trŏf´ ĭk)	somat/o troph -ic	body nourishment, development pertaining to	Pertaining to stimulation of body growth
superficial (sŭ″ pĕr-fĭsh´ ăl)			Pertaining to the surface, on or near the surface
systemic (sis-tĕm´ ĭk)	system -ic	composite, whole pertaining to	Pertaining to the body as a whole
topical (tŏp´ ĭ-kăl)	topic -al	place pertaining to	Pertaining to a place, definite locale
unilateral (ū″ nĭ-lăt´ ĕr-ăl)	uni- later -al	one side pertaining to	Pertaining to one side
ventral (vĕn´ trăl)	ventr -al	near the belly side pertaining to	Pertaining to the belly side, abdomen; front side of the body (same as anterior)
vertex (vĕr´ tĕks)			Top or highest point; top or crown of the head
visceral (vĭs´ ĕr-ăl)	viscer -al	body organs pertaining to	Pertaining to body organs enclosed within a cavity, especially abdominal organs

Study and Review II

Word Parts

Prefixes

Give the definitions of the following prefixes.

1. ambi- __________
2. ana- __________
3. bi- __________
4. chromo- __________
5. de- __________
6. dif- __________
7. ecto- __________
8. endo- __________
9. homeo- __________
10. meso- __________
11. per- __________
12. proto- __________
13. uni- __________

Combining Forms

Give the definitions of the following combining forms.

1. adip/o __________
2. andr/o __________
3. anter/o __________
4. bi/o __________
5. caud/o __________
6. cyt/o __________
7. dist/o __________
8. dors/o __________
9. hist/o __________
10. hydr/o __________
11. infer/o __________
12. inguin/o __________
13. kary/o __________
14. later/o __________
15. medi/o __________
16. organ/o __________
17. path/o __________
18. phen/o __________
19. physi/o __________
20. poster/o __________
21. proxim/o __________
22. somat/o __________
23. ventr/o __________
24. viscer/o __________

Suffixes

Give the definitions for the following suffixes.

1. -al ______________________
2. -ate ______________________
3. -genesis ______________________
4. -ic ______________________
5. -ion ______________________
6. -logy ______________________
7. -morph ______________________
8. -oid ______________________
9. -ose ______________________
10. -plasm ______________________
11. -some ______________________
12. -stasis ______________________
13. -tomy ______________________
14. -type ______________________

Identifying Medical Terms

In the spaces provided, write the medical terms for the following meanings.

1. ______________________ To resemble man
2. ______________________ Pertaining to two sides
3. ______________________ Study of cells
4. ______________________ Slender physical body form
5. ______________________ Formation of a cell's nucleus
6. ______________________ Pertaining to the stimulation of body growth
7. ______________________ Pertaining to one side

Matching

Select the appropriate lettered meaning for each of the following words.

________	1. ambilateral	a.	Hairlike processes that project from epithelial cells
________	2. anatomy	b.	Top or highest point
________	3. atom	c.	Pertaining to both sides
________	4. chromosome	d.	Study of the structure of an organism such as a human
________	5. cilia	e.	Smallest, most basic chemical unit of an element
________	6. homeostasis	f.	Microscopic bodies that carry the genes that determine hereditary characteristics
________	7. human genome	g.	Complete set of genes and chromosomes
________	8. phenotype	h.	Physical appearance or type of makeup of an individual
________	9. physiology	i.	State of equilibrium maintained in the body's internal environment
________	10. vertex	j.	Study of the nature of a living organism
		k.	Study of disease

Drug Highlights

A **drug** is a chemical substance that can alter or modify the functions of a living organism.

There are thousands of drugs that are available as over-the-counter (OTC) medicines and do not require a prescription. A prescription is a written legal document that gives directions for compounding, dispensing, and administering a medication to a patient.

In general, there are five medical uses for drugs:

- **Therapeutic use.** Used in the treatment of a disease or condition, such as an allergy, to relieve the symptoms or to sustain the patient until other measures are instituted.
- **Diagnostic use.** Certain drugs are used in conjunction with radiology to allow the physician to pinpoint the location of a disease process.
- **Curative use.** Certain drugs, such as antibiotics, kill or remove the causative agent of a disease.
- **Replacement use.** Certain drugs, such as hormones and vitamins, are used to replace or supplement substances normally found in the body.
- **Preventive** or **prophylactic use.** Certain drugs, such as immunizing agents, are used to ward off or lessen the severity of a disease.

Drug names

A drug can have multiple different names. The **chemical name** specifies the formula that denotes the composition of the drug. It is made up of letters and numbers that represent the drug's molecular structure. The **generic name** is the drug's official name and is descriptive of its chemical structure and is written in lowercase letters. A generic drug is generally more economical (costs less) than a brand name drug and is often preferred by insurance companies for patients. A generic drug can be manufactured by more than one pharmaceutical company. When this is the case, each company markets the drug under its own unique brand name. For example, the antibiotic drug amoxicillin (generic name) can have several brand names, such as Amoxil, Polymox, and Trimox. A **brand name** is the private property of the drug manufacturer that makes the drug and is registered by the U.S. Patent Office as well as approved by the U.S. Food and Drug Administration (FDA). A brand name is capitalized and is also called a *trade name*. See the following example of a nonsteroidal anti-inflammatory drug:

- *Chemical name: 4-hydroxyl-2-methyl-N-2-pyridinyl-2H-1, 2-benzothiazine3-carboxamide 1, 1-dioxide*
- *Generic name: piroxicam*
- *Brand or trade name: Feldene*

Undesirable actions of drugs

Most drugs have the potential for causing an action other than the intended action. A *side effect* is an undesirable action of a drug and may limit its usefulness. For example, antibiotics that are administered orally may disrupt the normal bacterial flora of the gastrointestinal (GI) tract and cause gastric discomfort.

An *adverse drug reaction (ADR)* is defined by the World Health Organization (WHO) as "any response to a drug which is noxious and unintended, and which occurs at doses normally used in man." For example, an adverse reaction to Demerol may be light-headedness, dizziness, sedation, nausea, and sweating. A *drug interaction* can occur when one drug potentiates (increases the action) or diminishes the action of another drug. Drugs can also interact with foods, alcohol, tobacco, and other substances.

An *adverse drug event (ADE)* can be a medication error, adverse drug reaction, allergic reaction, or overdose. With concurrent use of multiple medications the potential for adverse drug reactions and drug interactions increases.

insights In the ICD-10-CM, a significant classification change was made to include poisonings, adverse effects of drugs, underdosing of drugs, medicaments (substances used for medical treatment), and biological substances. This new classification category is T36–T50. Also, poisonings are further classified as accidental (unintentional), intentional (self-harm), assault, and undetermined. *Underdosing* is a new term that is defined as taking less of a medication than is prescribed by a physician or the manufacturer's instructions with a resulting negative health consequence.

Medication order and dosage

- The **medication order** is given for a specific patient and denotes the name of the drug, the dosage, the form of the drug, the time for or frequency of administration, and the route by which the drug is to be given.
- The **dosage** is the amount of medicine that is prescribed for administration. The form of the drug can be liquid, solid, semisolid, tablet, capsule, transdermal therapeutic patch, etc.
- The **route of administration** can be by mouth, by injection, into the eye(s), ear(s), nostril(s), rectum, vagina, etc. It is important for the patient to know when and how to take a medication.

Abbreviations

Abbreviation	Meaning	Abbreviation	Meaning
abd	abdomen	**FDA**	Food and Drug Administration
A&P	anatomy and physiology	**GI**	gastrointestinal
ADE	adverse drug event	**H_2O**	water
ADR	adverse drug reaction	**LAT, lat**	lateral
BMI	body mass index	**LLQ**	left lower quadrant
BP	blood pressure	**LUQ**	left upper quadrant
CO_2	carbon dioxide	**O or O_2**	oxygen
DNA	deoxyribonucleic acid	**OTC**	over-the-counter (drugs)
ER	endoplasmic reticulum (as used in this chapter); also means emergency room	**RLQ**	right lower quadrant
		RUQ	right upper quadrant
		T	temperature

Study and Review III

Building Medical Terms

Using the following word parts, fill in the blanks to build the correct medical terms.

bi-	inguin	-al
uni-	path/o	-ic
bi/o	physi/o	-logy

Definition	Medical Term
1. Pertaining to both sides	________lateral
2. Study of life	_________logy
3. Farthest from the point of origin	dist_________
4. Pertaining to the groin	___________al
5. Pertaining to the side	later________
6. Study of disease	_________logy
7. Study of the function of living organisms	_________logy
8. Pertaining to the body as a whole	system_______
9. Pertaining to one side	________lateral
10. Pertaining to body organs enclosed within a cavity	viscer________

Combining Form Challenge

Using the combining forms provided, write the medical term correctly.

adip/o	hist/o	phen/o
andr/o	kary/o	somat/o

1. Pertaining to fatty tissue throughout the body: __________ose
2. To resemble man: ___________oid
3. Study of tissue: ________ logy
4. Formation of a cell's nucleus: ___________genesis
5. Physical appearance or type of makeup of an individual: __________type
6. Pertaining to stimulation of body growth: ________trophic

Select the Right Term

Select the correct answer, and write it on the line provided.

1. Literally means *to cut up* or *to cut apart* is __________.

   physiology **anatomy** **homeostasis** **topical**

2. A surface or part situated toward the front of the body is __________.

   caudal **cranial** **anterior** **medical**

3. A well-proportioned body form is __________.

   endomorph **phenotype** **somatotrophic** **mesomorph**

4. The lower part or foundation of a structure is __________.

   apex **base** **dorsal** **vertex**

5. Nearest the center or point of origin is __________.

   superior **ventral** **topical** **proximal**

6. Pertaining to lying flat, even, level is __________.

   inguinal **horizontal** **medial** **dorsal**

Abbreviations

Place the correct word, phrase, or abbreviation in the space provided.

1. abd ____________________
2. A&P ____________________
3. DNA ____________________
4. body mass index ____________________
5. gastrointestinal ____________________
6. H_2O ____________________
7. LLQ ____________________
8. oxygen ____________________
9. over-the-counter (drugs) ____________________
10. RUQ ____________________

Practical Application

ICD-10-CM Terminology

Write your answers to the following questions.

1. In ICD-10-CM, morbid (severe) obesity (E66.01) is due to excess _______________.
2. The term _______________ is not recognized as a clinical term for high adiposity obesity.
3. __________ (side of the body affected) is a new coding convention added to the ICD-10-CM.
4. The term ________________ means "substances used for medical treatment."
5. The term ________________ means "taking less of a medication than is prescribed."

Chapter

5

Integumentary System

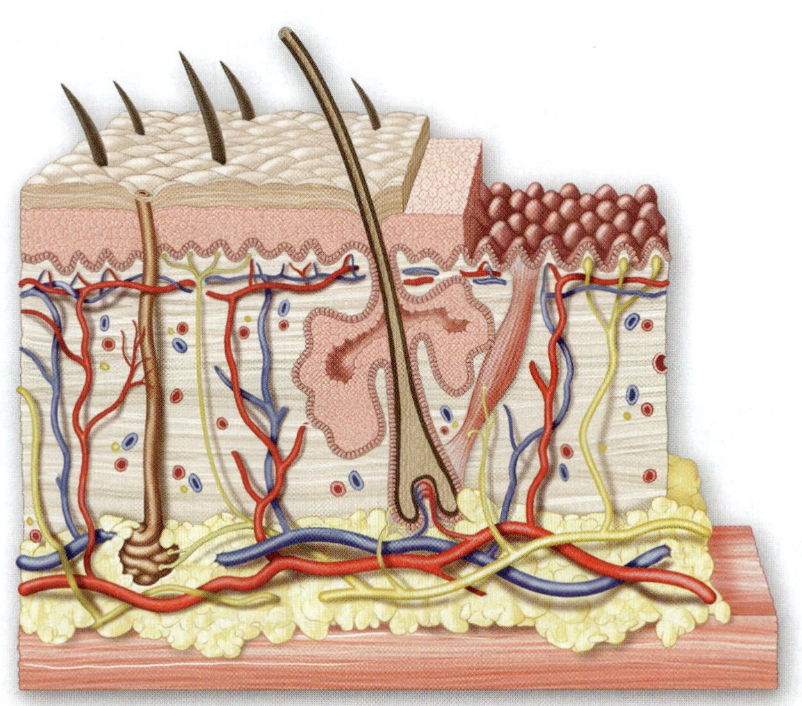

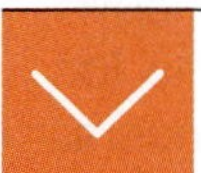

Learning Outcomes

On completion of this chapter, you will be able to:

1. Describe the integumentary system and its accessory structures.
2. List the functions of the skin.
3. Recognize terminology included in the ICD-10-CM.
4. Analyze, build, spell, and pronounce medical words.
5. Comprehend the drugs highlighted in this chapter.
6. Describe diagnostic and laboratory tests related to the integumentary system.
7. Identify and define selected abbreviations.
8. Apply your acquired knowledge of medical terms by successfully completing the *Practical Application* exercise.

Anatomy and Physiology

The integumentary system is composed of the skin, the largest organ of the body, and its accessory structures, the hair, nails, sebaceous glands, and sweat glands. Table 5.1 provides an at-a-glance look at the integumentary system.

Functions of the Skin

The **skin** is the external covering of the body. In an average adult, it covers more than 3,000 square inches of surface area, weighs more than 6 pounds, and is the largest organ of the body. The skin is well supplied with blood vessels and nerves and has four main functions: protection, regulation, sensation, and secretion.

Protection

The skin serves as a protective membrane against invasion by bacteria and other potentially harmful agents that could try to penetrate into deeper tissues. It protects against mechanical injury of delicate cells located beneath its epidermis or outer covering. The

Table 5.1 Integumentary System at-a-Glance

Organ/Structure	Primary Functions/Description
Skin	Protection, regulation, sensation, and secretion
Epidermis	Outer protective covering of the body that can be divided into five strata (*in order as the layers evolve and mature*)
stratum germinativum	Innermost epidermal layer responsible for regeneration of the epidermis. Damage to this layer, as in severe burns, necessitates the use of skin grafts (SG). **Melanin**, the pigment that gives color to the skin, is formed in this layer. The more abundant the melanin, the darker the color of the skin.
stratum spinosum	Means "spiny layer." Each time a stem cell divides, one of the daughter cells is pushed into this layer. Contains Langerhans cells, which are responsible for stimulating a defense against invading microorganisms and superficial skin cancers.
stratum granulosum	Large amounts of **keratin**, a protein substance, is made. In humans, keratin is the basic structural component of hair and nails.
stratum lucidum	Present in thick skin of the palms and soles. Cells are flattened, densely packed, and filled with keratin.
stratum corneum	Outermost, horny layer, consisting of dead cells. Cells are active in the **keratinization** process, during which the cells lose their nuclei and become hard or horny. Forms protective covering for the body.
Dermis	Nourishes the epidermis, provides strength, and supports blood vessels
Papillae	Produce ridges that are one's fingerprints
Subcutaneous tissue	Supports, nourishes, insulates, and cushions the skin
Hair	Provides sensation and some protection for the head. Hair around the eyes, in the nose, and in the ears filters out foreign particles.
Nails	Protects ends of fingers and toes
Sebaceous (oil) glands	Lubricates the hair and skin
Sudoriferous (sweat) glands	Secretes sweat or perspiration, which helps to cool the body by evaporation. Sweat also rids the body of waste.

skin also serves to inhibit excessive loss of water and electrolytes and provides a reservoir for storing food and water. The skin guards the body against excessive exposure to the sun's ultraviolet (UV) rays by producing a protective pigmentation, and it helps to produce the body's supply of vitamin D.

Regulation

The skin serves to raise or lower body temperature as necessary. When the body needs to lose heat, the blood vessels in the skin dilate, bringing more blood to the surface for cooling by **radiation**. At the same time, the sweat glands are secreting more sweat for cooling by means of **evaporation**. Conversely, when the body needs to conserve heat, the reflex actions of the nervous system cause the skin's blood vessels to constrict, thereby allowing more heat-carrying blood to circulate to the muscles and vital organs.

Sensation

The skin contains millions of microscopic nerve endings that act as **sensory receptors** for pain, touch, heat, cold, and pressure. When stimulation occurs, nerve impulses are sent to the cerebral cortex of the brain. The nerve endings in the skin are specialized according to the type of sensory information transmitted and, once this information reaches the brain, it triggers any necessary response. For example, touching a hot surface with the hand causes the brain to recognize the senses of *touch*, *heat*, and *pain* and results in the immediate removal of the hand from the hot surface.

Secretion

The skin contains millions of sweat glands, which secrete **perspiration** or **sweat**, and **sebaceous glands**, which secrete oil (sebum) for lubrication. Perspiration is largely water with a small amount of salt and other chemical compounds. This secretion, when left to accumulate, causes body odor, especially where it is trapped among hairs in the axillary region. **Sebum** is an oily secretion that acts to protect the body from dehydration and possible absorption of harmful substances.

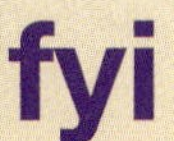

Before birth, **vernix caseosa**, a cheeselike substance, covers the fetus. At first, the fetal skin is transparent and blood vessels are clearly visible. In about 13–16 weeks, downy lanugo hair begins to develop, especially on the head. At 21–24 weeks, the skin is reddish and wrinkled and has little subcutaneous fat. At birth, the subcutaneous glands are developed, and the skin is smooth and pink. Newborns have less subcutaneous fat than adults; therefore, they are more sensitive to heat and cold.

Layers of the Skin

The skin is essentially composed of two layers, the epidermis and the dermis. See Figure 5.1.

Epidermis

The **epidermis** is the outer layer of skin. The thickness of the epidermis varies in different types of skin. It is the thinnest on the eyelids at 0.05 mm and the thickest on the palms and soles at 1.5 mm.

The epidermis can be divided into five strata: *stratum germinativum*, *stratum spinosum*, *stratum granulosum*, *stratum lucidum*, and *stratum corneum*. See Table 5.1 for the functions, descriptions, and locations of these strata within the epidermis.

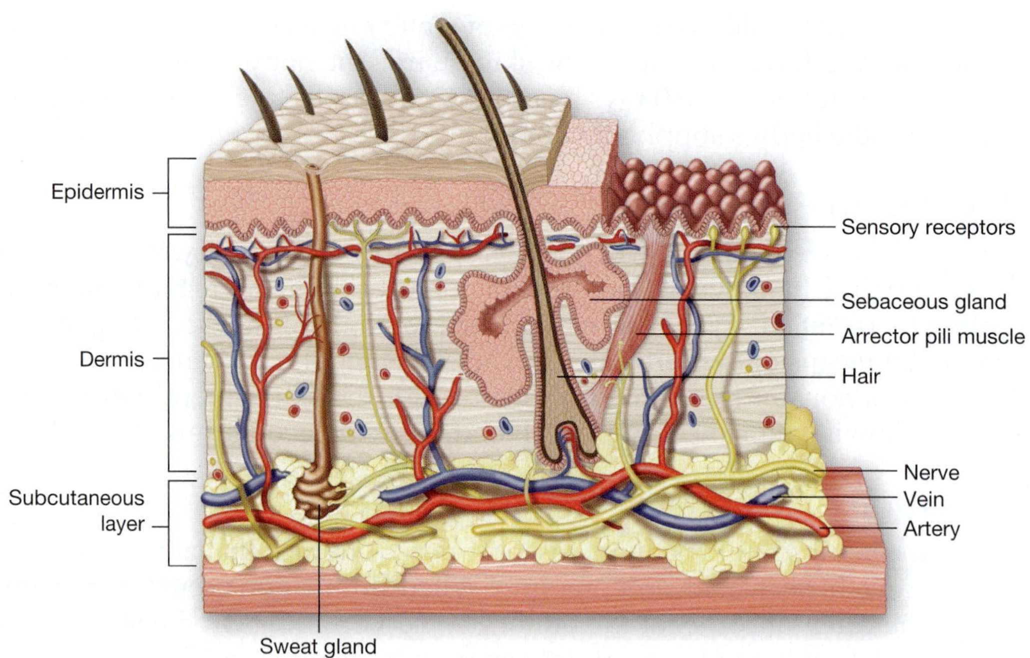

Figure 5.1 The integument: the epidermis, dermis, subcutaneous tissue, and its accessory structures.

Dermis

Sometimes called the **corium** or **true skin**, the **dermis** is composed of connective tissue containing lymphatics, nerves and nerve endings, blood vessels, sebaceous and sweat glands, elastic fibers, and hair follicles. It is divided into two layers: the *upper layer* or **papillary layer** and the *lower layer* or **reticular layer**. The papillary layer is arranged into parallel rows of microscopic structures called **papillae**, which produce the ridges of the skin that are one's fingerprints or footprints. The reticular layer is composed of white fibrous tissue that supports the blood vessels. The dermis is attached to underlying structures by the **subcutaneous tissue** (see Figure 5.1). This tissue supports, nourishes, insulates, and cushions the skin.

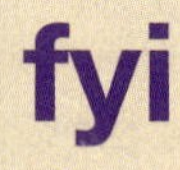

As a person ages, the skin becomes looser as the dermal papillae become thinner. Collagen and elastic fibers of the upper dermis decrease and skin loses its elastic tone and wrinkles more easily.

Accessory Structures of the Skin

The hair, nails, sebaceous glands, and sweat glands are the accessory structures of the skin.

Hair

A **hair** is a thin, threadlike structure formed by a group of cells that develop within a hair **follicle** or *socket*. See Figure 5.2. Each hair is composed of a **shaft**, which is the visible portion, and a **root**, which is embedded within the follicle. At the base of each follicle is a loop of capillaries enclosed within connective tissue called the **hair papilla**. The **pilomotor muscle** attaches to the side of each follicle. When the skin is cooled or the individual has an emotional reaction, the skin often forms "gooseflesh" as a result of contraction by these muscles. Hair is distributed over the whole body with the

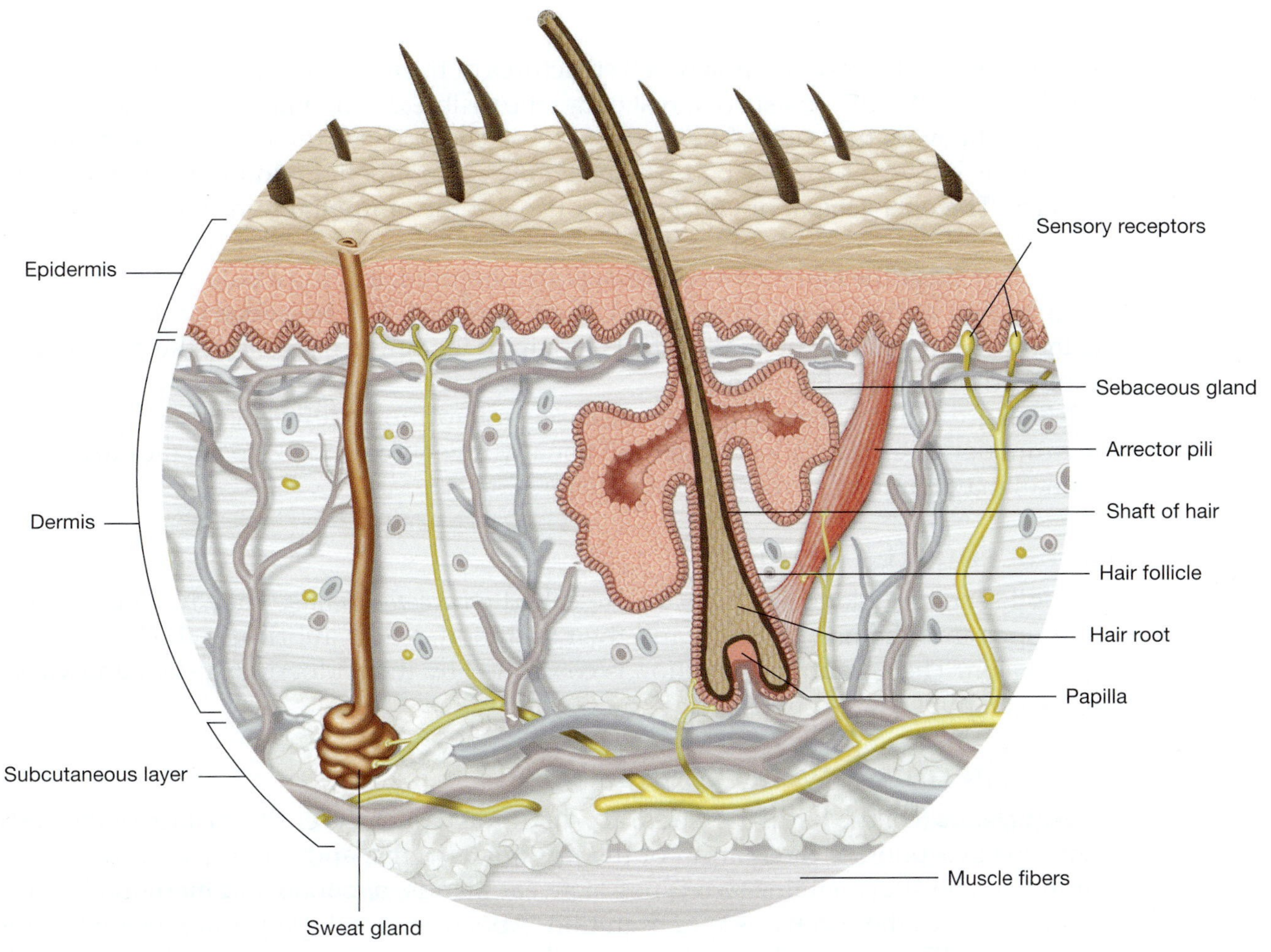

Figure 5.2 Cross-section of skin and a hair follicle. Note the shaft of the hair, the root, and papilla.

exception of the palms of the hands, soles of the feet, and the penis. It is thicker on the scalp and thinner on the other parts of the body. Hair around the eyes, in the nose, and in the ears serves to filter out foreign particles. Hair grows at approximately 0.5 inch a month, and its growth is not affected by cutting. Hair color is determined by the differences in the type and amount of melanin (pigment) produced by melanocytes at the hair papilla. Different types of melanin give dark-brown, yellow-brown, or red coloration to the hair. The color of hair is genetically determined, but the condition of the hair can be affected by hormonal or environmental factors. As pigment production decreases with age, the color of the hair lightens, and the process of graying occurs.

fyi By age 50, approximately half of all people have some gray hair. Scalp hair thins in women and men. The hair becomes dry and often brittle. Some older women may have an increase in facial hair due to hormonal changes. Some men may have an increase in hair of the nares (nostrils), eyebrows, or helix of the ear. In addition to the changes in the skin and hair, nails can flatten and become discolored, dry, and brittle.

Nails

Fingernails and **toenails** are horny cell structures of the epidermis and are composed of hard keratin. A nail consists of a **nail body** (the visible dense mass of dead keratinized cells) that covers the ends of fingers and toes. The body of the nail covers an area of epidermis known as the **nail bed**. The **nail root** is an epithelial fold not visible from the surface. The **eponychium** or *cuticle* is a portion of the epithelial fold that extends over the exposed nail adjacent to the root. The underlying blood vessels give the nail its pink color. Near the nail root these vessels are obscured, leaving a pale crescent-shaped area known as the **lunula** (from *luna*, Latin for moon). The **free edge** of the nail is the extension of the nail plate that protects the tip of the finger or toe. It is the portion that can be trimmed. See Figure 5.3.

Nail growth may vary with age, disease, and hormone deficiency. Average growth is 1 mm per week, and a lost fingernail usually regenerates in 3½ to 5½ months. A lost toenail may require 6–8 months for regeneration.

Sebaceous (Oil) Glands

The oil-secreting glands of the skin are called *sebaceous glands*. They have tiny ducts that open into the hair follicles, and their secretion, *sebum*, lubricates the hair as well as the skin. The amount of secretion is controlled by the endocrine system and varies with age, puberty, and pregnancy.

Sudoriferous (Sweat) Glands

Sweat glands (coiled, tubular glands) are distributed over the entire surface of the body with the exception of the margin of the lips, glans penis, and the inner surface of the prepuce. The skin contains two types of sweat glands, **apocrine** and **merocrine**. These names refer to the mechanism of secretion. Apocrine sweat glands are located in the armpits (axillae), around the nipples, and in the groin. They secrete their products into hair follicles. Apocrine sweat glands begin secreting at puberty. Merocrine sweat glands are coiled tubular glands that discharge their secretions directly onto the surface of the skin. The adult integument contains 2–5 million merocrine sweat glands, with the most numerous being in the palms of the hands and soles of the feet. Sweat glands secrete sweat or perspiration, which helps to cool the body by evaporation. Sweat also rids the body of waste through the pores of the skin. Left to accumulate, sweat becomes odorous by the action of bacteria. Under ordinary circumstances the body can lose about 0.5 L or more of fluid per day through sweat.

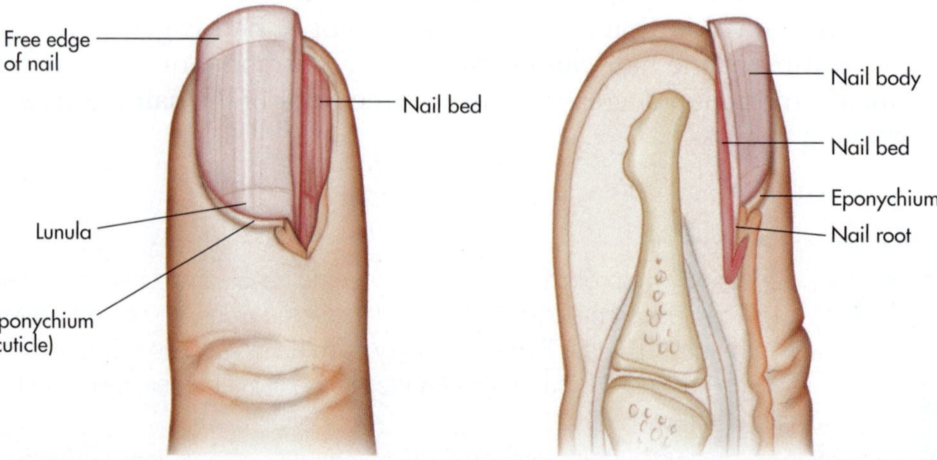

Figure 5.3 The fingernail, an appendage of the integument.

Study and Review I

Anatomy and Physiology

Write your answers to the following questions.

1. Name the primary organ of the integumentary system. ______________________

2. Name the four accessory structures of the integumentary system.

a. ______________________ **b.** ______________________

c. ______________________ **d.** ______________________

3. State the four main functions of the skin.

a. ______________________ **b.** ______________________

c. ______________________ **d.** ______________________

4. The skin is essentially composed of two layers, the ______________________ and the ______________________.

5. Name the five strata of the epidermis.

a. ______________________ **b.** ______________________

c. ______________________ **d.** ______________________

e. ______________________

6. ______________________ is a protein substance that is the basic structural component of hair and nails.

7. ______________________ is a pigment that gives color to the skin.

8. The ______________________ is known as the *corium* or *true skin*.

9. Name the two layers of the part of the skin described in question 8.

a. ______________________ **b.** ______________________

10. The crescent-shaped white area of the nail is the ______________________.

ANATOMY LABELING

Identify the structures shown below by filling in the blanks.

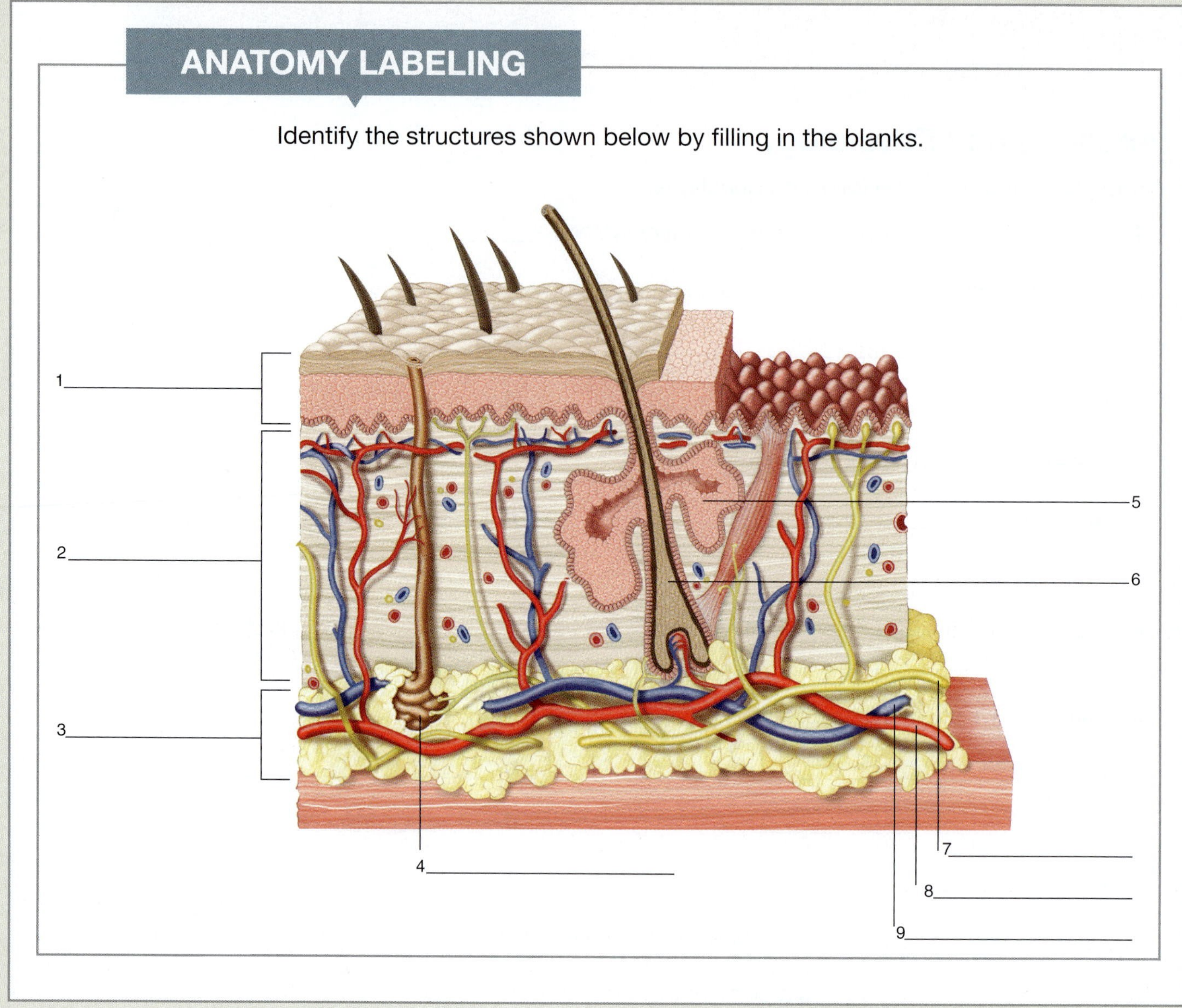

Building Your Medical Vocabulary

This section provides the foundation for learning medical terminology. Review the following alphabetized word list. Note how common prefixes and suffixes are repeatedly applied to word roots and combining forms to create different meanings. The word parts are color-coded: prefixes are yellow, suffixes are blue, roots/combining forms are red. A combining form is a word root plus a vowel. The chart below lists the combining forms for the word roots in this chapter and can help to strengthen your understanding of how medical words are built and spelled.

Remember These Guidelines

1. If the suffix begins with a vowel, drop the combining vowel from the combining form and add the suffix. For example, pedicul/o (a louse) + -osis (condition) becomes pediculosis.
2. If the suffix begins with a consonant, keep the combining vowel and add the suffix to the combining form. For example, dermat/o (skin) + -logy (study of) becomes dermatology.

You will find that some terms have not been divided into word parts. These are common words or specialized terms that are included to enhance your medical vocabulary.

Combining Forms of the Integumentary System			
acr/o	extremity	**leuk/o**	white
aden/o	gland	**melan/o**	black
albin/o	white	**myc/o**	fungus
ang/i	vessel	**onych/o**	nail
caus/o	burn; burning	**pachy/o**	thick
cellul/o	little cell	**pedicul/o**	a louse
cutane/o	skin	**plak/o**	plate
derm/a	skin	**prurit/o**	itching
derm/o	skin	**rhytid/o**	wrinkle
dermat/o	skin	**scler/o**	hard, hardening
erythr/o	red	**seb/o**	oil
follicul/o	little bag	**therm/o**	hot, heat
hidr/o	sweat	**trich/o**	hair
icter/o	jaundice	**vuls/o**	to pull
integument/o	a covering	**xanth/o**	yellow
kel/o	tumor	**xer/o**	dry
kerat/o	horn		

Medical Word	Word Parts		Definition
	Part	**Meaning**	
acne (ăk´ nē)			Inflammatory condition of the sebaceous glands and the hair follicles; *pimples*. See Figure 5.4.

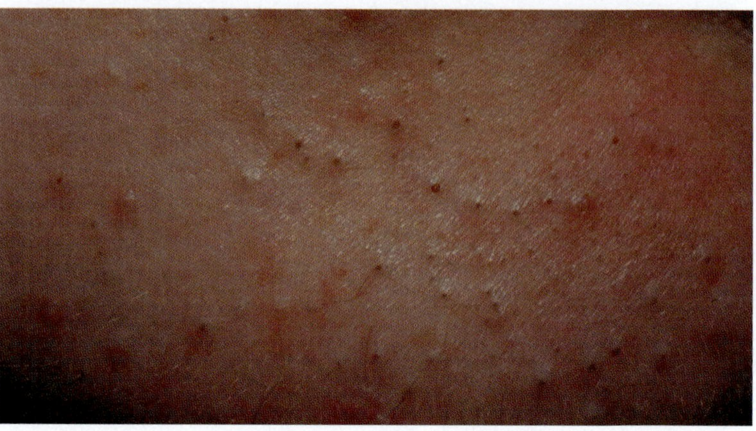

Figure 5.4 Acne.
(Courtesy of Jason L. Smith, MD)

fyi Acne fulminans is a rare type of acne in teenage boys, marked by inflamed, tender, ulcerative, and crusting lesions of the upper trunk and face. It has a sudden onset and is characterized by fever, leukocytosis (elevated white blood cells), and an elevated sedimentation rate. About 50% of the cases have inflammation of several joints. See Figure 5.5.

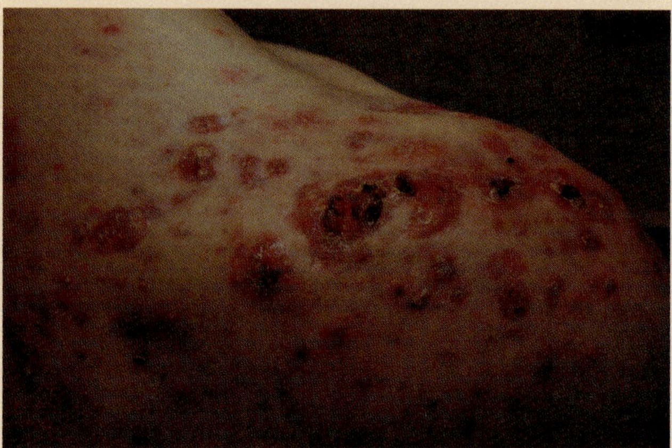

Figure 5.5 Acne fulminans.
(Courtesy of Jason L. Smith, MD)

Medical Word	Part	Meaning	Definition
acrochordon (ăk″ rō-kor´ dŏn)	acr/o chord -on	extremity cord pertaining to	Small outgrowth of epidermal and dermal tissue; *skin tags*

Medical Word	Word Parts: Part	Word Parts: Meaning	Definition
actinic dermatitis (ăk-tĭn´ ĭk dĕr″ mă-tī´ tĭs)	actin -ic dermat -itis	ray pertaining to skin inflammation	Inflammation of the skin caused by exposure to radiant energy, such as x-rays, ultraviolet light, and sunlight. See Figure 5.6.
albinism (ă l´ bĭn-ĭ sm)	albin -ism	white condition	Genetic condition in which there is partial or total absence of pigment in skin, hair, and eyes
alopecia (al″ ō-pē´ shē-ă)	a- lopec -ia	without, lack of fox mange condition	Absence or loss of hair, especially of the head; baldness; *alopecia areata* is loss of hair in defined patches usually involving the scalp. See Figure 5.7. Androgenetic (formerly called *male pattern*) alopecia begins in the frontal area and proceeds until only a horseshoe area of the hair remains in the back and temples. See Figure 5.8.

Figure 5.6 Photodermatitis.
(Courtesy of Jason L. Smith, MD)

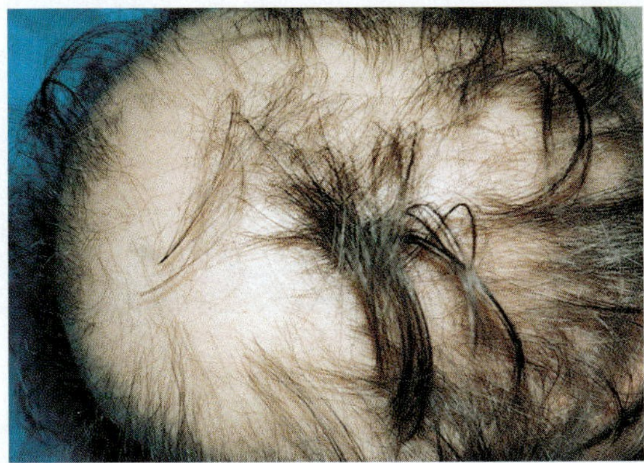

Figure 5.7 Alopecia areata.
(Courtesy of Jason L. Smith, MD)

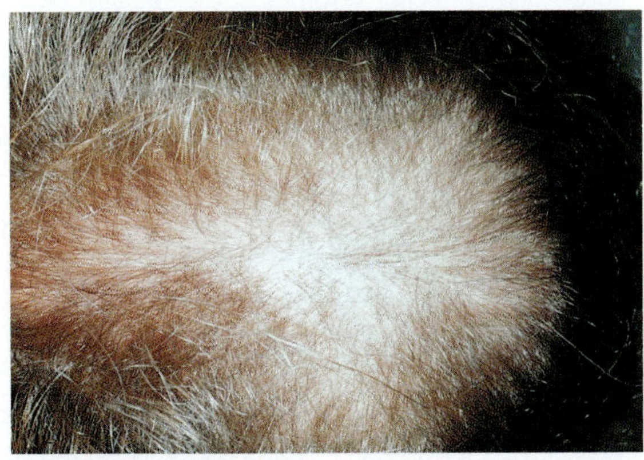

Figure 5.8 Androgenetic alopecia.
(Courtesy of Jason L. Smith, MD)

(*continued*)

Medical Word	Word Parts: Part	Word Parts: Meaning	Definition

insights In ICD-10-CM, the term **androgenetic alopecia** is used instead of *male-pattern baldness* because it is a common form of hair loss in both men and women. In men, hair is lost in a well-defined pattern, beginning above both temples and receding to form a characteristic "M″ shape over time. Hair also thins at the crown (near the top of the head), often progressing to partial or complete baldness. The pattern of hair loss in women differs from that of the male; the hair becomes thinner all over the head and the hairline does not recede. Androgenetic alopecia in women rarely leads to total baldness.

Medical Word	Part	Meaning	Definition
anhidrosis (ă n″ hī-drō´ sĭs)	an- hidr -osis	without, lack of sweat condition	Abnormal condition in which there is a lack of or complete absence of sweating. May be congenital or disease related, generalized or localized, temporary or permanent.
autograft (ŏ-tō-gră ft)	auto- -graft	self pencil, grafting knife	Graft taken from one part of the patient´s body and transferred to another part of that same patient
avulsion (ă-vŭl´ shŭn)	a- vuls -ion	away from to pull process	Process of forcibly tearing off a part or structure of the body, such as a finger or toe
basal cell carcinoma (BCC) (bā´ săl sĕl kăr″ sĭ-nō´ mă)	carcin -oma	cancer tumor	Epithelial malignant tumor of the skin that rarely metastasizes. It usually begins as a small, shiny papule and enlarges to form a whitish border around a central depression. See Figure 5.9.

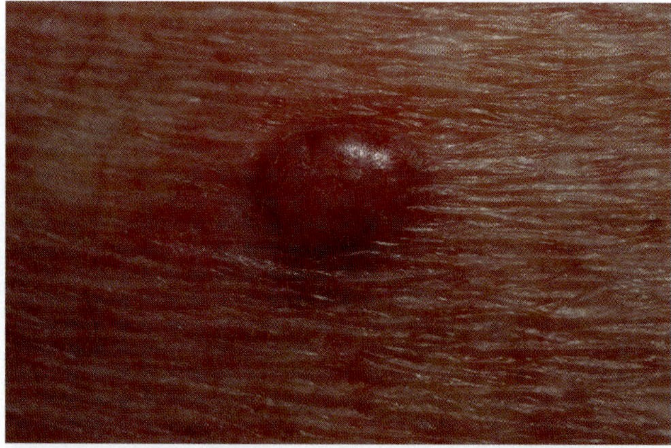

Figure 5.9 Basal cell carcinoma.
(Courtesy of Jason L. Smith, MD)

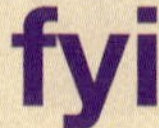

fyi Premalignant and malignant skin lesions increase with aging and with overexposure to the sun. Carcinomas appear frequently on the nose, eyelid, or cheek. Basal cell carcinomas (BCC) account for 80% of the skin cancers seen in the older adult. These cancers are generally slow growing but should be surgically removed as soon as possible.

Medical Word	Word Parts		Definition
	Part	**Meaning**	
bite			Injury in which a part of the skin is torn by an insect, animal, or human, resulting in a combination of an abrasion, puncture, or laceration. See Figures 5.10, 5.11, and 5.12.

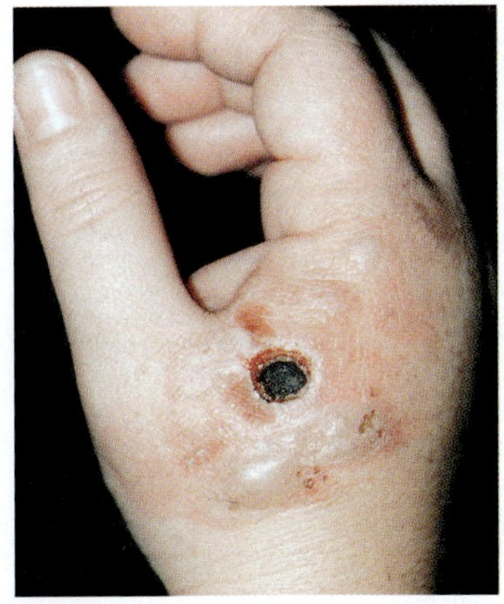

Figure 5.10 Brown recluse spider bites.
(Courtesy of Jason L. Smith, MD)

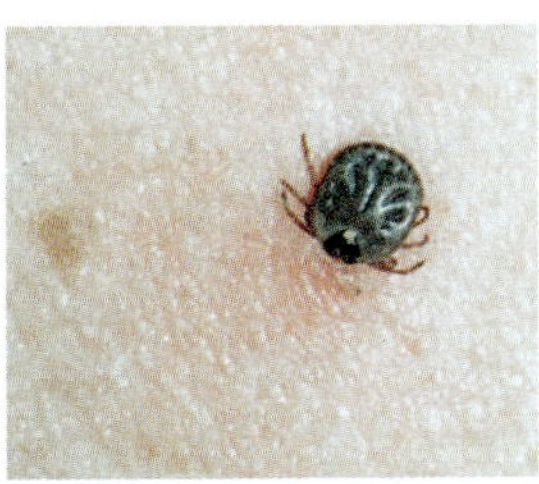

Figure 5.11 Tick bite.
(Courtesy of Jason L. Smith, MD)

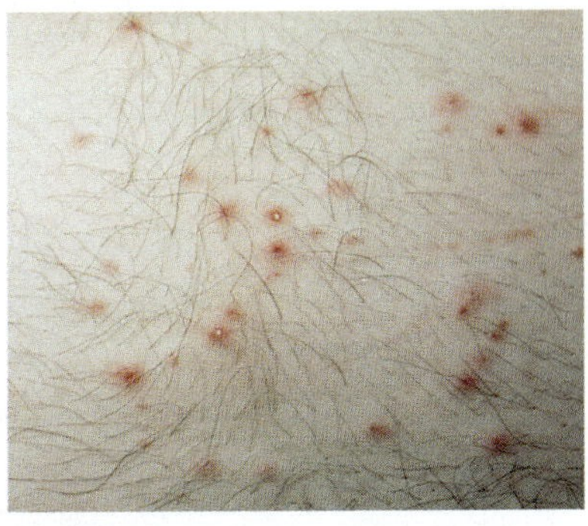

Figure 5.12 Flea bites.
(Courtesy of Jason L. Smith, MD)

Medical Word	Part	Meaning	Definition
boil			Acute, infected, painful nodule formed in the subcutaneous layers of the skin, gland, or hair follicle; most often caused by the invasion of staphylococci; *furuncle*
bulla (bŭl´ lă)			Larger blister; *bleb*. See Figure 5.13.

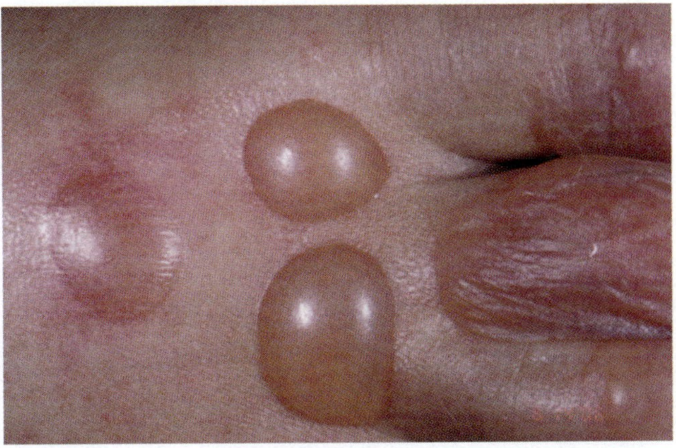

Figure 5.13 Bulla. (Courtesy of Jason L. Smith, MD)

Medical Word	Word Parts		Definition
	Part	Meaning	
burn			Injury to tissue caused by heat, fire, chemical agents, electricity, lightning, or radiation; classified according to degree or depth of skin damage. The three classifications are first degree, second degree, and third degree. See Figures 5.14 and 5.15.

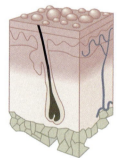

Figure 5.14 Burn, second degree.
(Courtesy of Jason L. Smith, MD)

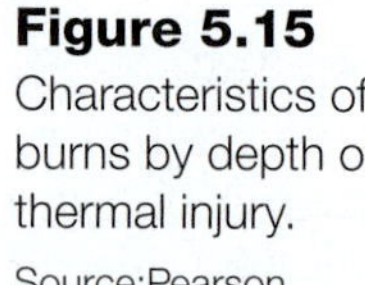
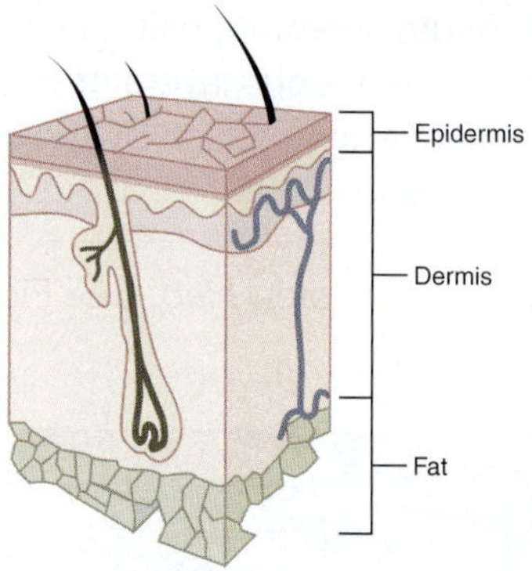
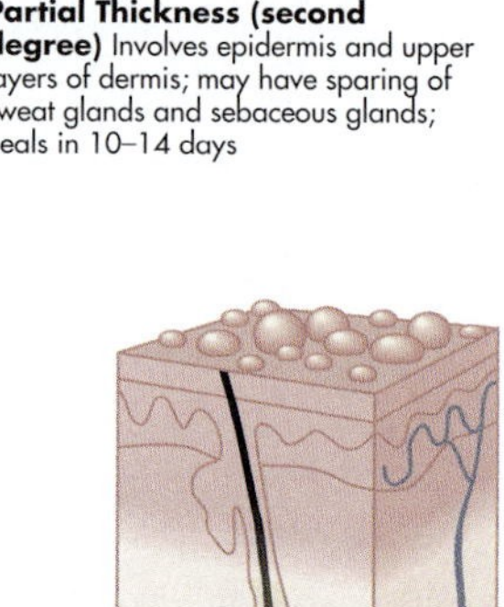
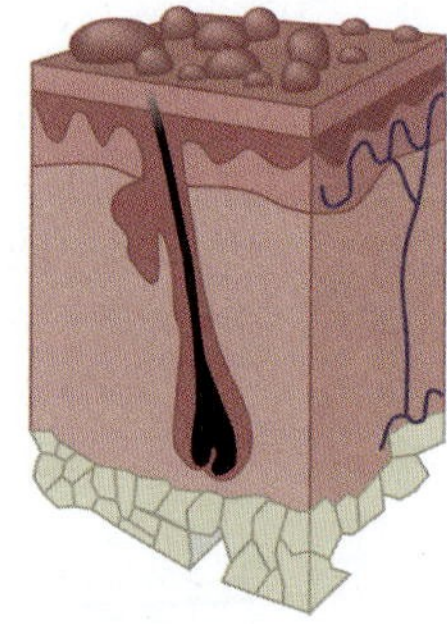

Superficial Partial Thickness (first degree) Damages only outer layer of skin; burn is painful and red; heals in a few days (e.g., sunburn)
Partial Thickness (second degree) Involves epidermis and upper layers of dermis; may have sparing of sweat glands and sebaceous glands; heals in 10–14 days
Full Thickness (third degree) Involves all of epidermis and dermis; may also involve underlying tissue; nerve ending usually destroyed; requires skin grafting
Epidermis
Dermis
Fat
Erythema, blanches on pressure, no bullae, peeling after a few days due to premature cell death
Blisters or bullae, erythema, blanches on pressure, pain and sensitivity to cold air, minimal scar formation
Skin may appear brown, black, deep cherry red, white to gray, waxy or translucent, usually no pain, injured area may appear sunken

Figure 5.15 Characteristics of burns by depth of thermal injury.
Source:Pearson Education, Inc.

insights In ICD-10-CM, there are distinct codes used for burns and corrosions. *Burn codes* apply to thermal burns (except sunburns) that come from a heat source, such as fire, a hot appliance, electricity, and radiation. **Corrosion** is a new term in ICD-10-CM and refers to burns due to chemicals. Burns and corrosions are classified by the body site, depth, encounter, laterality, extent (total body surface area [TBSA]), and external cause/agent. These classifications are needed to determine the correct code. *Note:* Burns of the eye and internal organs are classified by site, not by degree.

Medical Word	Word Parts		Definition
	Part	Meaning	
candidiasis (kă n″ dĭ-dī′ ă -sĭs)			Infection of the skin or mucous membranes with any species of *Candida* but chiefly *Candida albicans*. *Candida* is a genus of yeasts. See Figure 5.16. **Figure 5.16** Candidiasis. (Courtesy of Jason L. Smith, MD)
carbuncle (kăr′ bŭng″ kl)			Infection of the subcutaneous tissue, usually composed of a cluster of boils. See Figure 5.17. **Figure 5.17** Carbuncle. (Courtesy of Jason L. Smith, MD)
causalgia (kŏ-săl′ jē-ă)	caus -algia	burning pain	Intense burning pain associated with trophic skin changes such as thinning of hair and loss of sweat glands due to peripheral nerve damage
cellulitis (sĕl-ū-lī′ tĭs)	cellul -itis	little cell inflammation	An acute, diffuse inflammation of the skin and subcutaneous tissue characterized by local heat, redness, pain, and swelling. See Figure 5.18.

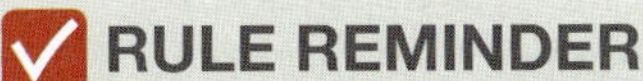

RULE REMINDER

The ***o*** has been removed from the combining form because the suffix begins with a vowel.

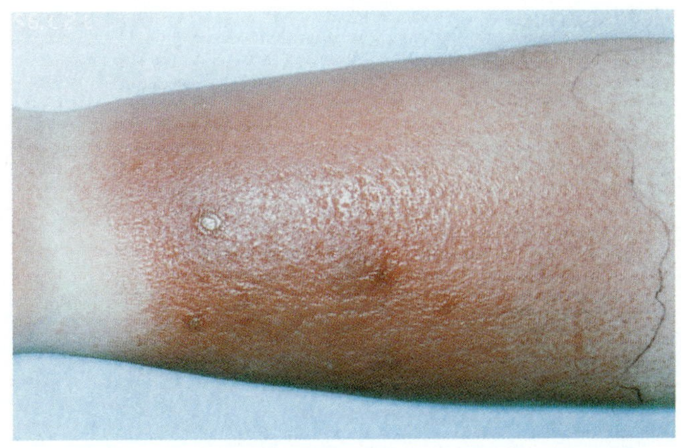

Figure 5.18 Cellulitis.
(Courtesy of Jason L. Smith, MD)

Medical Word	Word Parts: Part	Word Parts: Meaning	Definition
cicatrix (sĭk´ ă-trĭks)			Scar left after the healing of a wound
comedo (kŏm´ ē-dō)			Blackhead
corn (korn)			Condition of horny induration and thickening of the skin that may be soft or hard depending on location; caused by pressure, friction, or both from ill-fitting shoes
cryosurgery (krī˝ ō-sĕr´ jĕr-ē)			Technique of using subfreezing temperature (usually with liquid nitrogen) to produce well-demarcated areas of cell injury and destruction
cutaneous (kū-tā´ nē-ŭs)	cutane -ous	skin pertaining to	Pertaining to the skin
cyst (sĭst)			Closed sac that contains fluid, semifluid, or solid material
debridement (dā-brēd-mŏn´)			Removal of foreign material or damaged or dead tissue, especially in a wound. It is used to promote healing and to prevent infection.

insights In ICD-10-PCS, debridement is described as excision, extraction, irrigation, and extirpation. *Extirpation* is complete excision or surgical destruction of a body part. *Note:* Debridement is listed in ICD-10-*PCS*, not ICD-10-*CM*, because it is a procedure.

Medical Word	Word Parts: Part	Word Parts: Meaning	Definition
decubitus (decub) ulcer (dē-kū´ bĭ-tŭs ŭl´ sĕr)	de- cubit -us	down to lie pertaining to	An area of skin and tissue that becomes injured or broken down. Also known as a bedsore or pressure ulcer. The literal meaning of the word *decubitus* is *a lying down*. (See types of skin signs in Figure 5.39)
dehiscence (dē-hĭs´ ĕns)			Surgical complication where there is separation or bursting open of a surgical wound. See Figure 5.19.

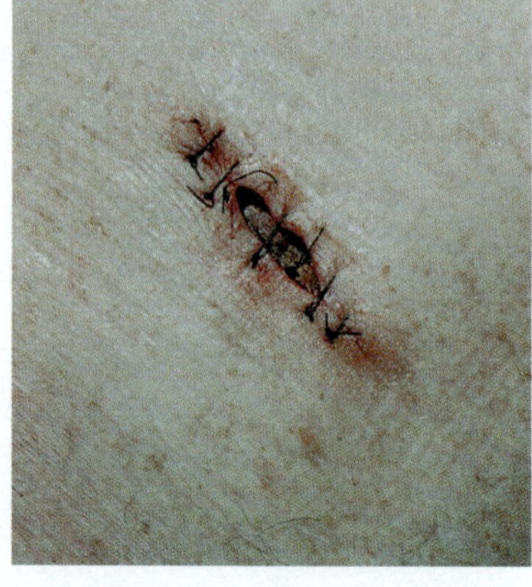

Figure 5.19 Wound dehiscence, back.
(Courtesy of Jason L. Smith, MD)

Medical Word	Word Parts		Definition
	Part	**Meaning**	
dermabrasion (dĕrm´ ă-brā˝ zhŭn)			Surgical procedure to remove acne scars, nevi, tattoos, or fine wrinkles on the skin by using sandpaper, wire brushes, or other abrasive materials on an anesthetized epidermis
dermatitis (dĕr˝ mă-ti´ tĭs)	dermat -itis	skin inflammation	Inflammation of the skin. See Figure 5.20.

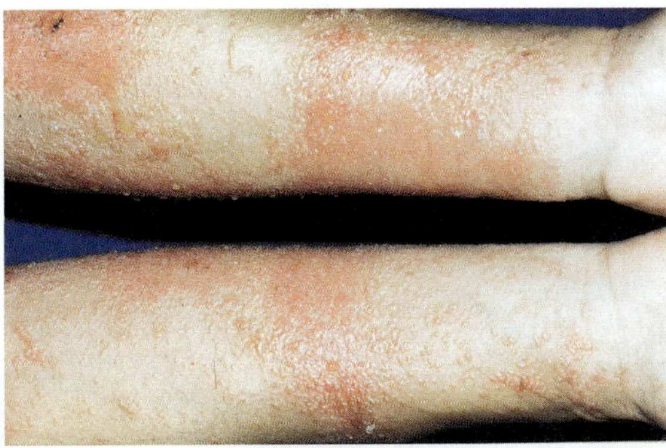

Figure 5.20 Dermatitis; poison ivy.
(Courtesy of Jason L. Smith, MD)

fyi

To help prevent contact dermatitis with poison ivy, learn to recognize and avoid poison ivy. One form of poison ivy is a low plant usually found in groups of many plants and looks like weeds growing from 6 to 30 inches high. The other form is a "hairy" vine that grows up a tree. Each form has stems with three leaves. See Figure 5.21. There is an old saying people should remember: "Leaflets three, let it be." If in contact with poison ivy, oak, or sumac, wash skin immediately with soap and water to remove oleoresin within 15 minutes of exposure. Also, wash all clothing including gloves, jackets, shoes, and shoelaces as soon as possible. Oleoresin, the extract of the plant, can be active for 6 months on surfaces such as clothing.

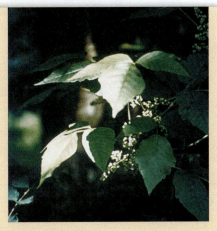

Figure 5.21 Poison ivy plant.
Source: Pearson Education, Inc.

Medical Word	Part	Meaning	Definition
dermatologist (dĕr´ mah-tol´ ŏ -jĭst)	dermat/o log -ist	skin study of one who specializes	Physician who specializes in the study of the skin
dermatology (Derm) (dĕr˝ mah-tol´ ŏ -jē)	dermat/o -logy	skin study of	Study of the skin
dermatome (dĕr´ mah-tōm)	derm/a -tome	skin instrument to cut	Surgical instrument used to cut the skin for grafting

Medical Word	Word Parts		Definition
	Part	**Meaning**	
dermomycosis (dĕr´ mō-mī-kō´ sĭs)	derm/o myc -osis	skin fungus condition	Skin condition caused by a fungus; also called *dermatomycosis* or *tinea*
ecchymosis (ĕk-ĭ-mō´ sĭs)	ec- chym -osis	out juice condition	Abnormal condition in which the blood seeps into the skin causing discolorations ranging from blue-black to greenish yellow; *bruise*
eczema (ĕk´ zĕ-mă)			An acute or chronic inflammatory skin disorder characterized by erythema, papules, vesicles, pustules, scales, crusts, or scabs alone or in combination. The most promising treatment involves nonsteroidal skin medications classified as topical immunomodulators (TIMS) or topical calcineurin (a protein phosphatase) inhibitor.
erythema (ĕr˝ ĭ-thē´ mă)	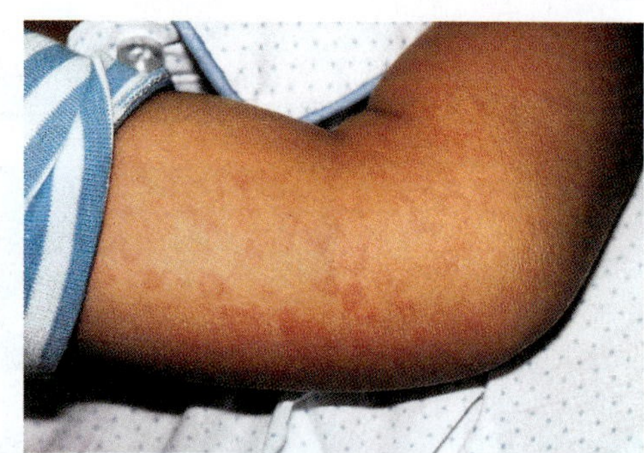 **Figure 5.22** Erythema infectiosum; fifth disease. (Courtesy of Jason L. Smith, MD)		Redness of the skin; may be caused by capillary congestion, inflammation, heat, sunlight, or cold temperature. *Erythema infectiosum* is known as fifth disease, a mild, moderately contagious disease caused by the human parvovirus B-19. It is most commonly seen in school-age children and is thought to be spread via respiratory secretions from infected persons. See Figure 5.22.
erythroderma (ĕ-rĭth˝ rō-dĕr´ -mă)	erythr/o -derma	red skin	Abnormal redness of the skin occurring over widespread areas of the body
eschar (ĕs´ kăr)			Slough, scab
excoriation (ĕks-kō˝ rē-ā´ shŭn)	ex- coriat -ion	out corium process	Abrasion of the epidermis by scratching, trauma, chemicals, or burns
exudate (ĕks´ ū-dāt)			An oozing of pus or serum

Medical Word	Word Parts		Definition
	Part	**Meaning**	
folliculitis (fō-lĭk″ ū-lī′ tĭs)	follicul -itis	little bag inflammation	Inflammation of a follicle or follicles. See Figure 5.23.
gangrene (gă ng′ grēn)			Literally means *an eating sore*. It is a necrosis, or death, of tissue or bone that usually results from a deficient or absent blood supply to the area.
herpes simplex (hĕr′ pēz sĭm′ plĕks)			An inflammatory skin disease caused by a herpes virus (type I); *cold sore* or *fever blister*. See Figure 5.24.
hidradenitis (hī-drăd-ĕ-nī′ tĭs)	hidr aden -itis	sweat gland inflammation	Inflammation of the sweat glands
hives (hīvz)			Eruption of itching and burning swellings on the skin; *urticaria*. See Figure 5.25.

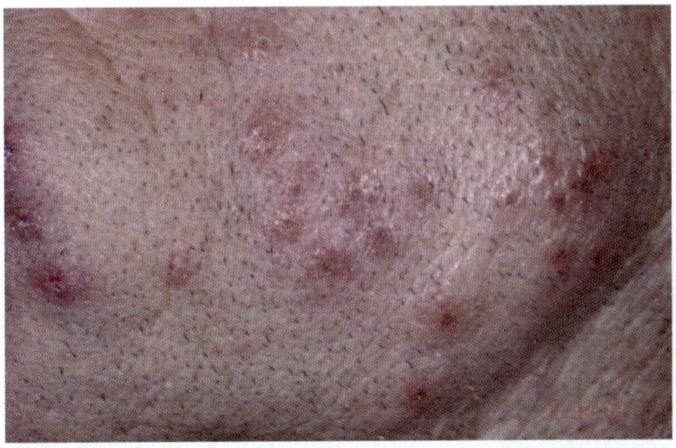

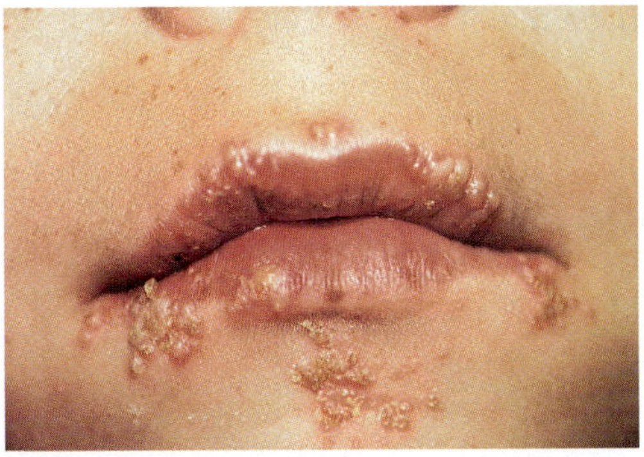

Figure 5.23 Staphylococcal folliculitis.
(Courtesy of Jason L. Smith, MD)

Figure 5.24 Herpes labialis.
(Courtesy of Jason L. Smith, MD)

(continued)

Medical Word	Word Parts		Definition
	Part	**Meaning**	
	Figure 5.25 Urticaria; hives. (Courtesy of Jason L. Smith, MD)		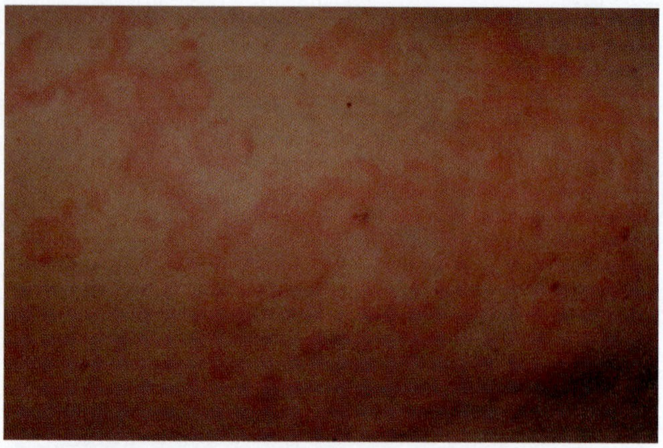
hyperhidrosis (hī″ pĕr-hī-drō′ sĭs)	hyper- hidr -osis	excessive sweat condition	Abnormal condition of excessive sweating
hypodermic (hī″ pō-dĕr′mĭk)	hypo- derm -ic	under skin pertaining to	Pertaining to under the skin or inserted under the skin, as a hypodermic injection
icteric (ik-tĕr′ ik)	icter -ic	jaundice pertaining to	Pertaining to jaundice
impetigo (ĭm″ pĕ-tī′ gō)			Skin infection marked by vesicles or bullae; usually caused by streptococcus (strep) or staphylococcus (staph). See Figure 5.26. 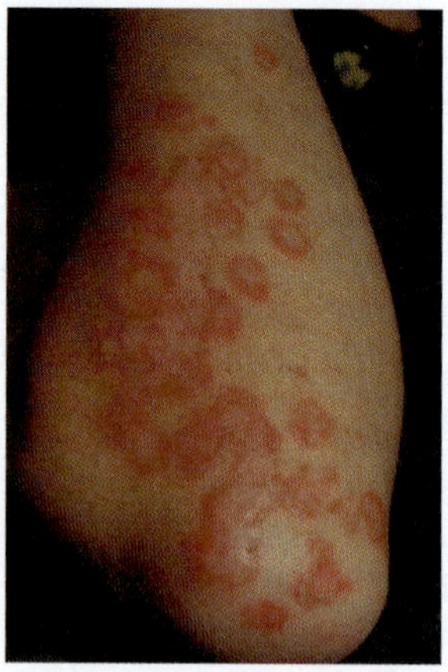 **Figure 5.26** Impetigo. (Courtesy of Jason L. Smith, MD)
integumentary (ĭn-tĕg″ ū-mĕn′ tă-rē)	integument -ary	a covering pertaining to	Covering; the skin, consisting of the dermis and the epidermis
intradermal (ID) (in″ trăh-dĕr′ măl)	intra- derm -al	within skin pertaining to	Pertaining to within the skin, as an intradermal injection

Medical Word	Word Parts		Definition
	Part	**Meaning**	
jaundice (jawn′ dĭs)	jaund -ic(e)	yellow pertaining to	Yellow; a symptom of a disease in which there is excessive bile in the blood; the skin, whites of the eyes, and mucous membranes are yellow; *icterus*
keloid (kē′ lō yd)	kel -oid	tumor resemble	Overgrowth of scar tissue caused by excessive collagen formation. See Figure 5.27. 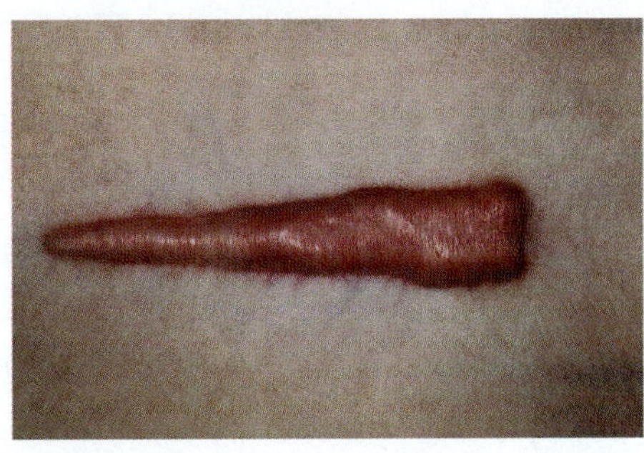 **Figure 5.27** Keloid. (Courtesy of Jason L. Smith, MD)
lentigo (lĕn-tī′ gō)			A flat, brownish spot on the skin sometimes caused by exposure to the sun and weather; *freckle*
leukoderma (lū″ kō-dĕr′ mă)	leuk/o -derma	white skin	Localized loss of pigmentation of the skin
leukoplakia (lū″ kō-plā′ kē-ă)	leuk/o plak -ia	white plate condition	White spots or patches formed on the mucous membrane of the tongue or cheek; the spots are smooth, hard, and irregular in shape and can become malignant
lupus (lū′ pŭs)			Originally used to describe a destructive type of skin lesion; current usage of the word is usually in combination with the words *vulgaris* or *erythematosus* (e.g., *lupus vulgaris* or *lupus erythematosus*)
melanoma (mĕl″ ă-nō′ mă)	melan -oma **Figure 5.28** Melanoma, forearm. (Courtesy of Jason L. Smith, MD)	black tumor	Cancer that develops in the pigment cells of the skin; malignant black mole or tumor. See Figure 5.28. Often the first sign of melanoma is change in the size, shape, or color of a mole. The ***ABCDs*** of melanoma describe the changes that can occur in a mole using the letters: ***A***—asymmetry; the shape of one half does not match the other. ***B***—border; the edges are ragged, notched, or blurred. ***C***—color; is uneven. Shades of black, brown, or tan are present. Areas of white, red, or blue may be seen. ***D***—diameter; there is a change in size.

(*continued*)

Medical Word	Word Parts		Definition
	Part	**Meaning**	

insights In ICD-10-CM, melanoma is classified as *melanoma* or *melanoma in situ*. Melanoma is reported with codes from category C43, while melanoma in situ is category D03.

Examples:

- C43.72 Malignant melanoma of left lower limb, including hip
- D03.71 Melanoma in situ of right lower limb, including hip. *Note:* Melanoma in situ is classified as *tumor in situ (TIS)*. The tumor is limited to the top layer of the epidermis with no evidence of invasion of dermis, surrounding tissues, lymph nodes, or distant sites.

Medical Word	Part	Meaning	Definition
miliaria (mĭl-ē-ā´ rē-ă)	miliar -ia	millet (tiny) condition	Rash with tiny pinhead-sized papules, vesicles, and/or pustules commonly seen in newborns and infants; *prickly heat*. It is caused by excessive body warmth. There is retention of sweat in the sweat glands, which have become blocked or inflamed, and then rupture or leak into the skin. See Figure 5.29.

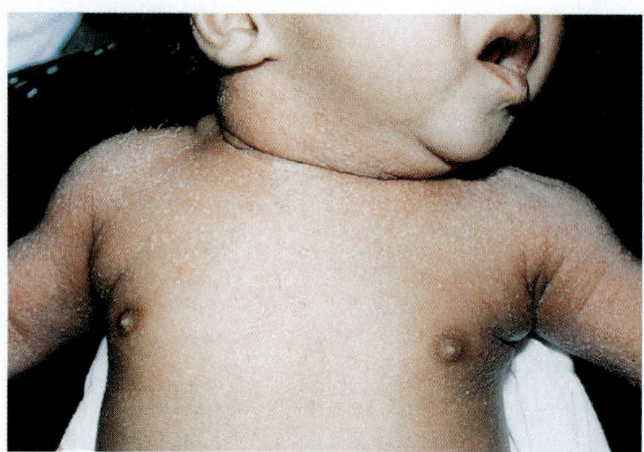

Figure 5.29 Miliaria.
(Courtesy of Jason L. Smith, MD)

Medical Word	Part	Meaning	Definition
mole (mōl)			Pigmented, elevated spot above the surface of the skin; *nevus*. See Figure 5.30.

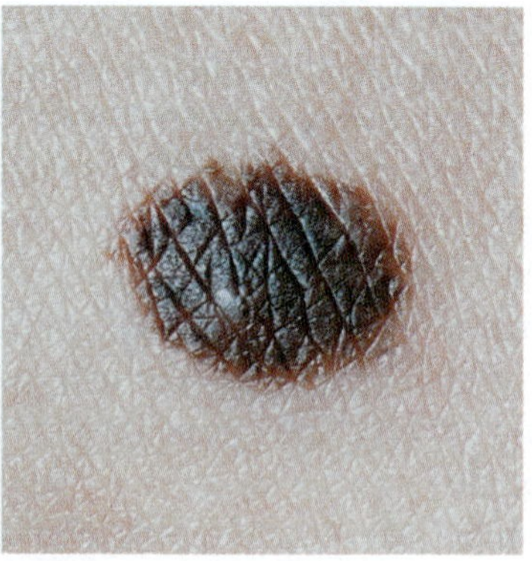

Figure 5.30 Nevus; mole.
(Courtesy of Jason L. Smith, MD)

Medical Word	Part	Meaning	Definition
onychia (ō- nĭk´ē-ă)	onych -ia	nail condition	Inflammation of the nail bed resulting in loss of nail

Medical Word	Word Parts		Definition
	Part	**Meaning**	
onychomycosis (ŏ n″ ĭ-kō-mī-kō′ sĭs)	onych/o myc -osis	nail fungus condition	A fungal infection of the nails. See Figure 5.31. **Figure 5.31** Onychomycosis. (Courtesy of Jason L. Smith, MD)
pachyderma (păk-ē-dĕr′ mă)	pachy -derma	thick skin	Thick skin; also called *pachydermia*
paronychia (păr″ ō-nĭk′ ĭ-ă)	par- onych -ia	around nail condition	Infectious condition of the marginal structures around the nail
pediculosis (pĕ-dĭk″ ū-lō′ sĭs)	pedicul -osis	a louse condition	Condition of infestation with lice. See Figure 5.32. **Figure 5.32** Pediculosis capitis. (Courtesy of Jason L. Smith, MD)
petechiae (pē-tē′ kē- ē)			Small, pinpoint, purplish hemorrhagic spots on the skin
pruritus (proo-rī′ tŭs)	prurit -us	itching pertaining to	Severe itching
psoriasis (sō-rī′ ă-sĭs)			Chronic skin condition characterized by frequent episodes of redness, itching, and thick, dry scales on the skin. See Figure 5.33.

(*continued*)

Medical Word	Word Parts		Definition
	Part	Meaning	

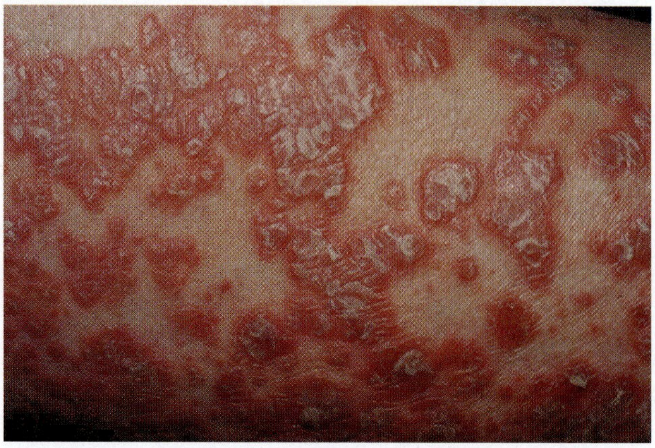

Figure 5.33 Psoriasis, lower extremities.
(Courtesy of Jason L. Smith, MD)

Medical Word	Part	Meaning	Definition
purpura (pŭr´ pū-ră)			Purplish discoloration of the skin caused by extravasation of blood into the tissues. See Figure 5.34.

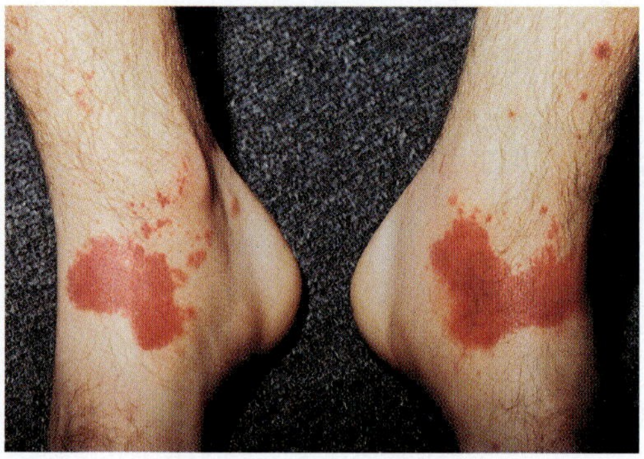

Figure 5.34 Purpura.
(Courtesy of Jason L. Smith, MD)

Medical Word	Part	Meaning	Definition
rhytidoplasty (rĭt´ ĭ-dō-plăs˝ tē)	rhytid/o -plasty	wrinkle surgical repair	Plastic surgery for the removal of wrinkles

RULE REMINDER

This term keeps the combining vowel ***o*** because the suffix begins with a consonant.

Medical Word	Part	Meaning	Definition
rosacea (rō-zā´ sē-ă)			A chronic disease of the skin of the face marked by varying degrees of papules, pustules, erythema, telangiectasia, and hyperplasia of the soft tissues of the nose; usually occurs in middle-aged and older people. See Figure 5.35.

(*continued*)

Medical Word	Word Parts		Definition
	Part	Meaning	
			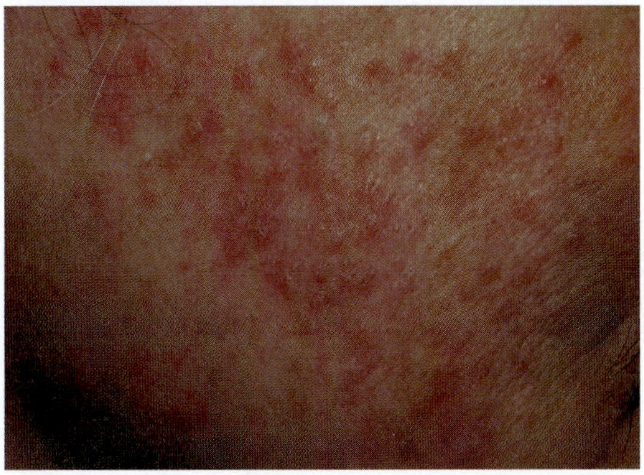 Figure 5.35 Rosacea. (Courtesy of Jason L. Smith, MD)
roseola (rō-zē´ ō-lă)			Any rose-colored rash marked by *maculae* or red spots on the skin. See Figure 5.36. 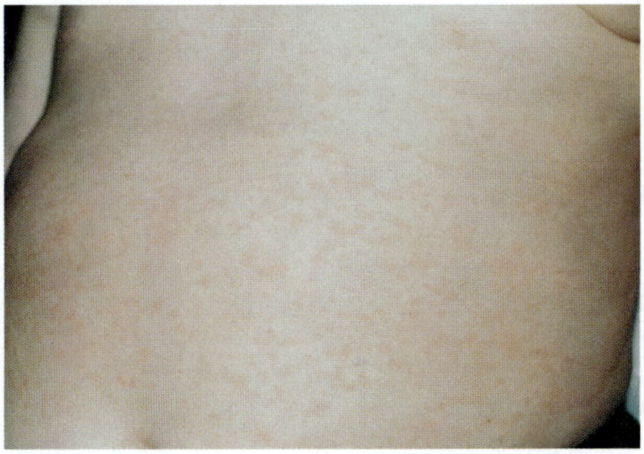 **Figure 5.36** Roseola. (Courtesy of Jason L. Smith, MD)
rubella (roo-bĕl´ lă)			Systemic disease caused by a virus and characterized by a rash and fever; also called *German measles* and *three-day measles*
rubeola (roo-bē´ ō-lă)			Contagious disease characterized by fever, inflammation of the mucous membranes, and rose-colored spots on the skin; also called *measles*
scabies (skā´ bēz)			Contagious skin disease characterized by papules, vesicles, pustules, burrows, and intense itching; it is caused by an arachnid, *Sarcoptes scabiei*, *variety hominis*, the itch mite; also called *the itch*. See Figure 5.37.

(continued)

Medical Word	Word Parts: Part	Word Parts: Meaning	Definition
			Figure 5.37 Scabies. (Courtesy of Jason L. Smith, MD)
scar			Mark left by the healing process of a wound, sore, or injury
scleroderma (sklĕr″ ă-dĕr′ mă)	scler/o -derma	hard, hardening skin	Chronic condition with hardening of the skin and other connective tissues of the body
seborrhea (sĕb″ or-ē′ ă)	seb/o -rrhea	oil flow	Excessive flow (secretion) of oil from the sebaceous glands
sebum (sē′ bŭm)			Fatty or oily secretion produced by the sebaceous glands
senile keratosis (sĕn′ ĭl kĕr″ ă-tō′ sĭs)	senile kerat -osis	old horn condition	Condition occurring in older people wherein there is dry skin and localized scaling caused by excessive exposure to the sun. See Figure 5.38.

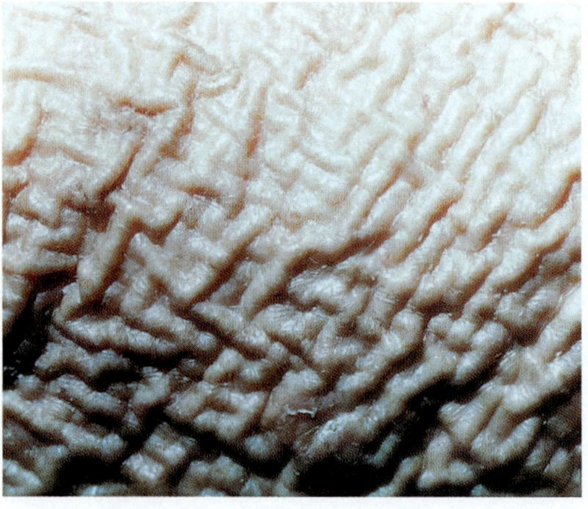

Figure 5.38 Photoaging solar elastosis; senile keratosis.
(Courtesy of Jason L. Smith, MD)

Medical Word	Word Parts		Definition
	Part	Meaning	
skin signs			Objective evidence of an illness or disorder. They can be seen, measured, or felt. Types of skin signs are shown and described in Figure 5.39.

A macule is a discolored spot on the skin; freckle

A pustule is a small, elevated, circumscribed lesion of the skin that is filled with pus; varicella (chickenpox)

A wheal is a localized, evanescent elevation of the skin that is often accompanied by itching; urticaria

An erosion or ulcer is an eating or gnawing away of tissue; decubitus ulcer

A papule is a solid, circumscribed, elevated area on the skin; pimple

A fissure is a crack-like sore or slit that extends through the epidermis into the dermis

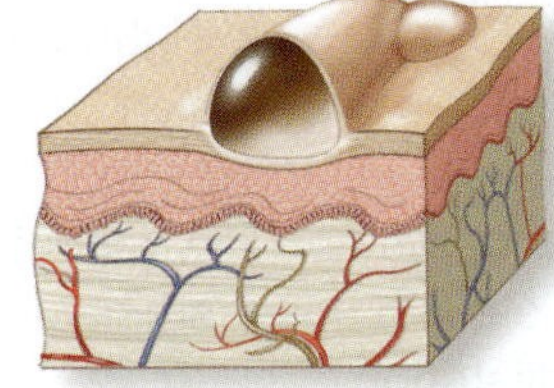

A vesicle is a small fluid-filled sac; blister. A bulla is a large vesicle.

Figure 5.39 Skin signs are objective evidence of an illness or disorder. They can be seen, measured, or felt.

squamous cell carcinoma (SCC) (skwā´ mŭs sĕl kăr″ sĭ-nō´ mă)			Malignant tumor of squamous epithelial tissue. See Figure 5.40.

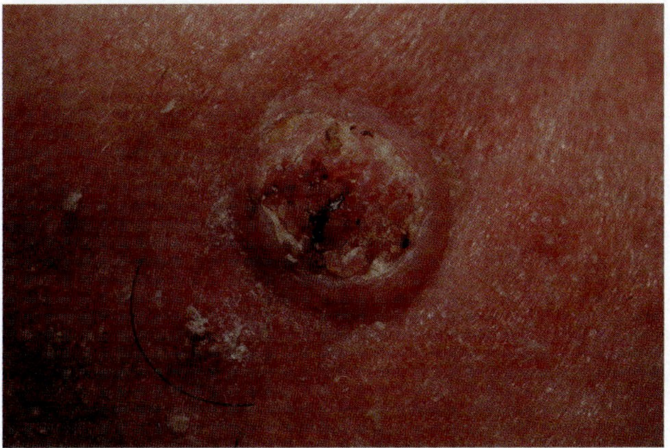

Figure 5.40 Squamous cell carcinoma.
(Courtesy of Jason L. Smith, MD)

Medical Word	Word Parts		Definition
	Part	**Meaning**	
striae *(plural)* (strī´ ē)			Streaks or lines on the breasts, thighs, abdomen, or buttocks caused by weakening of elastic tissue; can be caused by obesity or as a result of pregnancy. See Figure 5.41.
subcutaneous (sŭb″ kū-tā´ nē-ŭs)	sub- cutane -ous	below skin pertaining to	Pertaining to below the skin, as a subcutaneous injection
subungual (sŭb-ŭng´ gwăl)	sub- ungu -al	below nail pertaining to	Pertaining to below the nail
taut (tŏt)			Tight, firm; to pull or draw tight a surface, such as the skin
telangiectasia (tĕl-ăn″ jē-ĕk-tā´ zē-ă)	tel ang/i -ectasia	end, distant vessel dilatation	A vascular lesion formed by dilatation of a group of small blood vessels that may appear as a *birthmark*

Figure 5.41 Striae.
(Courtesy of Jason L. Smith, MD)

ALERT!

Note the spelling of *telangiectasia* and *thermoanesthesia*. The suffix ***-ectasia*** means *dilatation* and the suffix ***-esthesia*** means *sensation*.

Medical Word	Part	Meaning	Definition
thermoanesthesia (thĕr″ mō-ăn-ĕs-thē´ zē-ă)	therm/o an- -esthesia	hot, heat without, lack of sensation	Inability to distinguish between the sensations of heat and cold

Medical Word	Word Parts: Part	Word Parts: Meaning	Definition
tinea (tĭn′ē-ă)			Contagious skin diseases affecting both humans and domestic animals, caused by certain fungi and marked by the localized appearance of discolored, scaly patches on the skin; *ringworm*. See Figure 5.42. **Figure 5.42** Tinea corporis. (Courtesy of Jason L. Smith, MD)
trichomycosis (trĭk″ ō-mī-kō′ sĭs)	trich/o myc -osis	hair fungus condition	Fungal condition of the hair
ulcer (ŭl′ sĕr) **Figure 5.43** Leg ulcer radiation site. (Courtesy of Jason L. Smith, MD)			Open lesion or sore of the epidermis or mucous membrane. See Figure 5.43.
varicella (văr″ i-sĕl′ ă)	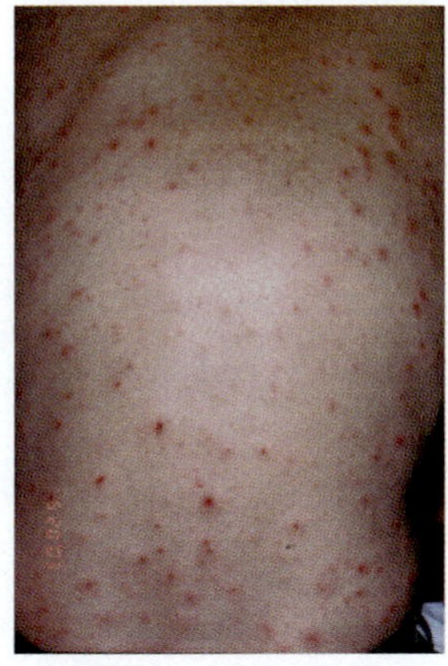		Contagious viral disease characterized by fever, headache, and a crop of red spots that become macules, papules, vesicles, and crusts; *chickenpox*. See Figure 5.44.

Figure 5.44 Varicella; chickenpox.
(Courtesy of Jason L. Smith, MD)

Medical Word	Word Parts		Definition
	Part	**Meaning**	
vitiligo (vĭt-ĭl ĭ´ gō)			Skin condition characterized by milk-white patches surrounded by areas of normal pigmentation
wart			A skin lesion with a rough papillomatous surface (of viral origin) on the epidermis; *verruca*. A plantar wart, *verruca plantaris*, that occurs on a pressure-bearing area, especially the sole of the foot. See Figure 5.45. **Figure 5.45** Plantar wart. (Courtesy of Jason L. Smith, MD)
wound (woond)			Injury to soft tissue caused by trauma; generally classified as open or closed
xanthoderma (zăn˝ thō-dĕr´ mă)	xanth/o -derma	yellow skin	Yellowness of the skin
xanthoma (zăn-thō´ mă)	xanth -oma	yellow tumor	Literally means *yellow tumor*; a soft, rounded plaque or nodule, usually on the eyelids, especially near the inner canthus
xeroderma (zē˝ rō-dĕr´ mă)	xer/o -derma	dry skin	Dry skin
xerosis (zē˝ rō´ sĭs)	xer -osis	dry condition	Abnormal dryness of skin, mucous membranes, or the conjunctiva

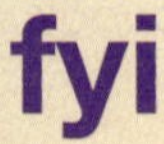

fyi Skin conditions can be acute or chronic, local or systemic. Dryness (*xerosis*) and itching (*pruritus*) are common in older adults. Certain children's skin conditions are associated with age, such as *miliaria* in babies and *acne* in adolescents.

Study and Review II

Word Parts

Prefixes

Give the definitions of the following prefixes.

1. a-, an-	______________	**2.** auto-	______________
3. ec-	______________	**4.** de-	______________
5. ex-	______________	**6.** hyper-	______________
7. hypo-	______________	**8.** intra-	______________
9. par-	______________	**10.** sub-	______________

Combining Forms

Give the definitions of the following combining forms.

1. albin/o	______________	**2.** caus/o	______________
3. cutane/o	______________	**4.** derm/o	______________
5. erythr/o	______________	**6.** hidr/o	______________
7. icter/o	______________	**8.** kel/o	______________
9. kerat/o	______________	**10.** leuk/o	______________
11. melan/o	______________	**12.** onych/o	______________
13. pachy/o	______________	**14.** pedicul/o	______________
15. plak/o	______________	**16.** prurit/o	______________
17. rhytid/o	______________	**18.** scler/o	______________
19. seb/o	______________	**20.** therm/o	______________
21. trich/o	______________	**22.** vuls/o	______________
23. xanth/o	______________	**24.** xer/o	______________

Suffixes

Give the definitions of the following suffixes.

1. -al ______________________ 2. -algia ______________________
3. -on ______________________ 4. -us ______________________
5. -derma ______________________ 6. -ary ______________________
7. -esthesia ______________________ 8. -graft ______________________
9. -ia ______________________ 10. -ic ______________________
11. -ion ______________________ 12. -ism ______________________
13. -ist ______________________ 14. -itis ______________________
15. -logy ______________________ 16. -ectasia ______________________
17. -oid ______________________ 18. -oma ______________________
19. -osis ______________________ 20. -ous ______________________
21. -plasty ______________________ 22. -rrhea ______________________
23. -tome ______________________

Identifying Medical Terms

In the spaces provided, write the medical terms for the following meanings.

1. ______________________ Inflammation of the skin caused by exposure to actinic rays
2. ______________________ Pertaining to the skin
3. ______________________ Inflammation of the skin
4. ______________________ Study of the skin
5. ______________________ Severe itching
6. ______________________ Condition of excessive sweating
7. ______________________ Pertaining to under the skin

8. ______________________ Pertaining to jaundice

9. ______________________ Inflammation of the nail

10. ______________________ Thick skin

11. ______________________ Inability to distinguish between the sensations of heat and cold

12. ______________________ Yellowness of the skin

Matching

Select the appropriate lettered meaning for each of the following words.

________	**1.** acne	**a.**	Small, pinpoint, purplish hemorrhagic spots on the skin
________	**2.** alopecia	**b.**	Production of pus or serum
________	**3.** cicatrix	**c.**	Severe itching
________	**4.** comedo	**d.**	Inflammatory condition of the sebaceous glands and the hair follicles
________	**5.** decubitus	**e.**	Scar left after the healing of a wound
________	**6.** dehiscence	**f.**	Loss of hair, baldness
________	**7.** exudate	**g.**	White spots or patches formed on the mucous membrane of the tongue or cheek
________	**8.** leukoplakia	**h.**	Blackhead
________	**9.** petechiae	**i.**	Separation or bursting open of a surgical wound
________	**10.** pruritus	**j.**	Bedsore
		k.	Slough, scab

Medical Case Snapshots

This learning activity provides an opportunity to relate the medical terminology you are learning to a precise patient case presentation. In the spaces provided, write in your answers.

Case 1

A 36-year-old male is concerned about noticeable loss of scalp hair. He states that his cousins on his mother's side have the same thing. The medical term for this condition is ____________ (loss of hair, especially on the scalp). The androgenetic type of this condition (formerly called *male-pattern baldness*) begins in the frontal area and progresses until only a horseshoe-shaped area of hair remains.

Case 2

When the 45-year-old female was asked about her chief complaint she said, "I would like something done to remove the wrinkles from around my eyes and mouth." Dr. Smith, a dermatologist, explained that he could either do a ___________ (surgical procedure to remove fine wrinkles) or he could perform a _______________ (type of plastic surgery).

Case 3

The 84-year-old bedridden patient is diagnosed with a large decubitus ulcer located on her right buttocks. The literal meaning of the word *decubitus* is ____________________.

Drug Highlights

Type of Drug	Description and Examples
emollients	Substances that are generally oily in nature. These substances are used for dry skin caused by aging, excessive bathing, and psoriasis. EXAMPLE: Desitin
keratolytics	Agents that cause or promote loosening of horny (keratin) layers of the skin. These agents may be used for acne, warts, psoriasis, corns, calluses (hardened skin), and fungal infections. EXAMPLES: Duofilm, Keralyt, and Compound W
local anesthetic agents	Agents that inhibit the conduction of nerve impulses from sensory nerves and thereby reduce pain and discomfort. These agents may be used topically to reduce discomfort associated with insect bites, burns, and poison ivy. EXAMPLES: Solarcaine and Xylocaine
antihistamine agents	Agents that act to prevent the action of histamine. Used to help relieve symptoms, such as itching, in allergic responses and contact dermatitis. EXAMPLE: Benadryl (diphenhydramine)
antipruritic agents	Agents that prevent or relieve itching EXAMPLES: Topical—tripelennamine HCl; Oral—Benadryl (diphenhydramine HCl) and hydroxyzine HCl
antibiotic agents	Agents that destroy or stop the growth of microorganisms (bacteria). These agents are used to prevent infection associated with minor skin abrasions and to treat superficial skin infections and acne. Several antibiotic agents are combined in a single product to take advantage of the different antimicrobial spectrum of each drug. EXAMPLES: Neosporin, Polysporin, and Mycitracin
antifungal agents	Agents that destroy or inhibit the growth of fungi and yeast. These agents are used to treat fungus and/or yeast infection of the skin, nails, and scalp. EXAMPLES: Equate antifungal cream (clotrimazole) and Lamisil (terbinafine)
antiviral agents	Agents that combat specific viral diseases. EXAMPLE: Zovirax (acyclovir) is used in the treatment of herpes simplex virus types 1 and 2, varicella zoster, Epstein–Barr, and cytomegalovirus
anti-inflammatory agents	Agents used to relieve the swelling, tenderness, redness, and pain of inflammation. Topically applied corticosteroids are used in the treatment of dermatitis and psoriasis. EXAMPLES: Carmol HC (hydrocortisone acetate; urea) and Temovate (clobetasol propionate) Oral corticosteroids are used in the treatment of contact dermatitis, such as in poison ivy, when the symptoms are severe. EXAMPLE: prednisone 12-day unipak

Study and Review III

Building Medical Terms

Using the following word parts, fill in the blanks to build the correct medical terms.

de-	xanth	-ic
melan	xanth/o	-rrhea
pachy	xer	
onych	-logy	

Definition	Medical Term
1. An area of skin and tissue that becomes broken down	________ cubitus
2. Study of the skin	dermato________
3. Pertaining to jaundice	icter__________
4. Cancer that develops in the pigment cells of the skin	__________ oma
5. Inflammation of the nail	___________ itis
6. Thick skin	_________derma
7. Excessive flow of oil from the sebaceous glands	sebo __________
8. Yellowness of the skin	_________ derma
9. Literally means yellow tumor	___________ oma
10. Abnormal dryness of skin	____________osis

Combining Form Challenge

Using the combining forms provided, write the medical term correctly.

albin/o	cutane/o	erythr/o
caus/o	dermat/o	integument/o

1. Genetic condition in which there is a partial or total absence of pigment in skin, hair, and eyes: _________ ism
2. Intense burning pain associated with trophic skin changes in the hand or foot after trauma to the part: __________ algia
3. Pertaining to the skin: _______ ous
4. Inflammation of the skin: __________ itis
5. Abnormal redness of the skin occurring over widespread areas of the body: _________derma
6. Covering; the skin, consisting of the dermis and epidermis: _______ ary

Select the Right Term

Select the correct answer and write it on the line provided.

1. Inflammatory condition of the sebaceous glands and hair follicles is ___________.

actinic dermatitis **bite** **boil** **acne**

2. The absence or loss of hair, especially of the head, is ________.

acrochordon **alopecia** **anhidrosis** **avulsion**

3. Scar left after the healing of a wound is _____________.

boil **burn** **corn** **cicatrix**

4. Slough, scab is _____________.

eschar **exudate** **folliculitis** **gangrene**

5. A flat, brownish spot on the skin; freckle is ____________.

keloid **lupus** **lentigo** **mole**

6. Any rose-colored rash marked by maculae or red spots on the skin is ______.

rosacea **roseola** **rubella** **robeola**

Diagnostic and Laboratory Tests

Select the best answer to each multiple-choice question. Circle the letter of your choice.

1. An intradermal test performed using a sterile, disposable, multiple-puncture lancet is called a ____________

a. sweat test.
b. Mantoux test.
c. tine test.
d. Tzanck test.

2. A test done on wound exudate to determine the presence of microorganisms is called a ______________

a. sweat test.
b. biopsy.
c. Tzanck test.
d. wound culture.

3. A microscopic examination of a small piece of tissue that has been surgically scraped from a pustule is called a ____________________

a. Tzanck test.
b. sweat test.
c. biopsy.
d. wound culture.

4. Tests performed to identify the presence of the *Tubercle bacilli* include the ______________________

a. tine, Heaf, and sweat tests.
b. tine, Heaf, and Mantoux tests.
c. tine, Tzanck, and Mantoux tests.
d. tine, Mantoux, and sweat tests.

5. The ____________________ test is used to determine the level of chloride concentration on the skin.

a. sweat
b. Tzanck
c. tine
d. Mantoux

Abbreviations

Place the correct word, phrase, or abbreviation in the space provided.

1. basal cell carcinoma ______________________________
2. Bx ______________________________
3. decub ______________________________
4. ID ______________________________
5. SCC ______________________________
6. PPD ______________________________
7. skin graft ______________________________
8. staph ______________________________
9. strep ______________________________
10. topical immunomodulators ______________________________

Practical Application

Medical Record Analysis

This exercise contains information, abbreviations, and medical terminology from an actual medical record or case study that has been adapted for this text. The names and any personal information have been created by the author. Read and study each form or case study and then answer the questions that follow. You may refer to Appendix III, *Abbreviations and Symbols*.

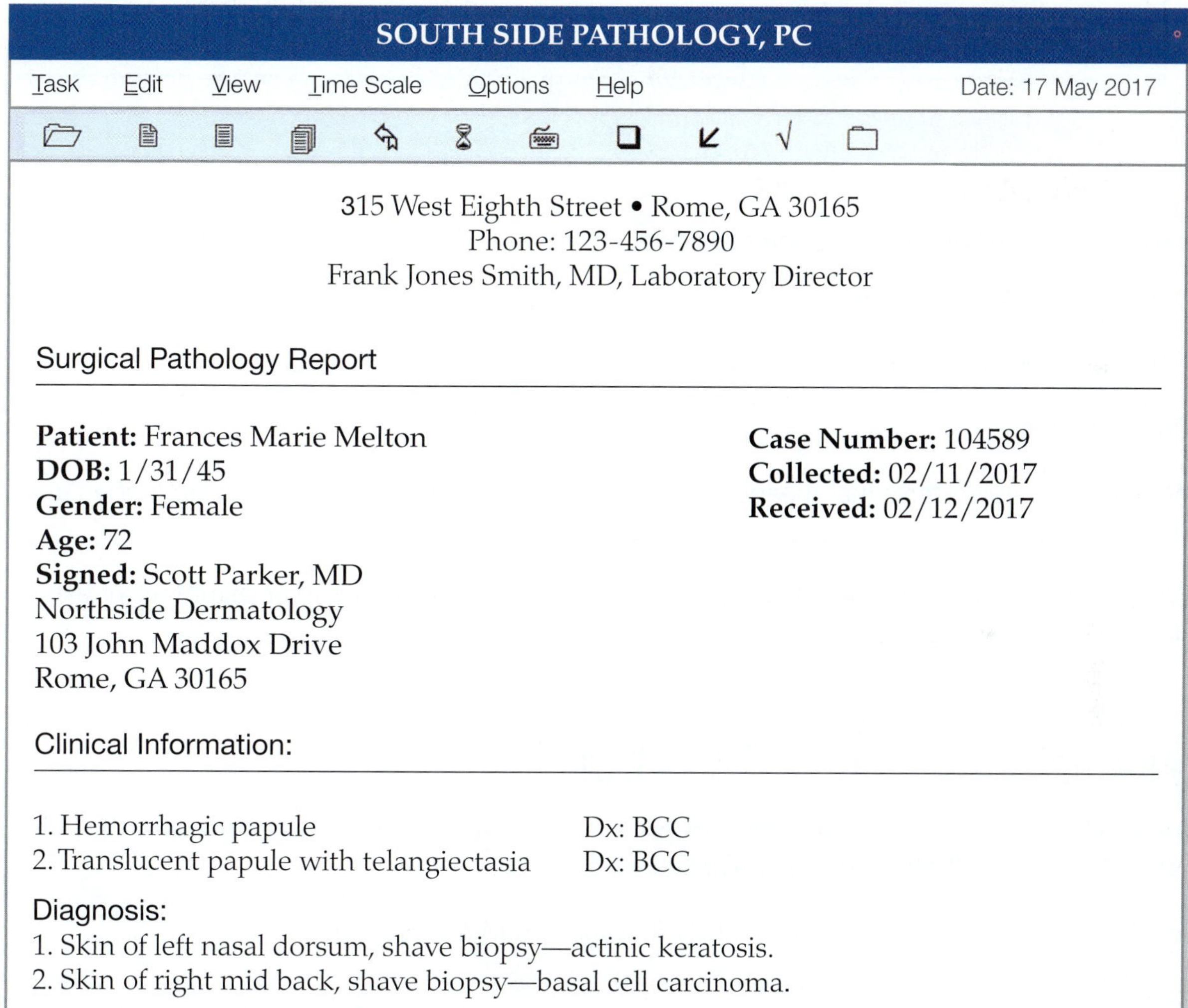

SOUTH SIDE PATHOLOGY, PC

Task Edit View Time Scale Options Help Date: 17 May 2017

315 West Eighth Street • Rome, GA 30165
Phone: 123-456-7890
Frank Jones Smith, MD, Laboratory Director

Surgical Pathology Report

Patient: Frances Marie Melton
DOB: 1/31/45
Gender: Female
Age: 72
Signed: Scott Parker, MD
Northside Dermatology
103 John Maddox Drive
Rome, GA 30165

Case Number: 104589
Collected: 02/11/2017
Received: 02/12/2017

Clinical Information:

1. Hemorrhagic papule Dx: BCC
2. Translucent papule with telangiectasia Dx: BCC

Diagnosis:

1. Skin of left nasal dorsum, shave biopsy—actinic keratosis.
2. Skin of right mid back, shave biopsy—basal cell carcinoma.

Gross Description:

1. Two containers, the first labeled "left nasal dorsum," have within a brown and white 4 × 5 mm superficial skin shave. With margins inked, this is bisected and entirely submitted.
2. The second, labeled "right mid back," has within a 0.5 × 0.7 cm superficial skin shave. With margins inked, this is trisected and entirely submitted.

Microscopic Description:

1. Sections show keratinocyte atypical involving the lower layers of the epidermis as well as solar elastosis (breakdown of elastic tissue due to apparent excessive sun exposure) and parakeratosis (incomplete keratinization due to apparent excessive sun exposure). The actinic keratosis has proliferative features.
2. Sections show a mixed superficial and micronodular form of basal cell carcinoma featuring focal pigmentation. The lesion extends to the base of the shave.

Frank Jones Smith, MD
Pathologist
(Case signed 02/14/2017)

Medical Record Questions

Place the correct answer in the space provided.

1. What is the abbreviation for diagnosis? ______________________
2. What does the abbreviation BCC mean? ______________________
3. Define papule. ______________________
4. What is the medical term that means dilatation of small blood vessels that may appear as a birthmark? ______________________
5. What is the medical term that means breakdown of elastic tissue due to apparent excessive sun exposure? ______________________

Chapter

6

Skeletal System

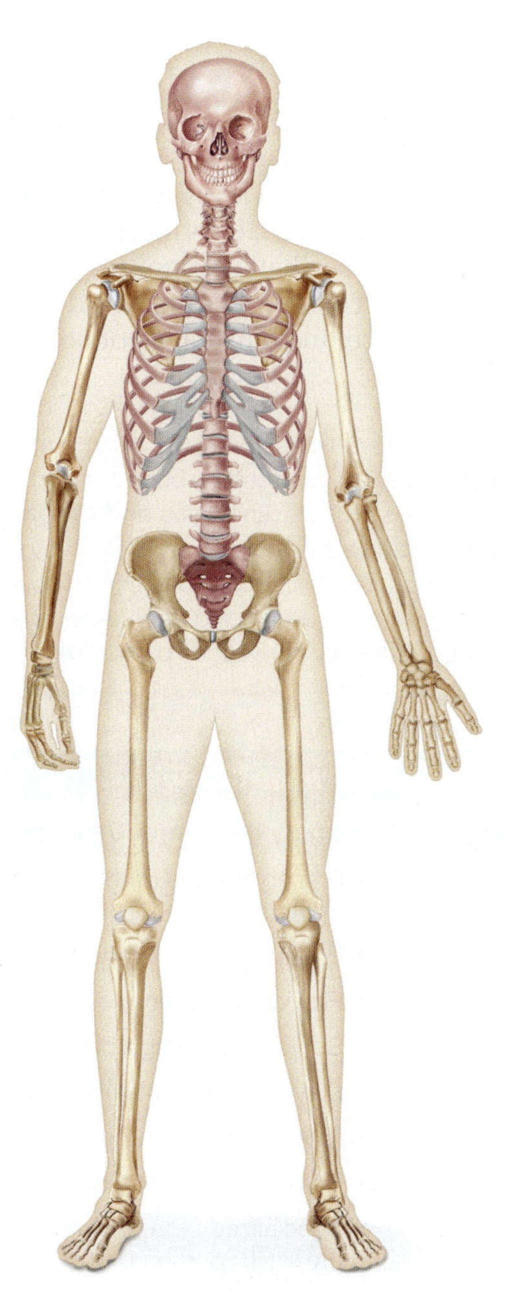

Learning Outcomes

On completion of this chapter, you will be able to:

1. List the primary functions of bones.
2. Explain various types of body movements that occur at the freely movable joints.
3. Contrast the male pelvis to the female pelvis.
4. Define fracture and state the various types.
5. Recognize terminology included in the ICD-10-CM.
6. Analyze, build, spell, and pronounce medical words.
7. Comprehend the drugs highlighted in this chapter.
8. Describe diagnostic and laboratory tests related to the skeletal system.
9. Identify and define selected abbreviations.
10. Apply your acquired knowledge of medical terms by successfully completing the *Practical Application* exercise.

Anatomy and Physiology

The human adult skeletal system is composed of 206 bones that, with **cartilage**, **tendons**, and **ligaments**, make up the **framework** or skeleton of the body. The skeleton can be divided into two main groups of bones: the **axial skeleton**, consisting of 80 bones, and the **appendicular skeleton**, with the remaining 126 bones. The principal bones of the axial skeleton are the skull, spine, ribs, and sternum. The shoulder girdle, arms, and hands and the pelvic girdle, legs, and feet are the primary bones of the appendicular skeleton. Table 6.1 provides an at-a-glance look at the skeletal system. See Figure 6.1 for an anterior view of the skeleton.

Bones

The **bones** are the primary organs of the skeletal system; they are composed of approximately 25% water and 75% solid matter. The solid matter in bone is a calcified, rigid substance known as **osseous tissue**. This tissue is a relatively hard and lightweight composite material, formed mostly of calcium phosphate. While bone is essentially brittle, it does have a significant degree of elasticity, contributed chiefly by collagen. All bones consist of living and dead cells embedded in the mineralized organic **matrix** (the intercellular substance of bone) that makes up the osseous tissue.

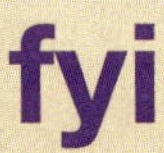

fyi Bone begins to develop during the second month of fetal life as cartilage cells enlarge, break down, disappear, and are replaced by bone-forming cells called **osteoblasts**. Most bones of the body are formed by this process, known as **endochondral ossification**. In this process, the bone cells deposit organic substances in the spaces vacated by cartilage to form bone matrix. As this process proceeds, blood vessels form within the bone and deposit salts such as calcium phosphate and phosphorus that serve to harden the developing bone. After age 35, both men and women will normally lose 0.3–0.5% of their bone density per year as part of the aging process.

Table 6.1 Skeletal System at-a-Glance

Organ/Structure	Primary Functions/Description
Bones	• Primary organs of the skeletal system, which are composed of water and solid matter • Provide shape, support, and the framework of the body • Provide protection for internal organs • Serve as a storage place for mineral salts, calcium, and phosphorus • Play an important role in the formation of blood cells (**hematopoiesis**) • Provide areas for the attachment of skeletal muscles • Help make movement possible through **articulation**
Cartilage	• Specialized type of fibrous connective tissue found at the ends of bones; forms the major portion of the embryonic skeleton and part of the skeleton in adults
Tendons	• Attach muscles to bones; consist of connective tissue
Ligaments	• Bands of fibrous connective tissue that connect bones, cartilages, and other structures; also serve as places for the attachment of fascia

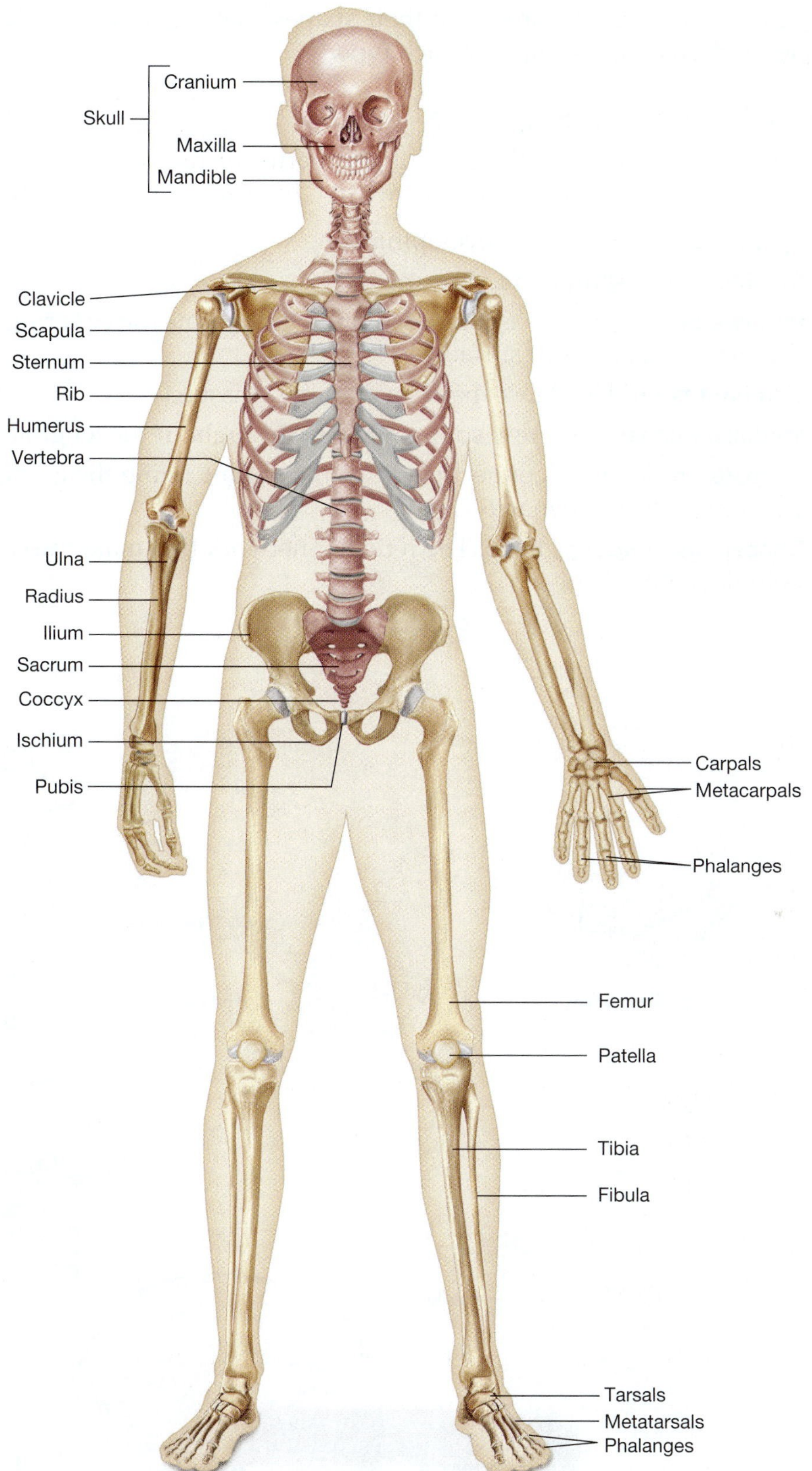

Figure 6.1 Anterior view of the human skeleton.

Classification of Bones

Bones are classified according to their shapes. See Figure 6.2. Table 6.2 classifies the bones and gives an example of each type.

Structure of a Long Bone

Long bones, such as the tibia, femur, humerus, or radius, have most of the features found in all bones. These features are listed here and shown in Figure 6.3.

- **Epiphysis**. The ends of a developing bone.
- **Diaphysis**. The shaft of a long bone.
- **Periosteum**. A fibrous vascular membrane that forms the covering of bones except at their articular (joint) surfaces.
- **Compact bone**. The dense, hard layer of bone tissue.
- **Medullary canal**. A narrow space or cavity throughout the length of the diaphysis.
- **Endosteum**. A tough, connective tissue membrane lining the medullary canal and containing the bone marrow.
- **Cancellous or spongy bone**. The reticular network that makes up most of the volume of bone.

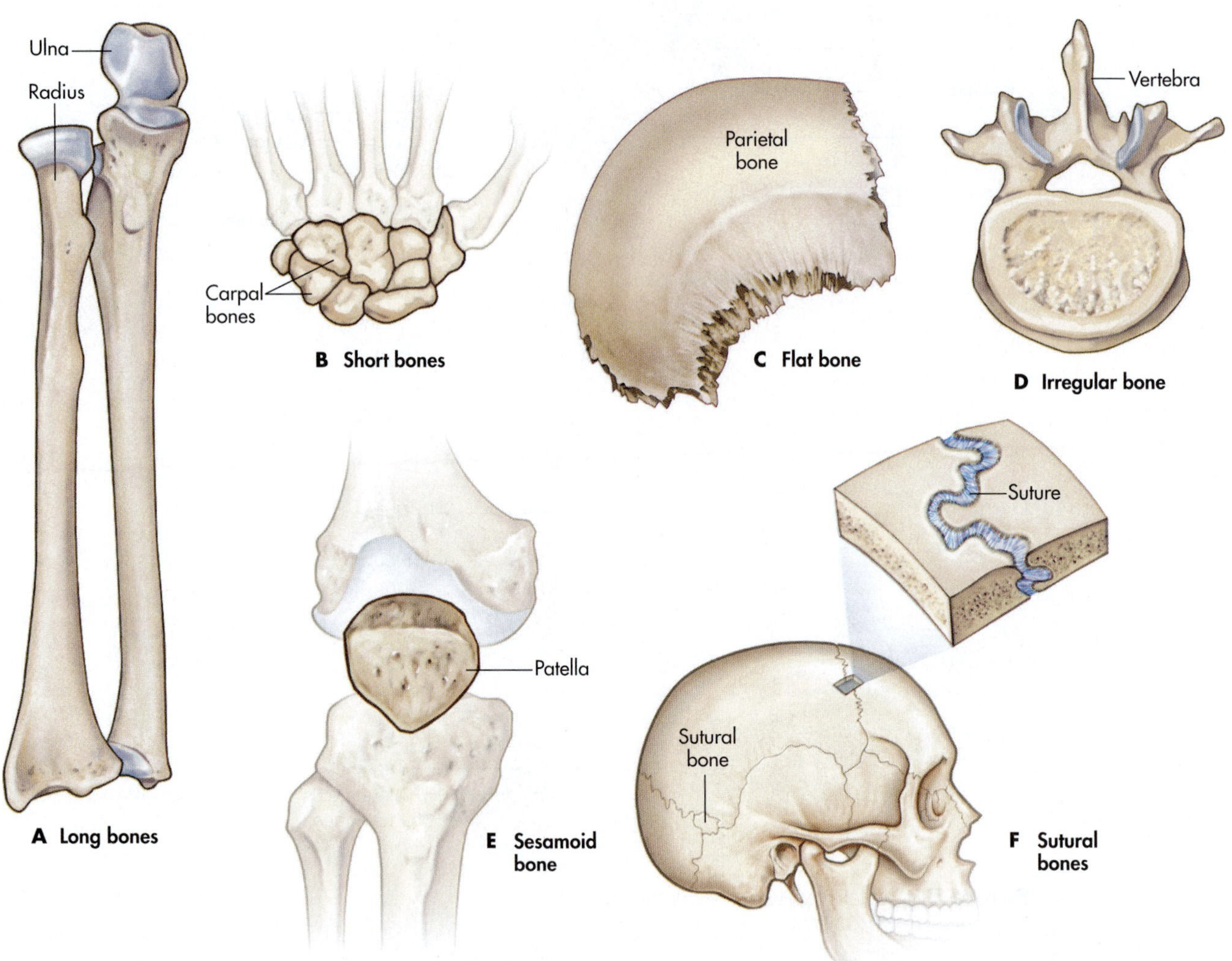

Figure 6.2 Classification of bones by shape.

Table 6.2 Classifications of Bone

Bone	Example
Flat	Ribs, scapula (shoulder blade), parts of the pelvic girdle, bones of the skull
Long	Tibia (shin bone), femur (thigh bone), humerus, radius
Short	Carpals, tarsals
Irregular	Vertebrae, ossicles of the ear
Sesamoid	Patella (kneecap)
Sutural or wormian	Between the flat bones of the skull

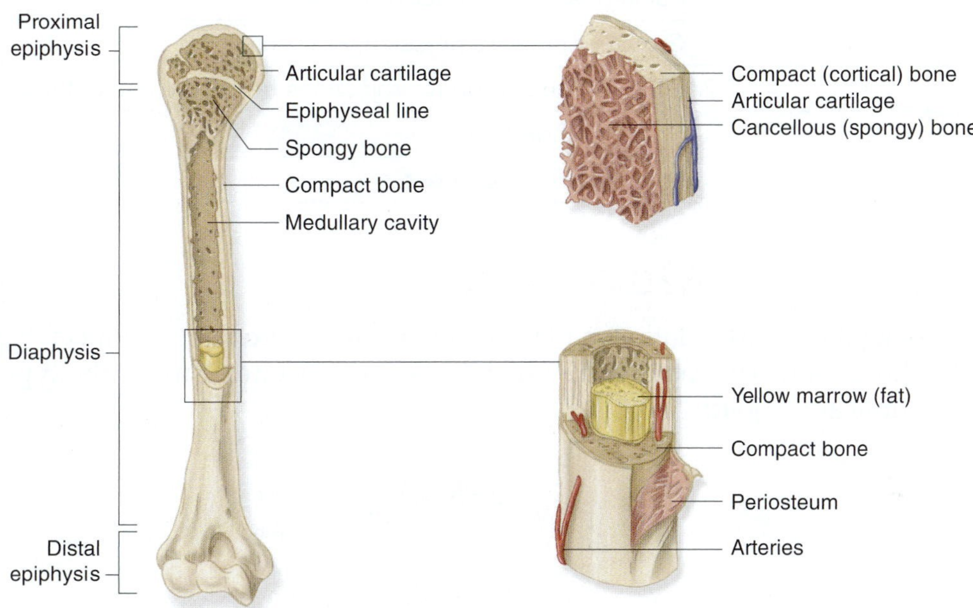

Figure 6.3 Features found in a long bone.

Bone Markings

Certain commonly used terms describe the **markings of bones**. These markings are listed and described in Table 6.3 so you can better understand their roles in joining bones together, providing areas for muscle attachments, and serving as a passageway for blood vessels, ligaments, and nerves.

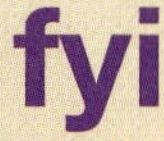

The **epiphyseal plate**, also known as the growth plate or physis, is a thin disc of hyaline cartilage (the type that makes up the embryonic skeleton) positioned between the epiphysis and diaphysis. In children, this is the center of longitudinal bone growth. It is possible to determine the biological age of a child from the development of epiphyseal ossification centers as shown radiographically. About 3 years after the onset of puberty, the ends of the long bones (*epiphyses*) knit securely to their shafts (*diaphysis*). Once growth is completed and an individual reaches full maturity and stature, the epiphyseal plate becomes the epiphyseal line.

Table 6.3 Bone Markings

Marking	Description of the Bone Structure
Condyle	Rounded projection that enters into the formation of a joint, articulation
Crest	Ridge on a bone
Fissure	Slitlike opening between two bones
Foramen	Opening in the bone for blood vessels, ligaments, and nerves
Fossa	Shallow depression in or on a bone
Head	Rounded end of a bone
Meatus	Tubelike passage or canal
Process	Enlargement or protrusion of a bone
Sinus	Air cavity within certain bones
Spine	Pointed, sharp, slender process
Sulcus	Groove, furrow, depression, or fissure
Trochanter	Either of the two bony projections below the neck of the femur
Tubercle	Small, rounded process
Tuberosity	Large, rounded process

Joints and Movement

A **joint (jt)** is an articulation, a place where two or more bones connect. Figure 6.4 shows the knee joint. The manner in which bones connect determines the type of movement possible at the joint.

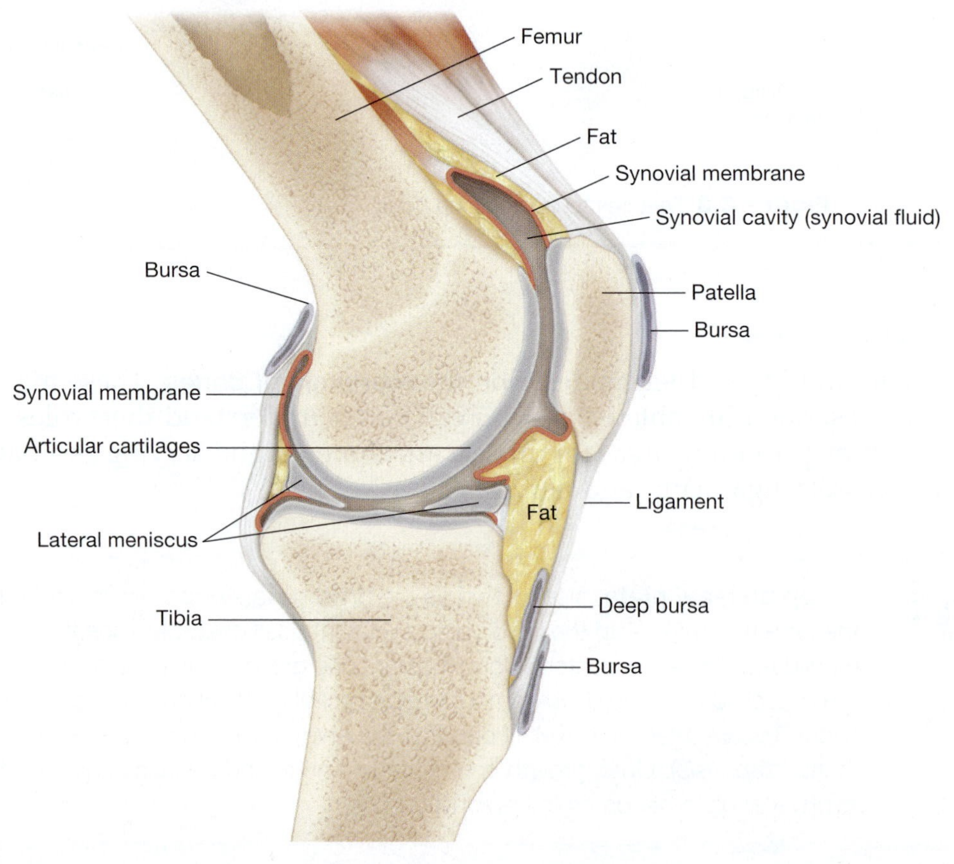

Figure 6.4 Knee joint.

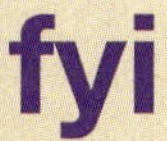

Various age-related joint changes that occur in the older person are due to diminished viscosity of the synovial fluid, degeneration of collagen and elastin cells, outgrowth of cartilaginous clusters in response to continuous wear and tear, and formation of scar tissues and calcification in the joint capsules.

Classification of Joints

Joints are classified as follows:

- **Synarthrosis (Fibrous)**. Does not permit movement. The bones are in close contact with each other, but there is no joint cavity. An example is a *cranial suture*.
- **Amphiarthrosis (Cartilaginous)**. Permits very slight movement. An example of this type of joint is a *vertebra*.
- **Diarthrosis (Synovial)**. Allows free movement in a variety of directions. A synovial membrane lines the joint and produces synovial fluid, which lubricates the joint. Examples of this type of joint are the *knee*, *hip*, *elbow*, *wrist*, and *foot*.

Joint Movements

The following terms describe types of body movement that occur at the **freely movable joints**. See Figure 6.5.

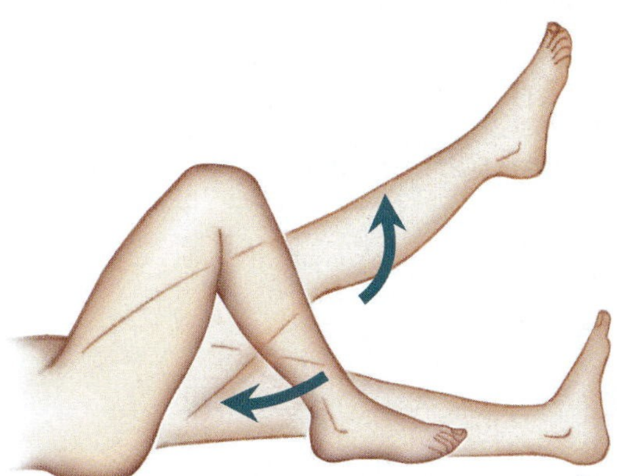

Figure 6.5A Flexion and extension
Flexion–Bending a limb.
Extension–Straightening a flexed limb.

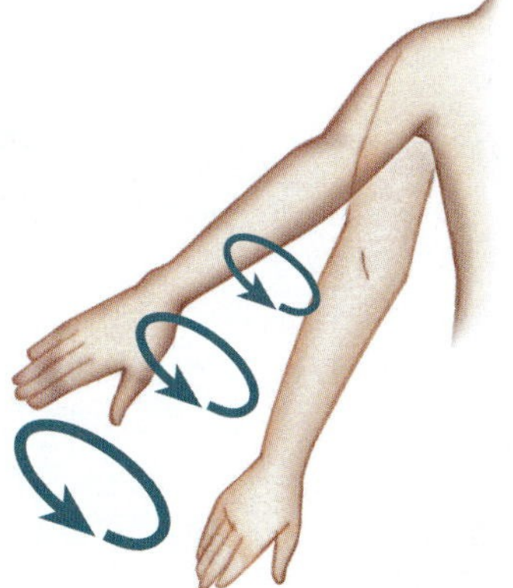

Figure 6.5B Circumduction
Circumduction–Moving a body part in a circular motion.

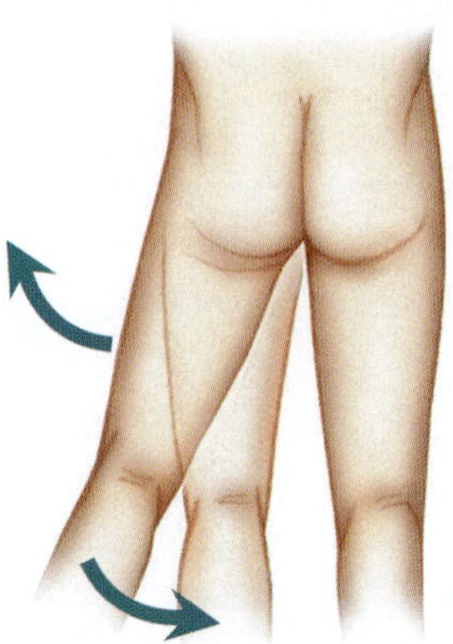

Figure 6.5C Abduction and adduction

Abduction–Moving a body part away from the middle.

Adduction–Moving a body part toward the middle.

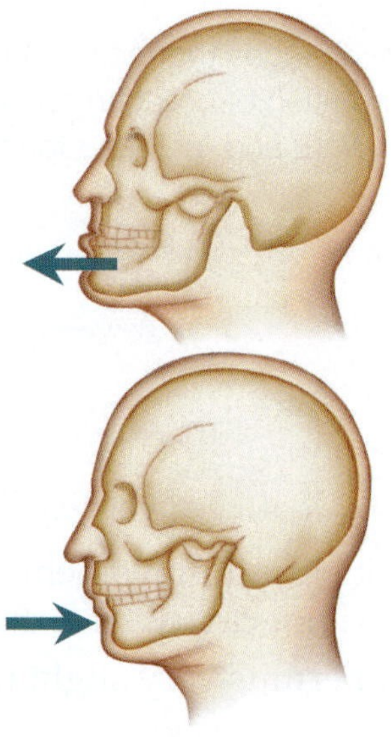

Figure 6.5D Protraction and retraction

Protraction–Moving a body part forward.

Retraction–Moving a body part backward.

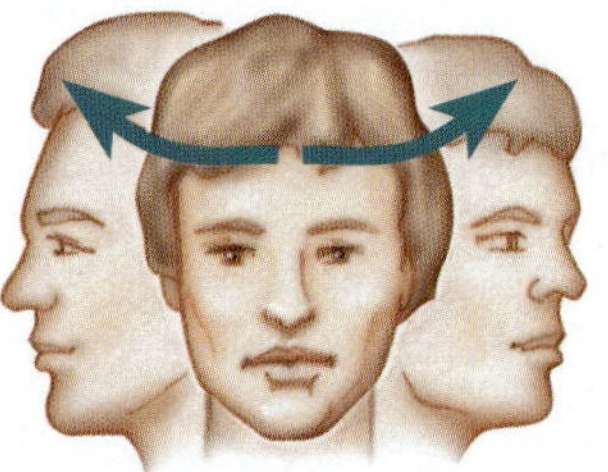

Figure 6.5E Rotation

Rotation–Moving a body part around a central axis.

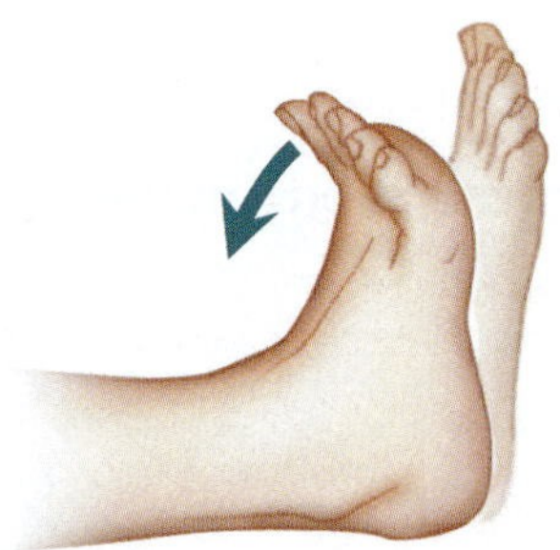

Figure 6.5F Dorsiflexion

Dorsiflexion–Bending a body part backward.

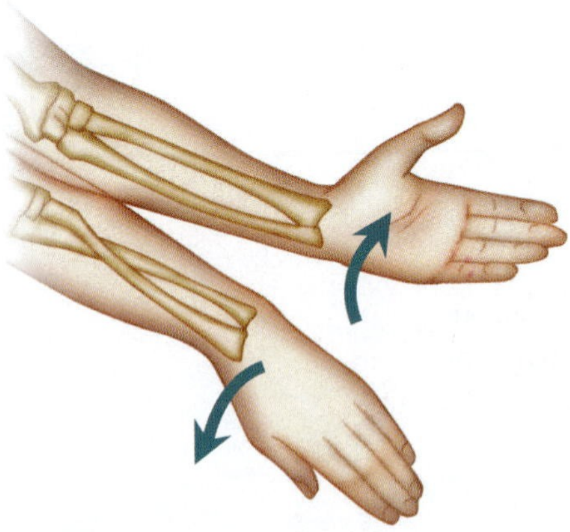

Figure 6.5G Pronation and supination

Pronation–Lying prone (face downward); also turning the palm downward.

Supination–Lying supine (face upward); also turning the palm or foot upward.

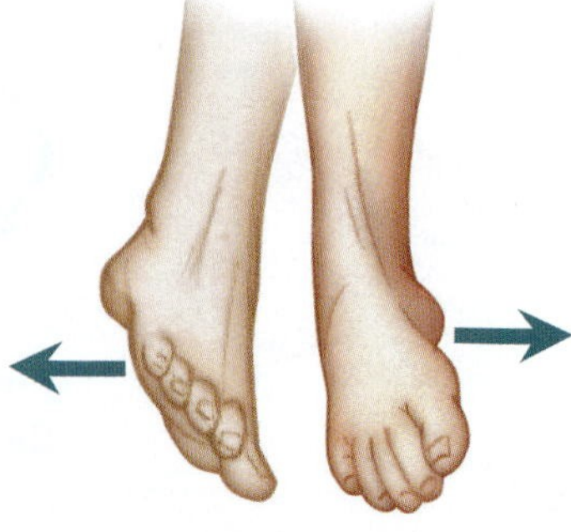

Figure 6.5H Eversion and inversion

Eversion–Turning outward.

Inversion–Turning inward.

Vertebral Column

The **vertebral column** is composed of a series of separate bones (**vertebrae**) connected in such a way as to form four spinal curves. These curves have been identified as the cervical, thoracic, lumbar, and sacral. The *cervical curve* consists of the first seven vertebrae, the *thoracic curve* consists of the next 12 vertebrae, the *lumbar curve* consists of the next five vertebrae, and the *sacral curve* consists of the sacrum and coccyx (tailbone). See Figure 6.6.

It is known that a curved structure has more strength than a straight structure. The spinal curves of the human body are most important because they help support the weight of the body and provide the balance that is necessary to walk on two feet.

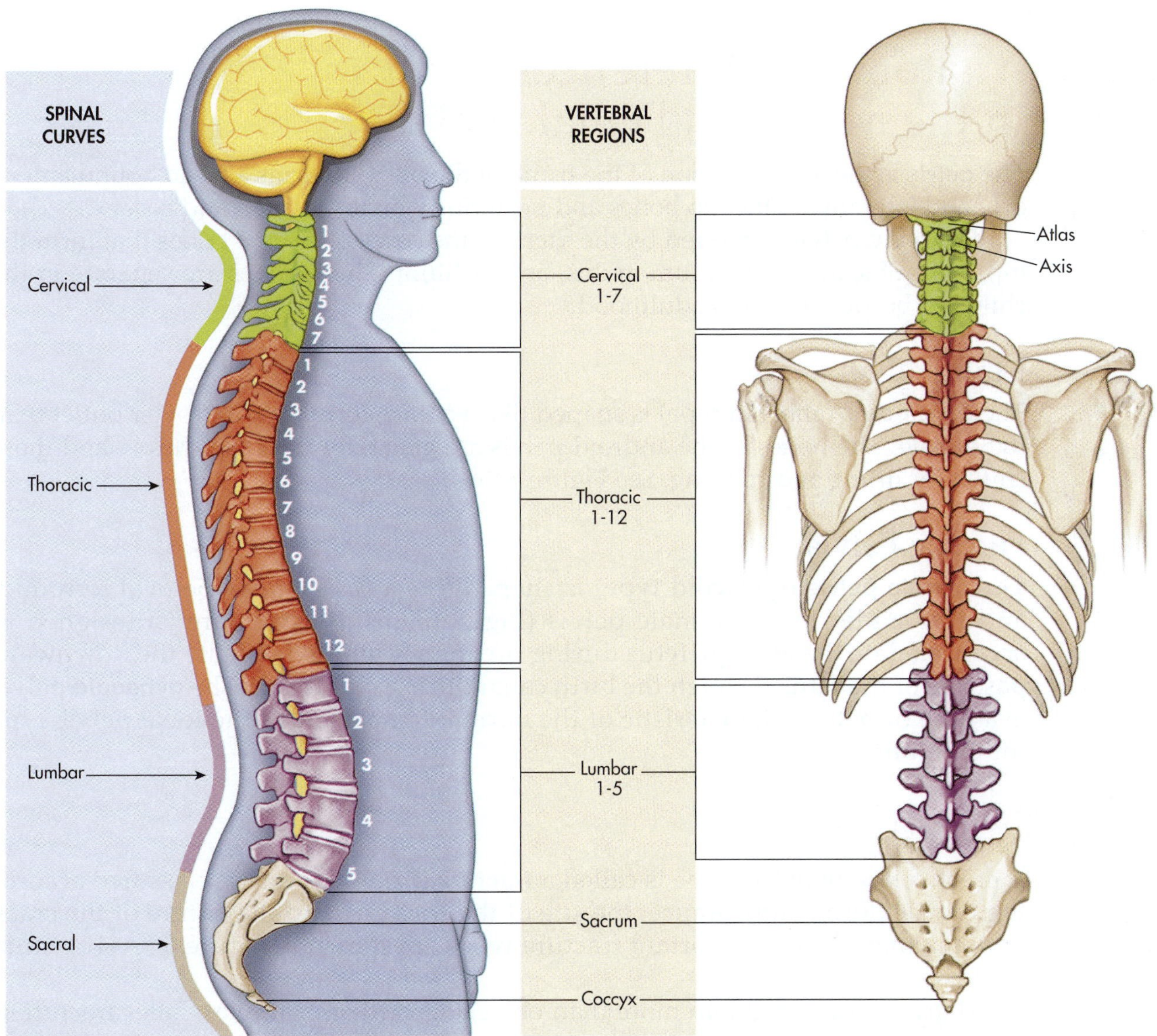

Figure 6.6 Vertebral (spinal) column.

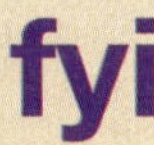

Young children who are beginning to walk often have a pot-bellied stance because of a lumbar lordosis. This posture usually disappears around 5 years of age. After 6 years of age, the spine has normal thoracic convex (arched; curved evenly) and lumbar concave (rounded; hollowed out) curves. See Figure 6.7.

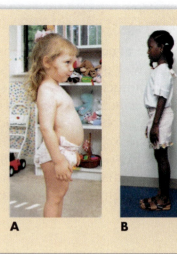

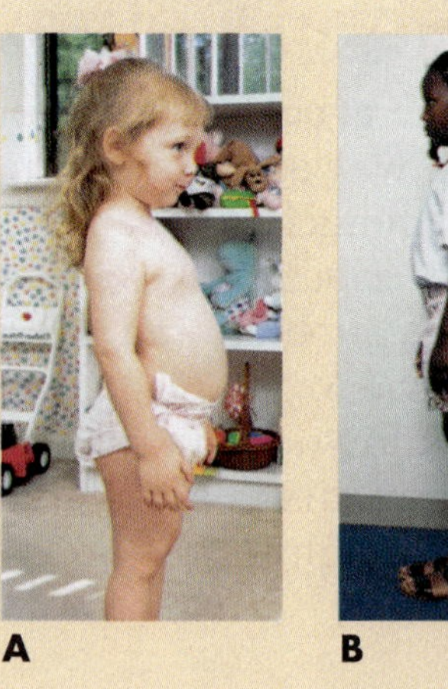

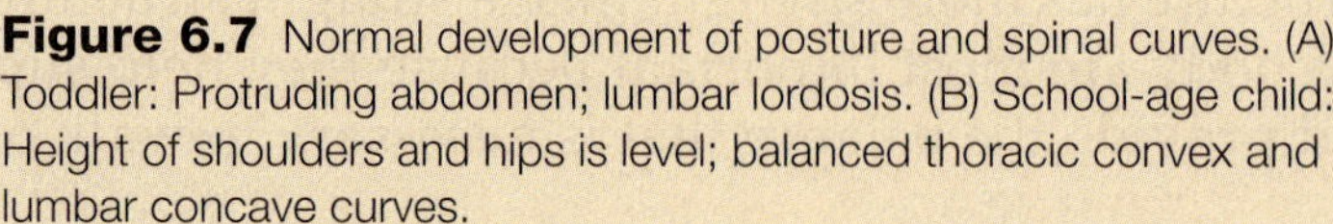

Figure 6.7 Normal development of posture and spinal curves. (A) Toddler: Protruding abdomen; lumbar lordosis. (B) School-age child: Height of shoulders and hips is level; balanced thoracic convex and lumbar concave curves.

Source: Pearson Education, Inc.

Anatomical Differences in the Male and Female Pelvis

The **pelvis** is the lower portion of the trunk of the body. It forms a basin bound anteriorly and laterally by the hip bones and posteriorly by the sacrum and coccyx.

The bony pelvis is formed by the sacrum, the coccyx, and the bones that form the hip and pubic arch—the ilium, pubis, and ischium. These bones are separate in the child but become fused in adulthood.

Male Pelvis

The **male pelvis** (android type) is shaped like a *funnel*, forming a narrower outlet than the female. The bones of the android pelvis are generally thick and heavy and more suited for lifting and running. See Figure 6.8A.

Female Pelvis

The **female pelvis** (gynecoid type) is shaped like a *basin*. It can be oval to round, and it is wider than the male pelvis (Figure 6.8B). Its structure is designed to accommodate the average fetus during pregnancy and to facilitate the downward passage of the fetus through the birth canal during childbirth. The **gynecoid** pelvis is a type of pelvis characteristic of the normal female and is the ideal pelvic type for childbirth.

Fractures

A crack or break in the bone is called a **fracture (Fx)**. A fracture is classified according to its external appearance, the site of the fracture, and the nature of the crack or break in the bone. Important fracture types are shown in Figure 6.9A–L, within Table 6.4.

Many fractures fall into more than one category. For example, Colles fracture is a transverse fracture, but depending on the injury, it can also be a comminuted fracture that can be either open or closed. Table 6.4 provides a summary of the types of fractures.

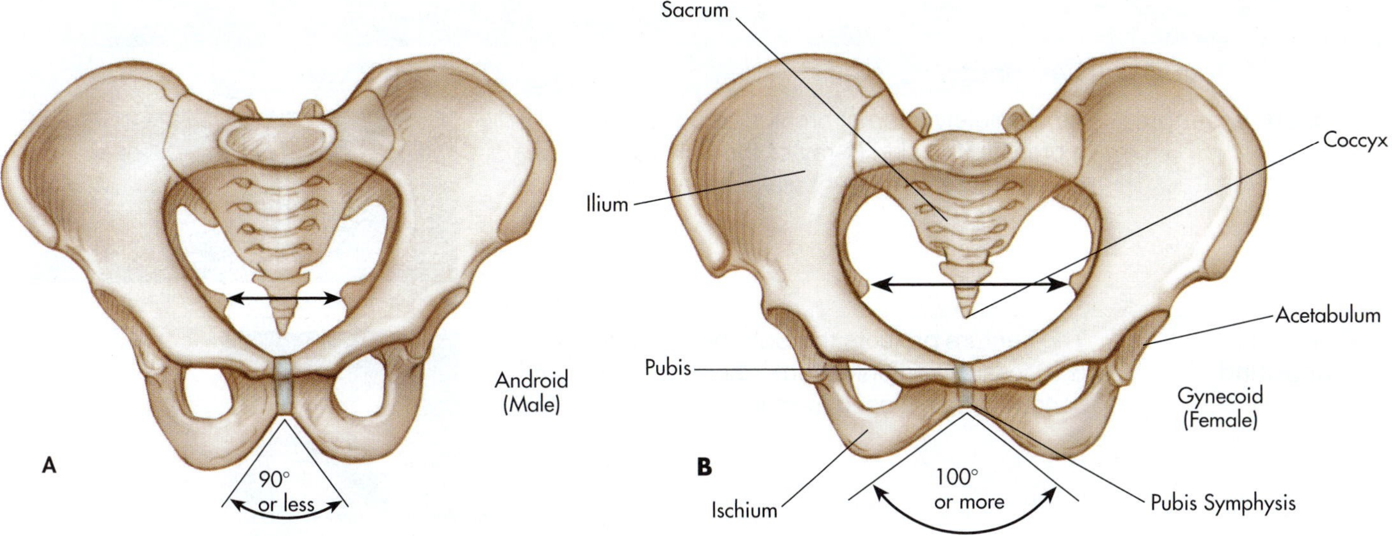

Figure 6.8 (A) The male pelvis (android) is shaped like a funnel, forming a narrower outlet than the female. (B) The female pelvis (gynecoid) is shaped like a basin.

insights The use of the seventh character extension in ICD-10-CM (i.e., A, B, C, etc., added after the code number) is designated to document the episode of care for fractures. When documenting fractures, the codes indicate the fracture type (greenstick, transverse, oblique, spiral, comminuted, open, closed), specific anatomical site, whether the fracture is displaced or not, laterality, routine versus delayed healing, nonunion, and malunion. *Nonunion* means the fragments of a broken bone have failed to heal (knit together). *Malunion* means the fractured bone has healed in an unacceptable or abnormal position. Laterality and type of encounter (initial, subsequent, sequela) are significant components of the code expansion. Documentation of pathological fractures will require the underlying cause of the fracture.

Examples:

- S42.001A Fracture of unspecified part of right clavicle, initial encounter for closed fracture
- S42.011B Anterior displaced fracture of sternal end of right clavicle, initial encounter for open fracture
- S42.014D Posterior displaced fracture of sternal end of right clavicle, subsequent encounter for fracture with routine healing

Note: There are multiple classification systems that exist for fracture. The Gustilo Open Fracture Classification is the most widely used system and is generally accepted as the primary classification for open fractures.

Table 6.4 Types of Fractures

Type of Fracture	Description	Figure 6.9A–L
Closed, or **simple**	A completely internal break that does not involve a break in the skin (x-ray of the tibia and fibula). Note the break in the fibula (smaller bone).	A 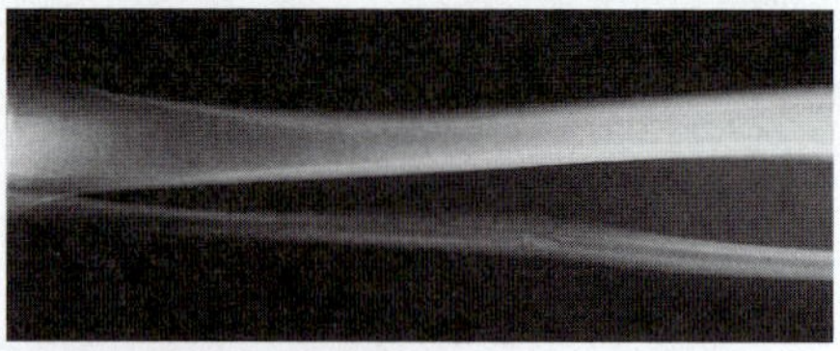 Source: Pearson Education, Inc.
Open, or **compound**	The fracture projects through the skin and there is a possibility of infection or hemorrhage; more serious than a closed fracture	B 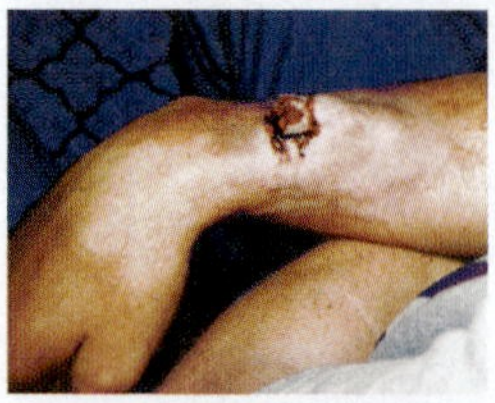 Source: Pearson Education, Inc.
Transverse	Breaks the shaft of a bone across its longitudinal axis; the break is in the fibula, the smaller bone (note that images A and C are the same)	C 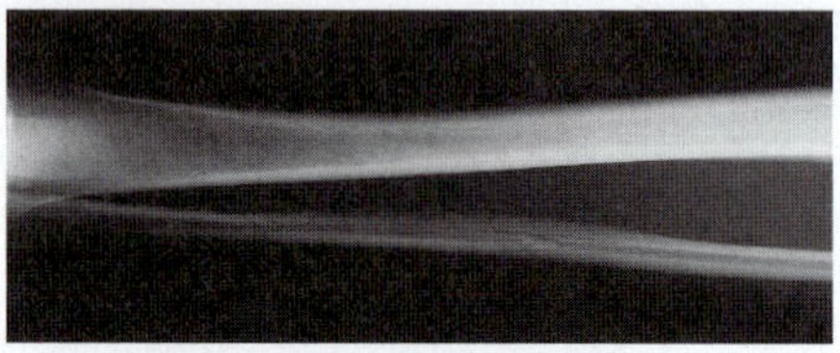 Source: Pearson Education, Inc.
Comminuted	Shatters the affected part into a multitude of bony fragments (x-ray of the femur bone)	D 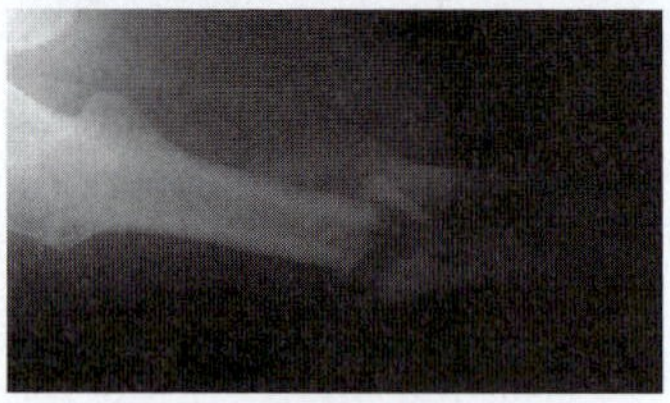 Source: Pearson Education, Inc.
Greenstick	Only one side of the shaft is broken, and the other is bent (like a green stick); usually occurs in children whose long bones have not fully ossified	E 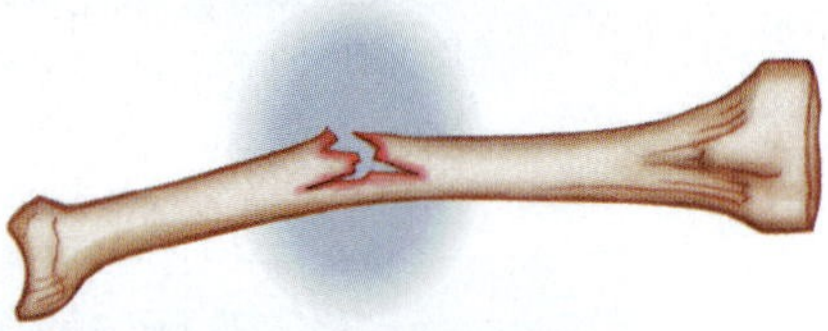
Spiral	Produced by twisting stresses that are spread along the length of a bone (note the break in the humerus)	F 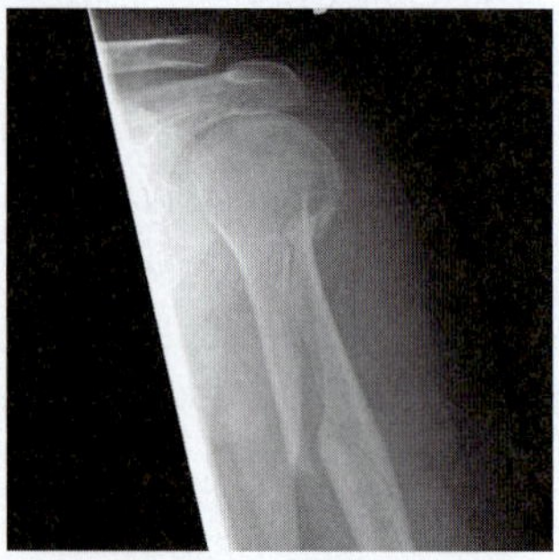 Source: Pearson Education, Inc.
Colles	A break in the distal portion of the radius; often the result of reaching out to cushion a fall	G 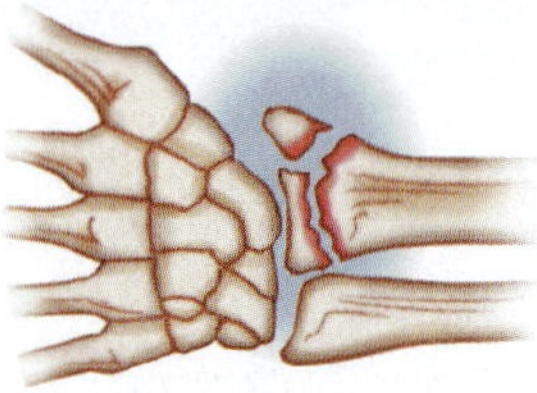

Table 6.4 Types of Fractures (*continued*)

Type of Fracture	Description	Figure 6.9A–L
Pott	Occurs at the ankle and affects both bones of the lower leg (fibula and tibia)	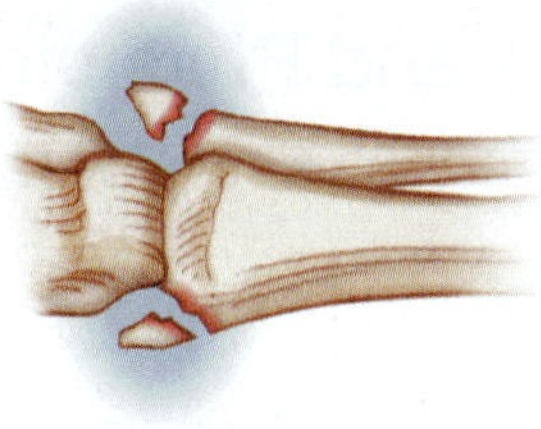 H
Compression	Due to the collapse of a vertebra. It may be caused by trauma or due to a weakening of the vertebra due to osteoporosis, tumors, or infection.	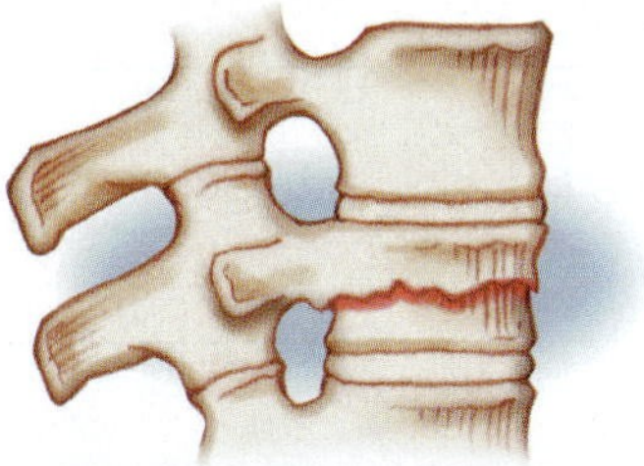 I
Vertebral compression	Fractures of the spine (vertebra) can cause severe "band-like" pain that radiates from the back to the sides of the body; often occur in patients with osteoporosis. Over the years, repeated spinal fractures can lead to chronic lower back pain as well as loss of height or curving of the spine due to collapse of the vertebrae. The collapse gives individuals a hunched-back appearance of the upper back, often called a "dowager's hump" because it is commonly seen in elderly women.	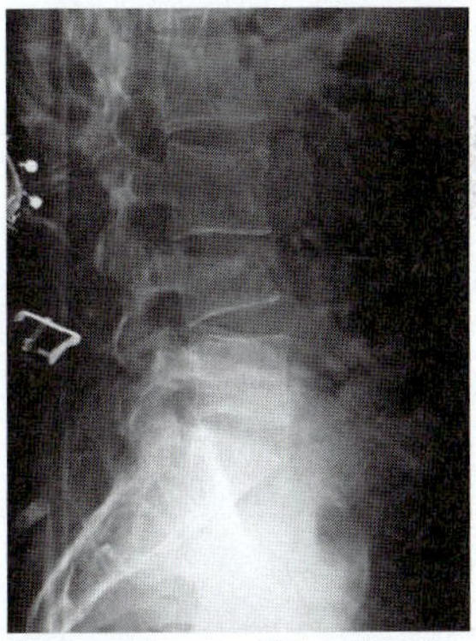 J Source: Pearson Education, Inc.
Epiphyseal	Usually occurs through the growth plate where the matrix is undergoing calcification and chondrocytes (cartilage cells) are dying; this type of fracture is seen in children	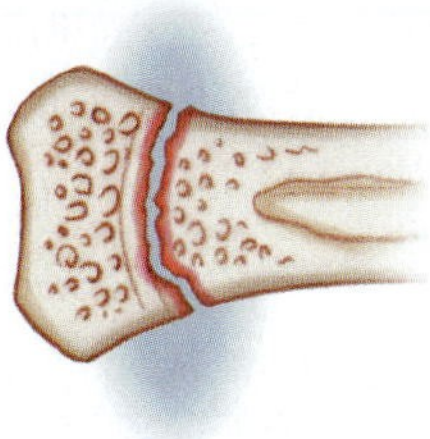 K
Stress	Usually occurs during the course of normal activity; some patients with osteoporosis develop stress fractures of the feet while walking or stepping off a curb	
Hip	Typically occurs as a result of a fall; with osteoporosis, hip fractures can occur as a result of the degenerative process	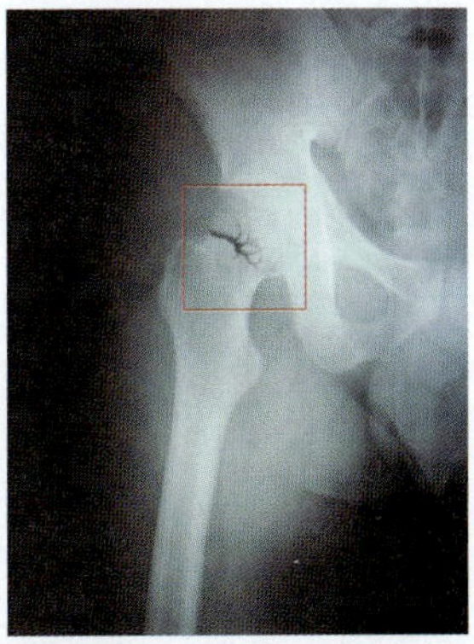 L Source: Muratart/Shutterstock

Study and Review I

Anatomy and Physiology

Write your answers to the following questions.

1. The skeletal system is composed of ____________________ bones.

2. Name the two main divisions of the skeletal system.

   a. ____________________ **b.** ____________________

3. Name five classifications of bone and give an example of each.

   a. ____________________ Example: ____________________

   b. ____________________ Example: ____________________

   c. ____________________ Example: ____________________

   d. ____________________ Example: ____________________

   e. ____________________ Example: ____________________

4. State the six main functions of bones.

   a. ____________________ **b.** ____________________

   c. ____________________ **d.** ____________________

   e. ____________________ **f.** ____________________

5. Define the following features of a long bone.

   a. Epiphysis ____________________

   b. Diaphysis ____________________

   c. Periosteum ____________________

   d. Compact bone ____________________

   e. Medullary canal ____________________

   f. Endosteum ____________________

   g. Cancellous or spongy bone ____________________

6. Match the term in the left column with its definition from the right. Place the correct letter from the right column in the space provided in the left column.

____________	1. meatus	a.	Air cavity within certain bones
____________	2. head	b.	Shallow depression in or on a bone
____________	3. tuberosity	c.	Pointed, sharp, slender process
____________	4. process	d.	Large, rounded process
____________	5. condyle	e.	Groove, furrow, depression, or fissure
____________	6. tubercle	f.	Tubelike passage or canal
____________	7. crest	g.	Opening in the bone for blood vessels, ligaments, and nerves
____________	8. trochanter	h.	Rounded projection that enters into the formation of a joint, articulation
____________	9. sinus	i.	Ridge on a bone
____________	10. fissure	j.	Small, rounded process
____________	11. fossa	k.	Rounded end of a bone
____________	12. spine	l.	Slitlike opening between two bones
____________	13. foramen	m.	Enlargement or protrusion of a bone
____________	14. sulcus	n.	Either of the two bony projections below the neck of the femur

7. Name the three classifications of joints.

a. ______________________________ b. ______________________________

c. ______________________________

8. ______________________________ is moving a body part away from the middle.

9. Adduction is ____.

10. ________________________ is moving a body part in a circular motion.

11. Dorsiflexion is ____.

12. ________________________ is turning outward.

13. Extension is ____.

14. ________________________ is bending a limb.

15. Inversion is ____.

16. ________________________ is lying face downward.

17. Protraction is ____.

18. ________________________ is moving a body part backward.

19. Rotation is ____.

20. ________________________ is lying face upward.

ANATOMY LABELING

Identify the structures shown below by filling in the blanks.

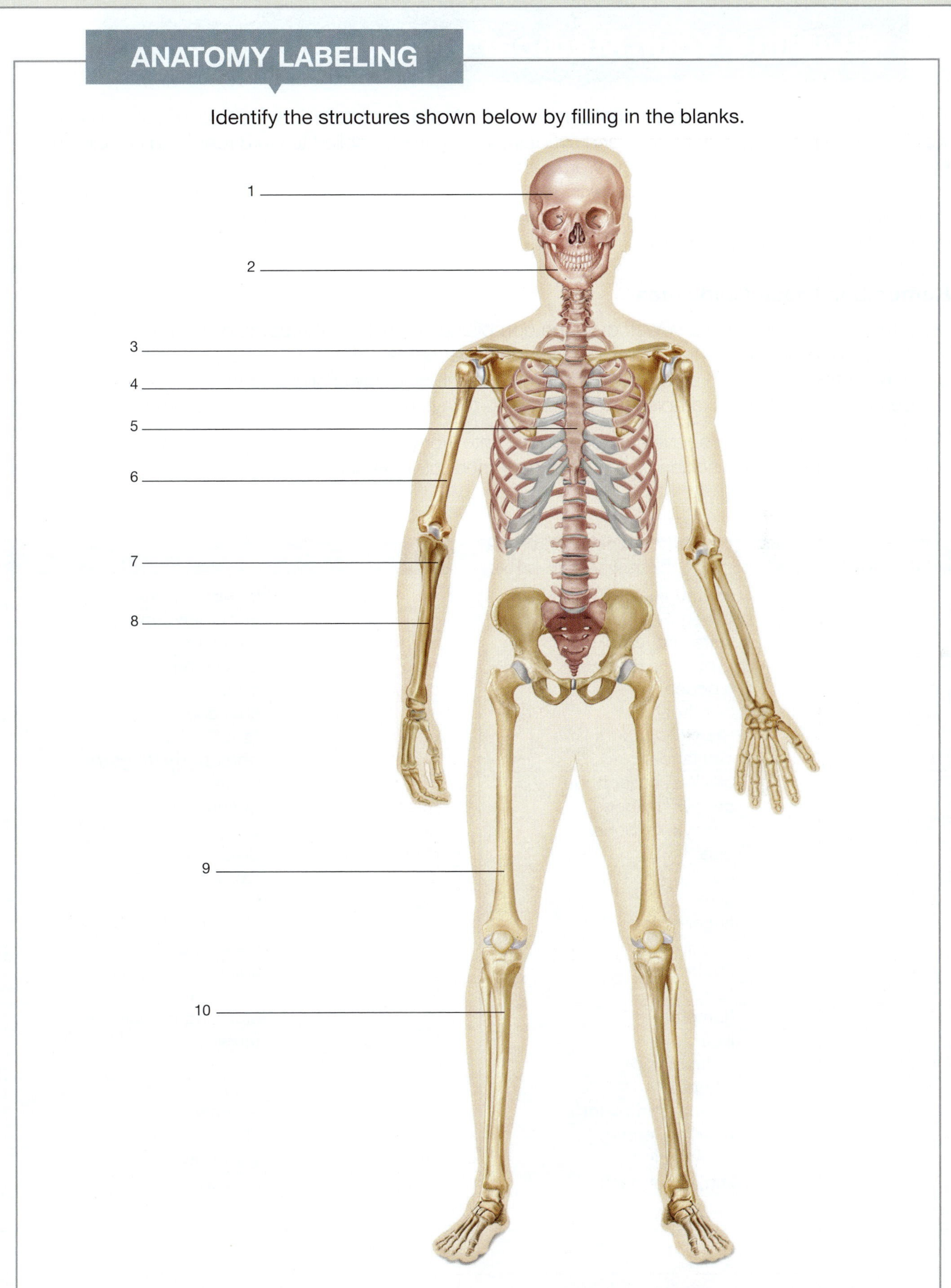

Building Your Medical Vocabulary

This section provides the foundation for learning medical terminology. Review the following alphabetized word list. Note how common prefixes and suffixes are repeatedly applied to word roots and combining forms to create different meanings. The word parts are color-coded: prefixes are yellow, suffixes are blue, roots/combining forms are red. A combining form is a word root plus a vowel. The chart below lists the combining forms for the word roots in this chapter and can help to strengthen your understanding of how medical words are built and spelled.

Remember These Guidelines

1. If the suffix begins with a vowel, drop the combining vowel from the combining form and add the suffix. For example, arthr/o (joint) + -algia (pain) becomes arthralgia.
2. If the suffix begins with a consonant, keep the combining vowel and add the suffix to the combining form. For example, crani/o (skull) + -tomy (incision) becomes craniotomy.

You will find that some terms have not been divided into word parts. These are common words or specialized terms that are included to enhance your medical vocabulary.

Combining Forms of the Skeletal System

acetabul/o	acetabulum	**mandibul/o**	lower jawbone
acr/o	extremity	**maxill/o**	upper jawbone
ankyl/o	stiffening, crooked	**menisc/i**	crescent
arthr/o	joint	**myel/o**	bone marrow
burs/o	a pouch	**oste/o**	bone
calcan/e	heel bone	**patell/o**	kneecap
carp/o	wrist	**ped/o**	foot
chondr/o	cartilage	**phalang/e** **phalang/o**	phalanges (finger/toe bones)
clavicul/o	clavicle, collar bone		
coccyg/e	coccyx, tailbone	**rad/i**	radius
coccyg/o	coccyx, tailbone	**radi/o**	x-ray
coll/a	glue	**rheumat/o**	discharge
cost/o	rib	**sacr/o**	sacrum
crani/o	skull	**sarc/o**	flesh
dactyl/o	finger or toe	**scapul/o**	shoulder blade
femor/o	femur	**scoli/o**	curvature
fibul/o	fibula	**spin/o**	spine
fixat/o	fastened	**spondyl/o**	vertebra
humer/o	humerus	**stern/o**	sternum, breastbone
ili/o	ilium	**tendin/o** **tendon/o**	tendon
isch/i	ischium, hip		
kyph/o	a hump	**tibi/o**	tibia
lamin/o	lamina (thin plate)	**tract/o**	to draw
lord/o	bending, curve, swayback	**uln/o**	ulna
		vertebr/o	vertebra
lumb/o	loin, lower back	**xiph/o**	sword

Medical Word	Word Parts		Definition
	Part	**Meaning**	
acetabulum (ăs″ ĕ-tăb′ ū-lŭm)	acetabul -um	acetabulum, hip socket structure, tissue	Cup-shaped socket of the innominate bone (hip bone) into which the head of the femur (thigh bone) fits
achondroplasia (ă -kŏn″ drō-plā′ sĭ-ă)	a- chondr/o -plasia	without cartilage formation	Defect in the formation of cartilage at the epiphyses of long bones
acroarthritis (ăk″ rō-ăr-thrī′ tĭs)	acr/o arthr -itis	extremity joint inflammation	Inflammation of the joints of the hands or feet (the extremities)
acromion (ă -krō′ mĭ-ŏn)	acr omion	extremity, point shoulder	Projection of the spine of the scapula that forms the point of the shoulder and articulates with the clavicle
ankylosis (ăng″ kĭ-lō′ sĭs)	ankyl -osis	stiffening, crooked condition	Abnormal condition of stiffening of a joint
arthralgia (ăr-thrăl′ jĭ-ă)	arthr -algia	joint pain	Joint pain
arthritis (ăr-thrī′ tĭs)	arthr -itis	joint inflammation	Inflammation of a joint that can result from various disease processes, such as injury to a joint (including fracture), an attack on the joints by the body itself (caused by an autoimmune disease, such as rheumatoid arthritis), or general wear and tear on joints (osteoarthritis)

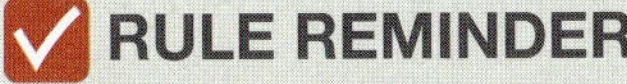

RULE REMINDER

The *o* has been removed from the combining form because the suffix begins with a vowel.

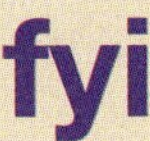

No matter the type of arthritis one has, the main symptoms are pain, swelling, and stiffness in the affected joint. Over time, the joint can become so stiff that movement is difficult or even impossible.

Total joint replacement is a surgical procedure in which parts of an arthritic or damaged joint are removed and replaced with a metal, plastic, or ceramic device called a *prosthesis*. The prosthesis is designed to replicate the movement of a normal, healthy joint.

In one year's time, almost 1 million total joint replacements are performed in the United States. Hip and knee replacements are the most commonly performed joint replacements, but replacement surgery can be performed on other joints, including the ankle, wrist, fingers, shoulder, and elbow.

Medical Word	Part	Meaning	Definition
arthrocentesis (ăr″ thrō-sĕn-tē′ sĭs)	arthr/o -centesis	joint surgical puncture	Surgical procedure to remove joint fluid; may be used as a diagnostic tool or as part of a treatment regimen
arthrodesis (ăr″ thrō-dē′ sĭs)	arthr/o -desis	joint binding	Surgical fusion of a joint

Medical Word	Word Parts		Definition
	Part	**Meaning**	
arthroplasty (ăr″ thrō-plăs′ tē)	arthr/o -plasty	joint surgical repair	Surgical procedure used to repair a joint
arthroscope (ăr′ thrō-scōp)	arthr/o -scope	joint instrument for examining	Surgical instrument used to examine the interior of a joint
bone marrow transplant			Surgical procedure used to transfer bone marrow from a donor to a patient
bursa (bŭr′ sah)			Padlike sac between muscles, tendons, and bones that is lined with synovial membrane and contains a fluid, *synovia*

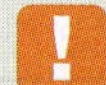

ALERT!

To change burs***a*** to its plural form, you change the ***a*** to ***ae*** to create *bursae*.

Medical Word	Part	Meaning	Definition
bursitis (bŭr-sī′ tĭs)	burs -itis	a pouch inflammation	Inflammation of a bursa
calcaneal (kăl-kā′ nē-ăl)	calcan/e -al	heel bone pertaining to	Pertaining to the heel bone
calcium (Ca) (kăl′ sē-ŭm)			Mineral that is essential for bone growth, teeth development, blood coagulation, and many other functions
carpal (kăr′ pəl)	carp -al	wrist pertaining to	Pertaining to the wrist bones; there are two rows of four bones in the wrist for a total of eight wrist bones.
carpal tunnel syndrome			Abnormal condition caused by compression of the median nerve by the carpal ligament due to injury or trauma to the area, including repetitive movement of the wrists; symptoms: soreness, tenderness, weakness, pain, tingling, and numbness at the wrist. See Figure 6.10.

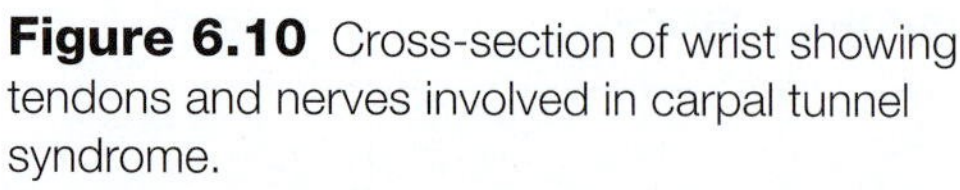

Figure 6.10 Cross-section of wrist showing tendons and nerves involved in carpal tunnel syndrome.

Medical Word	Word Parts		Definition
	Part	**Meaning**	
cast			Type of material made of plaster of Paris, fiberglass, sodium silicate, starch, or dextrin used to immobilize a fractured bone, a dislocation, a deformity, or a sprain. See Figure 6.11.
chondral (kŏn´ drăl)	chondr -al	cartilage pertaining to	Pertaining to cartilage
chondrocostal (kŏn″ drō-kŏs´ tăl)	chondr/o cost -al	cartilage rib pertaining to	Pertaining to the rib cartilage
clavicular (klă-vĭk´ ū-lăr)	clavicul -ar	clavicle, collar bone pertaining to	Pertaining to the clavicle (*collar bone*)
coccygeal (kŏk-sĭj´ ē-ăl)	coccyg/e -al	coccyx, tailbone pertaining to	Pertaining to the coccyx (*tailbone*)
coccygodynia (kŏk-sĭ-gō-dĭn´ ē-ă)	coccyg/o -dynia	coccyx, tailbone pain	Pain in the coccyx (*tailbone*)
collagen (kŏl´ ă-jĕn)	coll/a -gen	glue formation, produce	Fibrous insoluble protein found in the connective tissue, skin, ligaments, and cartilage
connective	connect -ive	to bind together nature of	Literally means *the nature of connecting or binding together*
costosternal (kŏs″ tō-stĕr´ năl)	cost/o stern -al	rib sternum pertaining to	Pertaining to rib and sternum
craniectomy (krā″ nē-ĕk´ tō-mē)	crani -ectomy	skull surgical excision	Surgical excision of a portion of the skull

Figure 6.11 This girl has a long leg cast, which was applied after surgery to correct her clubfoot.
Source: Pearson Education, Inc.

Medical Word	Word Parts		Definition
	Part	**Meaning**	
craniotomy (krā″ nē-ŏt′ ō-mē)	crani/o -tomy	skull incision	Surgical incision made into the skull

ALERT!

The word parts ***crani*** and ***crani/o*** build different terms by using the suffixes ***-ectomy*** (*surgical excision*) and ***-tomy*** (*incision*).

Medical Word	Part	Meaning	Definition
dactylic (dăk′ tĭl′ ĭk)	dactyl -ic	finger or toe pertaining to	Pertaining to the finger or toe
dactylogram (dăk-tĭl′ə grăm)	dactyl/o -gram	finger or toe mark, record	Medical term for fingerprint
dislocation (dĭs″ lō-kā′ shŭn)	dis- locat -ion	apart to place process	Displacement of a bone from a joint
femoral (fĕm′ ŏr-ăl)	femor -al	femur pertaining to	Pertaining to the femur; the *thigh bone*, the longest bone in the body
fibular (fĭb′ ū-lăr)	fibul -ar	fibula pertaining to	Pertaining to the fibula; the smaller of the two lower leg bones
fixation (fĭks-ā′ shŭn)	fixat -ion	fastened process	Process of holding or fastening in a fixed position; making rigid, immobilizing
flatfoot			Abnormal flatness of the sole and arch of the foot; also known as *pes planus*
genu valgum (jē′ nū văl gŭm)			Medical term for knock-knee. See Figure 6.12A.
genu varum (jē′ nū vā′ rŭm)			Medical term for bowleg. See Figure 6.12B.

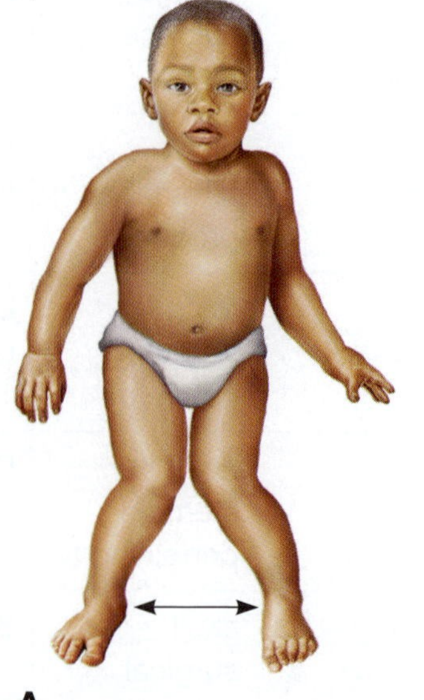

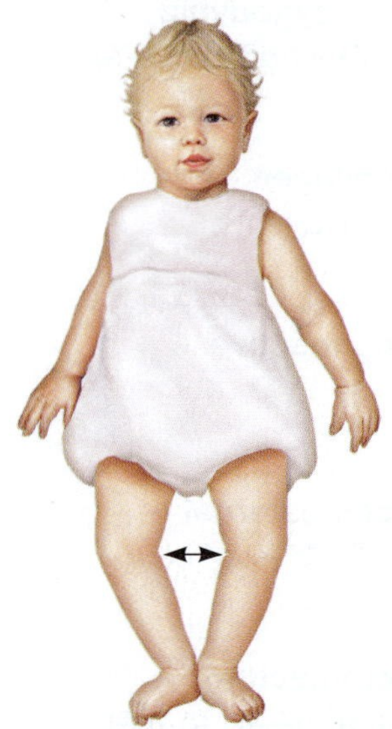

Figure 6.12 (A) Genu valgum, or knock-knee. Note that the ankles are far apart when the knees are together. (B) Genu varum, or bowleg. The legs are bowed so that the knees are far apart as the child stands.

Medical Word	Word Parts: Part	Word Parts: Meaning	Definition
gout (gowt)			Hereditary metabolic disease that is a form of acute arthritis, which is marked by joint inflammation. It is caused by hyperuricemia, excessive amounts of uric acid in the blood, and deposits of urates of sodium (uric acid crystals) in and around the joints. It usually affects the great toe first, but can be seen in the finger, knee, or foot joints.
hallux (hăl˝ ŭks)			Medical term for the big or great toe
hammertoe (hăm´ er-tō)			An acquired flexion deformity of the interphalangeal joint. See Figure 6.13.
humeral (hū´ mĕr-ăl)	humer -al	humerus pertaining to	Pertaining to the humerus (*upper arm bone*)
hydrarthrosis (hī˝ drăr-thrō´ sĭs)	hydr- arthr -osis	water joint condition	An abnormal condition in which there is an accumulation of watery fluid in the cavity of a joint
iliac (ĭl´ ē-ăk)	ili -ac	ilium pertaining to	Pertaining to the ilium
iliosacral (ĭl˝ ĭ-ō-sā´ krăl)	ili/o sacr -al	ilium sacrum pertaining to	Pertaining to the ilium and the sacrum
intercostal (ĭn˝ tĕr-kŏs´ tăl)	inter- cost -al	between rib pertaining to	Pertaining to the space between two ribs

Figure 6.13 Hammertoe.

Medical Word	Word Parts		Definition
	Part	**Meaning**	
ischial (ĭs´ kĭ-al)	isch/i -al	ischium, hip pertaining to	Pertaining to the ischium, hip
ischialgia (ĭs˝ kĭ-ăl´ jē-ă)	isch/i -algia	ischium, hip pain	Pain in the ischium, hip
kyphosis (kī-fō´ sĭs)	kyph -osis	a hump condition	Condition in which the normal thoracic curvature becomes exaggerated, producing a "humpback" appearance. It can be caused by a congenital defect, a disease process such as tuberculosis and/or syphilis, malignancy, compression fracture, faulty posture, osteoarthritis, rheumatoid arthritis, rickets, osteoporosis, or other conditions. See Figure 6.14A.

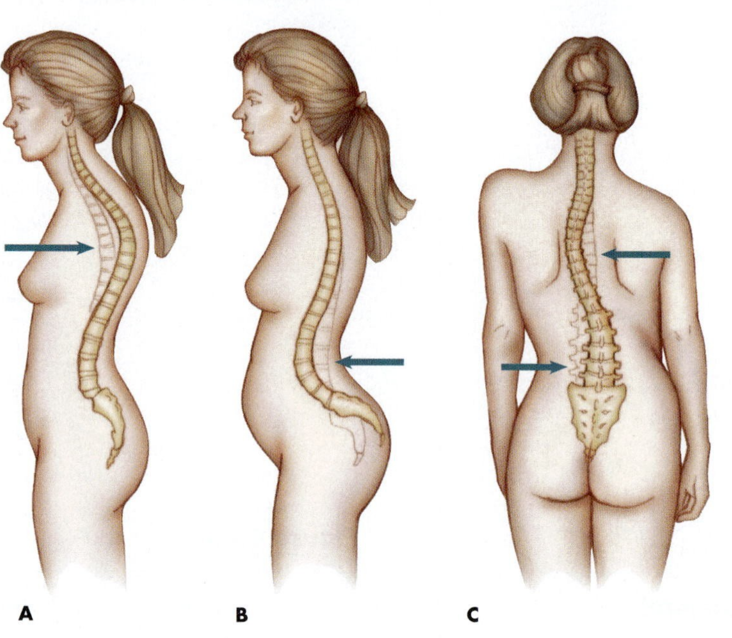

Figure 6.14 Abnormal curvatures of the spine: (A) kyphosis, (B) lordosis, and (C) scoliosis.

Medical Word	Part	Meaning	Definition
laminectomy (lăm˝ ĭ-nĕk´ tō-mē)	lamin -ectomy	lamina (thin plate) surgical excision	Surgical excision of a vertebral posterior arch
lordosis (lor-dō´ sĭs)	lord -osis	bending, curve, swayback condition	An abnormal anterior curvature of the lumbar spine. This condition can be referred to as *swayback* because the abdomen and buttocks protrude due to an exaggerated lumbar curvature. See Figure 6.14B.
lumbar (lŭm´ băr)	lumb -ar	loin, lower back pertaining to	Pertaining to the loins (lower back)

Medical Word	Word Parts		Definition
	Part	**Meaning**	
lumbodynia (lŭm″ bō-dĭn′ ē-ă)	lumb/o -dynia	loin, lower back pain	Pain in the loins (lower back)

RULE REMINDER

This term keeps the combining vowel ***o*** because the suffix begins with a consonant.

Medical Word	Part	Meaning	Definition
mandibular (măn-dĭb′ ū-lăr)	mandibul -ar	lower jawbone pertaining to	Pertaining to the lower jawbone
maxillary (măk′ sĭ-lĕr″ē)	maxill -ary	upper jawbone pertaining to	Pertaining to the upper jawbone
meniscus (mĕn-ĭs′ kŭs)	menisc -us	crescent structure	Crescent-shaped interarticular fibrocartilaginous structure found in certain joints, especially the lateral and medial *menisci* (semilunar cartilages) of the knee joint
metacarpals (mĕt″ ă-kär′ pəls)	meta- carp -al	beyond wrist pertaining to	Pertaining to the bones of the hand. There are five radiating bones in the fingers. *Note:* The bones of the foot are the *metatarsals*.
metacarpectomy (mĕt″ ă-kăr-pĕk′ tō-mē)	meta- carp -ectomy	beyond wrist surgical excision	Surgical excision of one or more bones of the hand
myelitis (mī-ĕ-lī′ tĭs)	myel -itis	bone marrow inflammation	Inflammation of the bone marrow
myeloma (mī-ĕ-lō′ mă)	myel -oma	bone marrow tumor	Tumor of the bone marrow
myelopoiesis (mī″ ĕl-ō-poy-ē′ sĭs)	myel/o -poiesis	bone marrow formation	Formation of bone marrow
olecranal (ō-lĕk′ răn-ăl)	olecran -al	elbow pertaining to	Pertaining to the elbow
orthopedics (Orth) (or″ thō-pē′ dĭks)	orth/o ped -ic	straight child pertaining to	Diseases and disorders involving locomotor structures of the body
orthopedist (or″ thō-pē′ dĭst)	orth/o ped -ist	straight child one who specializes	One who specializes in diseases and disorders involving locomotor structures of the body

Medical Word	Word Parts: Part	Word Parts: Meaning	Definition
osteoarthritis (OA) (ŏs″ tē-ō-ăr-thrī′ tĭs)	oste/o arthr -itis	bone joint inflammation	Inflammation of the bone and joint; the most common type of arthritis in the United States in people over 50 years of age. It is often called *wear-and-tear disease* because the cartilage that cushions a joint wears away as one ages, so that bone rubs against bone.

insights In ICD-10-CM, osteoarthritis is divided into primary, secondary, posttraumatic, and/or generalized.

Medical Word	Part	Meaning	Definition
osteoblast (ŏs′ tē-ō-blăst″)	oste/o -blast	bone immature cell, germ cell	Bone-forming cell
osteochondritis (ŏs″ tē-ō-kŏn-drī′ tĭs)	oste/o chondr -itis	bone cartilage inflammation	Inflammation of bone and cartilage
osteogenesis (ŏs″ tē-ō-jĕn′ ĕ-sĭs)	oste/o -genesis	bone formation	Formation of bone
osteomalacia (ŏs″ tē-ō-măl-ā′ shē-ă)	oste/o -malacia	bone softening	Softening of bones
osteomyelitis (ŏs″ tē-ō-mī″ ĕl-ī′ tĭs)	oste/o myel -itis	bone bone marrow inflammation	Inflammation of bone, especially the marrow, caused by a pathogenic organism. See Figure 6.15.

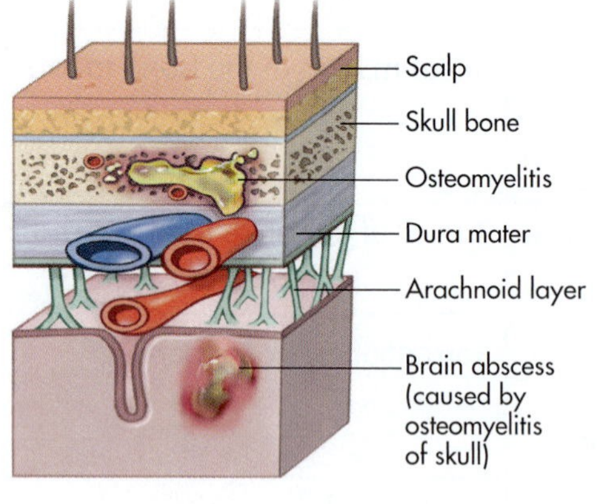

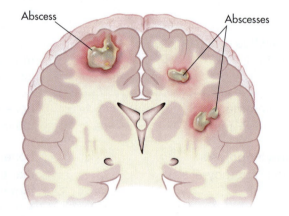

Figure 6.15
Abscess of the brain due to osteomyelitis.

Medical Word	Part	Meaning	Definition
osteopenia (ŏs″ tē-ō-pē′ nē-ă)	oste/o -penia	bone deficiency	Deficiency of bone tissue, regardless of the cause
osteoporosis (ŏs″ tē-ō-por-ō′ sĭs)	oste/o por -osis	bone passage condition	Abnormal condition characterized by a decrease in the density of bones, decreasing their strength and causing fragile bones, which can result in fractures. It is most common in women after menopause, when it is called postmenopausal osteoporosis, but may also develop in men. See Figure 6.16.

(*continued*)

Medical Word	Word Parts		Definition
	Part	Meaning	

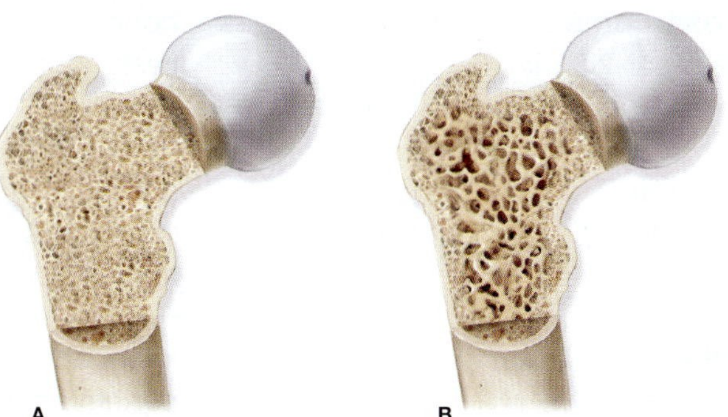

Figure 6.16 (A) Normal spongy bone. (B) Spongy bone with osteoporosis, which is characterized by a loss of bone density.

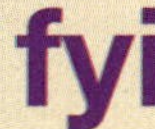

With normal aging, individuals can lose 1.0–1.5 inches in height. Loss of more than 1.5 inches in height can be related to vertebral compression fractures and other issues due to osteoporosis. See Figure 6.17.

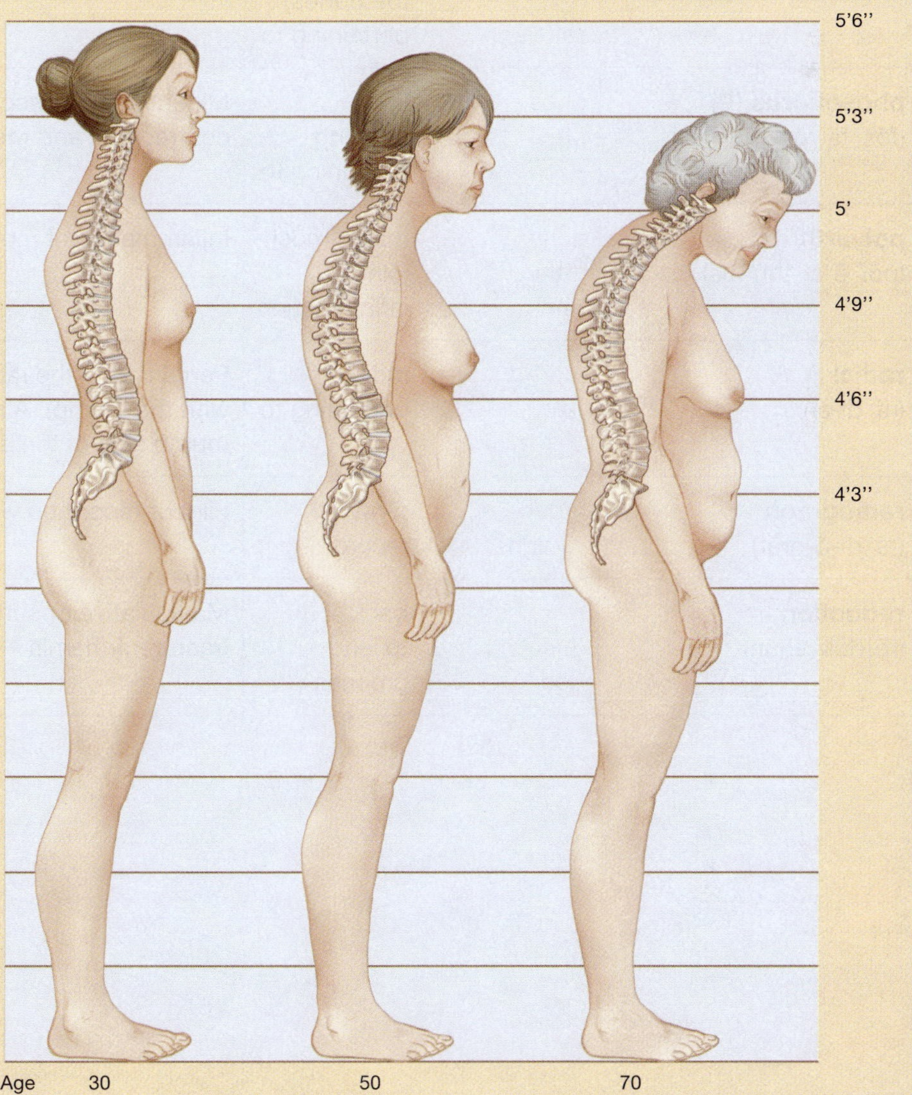

Figure 6.17 Spinal changes caused by osteoporosis.

Medical Word	Word Parts		Definition
	Part	Meaning	
osteosarcoma (ŏs″tē-ō-săr-kō′ mă)	oste/o sarc -oma	bone flesh tumor	Malignant tumor of the bone; cancer growing from cells of "fleshy" connective tissue such as bone or muscle
osteotome (ŏs′ tē-ō-tōm″)	oste/o -tome	bone instrument to cut	Surgical instrument used for cutting bone
patellar (pă-tĕl′ ăr)	patell -ar	kneecap pertaining to	Pertaining to the patella, the *kneecap*
pedal (pĕd′ l)	ped -al	foot pertaining to	Pertaining to the foot
phalangeal (fă-lăn′ jē-ăl)	phalang/e -al	phalanges (finger/toe bones) pertaining to	Pertaining to the bones of the fingers and the toes
phosphorus (P) (fŏs′ fă-rŭs)	phos phor -us	light carrying pertaining to	Mineral that is essential in bone formation, muscle contraction, and many other functions
polyarthritis (pŏl″ ē-ăr-thrī′ tĭs)	poly- arthr -itis	many, much joint inflammation	Inflammation of more than one joint
radial (rā′ dĭ-ăl)	rad/i -al	radius pertaining to	Pertaining to the radius (lateral lower arm bone in line with the thumb). A radial pulse can be found on the thumb side of the arm.
radiograph (rā′ dĭ-ō-grăf)	radi/o -graph	x-ray record	Film or record on which an x-ray image is produced
reduction (rē-dŭk′ shŭn)	re- duct -ion	back to lead process	Manipulative or surgical procedure used to correct a fracture or hernia

Medical Word	Word Parts		Definition
	Part	**Meaning**	
rheumatoid arthritis (RA) (roo´ mă-toyd ăr-thrī´ tĭs)	rheumat -oid arthr -itis	discharge resemble joint inflammation	Chronic autoimmune disease characterized by inflammation of the joints, stiffness, pain, and swelling, which results in crippling deformities. See Figure 6.18.

insights In ICD-10-CM, there are more specific categories for rheumatoid disease of organs with rheumatoid arthritis, such as lung, vasculitis, heart disease, myopathy, polyneuropathy, bursitis, and/or nodule.

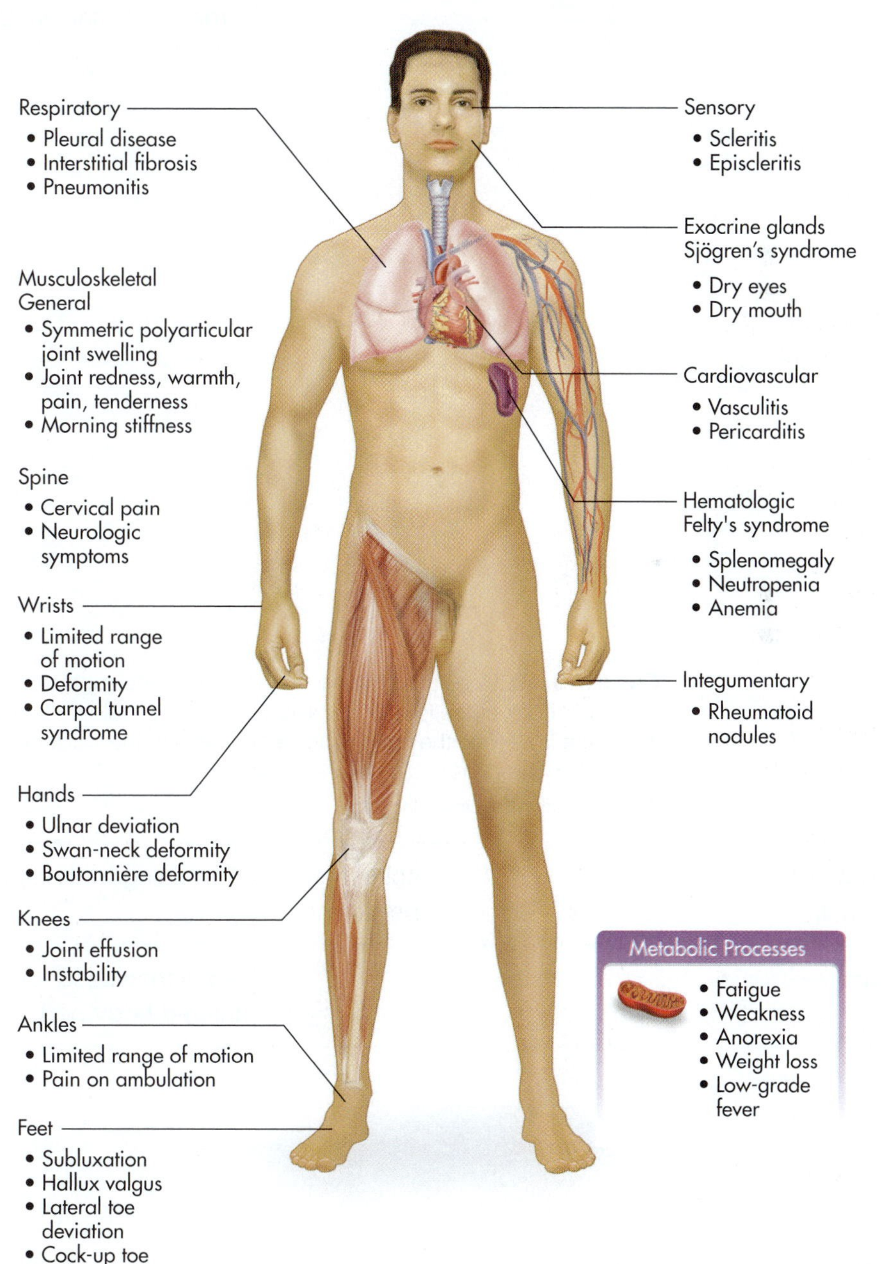

Figure 6.18 Multisystem effects of rheumatoid arthritis.

Medical Word	Word Parts		Definition
	Part	Meaning	
rickets (rĭk´ ĕts)			Abnormal condition that can occur in children; caused by a lack of vitamin D
scapular (skăp´ ū-lăr)	scapul -ar	shoulder blade pertaining to	Pertaining to the shoulder blade
scoliosis (skō˝ lĭ-ō´ sĭs)	scoli -osis	curvature condition	An abnormal lateral curvature of the spine. The characteristic signs include asymmetry of the trunk, uneven shoulders and hips, a one-sided rib hump, and a prominent scapula. See Figure 6.19 and Figure 6.14C.

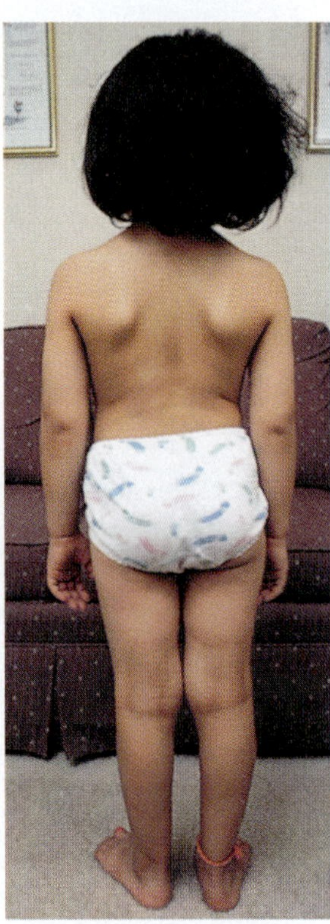

Figure 6.19 Does this child have legs of different lengths or scoliosis? Look at the level of the iliac crests and shoulders to see if they are level. See the more prominent crease at the waist on the right side? This child could have scoliosis.

Source: Pearson Education, Inc.

Medical Word	Part	Meaning	Definition
spinal (spī´ năl)	spin -al	spine pertaining to	Pertaining to the spine
splint			Appliance used for fixation, support, and rest of an injured body part

Medical Word	Word Parts		Definition
	Part	**Meaning**	
spondylodesis (spŏn-dĭ-lō-dĕ-sĭs)	spondyl/o -desis	vertebra binding	Surgery performed to permanently connect two or more vertebrae in the spine, eliminating motion between them. It involves techniques designed to mimic the normal healing process of broken bones. The surgeon places bone or a bonelike material within the space between two spinal vertebrae. Metal plates, screws, and rods may be used to hold the vertebrae together (binding), so they can heal into one solid unit. Also known as *spinal fusion* and *spondylo***syn***desis* (**syn-** *[P]*), meaning *together*.

! ALERT!

To change vertebr***a*** to its plural form, you change the ***a*** to ***ae*** to create *vertebrae*.

Medical Word	Part	Meaning	Definition
sprain			A traumatic injury to the tendons, muscles, or ligaments around a joint characterized by pain, swelling, and discoloration
spur			Sharp or pointed projection, as on a bone
sternal (stĕr´ năl)	stern -al	sternum, breastbone pertaining to	Pertaining to the sternum, the *breastbone*
sternotomy (stĕr-nŏt´ ō-mē)	stern/o -tomy	sternum, breastbone incision	Surgical incision of the sternum, the *breastbone*
subclavicular (sŭb˝ klă-vĭk´ ū-lăr)	sub- clavicul -ar	under, beneath clavicle, collar bone pertaining to	Pertaining to beneath the clavicle (*collar bone*)
subcostal (sŭb-kŏs´ tăl)	sub- cost -al	under, beneath rib pertaining to	Pertaining to beneath the ribs
submaxilla (sŭb˝ măk-sĭl´ă)	sub- maxilla	under, beneath jaw	Below the jaw or mandible
symphysis (sĭm´ fĭ-sĭs)	sym- -physis	together growth	Literally means *growing together*; a joint in which adjacent bony surfaces are firmly united by fibrocartilage. An example is the *symphysis pubis*, where the bones of the pelvis have grown together.
tendinitis (tĕn˝ dĭn-ī´tĭs)	tendin -itis	tendon inflammation	Inflammation of a tendon

Medical Word	Word Parts		Definition
	Part	**Meaning**	
tennis elbow			Chronic condition characterized by elbow pain caused by excessive pronation and supination activities of the forearm; usually caused by strain, as in playing tennis

fyi The medical term used to denote tennis elbow is *lateral humeral epicondylitis*. Epi/condyl/itis is divided into epi- (*upon*) + condyl (*knuckle*) + -itis (*inflammation*). A "knuckle" is a rounded protuberance formed by the bones in a joint.

Medical Word	Part	Meaning	Definition
tibial (tĭb′ ē-ăl)	tibi -al	tibia pertaining to	Pertaining to the tibia; the *shin bone*. Larger of the two bones of the lower leg.
traction (Tx) (trăk′ shĭn)	tract -ion	to draw process	Process of drawing or pulling on bones or muscles to relieve displacement and facilitate healing. See Figure 6.20.

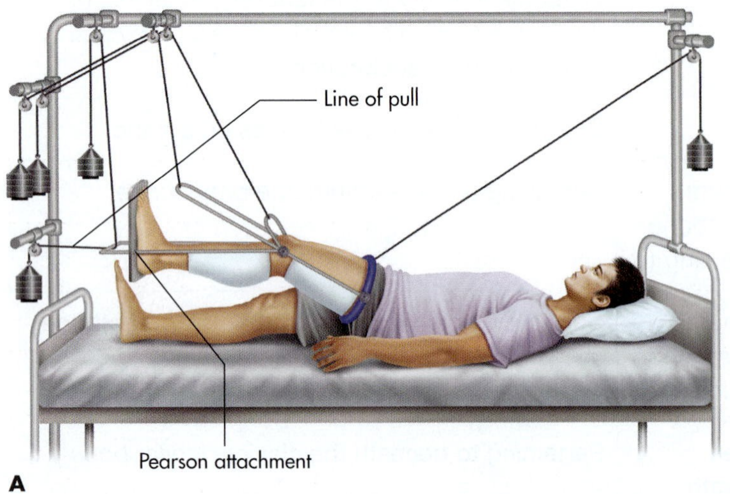

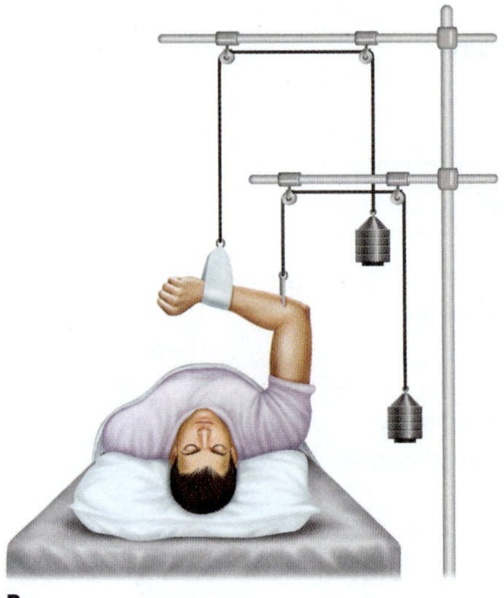

Figure 6.20 Traction is the application of a pulling force to maintain bone alignment during fracture healing. Different fractures require different types of traction. (A) Balanced suspension traction is commonly used for fractures of the femur. (B) Skeletal traction, in which the pulling force is applied directly to the bone, may be used to treat fractures of the humerus.

Medical Word	Part	Meaning	Definition
ulnar (ŭl′ năr)	uln -ar	ulna pertaining to	Pertaining to the ulna (the longer bone of the forearm between the wrist and elbow), or to the nerve or artery named from it. The ulna is located on the little-finger side of the arm.
ulnocarpal (ŭl″ nō-kăr′ păl)	uln/o carp -al	ulna wrist pertaining to	Pertaining to the ulna side of the wrist
vertebral (vĕr′ tĕ-brăl)	vertebr -al	vertebra pertaining to	Pertaining to a vertebra (any of the small bones linked together to form the backbone)
xiphoid (zĭf′ oyd)	xiph -oid	sword resemble	Literally means *resembling a sword*. The xiphoid process is the lowest portion of the sternum; a sword-shaped cartilaginous process supported by bone.

Study and Review II

Word Parts

Prefixes

Give the definitions of the following prefixes.

1. a- ______________________
2. dis- ______________________
3. hydr- ______________________
4. inter- ______________________
5. meta- ______________________
6. peri- ______________________
7. poly- ______________________
8. sub- ______________________
9. sym- ______________________
10. re- ______________________

Combining Forms

Give the definitions of the following combining forms.

1. acr/o ______________________
2. ankyl/o ______________________
3. arthr/o ______________________
4. burs/o ______________________
5. calcan/e ______________________
6. carp/o ______________________
7. chondr/o ______________________
8. coccyg/o ______________________
9. cost/o ______________________
10. crani/o ______________________
11. dactyl/o ______________________
12. isch/i ______________________
13. kyph/o ______________________
14. lord/o ______________________
15. lumb/o ______________________
16. oste/o ______________________
17. patell/o ______________________
18. ped/o ______________________
19. sacr/o ______________________
20. scoli/o ______________________
21. spin/o ______________________
22. stern/o ______________________
23. uln/o ______________________
24. xiph/o ______________________

Suffixes

Give the definitions of the following suffixes.

1. -ac ______________________
2. -al ______________________
3. -algia ______________________
4. -ar ______________________
5. -ary ______________________
6. -blast ______________________
7. -centesis ______________________
8. -age ______________________
9. -ion ______________________
10. -dynia ______________________
11. -ectomy ______________________
12. -edema ______________________
13. -gen ______________________
14. -genesis ______________________
15. -gram ______________________
16. -graph ______________________
17. -ic ______________________
18. -itis ______________________
19. -ive ______________________
20. -scope ______________________
21. -malacia ______________________
22. -us ______________________
23. -oid ______________________
24. -oma ______________________
25. -osis ______________________
26. -penia ______________________
27. -physis ______________________
28. -plasia ______________________
29. -plasty ______________________
30. -poiesis ______________________
31. -tome ______________________
32. -tomy ______________________
33. -um ______________________

Identifying Medical Terms

In the spaces provided, write the medical terms for the following meanings.

1. ______________________ Inflammation of the joints of the hands or feet
2. ______________________ Abnormal condition of stiffening of a joint
3. ______________________ Inflammation of a joint
4. ______________________ Pertaining to the heel bone
5. ______________________ Pertaining to cartilage
6. ______________________ Pain in the coccyx

7. ______________________ Pertaining to the rib cartilage

8. ______________________ Surgical excision of a portion of the skull

9. ______________________ Pertaining to the finger or toe

10. ______________________ Surgical instrument used for cutting bone

11. ______________________ Pertaining to the space between two ribs

12. ______________________ Pain in the hip

13. ______________________ Pertaining to the loins

14. ______________________ Tumor of the bone marrow

15. ______________________ Inflammation of the bone and joint

16. ______________________ Inflammation of the bone marrow

17. ______________________ Deficiency of bone tissue

18. ______________________ Pertaining to the foot

19. ______________________ Literally means resembling a sword

Matching

Select the appropriate lettered meaning for each of the following words.

______ **1.** arthroscope

______ **2.** carpal tunnel syndrome

______ **3.** fixation

______ **4.** gout

______ **5.** hammertoe

______ **6.** kyphosis

______ **7.** metacarpal

______ **8.** rickets

______ **9.** tennis elbow

______ **10.** ulnar

a. Abnormal condition that can occur in children and is caused by a lack of vitamin D

b. An acquired flexion deformity of the interphalangeal joint

c. Hereditary metabolic disease that is a form of acute arthritis

d. Chronic condition characterized by elbow pain that is caused by excessive pronation and supination activities of the forearm

e. Making rigid, immobilizing

f. Pertaining to the ulna (long bone of the forearm between the wrist and elbow), or to the nerve or artery named for it

g. Pertaining to the bones of the hand

h. In this condition, the normal thoracic curvature becomes exaggerated, producing a "humpback" appearance

i. Surgical instrument used to examine the interior of a joint

j. Abnormal condition caused by compression of the median nerve by the carpal ligament

k. Pertaining to the knee

Medical Case Snapshots

This learning activity provides an opportunity to relate the medical terminology you are learning to a precise patient case presentation. In the spaces provided, write in your answers.

Case 1

A 66-year-old female is scheduled for a dual-energy x-ray absorptiometry (DXA) scan, to measure her bone mineral density. She is diagnosed with osteoarthritis. The results of her test show ______________ (deficiency of bone tissue) and ____________ (which is characterized by a decrease in bone density).

Case 2

A 4-year-old female is seen by an orthopedic specialist. Upon physical examination an abnormal lateral curvature of the spine, known as ____________, was noted. The characteristic signs of this condition include _____________ of the trunk, uneven shoulders and hips, a one-sided rib hump, and a prominent __________.

Case 3

Upon a return visit to her physician, Ms. Anita Sinclair presented with symptoms of inflammation of the joints, stiffness, pain, and swelling, especially of both hands. This condition is referred to as ______________ ______________ (RA). The multisystem effects of this condition are varied. See Figure 6.18.

Drug Highlights

Type of Drug	Description and Examples
anti-inflammatory agents	Relieves the swelling, tenderness, redness, and pain of inflammation. Such agents can be classified as steroidal (corticosteroids) and nonsteroidal.
corticosteroids (glucocorticoids)	Steroid substances that have potent anti-inflammatory effects in disorders of many organ systems. Steroids have an array of serious side effects that may be caused by long-term use. EXAMPLES: Depo-Medrol (methylprednisolone acetate) and prednisone
nonsteroidal anti-inflammatory drugs (NSAIDs)	Agents used in the treatment of arthritis and related disorders EXAMPLES: Bayer aspirin (acetylsalicylic acid), Motrin IB (ibuprofen), Feldene (piroxicam), ketoprofen, and Naprosyn (naproxen)
disease-modifying antirheumatic drugs (DMARDs)	Can influence the course of the disease progression; therefore, their introduction in early rheumatoid arthritis is recommended to limit irreversible joint damage. EXAMPLES: gold preparation Ridaura (auranofin); antimalarial Plaquenil (hydroxychloroquine sulfate); a chelating agent Cuprimine (penicillamine); and the immunosuppressants Trexall (methotrexate sodium), Imuran (azathioprine), and Cytoxan (cyclophosphamide)
COX-2 inhibitors	Cyclooxygenase (COX) is an enzyme involved in many aspects of normal cellular function and in the inflammatory response. COX-2 is found in joints and other areas affected by inflammation as occurs with osteoarthritis and rheumatoid arthritis. Inhibition of COX-2 reduces the production of compounds associated with inflammation and pain. EXAMPLES: Celebrex (celecoxib) and Mobic (meloxicam)
biologics	Includes a wide range of medicinal products such as vaccines, blood and blood components, and drugs made from recombinant DNA technology. EXAMPLES: Humira (adalimumab), Enbrel (etanercept), Remicade (infliximab), and Orencia (abatacept)
agents used to treat gout	Acute attacks of gout are treated with colchicine. Once the acute attack of gout has been controlled, drug therapy to control hyperuricemia can be initiated. EXAMPLES: Zyloprim (allopurinol) and probenecid
agents used to treat or prevent postmenopausal osteoporosis	
antiresorptive agents	Antiresorptive agents decrease the removal of calcium from bones. *Fosamax* reduces the activity of the cells that cause bone loss and increases the amount of bone in most patients. *Actonel* inhibits osteoclast-mediated bone resorption and modulates bone metabolism. To receive the clinical benefits of either of these drugs, the patient must be informed and follow the prescribed drug regimen. EXAMPLES: Fosamax (alendronate), Actonel (risedronate), Evista (raloxifene), Boniva (ibandronate), Reclast (zoledronate), and calcitonin

Chapter

7 Muscular System

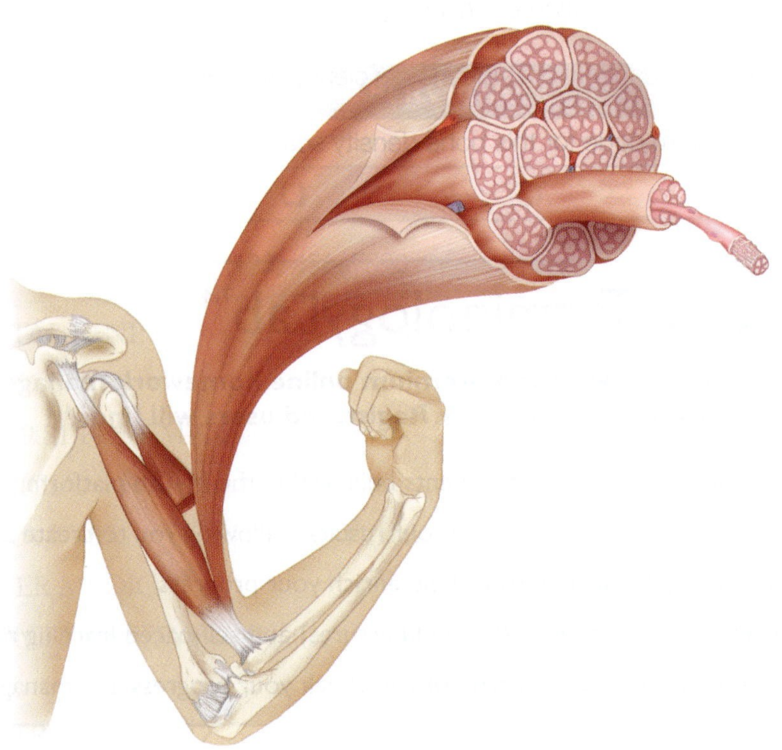

Learning Outcomes

On completion of this chapter, you will be able to:

1. Describe the muscular system.
2. Describe the three basic types of muscle tissue.
3. Explain the primary functions of muscles.
4. Recognize terminology included in the ICD-10-CM.
5. Analyze, build, spell, and pronounce medical words.
6. Comprehend the drugs highlighted in this chapter.
7. Describe diagnostic and laboratory tests related to the muscular system.
8. Identify and define selected abbreviations.
9. Apply your acquired knowledge of medical terms by successfully completing the *Practical Application* exercise.

Anatomy and Physiology

The muscular system is composed of all the **muscles** in the body and works in coordination with the skeletal and nervous systems. Muscles provide the mechanism for movement of the body and locomotion from one place to another. In addition to causing movement, muscles produce heat and help the body maintain posture and stability. There are three basic types of muscles: skeletal, smooth, and cardiac. Table 7.1 provides an at-a-glance look at the muscular system.

The muscles are the primary tissues of the system. They make up approximately 42% of a person's body weight and are composed of long, slender cells known as **fibers**. Muscle fibers are of different lengths and shapes and vary in color from white to deep red. Each muscle consists of a group of fibers held together by connective tissue and enclosed in a fibrous sheath or **fascia**. See Figure 7.1.

Each fiber within a muscle receives its own nerve impulses and has its own stored supply of glycogen, which it uses as fuel for energy. Muscle must be supplied with proper nutrition and oxygen to perform properly; therefore, blood and lymphatic vessels permeate its tissues.

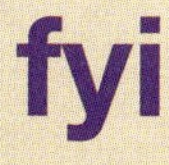

As a person grows older, the number and size of muscle fibers diminish and the water content of tendons is reduced. Decrease in handgrip strength can make performing routine activities such as opening a jar or turning a key more difficult.

Types of Muscles

Skeletal muscle, smooth muscle, and cardiac muscle are the three basic types of muscles in the body. They are composed of different types of muscle tissue (e.g., striated or smooth) and classified according to their functions and appearance. See Figure 7.2.

Skeletal Muscle

Also known as **voluntary** or **striated** muscles, **skeletal muscles** are controlled by the conscious part of the brain and attach to the bones. These muscles have a cross-striped appearance (striated) and vary in size, shape, arrangement of fibers, and means of attachment to bones. Selected skeletal muscles are listed with their functions in Table 7.2 and are shown in Figure 7.3.

Table 7.1 Muscular System at-a-Glance

Organ/Structure	Primary Functions/Description
Muscles	Cause movement, help to maintain posture, and produce heat
Skeletal muscles	Produce various types of body movement through contractility, extensibility, and elasticity
Smooth muscles	Produce relatively slow contraction with greater degree of extensibility in the internal organs, especially organs of the digestive, respiratory, and urinary tract, plus certain muscles of the eye and skin, and walls of blood vessels
Cardiac muscle	Contraction of the myocardium, which is controlled by the autonomic nervous system and specialized neuromuscular tissue located within the right atrium
Tendons	Bands of connective tissue that attach muscles to bones

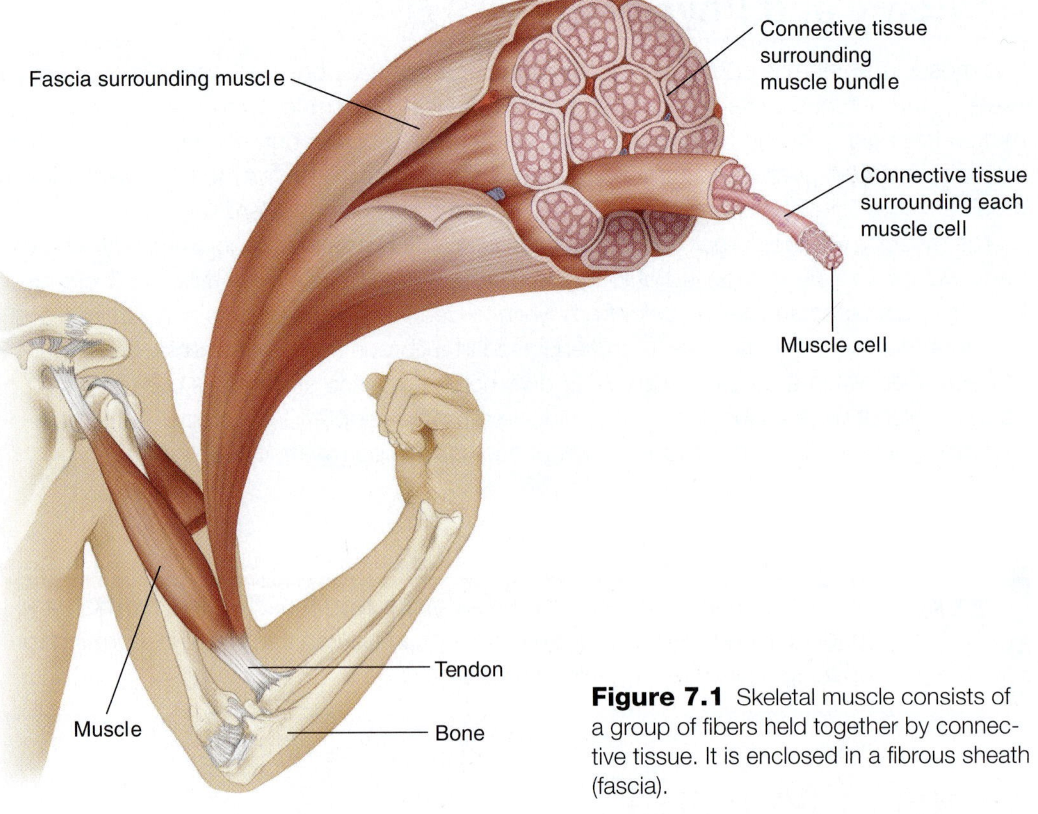

Figure 7.1 Skeletal muscle consists of a group of fibers held together by connective tissue. It is enclosed in a fibrous sheath (fascia).

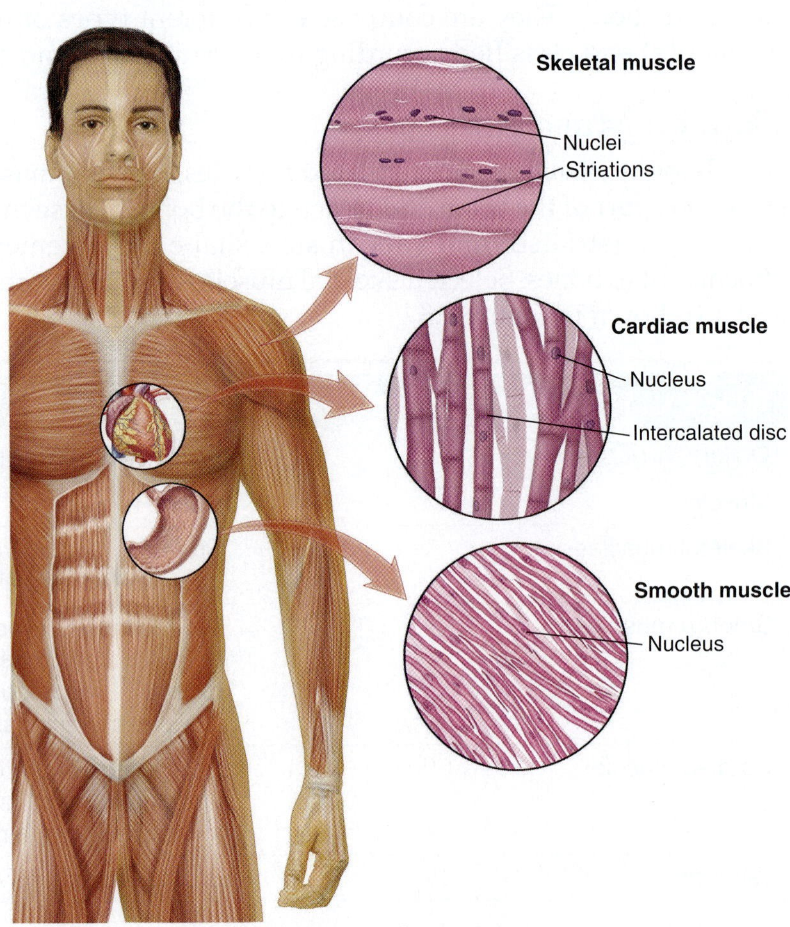

Figure 7.2 Types of muscle tissue.

Table 7.2 Selected Skeletal Muscles

Muscle	Direction	Action
Sternocleidomastoid	Anterior	Rotates and laterally flexes neck
Trapezius	Anterior/posterior	Draws head back and to the side; rotates scapula
Deltoid	Anterior/posterior	Raises and rotates arm
Rectus femoris	Anterior	Extends leg and assists flexion of thigh
Sartorius	Anterior	Flexes and rotates the thigh and leg
Tibialis anterior	Anterior	Dorsiflexes foot and increases the arch in the beginning process of walking
Pectoralis major	Anterior	Flexes, adducts, and rotates arm
Biceps brachii	Anterior	Flexes arm and forearm and supinates forearm
External oblique	Anterior	Contracts abdomen and viscera (internal organs)
Rectus abdominis	Anterior	Compresses or flattens abdomen
Gastrocnemius	Anterior/posterior	Plantar flexes foot and flexes knee
Soleus	Anterior	Plantar flexes foot
Triceps	Posterior	Extends forearm
Latissimus dorsi	Posterior	Adducts, extends, and rotates arm; used during swimming
Gluteus medius	Posterior	Abducts and rotates thigh
Gluteus maximus	Posterior	Extends and rotates thigh
Biceps femoris	Posterior	Flexes knee and rotates it outward
Semitendinosus	Posterior	Flexes and rotates leg; extends thigh
Semimembranosus	Posterior	Flexes and rotates leg; extends thigh
Achilles tendon	Posterior	Plantar (sole of the foot) flexion and extension of ankle

There are over 600 skeletal muscles in the body that, through contractility, extensibility, excitability, and elasticity, are responsible for the movement of the body. **Contractility** allows muscles to change shape to become shorter and thicker. With **extensibility**, living muscle cells can be stretched and extended. They become longer and thinner. In **excitability**, muscles receive and respond to stimulation. With **elasticity**, once the stretching force is removed, a living muscle cell returns to its original shape.

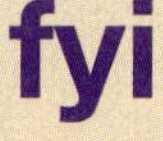

The movements of a newborn are uncoordinated and random. Muscular development proceeds from head to foot and from the center of the body to the periphery. Head and neck muscles are the first ones that a baby can control. A baby can hold his or her head up before he or she can sit erect.

Muscles have three distinguishable parts: the **body** or main portion, an **origin**, and an **insertion**. The origin is the more fixed attachment of the muscle to the stationary bone and the insertion is the point of attachment of a muscle to the bone that it moves.

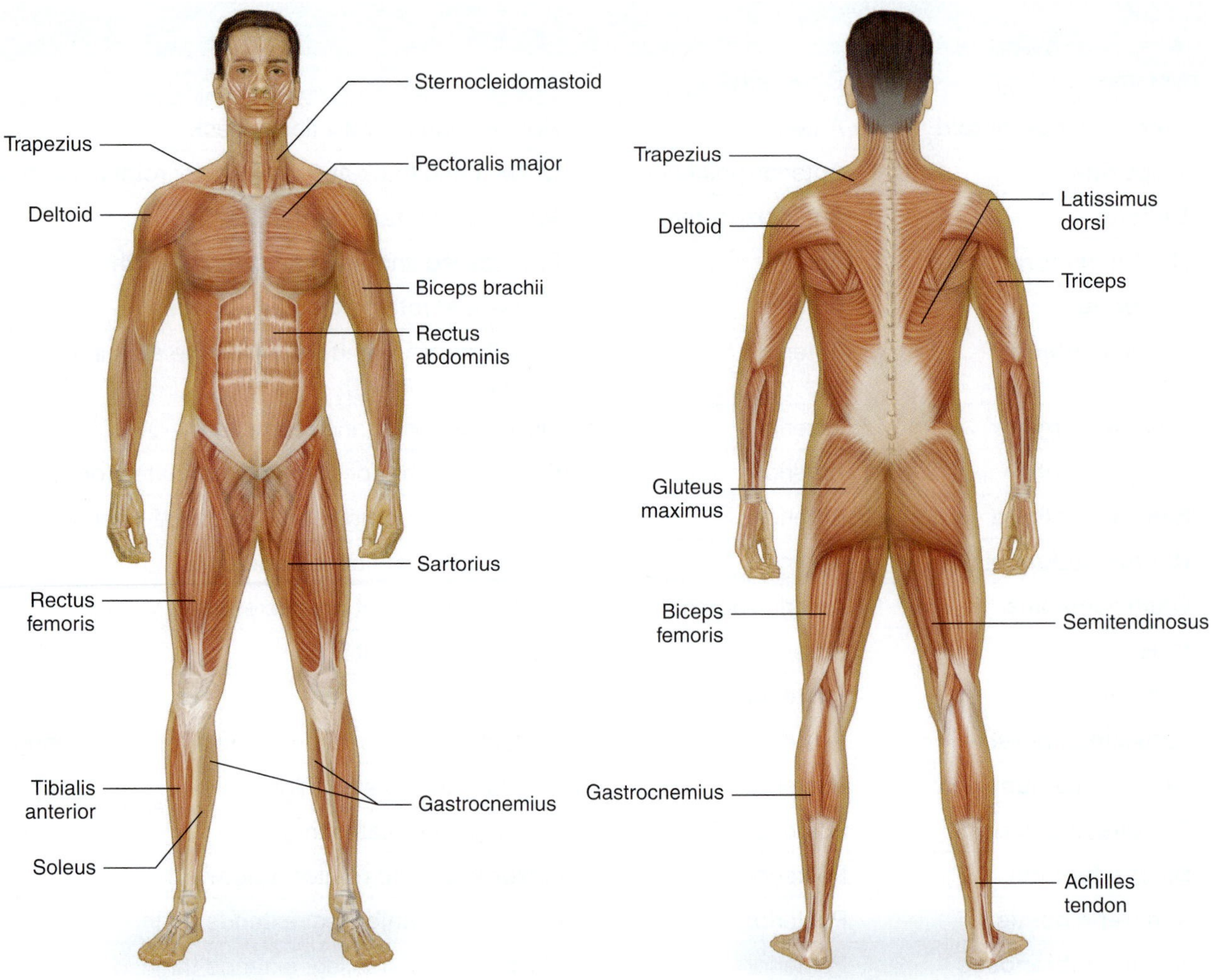

Figure 7.3 Selected skeletal muscles and the Achilles tendon (anterior and posterior views).

The means of attachment is a band of connective tissue called a **tendon**, which can vary in length from less than 1 inch to more than 1 foot. Some muscles, such as those in the abdominal region, the dorsal lumbar region, and the palmar region, form attachments using a wide, thin, sheetlike tendon known as an **aponeurosis**.

Skeletal muscles move body parts by pulling from one bone across its joint to another bone, with movement occurring at the freely movable (diarthrosis/synovial) joint. The types of body movement occurring at the freely movable joints are described in Chapter 6.

Muscles and nerves function together as a motor unit. For skeletal muscles to contract, it is necessary to have stimulation by impulses from motor nerves. Skeletal muscles perform in groups and are classified as follows:

- **Antagonist**. Muscle that counteracts the action of another muscle; when one contracts, the other relaxes
- **Prime mover or agonist**. Muscle that is primary in a given movement; the movement is produced by its contraction
- **Synergist**. Muscle that acts with another muscle to produce and assist movement

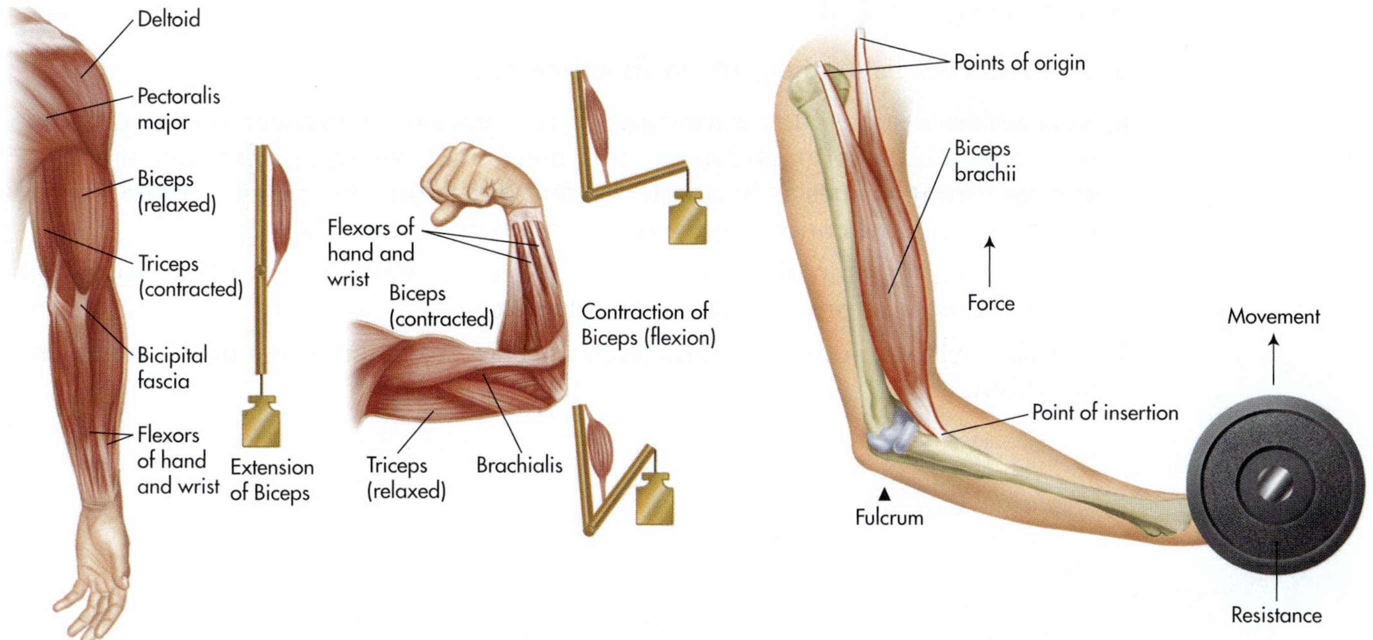

Figure 7.4 Coordination of antagonist muscles to perform movement.

All movement is a result of the contraction of a prime mover (agonist) and the relaxation of the opposing muscle (antagonist). See Figure 7.4.

Smooth Muscle

Also called *involuntary*, *visceral*, or *unstriated*, **smooth muscles** are not controlled by the conscious part of the brain. They are under the control of the autonomic nervous system and, in most cases, produce relatively slow contraction with a greater degree of extensibility. These muscles lack the cross-striped appearance of skeletal muscle and are smooth. Included in this type are the muscles of internal organs of the digestive, respiratory, and urinary tract plus certain muscles of the eye and skin.

Cardiac Muscle

The muscle of the heart, the **cardiac muscle** (**myocardium**), is *involuntary* but *striated* in appearance. It is under the control of the autonomic nervous system and has specialized neuromuscular tissue located within the right atrium. Cardiac muscle differs from the other two muscle types in that contraction can occur even without an initial nervous input. The cells that produce the stimulation for contraction without nervous input are called the **pacemaker cells**. Coordinated contraction of cardiac muscle cells in the heart propels blood from the atria and ventricles to the blood vessels of the circulatory system. Cardiac muscle cells, like all tissues in the body, rely on an ample blood supply to deliver oxygen and nutrients and to remove waste products such as carbon dioxide. The coronary arteries fulfill this function.

fyi In the older adult, the heart muscle becomes less able to propel the large amount of blood that is needed by the body. This makes a person feel tired more quickly and takes longer for recovery to occur.

Functions of Muscles

The following is a list of the primary functions of muscles:

1. Muscles are responsible for movement. The types of movement are locomotion where chemical energy is changed into mechanical energy, propulsion of substances through tubes as in circulation and digestion, and changes in the size of openings as in the contraction and relaxation of the iris of the eye.
2. Muscles help to maintain posture through a continual partial contraction of skeletal muscles. This process is known as **tonicity**.
3. Muscles help to produce heat through the chemical changes involved in muscular action.

Study and Review I

Anatomy and Physiology

Write your answers to the following questions.

1. The muscular system is made up of three types of muscle tissue. Name the three types.

   a. ______________________ **b.** ______________________

   c. ______________________

2. Muscles make up approximately ______________ percent of a person's body weight.

3. Name the two essential ingredients that are needed for a muscle to perform properly.

   a. ______________________ **b.** ______________________

4. Name the two points of attachment for a skeletal muscle.

   a. ______________________ **b.** ______________________

5. Skeletal muscle is also known as ______________________ or ______________________.

6. A wide, thin, sheetlike tendon is known as an ______________________.

7. Name the three distinguishable parts of a muscle.

   a. ______________________ **b.** ______________________

   c. ______________________

8. Define the following:

a. Antagonist ____________________

b. Prime mover ____________________

c. Synergist ____________________

9. Smooth muscle is also called ____________, ____________, or ____________.

10. Smooth muscles are found in the internal organs. Name five examples of these locations.

a. ____________ **b.** ____________

c. ____________ **d.** ____________

e. ____________

11. ____________ is the muscle of the heart.

12. Name the three primary functions of the muscular system.

a. ____________ **b.** ____________

c. ____________

ANATOMY LABELING

Identify the structures shown below by filling in the blanks.

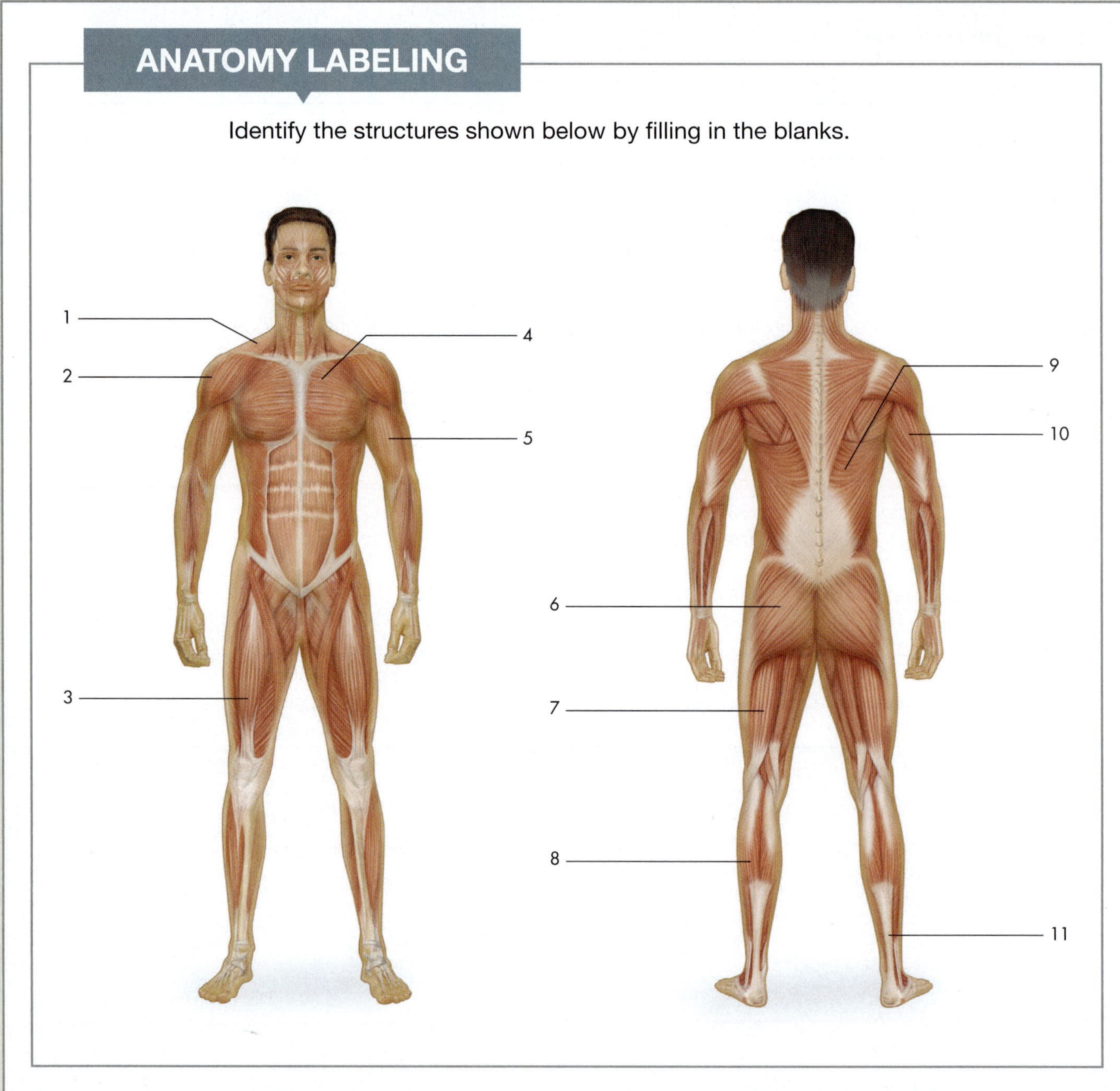

Building Your Medical Vocabulary

This section provides the foundation for learning medical terminology. Review the following alphabetized word list. Note how common prefixes and suffixes are repeatedly applied to word roots and combining forms to create different meanings. The word parts are color-coded: prefixes are yellow, suffixes are blue, roots/combining forms are red. A combining form is a word root plus a vowel. The chart below lists the combining forms for the word roots in this chapter and can help to strengthen your understanding of how medical words are built and spelled.

Remember These Guidelines

1. If the suffix begins with a vowel, drop the combining vowel from the combining form and add the suffix. For example, rheumat/o (*discharge*) + -ism (*condition*) becomes rheumatism.
2. If the suffix begins with a consonant, keep the combining vowel and add the suffix to the combining form. For example, my/o (*muscle*) + -plasty (*surgical repair*) becomes myoplasty.

You will find that some terms have not been divided into word parts. These are common words or specialized terms that are included to enhance your medical vocabulary.

Combining Forms of the Muscular System

agon/o	agony, a contest	**prosth/e**	an addition
amputat/o	to cut through	**rhabd/o**	rod
brach/i, brachi/o	arm	**rheumat/o**	discharge
cleid/o	clavicle	**rotat/o**	to turn
clon/o	turmoil	**sarc/o**	flesh
dactyl/o	finger or toe	**scler/o**	hardening
dermat/o	skin	**stern/o**	sternum
duct/o	to lead	**synov/o**	synovial
fasci/o	a band	**ten/o**	tendon
fibr/o	fiber	**therm/o**	hot, heat
is/o	equal	**ton/o**	tone, tension
metr/o	to measure	**tors/o**	twisted
muscul/o	muscle	**tort/i**	twisted
my/o(s)	muscle	**troph/o**	nourishment; development
neur/o	nerve	**volunt/o**	will
path/o	disease		

Medical Word	Word Parts		Definition
	Part	**Meaning**	
abductor (ăb-dŭk´ tōr)	ab- duct -or	away from to lead a doer	Muscle that on contraction draws *away from* the middle
adductor (ă-dŭk´ tōr)	ad- duct -or	toward to lead a doer	Muscle that draws a part *toward* the middle

ALERT!

The only difference in the terms **ab**/duct/or and **ad**/duct/or are the prefixes **ab-** (away from) and **ad-** (toward). What a difference a couple of letters can make!

Medical Word	Part	Meaning	Definition
amputation (ăm″ pū-tā´ shŭn)	amputat -ion	to cut through process	Surgical or traumatic removal of a limb, part, or other appendage. See Figure 7.5.

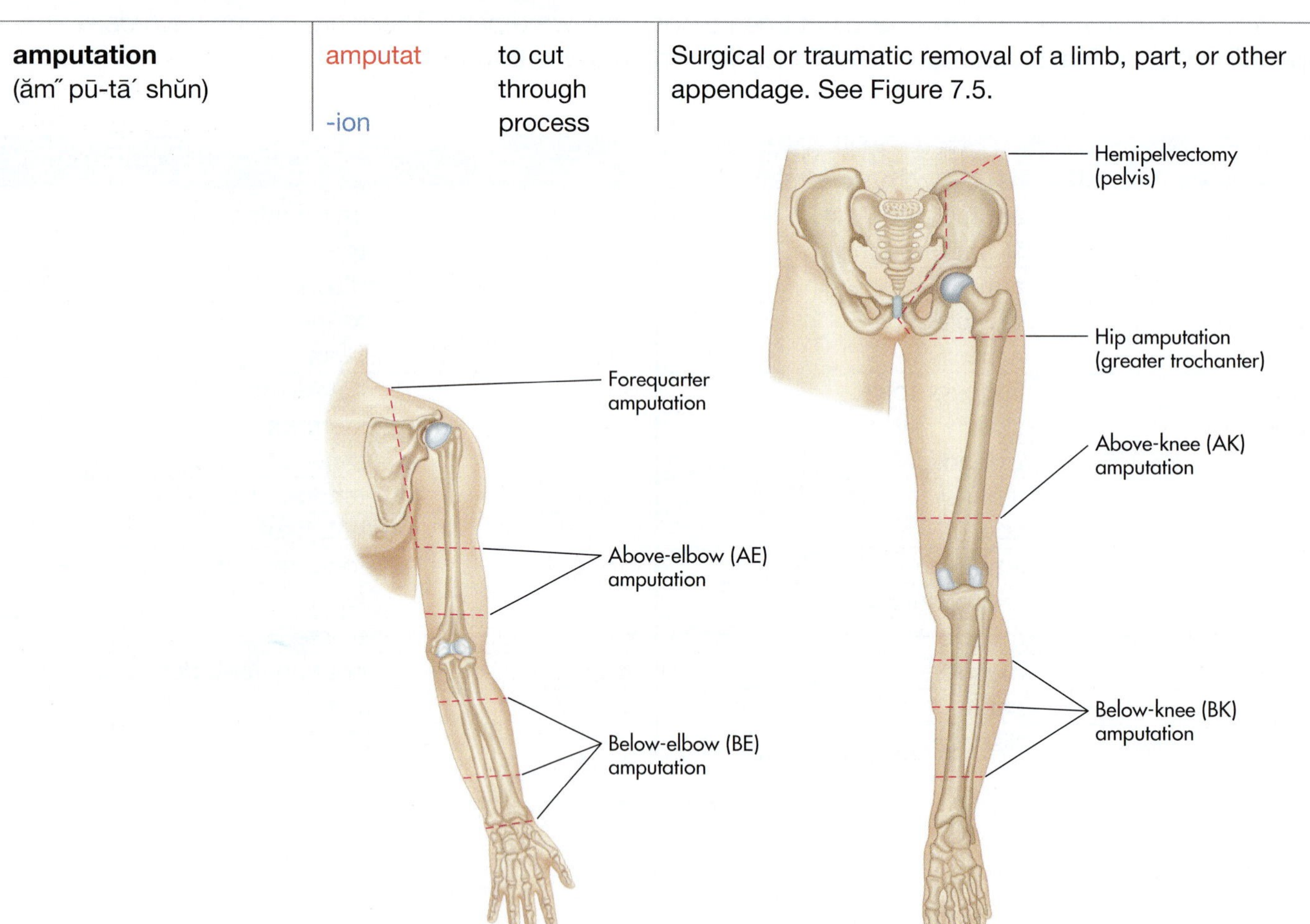

Figure 7.5 Common sites of amputation. (A) Upper extremities. (B) Lower extremities. The surgeon determines the level of amputation based on blood supply and tissue condition.

Medical Word	Part	Meaning	Definition
antagonist (ăn-tăg´ ō-nĭst)	ant- agon -ist	against agony, a contest agent	Muscle that counteracts the action of another muscle; when one contracts, the other relaxes (see Figure 7.4)

Medical Word	Word Parts		Definition
	Part	**Meaning**	
aponeurosis (ăp″ ō-nū-rō´ sĭs)			A strong, flat sheet of fibrous connective tissue that serves as a tendon to attach muscles to bone or as fascia to bind muscles together or to other tissues at their origin or insertion
ataxia (ă-tăk´ sē-ă)	a- -taxia	lack of order	Lack of muscular coordination; an inability to coordinate voluntary muscular movements that is symptomatic of some nervous disorders
atonic (ă-tŏn´ ĭk)	a- ton -ic	lack of tone, tension pertaining to	Pertaining to a lack of normal tone or tension; the lack of normal muscle tone
atrophy (ăt´ rō-fē)	a- -trophy	lack of nourishment, development	Literally means *a lack of nourishment*; wasting away of muscular tissue that may be caused by lack of use or lack of nerve stimulation of the muscle. *Lipoatrophy* (also called *lipodystrophy*) is atrophy of fat tissue. This condition can occur at the site of an insulin and/or corticosteroid injection. See Figure 7.6.

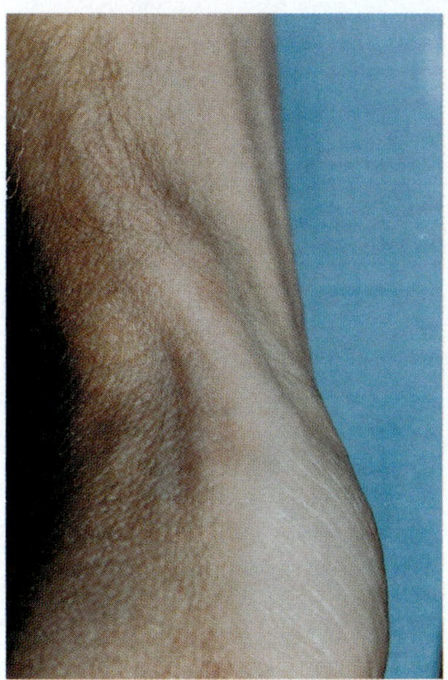

Figure 7.6 Lipoatrophy, wrist.
(Courtesy of Jason L. Smith, MD)

Medical Word	Part	Meaning	Definition
biceps (bī´ sĕps)	bi- -ceps	two head	Muscle with two heads or points of origin
brachialgia (brā″ kē-ăl´ jē-ă)	brach/i -algia	arm pain	Pain in the arm
bradykinesia (brăd″ ĭ-kĭ-nē´ sĭ-ă)	brady- -kinesia	slow motion	Slowness of motion or movement

Medical Word	Word Parts		Definition
	Part	Meaning	
clonic (klŏn´ ĭk)	clon -ic	turmoil pertaining to	Pertaining to alternate contraction and relaxation of muscles
contraction (kŏn-trăk´ shŭn)	con- tract -ion	with, together to draw process	Process of drawing up and thickening of a muscle fiber
contracture (kŏn-trăk´ chūr)	con- tract -ure	with, together to draw process	Condition in which a muscle shortens and renders the muscle resistant to the normal stretching process. For example, *Dupuytren contracture* is a thickening and tightening of subcutaneous tissue of the palm, causing the ring and little fingers to bend into the palm so that they cannot be extended. See Figure 7.7.

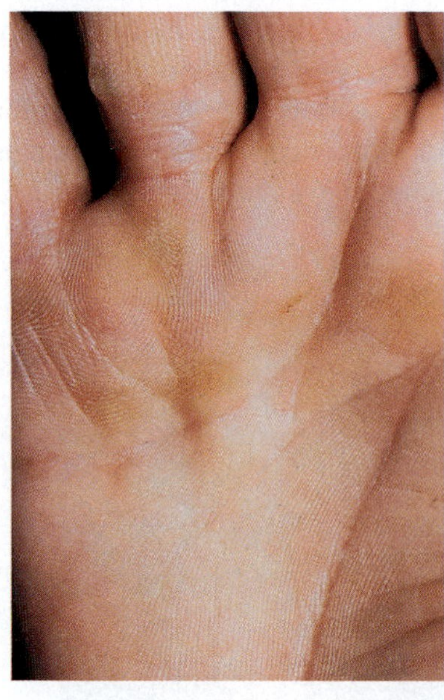

Figure 7.7 Dupuytren contracture.
(Courtesy of Jason L. Smith, MD)

Medical Word	Part	Meaning	Definition
dactylospasm (dăk´ tĭ-lō-spăzm)	dactyl/o -spasm	finger or toe tension, spasm	Medical term for cramp of a finger or toe

 **RULE REMINDER**

This term keeps the combining vowel ***o*** because the suffix begins with a consonant.

Medical Word	Word Parts		Definition
	Part	**Meaning**	
dermatomyositis (dĕr″ mă-tō-mī″ ō-sī′ tĭs)	dermat/o my/o(s) -itis	skin muscle inflammation	Acute or chronic disease with systemic pathology; inflammation of the muscles and the skin; a connective tissue disease characterized by edema, dermatitis, and inflammation of the muscles. Occurs in children and adults, and in the latter may be associated with neoplastic disease (cancer) or other disorders of connective tissue. Also referred to as *dermatopolymyositis*. See Figure 7.8.

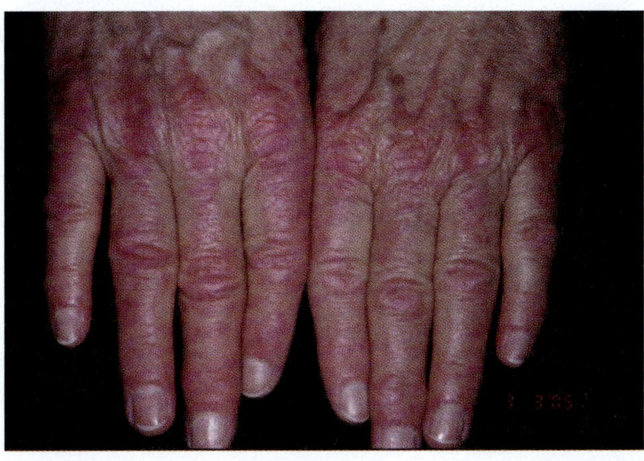

Figure 7.8 Dermatomyositis.
(Courtesy of Jason L. Smith, MD)

insights In ICD-10-CM, the code used for dermatopolymyositis is M33.90, followed by more specific categories for types: ***with myopathy*** (M33.92), *respiratory involvement* (M33.91), *juvenile* (M33.00), and many more.

Medical Word	Part	Meaning	Definition
diaphragm (dī′ ă-frăm)	dia- -phragm	through a fence, partition	Partition of muscles and membranes that separates the chest cavity and the abdominal cavity. It is the major muscle of breathing. See Figure 7.9.

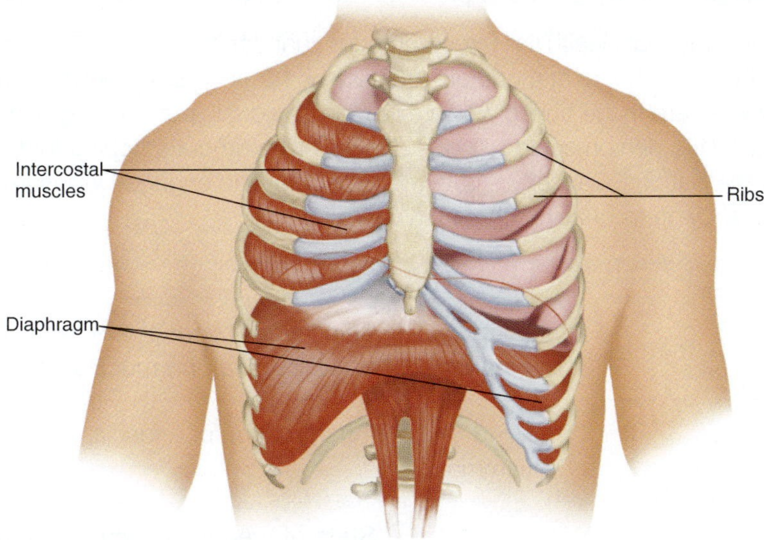

Figure 7.9 Diaphragm, the major muscle of breathing.

Medical Word	Word Parts		Definition
	Part	Meaning	
diathermy (dī´ ă-thĕr˝ mē)	dia- therm -y	through hot, heat pertaining to	Treatment using high-frequency current to produce heat within a part of the body; used to increase blood flow but should not be used in acute stage of recovery from trauma
dystonia (dĭs-tō´ nē-ă)	dys- ton -ia	difficult tone, tension condition	Condition of impaired muscle tone
dystrophin (dĭs-trōf´ ĭn)	dys- troph -in	difficult nourishment, development chemical	Protein found in muscle cells. When the gene that is responsible for this protein is defective and sufficient dystrophin is not produced, muscle wasting occurs. For example, in *Duchenne muscular dystrophy*, this protein is absent.
dystrophy (dĭs´ trō-fē)	dys- -trophy	difficult nourishment, development	Any condition of abnormal development caused by defective nourishment, often noted by the degeneration of muscles
exercise			Performed activity of the muscles for improvement of health or correction of deformity

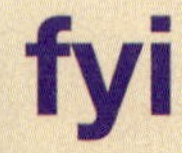

Types of exercise include:

Active. Muscular contraction and relaxation by patient

Assistive. Muscular contraction and relaxation with the assistance of a therapist

Isometric. Active muscular contraction performed against stable resistance, thereby not shortening muscle length

Passive. Exercise performed by another individual without patient assistance

Range of motion (ROM). Movement of each joint through its full range of motion (FROM); used to prevent loss of mobility or to regain usage after an injury or fracture

Relief of tension. Technique used to promote relaxation of the muscles and provide relief from tension

The National Institutes of Health (NIH) recommends that adults ages 18–64 engage in regular aerobic physical activity for 2.5 hours at moderate intensity or 1.25 hours at vigorous intensity each week. Moderate activities are those during which a person could talk but not sing. Vigorous activities are those during which a person could say only a few words without stopping for breath. *Note:* According to a study by the National Cancer Institute (NCI), people who engaged in leisure-time physical activity had life expectancy gains of as much as 4.5 years.

Medical Word	Part	Meaning	Definition
fascia (făsh´ĭ-ă)	fasc -ia	a band condition	Thin layer of connective tissue covering, supporting, or connecting the muscles or inner organs of the body
fasciitis (făs˝-ē-ī´ tĭs)	fasci -itis	a band inflammation	Inflammation of a fascia
fatigue (fă-tēg´)			State of tiredness occurring in a muscle as a result of repeated contractions

Medical Word	Word Parts		Definition
	Part	**Meaning**	
fibromyalgia syndrome (FMS) (fī″ brō-mī-ăl′ jē-ă sĭn′ drōm)	fibr/o my -algia	fiber muscle pain	Disorder with chronic, widespread musculoskeletal (MS) pain and fatigue. Other symptoms include sleep disorders, irritable bowel syndrome, depression, and chronic headaches. Although the exact cause is still unknown, fibromyalgia is often traced to an injury or physical or emotional trauma. The American College of Rheumatology (ACR) classifies a patient with fibromyalgia if at least 11 of 18 specific areas of the body (called *trigger points*) are painful under pressure. See Figure 7.10. The location of some of these trigger points includes the inside of the elbow joint, the front of the collarbone, and the base of the skull. Treatments for fibromyalgia are geared toward improving the quality of sleep, as well as reducing pain.

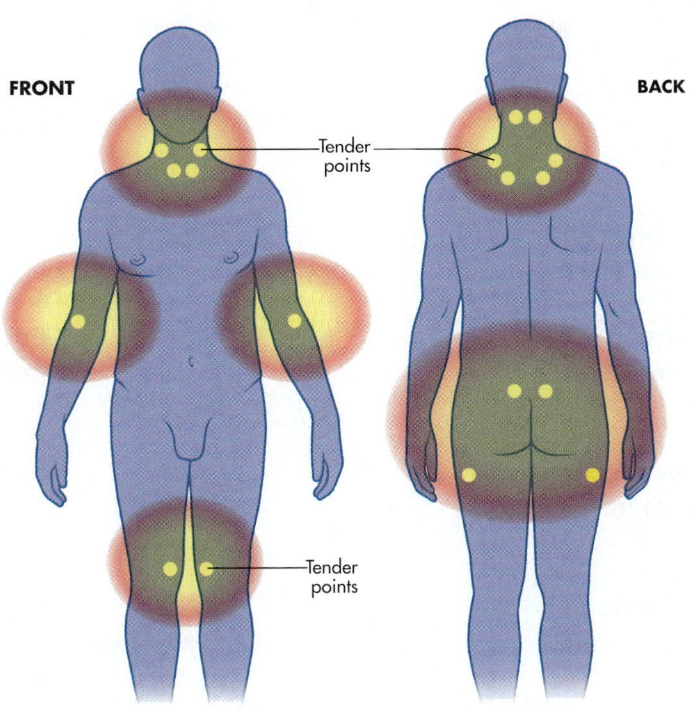

Figure 7.10 The 18 tender points of fibromyalgia.

Medical Word	Part	Meaning	Definition
fibromyitis (fī″ brō-mī-ī′ tĭs)	fibr/o my -itis	fiber muscle inflammation	Inflammation of muscle and fibrous tissue; also known as *fibromyositis*

Medical Word	Word Parts		Definition
	Part	**Meaning**	
First Aid Treatment—RICE (Rest Ice Compression Elevation)			**Cryotherapy** (use of cold) is the treatment of choice for soft-tissue and muscle injuries. It causes vasoconstriction of blood vessels and is effective in diminishing bleeding and edema. Ice should not be placed directly onto the skin. **Compression** by an elastic bandage is generally determined by the type of injury and physician preference. Some experts disagree on the use of elastic bandages. When used, the bandage should be 3–4 inches wide and applied firmly. Toes or fingers should be periodically checked for blue or white discoloration, indicating that the bandage is too tight. **Elevation** is used to reduce swelling. The injured part should be elevated above the level of the heart.
flaccid (flăk´ sĭd)			Lacking muscle tone; *weak*, *soft*, *flabby*
heat			Thermotherapy; treatment using scientific application of heat can be used 48–72 hours after the injury. Types: heating pad, hot water bottle, hot packs, infrared light, and immersion of body part in warm water.
hydrotherapy (hī-drō-thĕr´ ă-pē)	hydro- -therapy	water treatment	Treatment using scientific application of water; types: hot tub, cold bath, whirlpool, and vapor bath
insertion (ĭn-sĕr´ shŭn)	in- sert -ion	into to gain process	Point of attachment of a muscle to the part that it moves
intramuscular (IM) (ĭn″ tră-mŭs´ kū-lăr)	intra- muscul -ar	within muscle pertaining to	Pertaining to within a muscle, such as an IM injection
isometric (ī″ sō-mĕ´ trĭk)	is/o metr -ic	equal to measure pertaining to	Literally means *pertaining to having equal measure*; increasing tension of muscle while maintaining equal length
isotonic (ī″ sō-tŏn´ ĭk)	is/o ton -ic	equal tone, tension pertaining to	Pertaining to having the same tone or tension
levator (lē-vā´ tor)	levat -or	lifter a doer	Muscle that raises or elevates a part
massage (măh-săhzh)			Kneading that applies pressure and friction to external body tissues
muscle spasm (mŭs´ ĕl spăzm)			Involuntary contraction of one or more muscles; usually accompanied by pain and the limitation of function

Medical Word	Word Parts		Definition
	Part	Meaning	
muscular dystrophy (MD) (mŭs´ kū-lăr dĭs´ trō-fē)			Refers to a group of genetic diseases characterized by progressive weakness and degeneration of the skeletal or voluntary muscles that control movement. The muscles of the heart and some other involuntary muscles are also affected in some forms of MD, and a few forms involve other organs as well.

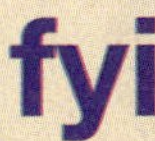

fyi MD can affect people of all ages, with some forms apparent in infancy or childhood and others not appearing until middle age or later. Duchenne muscular dystrophy, the most common form of MD affecting children, is an X-linked disorder seen mostly in males. In this disorder, the protein dystrophin is absent from muscle cells, leading to necrosis in muscle fibers and their replacement with connective tissue and fat. Myotonic MD is the most common form affecting adults. There is no specific treatment for any of the forms of MD. Physical therapy to prevent ***contractures*** (a condition in which shortened muscles around joints cause abnormal and sometimes painful positioning of the joints), ***orthoses*** (orthopedic appliances used for support), and corrective orthopedic surgery could be needed to improve the quality of life in some cases. Some cases of MD are mild and other cases have marked progressions of muscle weakness, functional disability, and loss of ambulation. See Figure 7.11.

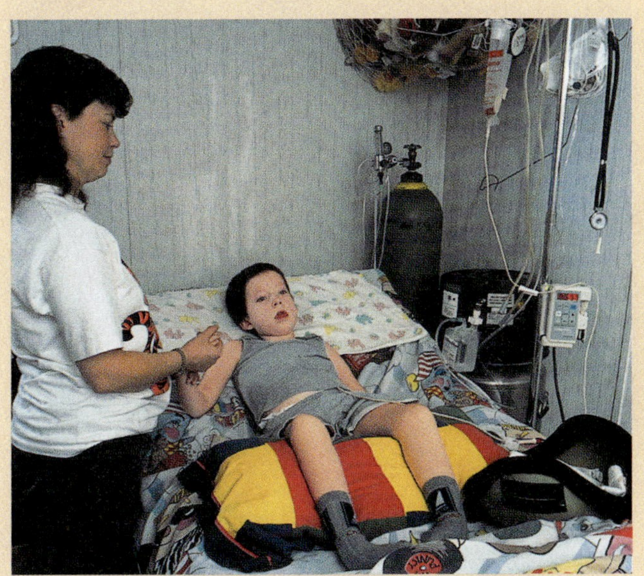

Figure 7.11 This young boy with muscular dystrophy needs to receive tube feedings and home nursing care. He attends school when possible and is able to use an adapted computer.

Source: Pearson Education, Inc.

Medical Word	Word Parts		Definition
	Part	Meaning	

fyi The **Gowers maneuver**, as seen in Figure 7.12, is the use of the upper extremity muscles to raise oneself to a standing position. This is a good indicator of muscle weakness of the legs caused by muscular dystrophy. Early in the diagnostic process, a serum creatine kinase (CK) test, an electromyography (EMG), and a muscle biopsy are ordered.

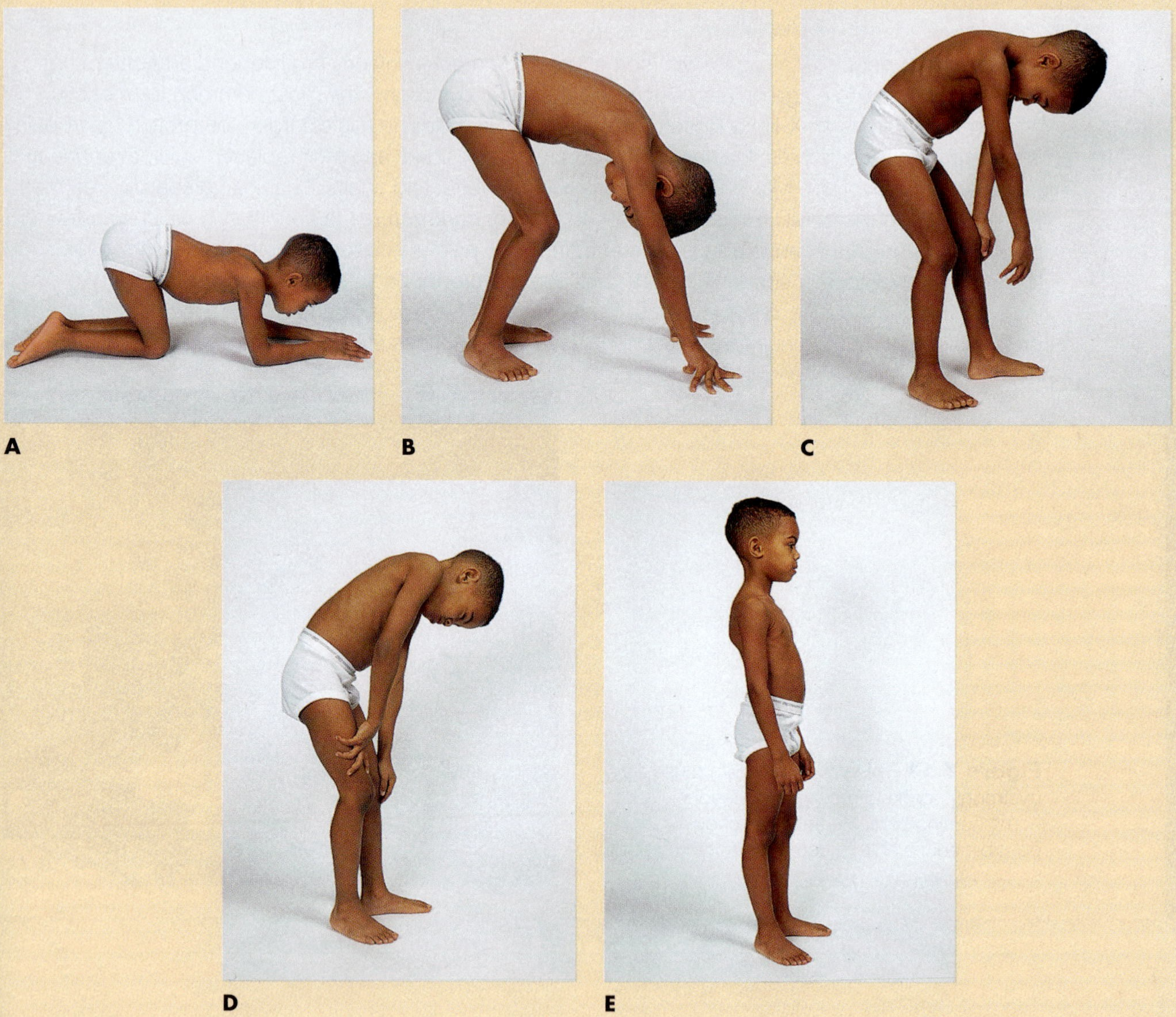

A B C

D E

Figure 7.12 Because the leg muscles of children with muscular dystrophy are weak, they must perform the Gowers maneuver to rise to a standing position. (A) and (B) The child first maneuvers to a position supported by arms and legs. (C) The child next pushes off the floor and rests one hand on the knee. (D) and (E) The child then pushes himself upright.

Source: Pearson Education, Inc.

Medical Word	Word Parts		Definition
	Part	**Meaning**	
myalgia (mī-ăl′ jĭ-ă)	my -algia	muscle pain	Pain in the muscle

insights Most of the codes within ICD-10-CM, Chapter 13, *Diseases of the Musculoskeletal System and Connective Tissue (M00-M99)*, have site and laterality designations. For conditions in which more than one bone, joint, or muscle is involved, such as osteoarthritis, there is a *multiple sites* code available. Many musculoskeletal conditions are a result of previous injury or trauma to a site, or are recurrent conditions. Bone, joint, or muscle conditions that are the result of a healed injury are usually found here as well. *Disorders of muscles* are coded M60–M63, *disorders of synovium and tendon* are coded M65–M67, and other *soft tissue disorders* are coded M70–M79.

Medical Word	Part	Meaning	Definition
myasthenia gravis (MG) (mī-ăs-thē′ nĭ-ă gră vĭs)	my -asthenia gravis	muscle weakness grave	Chronic autoimmune neuromuscular disease characterized by varying degrees of weakness of the skeletal (voluntary) muscles of the body. Its name, which is Latin and Greek in origin, literally means *grave muscle weakness*. The primary symptom is muscle weakness that increases during periods of activity and improves after periods of rest.
myoblast (mī′ ō blăst)	my/o -blast	muscle immature cell, germ cell	Embryonic cell that develops into a cell of muscle fiber
myofibroma (mī″ ō fī-brō′ mă)	my/o fibr -oma	muscle fiber tumor	Tumor that contains muscle and fiber
myograph (mī′ ō-grăf)	my/o -graph	muscle instrument for recording	Instrument used to record muscular contractions
myokinesis (mī″ ō-kĭn-ē′ sĭs)	my/o -kinesis	muscle motion	Muscular motion or activity
myoma (mī-ō′ mă)	my -oma	muscle tumor	Tumor containing muscle tissue

RULE REMINDER

The *o* has been removed from the combining form because the suffix begins with a vowel.

Medical Word	Part	Meaning	Definition
myomalacia (mī″ ō-mă-lā′ sĭ-ă)	my/o -malacia	muscle softening	Softening of muscle tissue
myoparesis (mī″ ō-păr′ ĕ-sĭs)	my/o -paresis	muscle weakness	Weakness or slight paralysis of a muscle

Medical Word	Word Parts		Definition
	Part	**Meaning**	
myopathy (mī-ŏp′ ă-thē)	my/o -pathy	muscle disease	Muscle disease

insights In ICD-10-CM, the code used for myopathy is G72.9 followed by more specific categories for types: *acute-necrotizing* (G72.81), *alcoholic* (G72.1), *benign congenital* (G71.2), and many more.

Medical Word	Part	Meaning	Definition
myoplasty (mī′ ō-plăs″ tē)	my/o -plasty	muscle surgical repair	Surgical repair of a muscle
myorrhaphy (mī-ŏr′ ă-fē)	my/o -rrhaphy	muscle suture	Surgical suture of a muscle wound
myosarcoma (mī″ ō-săr-kō′ mă)	my/o sarc -oma	muscle flesh tumor	Malignant tumor derived from muscle tissue
myosclerosis (mī″ ō-sklĕr-ō′ sĭs)	my/o scler -osis	muscle hardening condition	Abnormal condition of hardening of muscle
myositis (mī″ ō-sī′ tĭs)	my/o(s) -itis	muscle inflammation	Inflammation of muscle tissue, especially skeletal muscles; may be caused by infection, trauma, or parasitic infestation
myospasm (mī″ ō-spăzm)	my/o -spasm	muscle tension, spasm	Spasmodic contraction of a muscle
myotome (mī′ ō-tōm)	my/o -tome	muscle instrument to cut	Surgical instrument used to cut muscle
myotomy (mī″ ŏt′ ō-mē)	my/o -tomy	muscle incision	Surgical incision into a muscle
neuromuscular (nū″ rō-mŭs′ kū-lăr)	neur/o muscul -ar	nerve muscle pertaining to	Pertaining to both nerves and muscles
neuromyopathic (nū″ rō-mī″ ō-păth′ ĭk)	neur/o my/o path -ic	nerve muscle disease pertaining to	Pertaining to a disease condition involving both nerves and muscles
polyplegia (pŏl″ ē-plē′ jĭ-ă)	poly- -plegia	many stroke, paralysis	Paralysis affecting many muscles

Medical Word	Word Parts		Definition
	Part	Meaning	
position			Bodily posture or attitude; the manner in which a patient's body may be arranged for examination. See Table 7.3.

Table 7.3 Types of Patient Positions

Position	Description
anatomic	Body erect, head facing forward, arms by the sides with palms to the front; used as a standard anatomical position of reference
dorsal recumbent	On back with lower extremities flexed and rotated outward; used in application of obstetric forceps, vaginal and rectal examination, and bimanual palpation
Fowler	Head of the bed or examining table is raised about 18 inches or 46 cm; patient sitting up with knees also elevated Fowler position
knee-chest	On knees, thighs upright, head and upper part of chest resting on bed or examining table, arms crossed and above head; used in sigmoidoscopy, displacement of prolapsed uterus, rectal exams, and flushing of intestinal canal
lithotomy	On back with lower extremities flexed and feet placed in stirrups; used in vaginal examination, Pap smear, vaginal operations, and diagnosis and treatment of diseases of the urethra and bladder Lithotomy position
orthopneic	Sitting upright or erect; used for patients with dyspnea, shortness of breath (SOB)
prone	Lying face downward; used in examination of the back, injections, and massage Prone position
Sims	Lying on left side, right knee and thigh flexed well up above left leg that is slightly flexed, left arm behind the body, and right arm forward, flexed at elbow; used in examination of rectum, sigmoidoscopy, enema, and intrauterine irrigation after labor

(*continued*)

Medical Word	Word Parts		Definition
	Part	**Meaning**	

Table 7.3 Types of Patient Positions (*continued*)

Position	Description
supine	Lying flat on back with face upward and arms at the sides; used in examining the head, neck, chest, abdomen, and extremities and in assessing vital signs Supine position
Trendelenburg	Body supine on a bed or examining table that is tilted at about a 45° angle with the head lower than the feet; used to displace abdominal organs during surgery and in treating cardiovascular shock Trendelenburg position

Medical Word	Part	Meaning	Definition
prosthesis (prŏs´ thē-sĭs)	prosth/e -sis	an addition condition	Artificial device used to replace an organ or body part, such as a hand, arm, leg, or hip. See Figure 7.13.

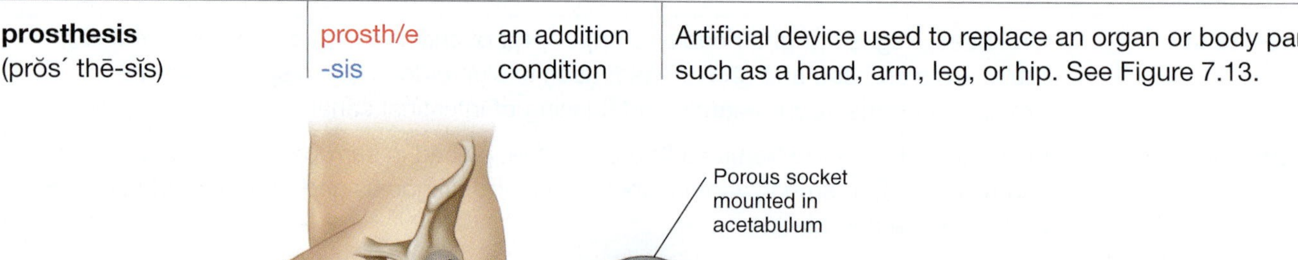

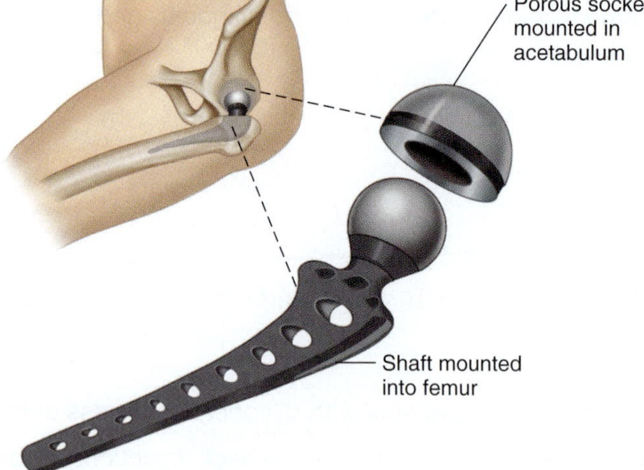

Figure 7.13 Total hip prosthesis.

Medical Word	Part	Meaning	Definition
quadriceps (kwŏd´ rĭ-sĕps)	quadri- -ceps	four head	Muscle that has four heads or points of origin
relaxation (rē-lăk-sā´ shŭn)	relaxat -ion	to loosen process	Process in which a muscle loosens and returns to a resting stage
rhabdomyoma (răb˝ dō-mī-ō´ mă)	rhabd/o my -oma	rod muscle tumor	Tumor of striated muscle tissue

Medical Word	Word Parts: Part	Word Parts: Meaning	Definition
rheumatism (roo´ mă-tĭzm)	rheumat -ism	discharge condition	General term used to describe conditions characterized by inflammation, soreness, and stiffness of muscles and pain in joints

RULE REMINDER

The *o* has been removed from the combining form because the suffix begins with a vowel.

Medical Word	Word Parts: Part	Word Parts: Meaning	Definition
rheumatology (roo″mă-tŏl´ ō-jē)	rheumat/o -logy	discharge study of	Study of rheumatic diseases
rheumatologist (roo″mă-tŏl´-ō-jĭst)	rheumat/o -log -ist	discharge study of one who specializes	One who specializes in rheumatic diseases
rigor mortis (rĭg´ ur mōr tĭs)			Stiffness of skeletal muscles seen in death; develops between the 4th and 24th hour after death, then ceases
rotation (rō-tā´ shŭn)	rotat -ion	to turn process	Process of moving a body part around a central axis
rotator cuff (rō-tā´ tor kŭf)			Group of muscles and their tendons that act to stabilize the shoulder

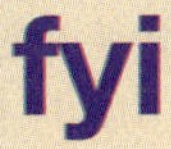

fyi The rotator cuff is the area that enables people to reach above their heads and lift with the arms. Rotator cuff injuries and/or tears can occur as the result of years of overuse of the muscles and tendons or from a single traumatic injury. The four muscles of the rotator cuff (subscapularis, supraspinatus, infraspinatus, and teres minor), along with the teres major and the deltoid, make up the six **scapulohumeral** muscles (those that connect to the humerus and scapula and act on the glenohumeral joint) of the human body.

Medical Word	Word Parts: Part	Word Parts: Meaning	Definition
sarcolemma (săr″ kō-lĕm´ ă)	sarc/o -lemma	flesh a rind	Plasma membrane surrounding each striated muscle fiber
spasticity (spăs-tĭs´ ĭ-tē)	spastic -ity	convulsive condition	Condition of increased muscular tone causing stiff and awkward movements
sternocleidomastoid (stur″ nō-klī″ dō-măs´ toyd)	stern/o cleid/o mast -oid	sternum clavicle breast resemble	Muscle arising from the sternum and clavicle with its insertion in the mastoid process
strain			Excessive, forcible stretching of a muscle or the musculotendinous unit
synergetic (sĭn″ ĕr-jĕt´ ĭk)	syn- erget -ic	with, together work pertaining to	Pertaining to certain muscles that work together

Medical Word	Word Parts		Definition
	Part	**Meaning**	
synovitis (sĭn″ ō-vī′ tĭs)	synov -itis	synovial membrane inflammation	Inflammation of a synovial membrane
tendon (tĕn′ dŭn)	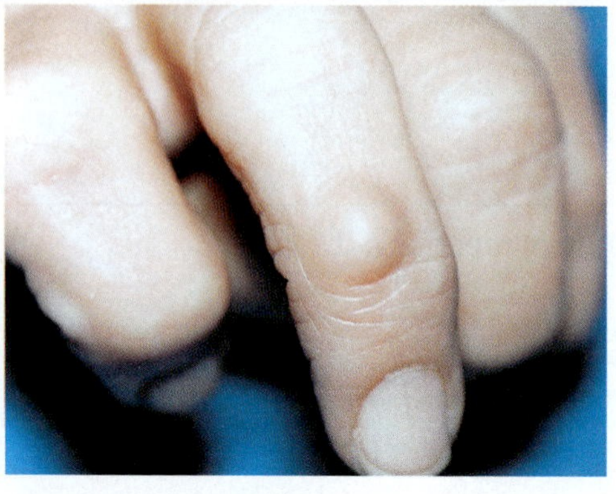 **Figure 7.14** Giant cell tumor of tendon sheath. (Courtesy of Jason L. Smith, MD)		Band of fibrous connective tissue serving for the attachment of muscles to bones; a giant cell tumor of a tendon sheath is a benign, small, yellow, tumorlike nodule. See Figure 7.14.
tenodesis (tĕn-ŏd′ ĕ-sĭs)	ten/o -desis	tendon binding	Surgical binding of a tendon
tenodynia (tĕn″ ō-dĭn-ĭ-ă)	ten/o -dynia	tendon pain	Pain in a tendon
tetany (tĕt′ ă-nē)			Condition characterized by cramps, convulsions, twitching of the muscles, and sharp flexion of the wrist and ankle joints; generally caused by an abnormality in calcium (Ca) metabolism
tonic (tŏn′ ĭk)	ton -ic	tone, tension pertaining to	Pertaining to tone, especially muscular tension
torsion (tor′ shŭn)	tors -ion	twisted process	Process of being twisted
torticollis (tor″ tĭ-kŏl′ ĭs)	tort/i -collis	twisted neck	Stiff neck caused by spasmodic contraction of the muscles of the neck; sometimes called *wryneck*

insights In the ICD-10-CM, the code used for torticollis is M43.6, followed by more specific categories for types: *congenital sternomastoid deformity* (Q68.0), *sternomastoid injury due to birth injury* (P15.8), ***spasmodic torticollis*** (G24.3), and many others.

Medical Word	Part	Meaning	Definition
triceps (trī′ sĕps)	tri- -ceps	three head	Muscle having three heads with a single insertion
voluntary (vŏl′ ŭn-tĕr″ ē)	volunt -ary	will pertaining to	Under the control of one's will

Study and Review II

Word Parts

Prefixes

Give the definitions of the following prefixes.

1. a- ______________________
2. ab- ______________________
3. ad- ______________________
4. ant- ______________________
5. bi- ______________________
6. brady- ______________________
7. con- ______________________
8. dia- ______________________
9. dys- ______________________
10. in- ______________________
11. intra- ______________________
12. hydro- ______________________
13. quadri- ______________________
14. syn- ______________________
15. tri- ______________________

Combining Forms

Give the definitions of the following combining forms.

1. agon/o ______________________
2. amputat/o ______________________
3. brach/i ______________________
4. cleid/o ______________________
5. clon/o ______________________
6. duct/o ______________________
7. fasci/o ______________________
8. fibr/o ______________________
9. is/o ______________________
10. metr/o ______________________
11. muscul/o ______________________
12. my/o ______________________
13. neur/o ______________________
14. path/o ______________________
15. prosth/e ______________________
16. rhabd/o ______________________
17. rotat/o ______________________
18. sarc/o ______________________
19. synov/o ______________________
20. ten/o ______________________
21. ton/o ______________________
22. tors/o ______________________
23. troph/o ______________________
24. volunt/o ______________________

Suffixes

Give the definitions of the following suffixes.

1. -algia ____________________
2. -ar ____________________
3. -ary ____________________
4. -asthenia ____________________
5. -blast ____________________
6. -ceps ____________________
7. -desis ____________________
8. -dynia ____________________
9. -in ____________________
10. -therapy ____________________
11. -graph ____________________
12. -ia ____________________
13. -ic ____________________
14. -ion ____________________
15. -ist ____________________
16. -itis ____________________
17. -ity ____________________
18. -kinesia ____________________
19. -kinesis ____________________
20. -logy ____________________
21. -ure ____________________
22. -malacia ____________________
23. -oid ____________________
24. -oma ____________________
25. -or ____________________
26. -osis ____________________
27. -paresis ____________________
28. -pathy ____________________
29. -phragm ____________________
30. -plasty ____________________
31. -plegia ____________________
32. -rrhaphy ____________________
33. -y ____________________
34. -spasm ____________________
35. -taxia ____________________
36. -tome ____________________
37. -tomy ____________________
38. -trophy ____________________
39. -sis ____________________
40. -ism ____________________

Identifying Medical Terms

In the spaces provided, write the medical terms for the following meanings.

1. ____________________ Pertaining to a lack of normal tone or tension
2. ____________________ Slowness of motion or movement
3. ____________________ Medical term for cramp of a finger or toe

4. ______________________________ Any condition of abnormal development caused by defective nourishment, often noted by the degeneration of muscles

5. ______________________________ Pertaining to within a muscle, such as an IM injection

6. ______________________________ Muscle that raises or elevates a part

7. ______________________________ Chronic autoimmune neuromuscular disease characterized by varying degrees of weakness of the skeletal (voluntary) muscles of the body

8. ______________________________ Weakness or slight paralysis of a muscle

9. ______________________________ Surgical repair of a muscle

10. ______________________________ Malignant tumor derived from muscle tissue

11. ______________________________ Surgical incision into a muscle

12. ______________________________ Paralysis affecting many muscles

13. ______________________________ Surgical binding of a tendon

14. ______________________________ Pertaining to certain muscles that work together

15. ______________________________ Muscle having three heads with a single insertion

Matching

Select the appropriate lettered meaning for each of the following words.

__________ **1.** dermatomyositis

__________ **2.** fibromyalgia

__________ **3.** muscular dystrophy

__________ **4.** flaccid

__________ **5.** prosthesis

__________ **6.** rotator cuff

__________ **7.** strain

__________ **8.** tenodynia

__________ **9.** torsion

__________ **10.** voluntary

a. Group of muscles and their tendons that act to stabilize the shoulder

b. Process of being twisted

c. Pain in a tendon

d. Chronic immunological disease with systemic pathology

e. Lacking muscle tone; *weak*, *soft*, and *flabby*

f. Under the control of one's will

g. Refers to a group of genetic diseases characterized by progressive weakness and degeneration of the skeletal or voluntary muscles that control movement

h. Excessive, forcible stretching of a muscle or the musculotendinous unit

i. A chronic widespread musculoskeletal pain and fatigue disorder

j. Artificial device used to replace an organ or a body part, such as a hand, arm, leg, or hip

k. Pain in a joint

Medical Case Snapshots

This learning activity provides an opportunity to relate the medical terminology you are learning to a precise patient case presentation. In the spaces provided, write in your answers.

Case 1

The 30-year-old female states, "I feel so tired all the time. I can't sleep at night and my muscles ache." The diagnosis is abbreviated FMS. The American College of Rheumatology classifies a patient with ____________ (FMS) if at least 11 of 18 trigger points are painful under pressure. This patient had 12 trigger points including tiredness or fatigue, and muscle pain or ____________.

Case 2

The mother of a 3-year-old boy states that her son is beginning to appear "clumsy" with increasing episodes of falling. He has trouble getting back up to his feet and has to use his upper body to arise. The physician suspects early onset of ____________ ____________, a term for a group of genetic diseases characterized by progressive weakness and degeneration of the skeletal muscles. The ____________ maneuver is the use of the upper extremity muscles to raise oneself to a standing position. (See Figure 7.12.)

Case 3

The instructor thought it would be a fun and educational experience to ask her students to stand and demonstrate the standard anatomic position. The student should stand with his or her ____________ ____________, head facing ____________, arms by the sides with ____________ to the front. (See Table 7.3.)

Drug Highlights

Type of Drug	Description and Examples
skeletal muscle relaxants	Used to treat painful muscle spasms that can result from strains, sprains, and musculoskeletal trauma or disease. Centrally acting muscle relaxants depress the central nervous system (CNS) and can be administered orally or by injection. The patient must be informed of the sedative effect produced by these drugs. Drowsiness, dizziness, and blurred vision can diminish the patient's ability to drive a vehicle, operate equipment, or climb stairs. EXAMPLES: Flexeril (cyclobenzaprine HCl), and Robaxin (methocarbamol)
anti-inflammatory agents and analgesics	(See *Drug Highlights* in Chapter 6 for a description of anti-inflammatory agents and analgesics.)

Diagnostic and Laboratory Tests

Test	Description
aldolase (ALD) blood test (ăl´ dō-lāz)	Test performed on serum that measures ALD enzyme present in skeletal and heart muscle; helpful in the diagnosis of Duchenne muscular dystrophy before symptoms appear.
calcium blood test (kăl´ sē-ŭm)	Test performed on serum to determine levels of calcium, which is essential for muscular contraction, nerve transmission, and blood clotting.
creatine kinase (CK) (krē´ ă-tĭn kĭn´ āz)	Blood test to determine the level of CK, which is increased in necrosis or atrophy of skeletal muscle, traumatic muscle injury, strenuous exercise, and progressive muscular dystrophy.
electromyography (EMG) (ē-lĕk˝ trō-mī-ŏg´ ră-fē)	Test to measure electrical activity across muscle membranes by means of electrodes attached to a needle that is inserted into the muscle. Electrical activity can be heard over a loudspeaker, viewed on an oscilloscope, or printed on a graph (electromyogram). Abnormal results can indicate myasthenia gravis, amyotrophic lateral sclerosis, muscular dystrophy, peripheral neuropathy, and anterior poliomyelitis.
lactic dehydrogenase (LDH, LD) (lăk´ tĭk dē-hī-drŏj´ ĕ-nāz)	Blood test to determine the level of LDH enzyme, which is increased in muscular dystrophy, damage to skeletal muscles, after a pulmonary embolism, and during skeletal muscle malignancy.

Test	Description
muscle biopsy	Surgical removal of a small piece of muscle tissue for examination. There are two types. A *needle biopsy* involves inserting a needle into the muscle. When the needle is removed, a small piece of tissue remains in the needle. The tissue is sent to a laboratory for examination. An *open biopsy* involves making a small cut in the skin and into the muscle. The muscle tissue is then removed. A muscle biopsy may be done to identify or detect diseases of the connective tissue and blood vessels (e.g., polyarteritis nodosa); infections that affect the muscles (e.g., trichinosis or toxoplasmosis); muscular disorders such as muscular dystrophy or congenital myopathy; and metabolic defects of the muscle.
aspartate aminotransferase (AST) (ă-spăr-´tāt˝ ă-mē˝ nō-trăns´fĕr-ās)	Blood test to determine the level of AST enzyme, which is increased in skeletal muscle damage and muscular dystrophy
alanine aminotransferase (ALT) (ăl´ăh-nēn ă-mē´nō-trăns´fĕr-ās)	Blood test to determine the level of ALT enzyme, which is increased in skeletal muscle damage

Abbreviations

Abbreviation	Meaning	Abbreviation	Meaning
ACR	American College of Rheumatology	**FMS**	fibromyalgia syndrome
AE	above elbow	**FROM**	full range of motion
AK	above knee	**IM**	intramuscular
ALD	aldolase	**LDH, LD**	lactic dehydrogenase
ALT	alanine aminotransferase	**MD**	muscular dystrophy
AST	aspartate aminotransferase	**MG**	myasthenia gravis
BE	below elbow	**MS**	musculoskeletal
BK	below knee	**NCI**	National Cancer Institute
Ca	calcium	**NIH**	National Institutes of Health
CK	creatine kinase	**ROM**	range of motion
EMG	electromyography	**SOB**	shortness of breath

Study and Review III

Building Medical Terms

Using the following word parts, fill in the blanks to build the correct medical terms.

a-	ten/o	-graph
bi-	-ion	-lemma
poly-	-ary	
rhabd/o	-or	

Definition	Medical Term
1. Surgical removal of a limb, part, or other appendage	amputat______
2. Lack of muscular coordination	_________taxia
3. Muscle with two points of origin	_________ceps
4. Muscle that raises or elevates a part	levat_________
5. Instrument used to record muscular contractions	myo_________
6. Paralysis affecting many muscles	_________plegia
7. Tumor of striated muscle tissue	_______myoma
8. Plasma membrane surrounding each striated muscle fiber	sarco_________
9. Pain in a tendon	_________dynia
10. Under the control of one's will	volunt________

Combining Form Challenge

Using the combining forms provided, write the medical term correctly.

brach/i	fasci/o	my/o
dactyl/o	is/o	sarc/o

1. Pain in the arm: __________algia
2. Medical term for cramp of a finger or toe: ______________spasm
3. Inflammation of a fascia: ______________itis
4. Literally means pertaining to having equal measure: _____________metric
5. Weakness or slight paralysis of a muscle: ______________paresis
6. Plasma membrane surrounding each striated muscle fiber: _____________lemma

Select the Right Term

Select the correct answer, and write it on the line provided.

1. Muscle that counteracts the action of another muscle is _______________.

   adductor **aponeurosis** **antagonist** **atrophy**

2. Pertains to alternate contraction and relaxation of muscles is ____________.

   bradykinesia **clonic** **contracture** **dystonia**

3. Lacking muscle tone; weak, soft, and flabby is ______________.

   isotonic **myokinesis** **flaccid** **relaxation**

4. Surgical repair of a muscle is _______________.

   myopathy **myoplasty** **myorrhaphy** **myotome**

5. Pertaining to certain muscles that work together is ______________.

   synergetic **synovitis** **adductor** **tetany**

6. Process of being twisted is _______________.

   triceps **torticollis** **tonic** **tenodesis**

Diagnostic and Laboratory Tests

Select the best answer to each multiple-choice question. Circle the letter of your choice.

1. Diagnostic test to help diagnose Duchenne muscular dystrophy before symptoms appear.
   a. creatine kinase
   b. aldolase blood test
   c. calcium blood test
   d. muscle biopsy

2. Test to measure electrical activity across muscle membranes by means of electrodes that are attached to a needle that is inserted into the muscle.
   a. muscle biopsy
   b. lactic dehydrogenase
   c. creatine kinase
   d. electromyography

3. Blood test to determine the level of _________ enzyme, which is increased in skeletal muscle damage and muscular dystrophy, is:
   a. lactic dehydrogenase
   b. aspartate aminotransferase
   c. aldolase
   d. creatine kinase

4. Blood test to determine the level of _____________ enzyme, which is increased in skeletal muscle damage is:
   a. lactic dehydrogenase
   b. aldolase
   c. alanine aminotransferase
   d. creatine kinase

5. A/an _________________________________ is the surgical removal of a small piece of muscle tissue for examination.
   a. muscle biopsy
   b. electromyography
   c. bone biopsy
   d. electrocardiography

Abbreviations

Place the correct word, phrase, or abbreviation in the space provided.

1. AE ________________________________
2. AST ________________________________
3. calcium ________________________________
4. electromyography ________________________________
5. FROM ________________________________
6. MS ________________________________
7. range of motion ________________________________
8. MG ________________________________
9. MD ________________________________
10. FMS ________________________________

Practical Application

Medical Record Analysis

This exercise contains information, abbreviations, and medical terminology from an actual medical record or case study that has been adapted for this text. The names and any personal information have been created by the author. Read and study each form or case study and then answer the questions that follow. You may refer to Appendix III, *Abbreviations and Symbols*.

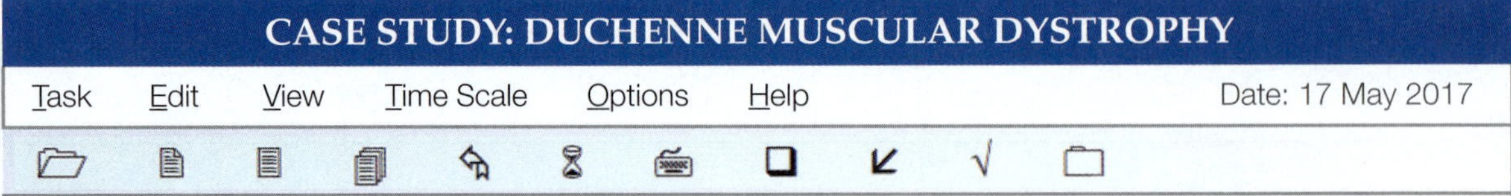

A 3-year-old male child was seen by a physician; the following is a synopsis of the visit.

Present History: The mother states that she noticed that her son has been falling a lot and seems to be very clumsy. She says that he has a waddling gait, is very slow in running and climbing, and walks on his toes. She is most concerned as she is at risk for carrying the gene that causes muscular dystrophy (MD).

Signs and Symptoms: A waddling gait, very slow in running and climbing, walks on his toes, frequent falling, clumsy.

Diagnosis: Duchenne muscular dystrophy. The diagnosis was determined by the characteristic symptoms, family history, a muscle biopsy, an electromyography (EMG), and an elevated serum creatine kinase (CK) level.

Treatment: Physical therapy, deep breathing exercises to help delay muscular weakness, supportive measures such as splints and braces to help minimize deformities and to preserve mobility. Counseling and referral services are essential. For more information and resources, the family may visit the website of the Muscular Dystrophy Association at *www.mda.org*.

Case Study Questions

Place the correct answer in the space provided.

1. Signs and symptoms of Duchenne muscular dystrophy include a ______________________ gait, frequent falls, clumsiness, slowness in running and climbing, and walking on toes.

2. The diagnosis was determined by the characteristic symptoms, family history, a muscle biopsy, an ______________________, and an elevated serum creatine kinase level.

3. As part of the treatment for Duchenne muscular dystrophy, the use of splints and braces help to (a) ______________________ and (b) ______________________.

4. Define electromyography. ____

5. Define muscle biopsy. ____

Chapter

8 Digestive System

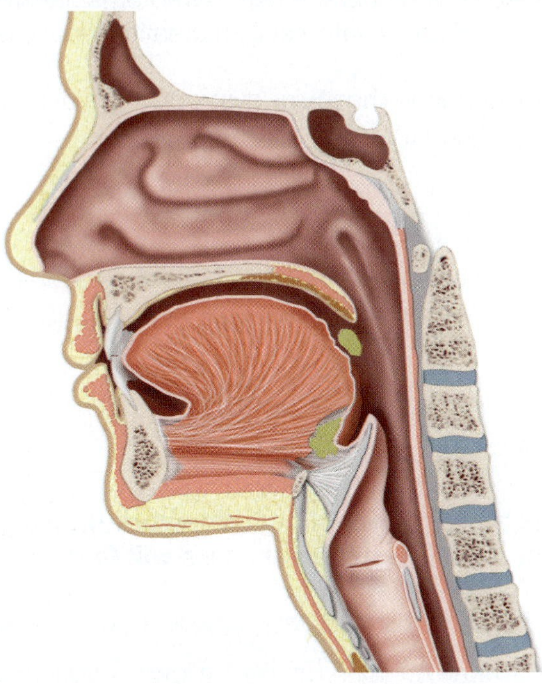

Learning Outcomes

On completion of this chapter, you will be able to:

1. Describe the digestive system.
2. Explain the primary functions of the organs of the digestive system.
3. Describe the two sets of teeth found in humans.
4. Identify the three main portions of a tooth.
5. Discuss the accessory organs of the digestive system and state their functions.
6. Recognize terminology included in the ICD-10-CM.
7. Analyze, build, spell, and pronounce medical words.
8. Comprehend the drugs highlighted in this chapter.
9. Describe diagnostic and laboratory tests related to the digestive system.
10. Identify and define selected abbreviations.
11. Apply your acquired knowledge of medical terms by successfully completing the *Practical Application* exercise.

Anatomy and Physiology

A general description of the digestive or gastrointestinal (GI) system is that of a continuous tube beginning with the mouth and ending at the anus. This tube is known as the **alimentary canal** and/or **gastrointestinal tract**. It measures about 30 feet in adults and contains both primary and accessory organs for the conversion of food and fluids into a semiliquid that can be absorbed for the body to use.

The three main functions of the digestive system are digestion, absorption, and elimination. **Digestion** is the process by which food is changed in the mouth, stomach, and intestines by chemical, mechanical, and physical action, so that the body can absorb it. Digestive enzymes increase chemical reactions and, in so doing, break down complex nutrients. See further discussion of chemical digestion in Table 8.2. **Absorption** is the process by which nutrient material is taken into the bloodstream or lymph and travels to all cells of the body. Valuable nutrients such as amino acids, glucose, fatty acids, and glycerol can then be utilized for energy, growth, and development of the body. **Elimination** is the process whereby the solid waste (end) products of digestion are excreted. Each of the various organs commonly associated with digestion is described in this chapter. See Table 8.1 for the digestive system at-a-glance. The organs of digestion are shown in Figure 8.1.

Table 8.1 Digestive System at-a-Glance

Organ/Structure	Primary Functions/Description
Mouth	Mechanically breaks food apart by the action of the teeth; moistens and lubricates food with saliva; food formed into a **bolus**, a soft mass of chewed food ready to be swallowed
Teeth	Used in mastication (chewing)
Salivary glands	Secrete saliva to moisten and lubricate food
Pharynx	Common passageway for both respiration and digestion; muscular constrictions move the swallowed bolus into the esophagus
Esophagus	Moves the bolus by peristalsis (wavelike contractions) down the esophagus into the stomach
Stomach	Reduces food to a digestible state; converts the food to a semiliquid state called **chyme** (mixture of partly digested food and digestive secretions)
Small intestine	Digestion and absorption take place chiefly in the small intestine; nutrients are absorbed and transferred to body cells by the circulatory system
Large intestine	Reabsorbs water from the fecal material, stores, and then eliminates waste from the body via the rectum and anus
Liver	Changes glucose to glycogen and stores it until needed; changes glycogen back to glucose; desaturates fats; assists in protein catabolism (the breaking down of molecules to form simpler ones); manufactures bile, fibrinogen, prothrombin, heparin, and blood proteins; stores vitamins; produces heat; and detoxifies toxins
Gallbladder	Stores and concentrates bile that has been produced by the liver
Pancreas	Secretes pancreatic juice into the small intestine, contains cells that produce digestive enzymes, produces the hormones insulin and glucagon

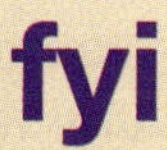

With aging, the digestive system becomes less motile, as muscle contractions become weaker. Glandular secretions decrease, thus causing a drier mouth and a lower volume of gastric juices. Nutrient absorption is mildly reduced due to **atrophy** of the mucosal lining. The teeth are mechanically worn down with age, and the gums begin to recede from the teeth. There is a loss of taste buds, and food preferences change. Gastric motor activity slows; as a result, gastric emptying is delayed and hunger contractions diminish.

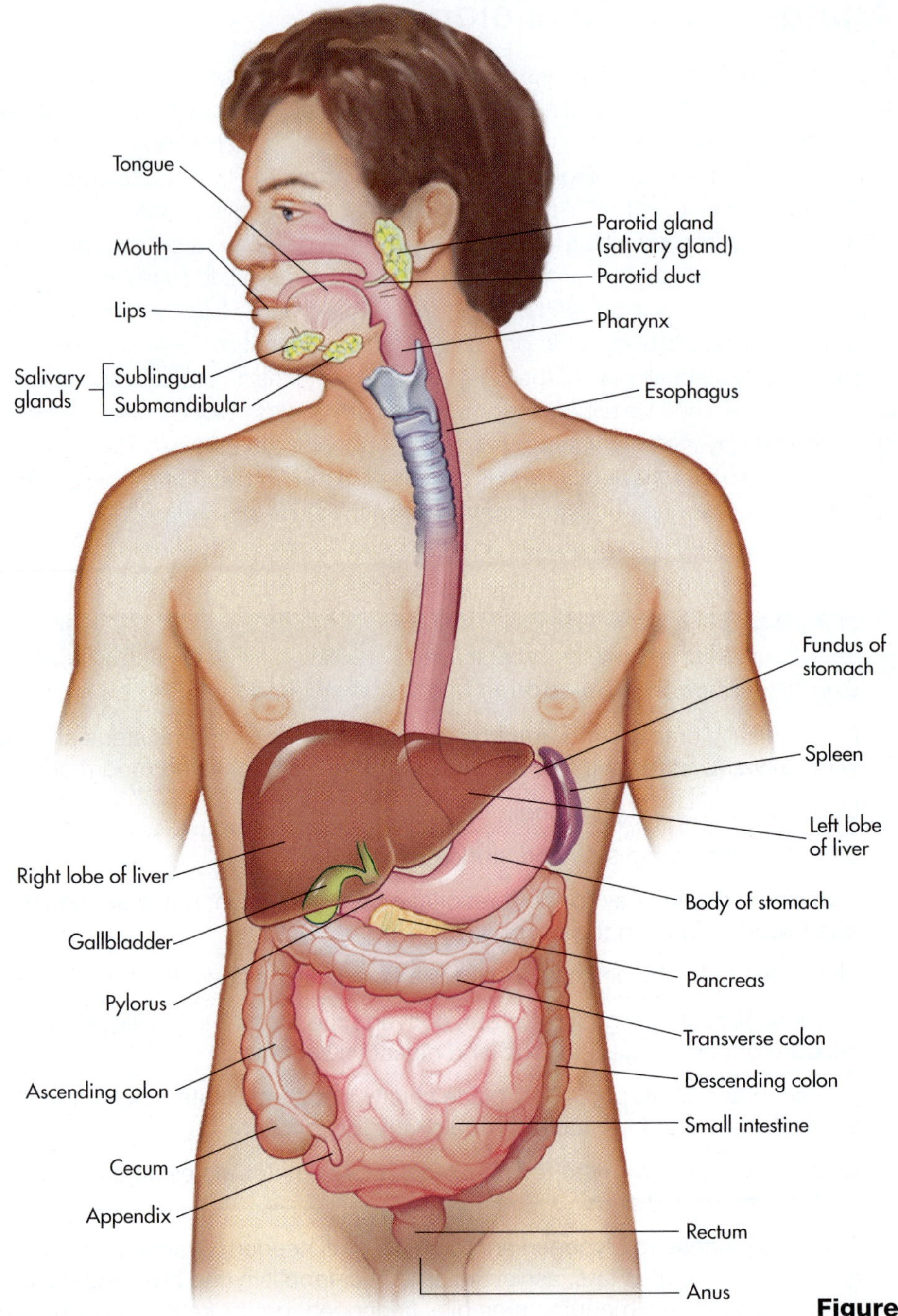

Figure 8.1 Digestive system.

Mouth

The **mouth** or oral cavity is formed by the hard and soft palates at the top or roof, the cheeks on the sides, the tongue at the floor, and the lips that frame the opening to the cavity. Contained within are the teeth and salivary glands. The vestibule includes the space between the cheeks and the teeth. The **gingivae** (gums) surround the necks of the teeth. See Figures 8.2A and 8.4A. The free portion of the tongue is connected to the underlying epithelium by a thin fold of mucous membrane, the **lingual frenulum**, which prevents extreme movement of the tongue. See Figure 8.2B.

The **tongue** is made of skeletal muscle and is covered with mucous membrane. It manipulates food during chewing and assists in swallowing. The tongue can be divided into a blunt rear portion called the **root**, a pointed **tip**, and a central **body**. Located on the surface of the tongue are **papillae** (elevations) and **taste buds** (sweet, salt, sour, and bitter). Three pairs of salivary glands secrete saliva into the oral cavity. The posterior margin

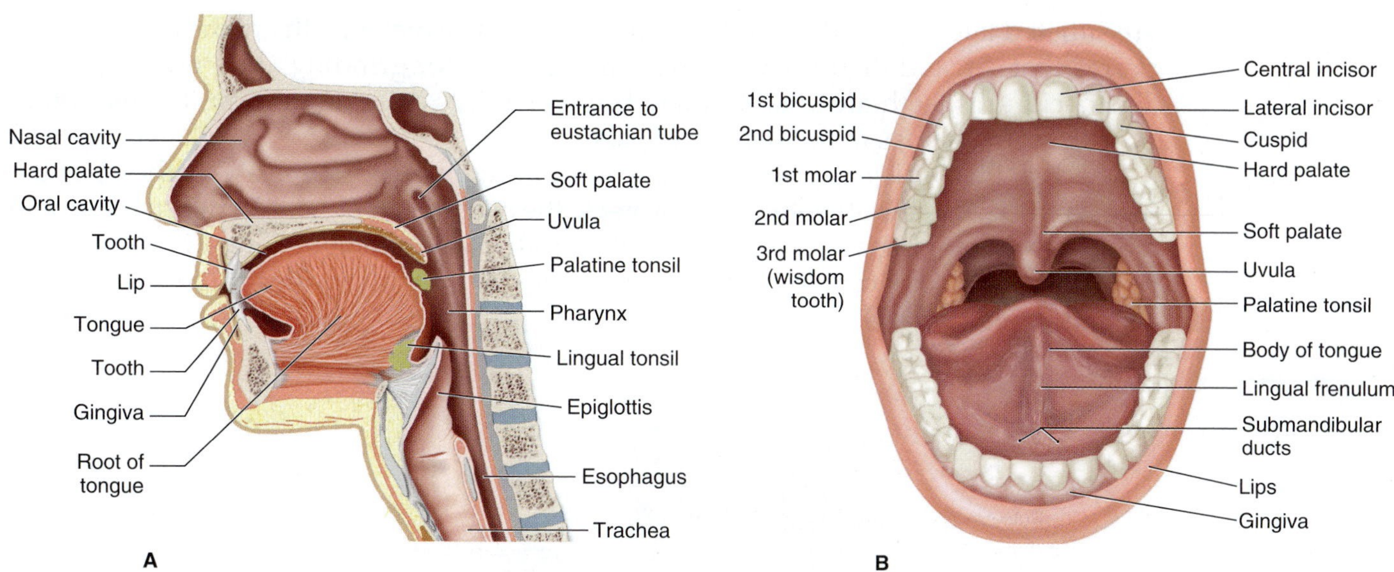

Figure 8.2 Oral cavity: (A) sagittal section; (B) anterior view as seen through the open mouth.

of the soft palate supports the dangling uvula and two pairs of muscular pharyngeal arches. On either side, a palatine tonsil lies between an anterior glossopalatine arch and a posterior pharyngopalatine arch. A curving line that connects the palatine arches and uvula forms the boundaries of the fauces, the passageway between the oral cavity and the pharynx. See Figure 8.2A. Digestion begins as food is broken apart by the action of the teeth, moistened and lubricated by saliva, and formed into a bolus. See Figure 8.3.

Teeth

Human beings are provided two sets of teeth. The 20 **deciduous teeth**, the temporary teeth of the primary dentition, include eight incisors, four canines (cuspids), and eight molars. Deciduous teeth are also referred to as *milk teeth* or *baby teeth*. There are 32 **permanent** or **secondary dentition teeth**: eight incisors, four canines, eight premolars, and 12 molars.

The **incisors** are so named because they present a sharp cutting edge, adapted for biting into food. They form the four front teeth in each dental arch. The **canine** or **cuspid** teeth are larger and stronger than the incisors. Their roots sink deeply into the bones and cause well-marked prominences upon the surface. The **premolars** or **bicuspid** teeth

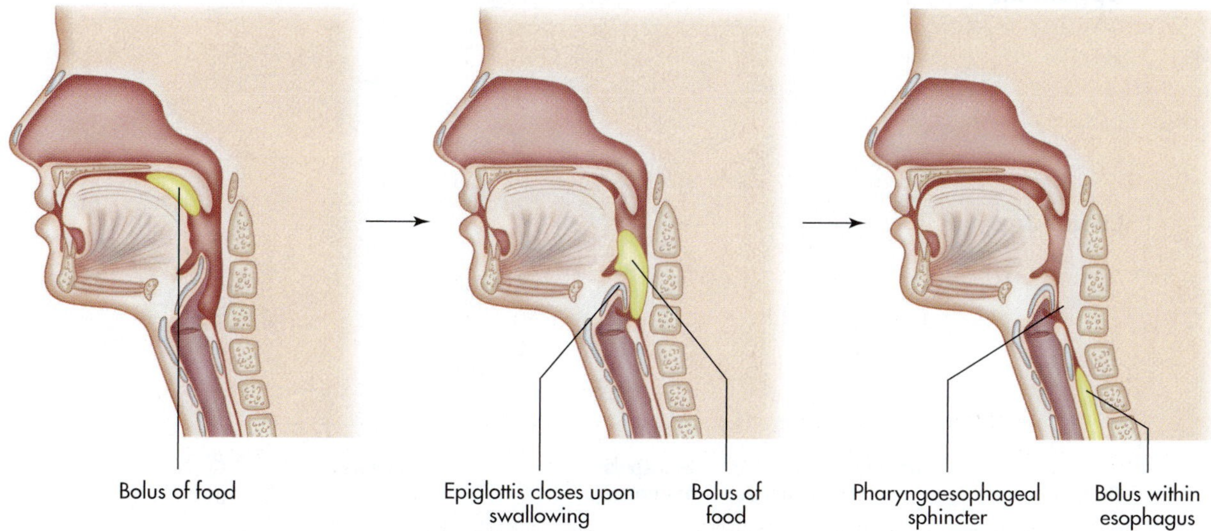

Figure 8.3 Movement of a bolus of food from the mouth to the esophagus. The bolus then travels to the stomach.

are situated lateral to and behind the canine teeth. The **molar** teeth are the largest of the permanent set, and their broad crowns are adapted for grinding and pounding food. The deciduous teeth are smaller than, but generally resemble in form, the teeth that bear the same names in the permanent set.

Each tooth consists of three main portions: the **crown**, projecting above the gum; the *root*, embedded in the alveolus; and the **neck**, the constricted portion between the crown and root. On making a vertical section of a tooth, a cavity will be found in the interior of the crown and the center of each root; it opens by a minute orifice at the extremity of the latter. See Figure 8.4.

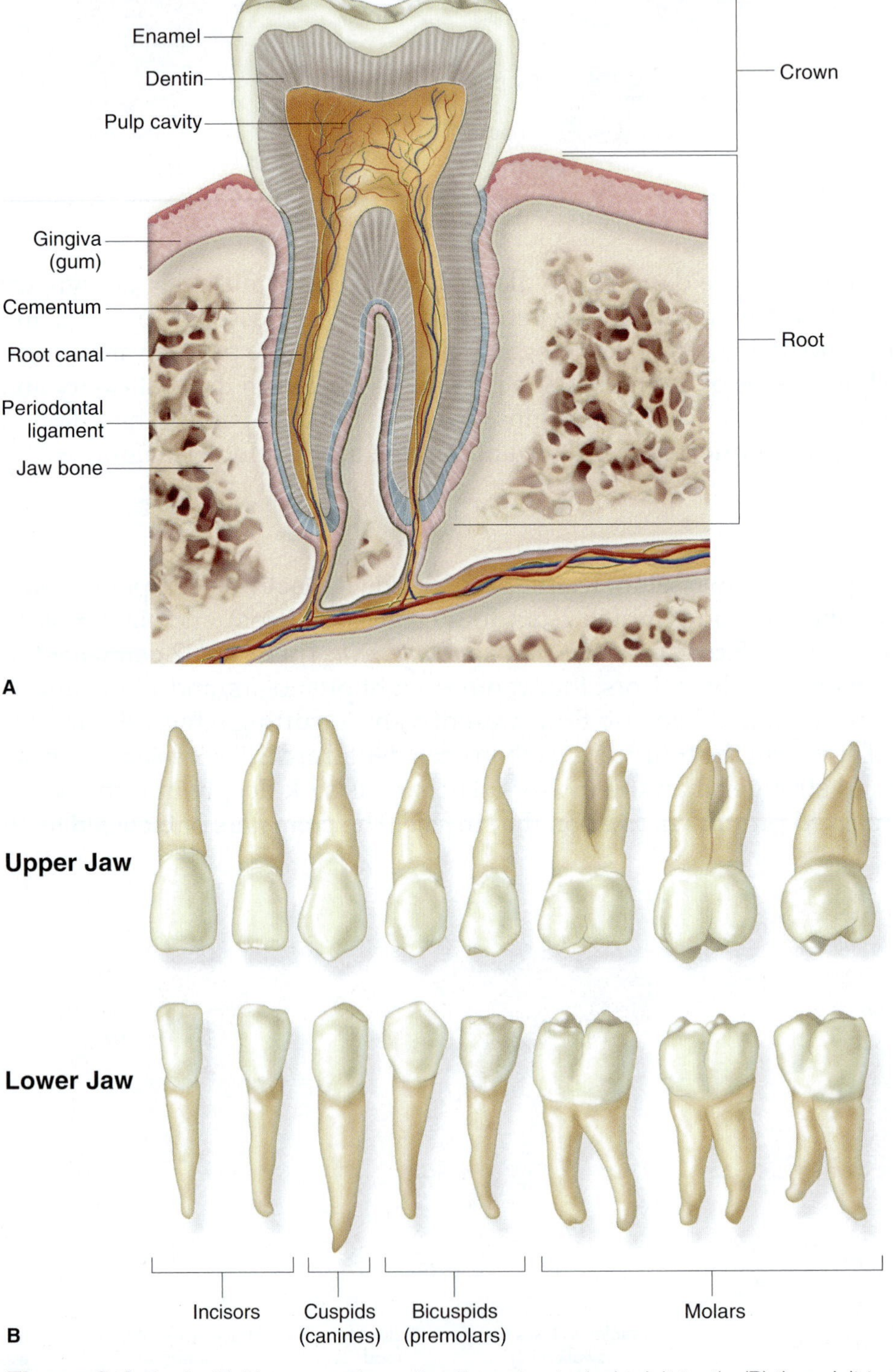

Figure 8.4 Teeth. (A) Diagrammatic section through a typical adult tooth; (B) the adult teeth.

This cavity is called the **pulp cavity**, which contains the dental pulp, a loose connective tissue richly supplied with vessels and nerves that enter the cavity through the small aperture at the point of each root. The pulp cavity receives blood vessels and nerves from the **root canal**, a narrow tunnel located at the root, or base, of the tooth. Blood vessels and nerves enter the root canal through an opening called the **apical foramen** to supply the pulp cavity.

The root of each tooth sits in a bony socket called an *alveolus*. Collagen fibers of the **periodontal ligament** extend from the dentin of the root to the bone of the alveolus, creating a strong articulation known as a *gomphosis*, which binds the teeth to bony sockets in the maxillary bone and mandible. A layer of **cementum** (a thin layer of bone) covers the dentin of the root, providing protection and firmly anchoring the periodontal ligament.

The solid portion of the tooth consists of the **dentin**, which forms the bulk of the tooth; the **enamel**, which covers the exposed part of the crown and is the hardest and most compact part of a tooth; and the cementum, which is deposited on the surface of the root.

The neck of the tooth marks the boundary between the root and the crown, the exposed portion of the tooth that projects above the soft tissue of the *gingiva*. A shallow groove called the **gingival sulcus** surrounds the neck of each tooth.

Pharynx

The **pharynx**, or throat, is a chamber that extends between the internal nares and the entrance to the larynx and esophagus (Figure 8.1). Its three subdivisions are the nasopharynx, oropharynx, and laryngopharynx. The upper portion, the **nasopharynx**, is above the soft palate. The middle portion, the **oropharynx**, lies between the palate and the hyoid bone and has an opening to the oral cavity. The lowest portion, the **laryngopharynx**, is below the hyoid bone and opens inferiorly to the larynx anteriorly and the esophagus posteriorly.

The pharynx is a common passageway for both respiration and digestion. Both the **larynx**, or voice box, and the esophagus begin in the pharynx. Food that is swallowed passes through the pharynx into the esophagus reflexively. Muscular contractions move the bolus into the esophagus and the **epiglottis** (a flap of tissue) blocks the opening of the larynx, preventing food from entering the airway leading to the trachea (windpipe).

Esophagus

The **esophagus** is a muscular tube about 10 inches long that leads from the pharynx to the stomach (Figure 8.1). Food and liquids pass down the esophagus and into the stomach. At the junction with the stomach is the lower esophageal sphincter (LES) or **cardiac sphincter**. This sphincter relaxes to permit passage of food and then contracts to prevent the backup of stomach contents. Food is carried along the esophagus by a series of wavelike muscular contractions called **peristalsis**.

Stomach

The **stomach** is a muscular, distensible saclike portion of the alimentary canal between the esophagus and duodenum. See Figure 8.5. The upper region of the stomach is called the *fundus*, the main portion is called the *body*, and the lower region is the *antrum*. There are folds in the mucous membrane lining the stomach called *rugae* that stretch when the stomach fills with food and contain glands that produce digestive juices.

Food and liquids pass from the esophagus into the stomach. Here food is reduced to a digestible state by mechanical churning and the release of chemicals such as

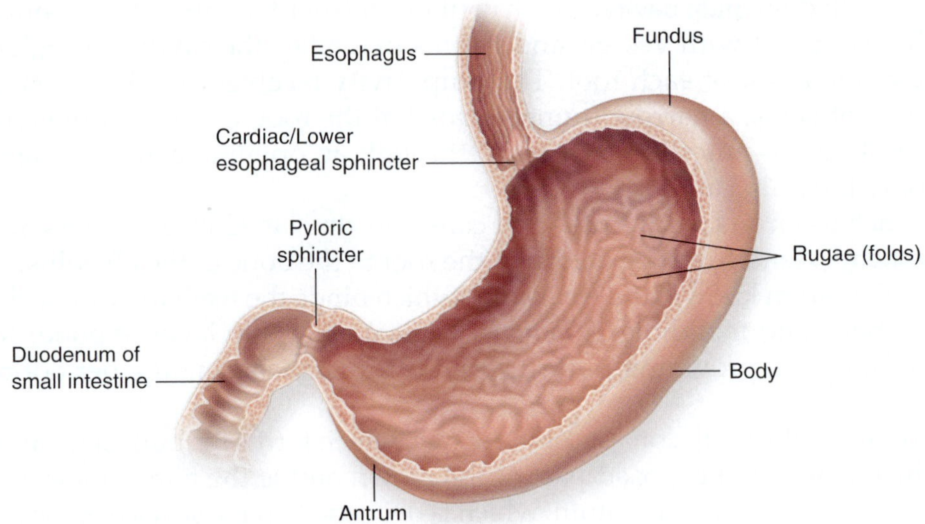

Figure 8.5 Stomach.

hydrochloric acid, digestive hormones, and enzymes. Gastric juices help convert the food to a semiliquid state called chyme, which is passed at intervals through a valve called the pyloric sphincter into the small intestine. An empty stomach has a volume of about 50 mL. Typically after a meal, its capacity can expand to about 1 liter and may expand to hold as much as 4 liters.

Small Intestine

The **small intestine** is about 21 feet long and 1 inch in diameter. It extends from the pyloric sphincter at the base of the stomach to the entrance of the large intestine. The small intestine is divided into three parts: the **duodenum**, the **jejunum**, and the **ileum**. The duodenum is the first 12 inches just beyond the stomach. The jejunum is the next 8 feet or so, and the ileum is the remaining 12 feet of the tube. See Figure 8.6.

Digestion and absorption take place chiefly in the small intestine. Chyme is received from the stomach through the pylorus and is mixed with bile from the liver and gallbladder along with pancreatic juice from the pancreas. Intestinal villi, the tiny, finger-like projections in the wall of the small intestine, increase the surface area and thus the absorptive area of the intestinal wall, providing more places for food to be absorbed. It is important that food is absorbed at a considerably fast rate so as to allow more food to be absorbed.

Digested nutrients (including sugars and amino acids) pass into the villi through diffusion. Complex proteins are broken down into simple amino acids, complicated sugars are reduced to simple sugars (glucose), and large fat molecules (triglycerides) are broken down to fatty acids and glycerol. Circulating blood then transmits these nutrients to body cells. Enzymes within the villi capillaries collect amino acids and simple sugars, which are taken up by the villi and sent into the bloodstream. Villus lacteals (lymph capillary) collect absorbed lipoproteins and are taken to the rest of the body through the lymph fluid. See Table 8.2 for a general description of chemical digestion.

Large Intestine

The **large intestine** is about 5 feet long and 2½ inches in diameter. It extends from the ileocecal valve at the small intestine to the anus. The large intestine is divided into the **cecum**, the **colon**, the **rectum**, and the **anal canal**. The cecum is a pouchlike structure forming the beginning of the large intestine. It is about 3 inches long and has

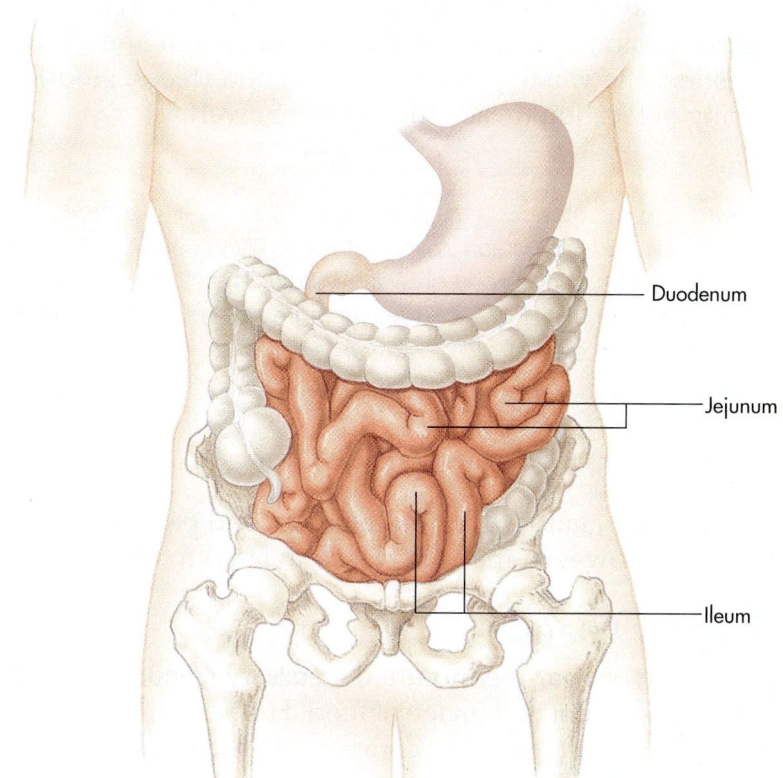

Figure 8.6 Small intestine.

Table 8.2 Components of Chemical Digestion

Digestive Juices and Enzymes	Food Enzyme Digests	Resulting Product
1. Saliva		
a. Ptyalin (salivary amylase)	Starch and sugar	Maltose (a disaccharide, or double sugar)
2. Gastric juice		
a. Rennin	Caseinogen (milk products)	Casein (curds)
b. Pepsin, plus hydrochloric acid (HCl)	Proteins, including casein	Proteoses and peptones (partially digested proteins)
c. Lipase	Emulsified fats (butter, cream)	Fatty acids and glycerol
3. Bile (contains no enzymes)	Large fat droplets (unemulsified fats)	Small fat droplets, or emulsified fats
4. Pancreatic juice		
a. Trypsin (protease)	Proteins	Peptones, peptides, amino acids
b. Steapsin (lipase)	Bile-emulsified fats	Fatty acids and glycerol
c. Amylopsin (pancreatic amylase)	Starch	Maltose
5. Intestinal juice		
a. Sucrase	Sucrose (cane sugar)	Glucose and fructose
b. Lactase	Lactose (milk sugar)	Glucose and galactose
c. Maltase	Maltose (malt sugar)	Glucose

the **appendix** attached to it. The colon makes up the bulk of the large intestine and is divided into the ascending colon, the transverse colon, the descending colon, and the sigmoid colon (see Figure 8.7). With digestion and absorption completed in the large intestine, the waste product of digestion (feces, stool) is expelled through the anus during defecation (evacuation of the bowel).

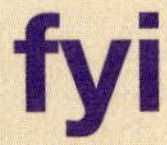

Meconium, the first stool, is a mixture of amniotic fluid and secretions of the intestinal glands. It is thick and sticky, and dark green in color. It is usually passed 8–24 hours following birth. The stool during the first week is loose and greenish-yellow. The stool of a breast-fed baby is bright yellow, soft, and pasty. The stool of a bottle-fed baby is more solid than that of a breast-fed baby, and the color varies from yellow to brown.

Accessory Organs

The salivary glands, liver, gallbladder, and pancreas are not actually part of the digestive tube; however, they are closely related to the digestive process.

Salivary Glands

Located in or near the mouth, the **salivary glands** secrete **saliva** in response to the sight, smell, taste, or mental image of food. Human saliva is composed of 98% water, while the other 2% consists of other compounds such as electrolytes, mucus, antibacterial compounds, and various enzymes that help start the process of digestion. The various salivary glands are the **parotid**, located on either side of the face slightly below the ear; the

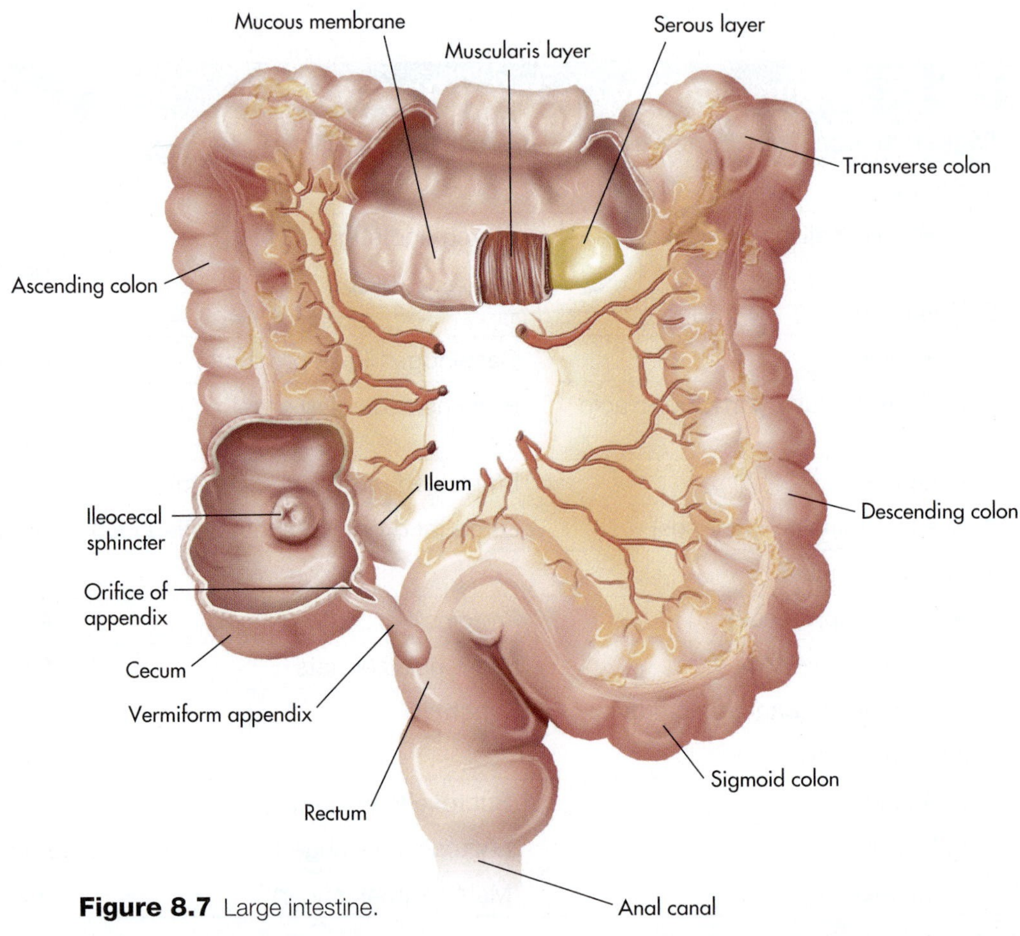

Figure 8.7 Large intestine.

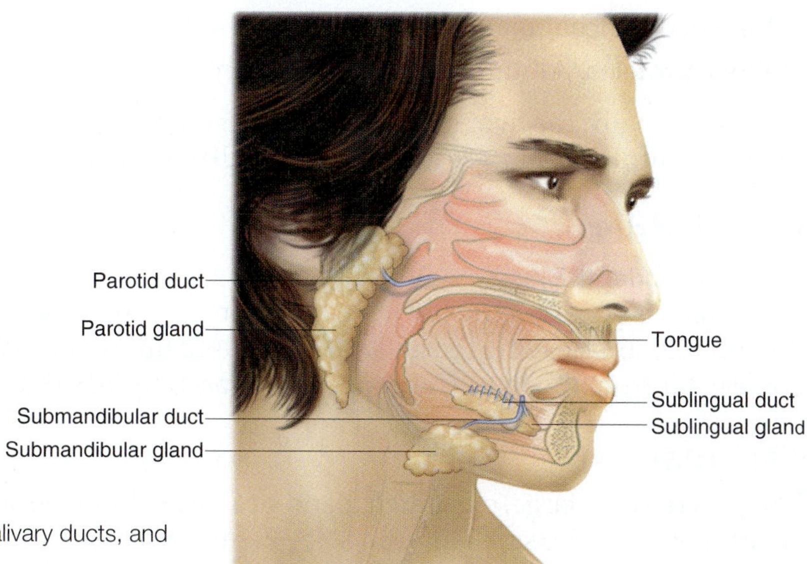

Figure 8.8 Salivary glands, salivary ducts, and the tongue.

submandibular, located in the floor of the mouth; and the **sublingual**, located below the tongue (see Figure 8.1). All salivary glands secrete through openings (salivary ducts) into the mouth to lubricate food and begin the digestion of carbohydrates. See Figure 8.8.

Liver

The largest glandular organ in the body, the **liver** weighs about 3½ lbs and is located in the upper right part of the abdomen. See Figure 8.9. The liver plays an essential role in the normal metabolism of carbohydrates, fats, and proteins. In carbohydrate (CHO) metabolism, it changes glucose to glycogen and stores the glycogen until needed by body cells. When required, glycogen is converted back to glucose. In fat metabolism, the liver serves as a storage place and acts to desaturate fats before releasing them into the bloodstream. In protein metabolism, the liver acts as a storage place and assists in both protein **catabolism** (metabolic breaking down of complex substances into more basic elements) and **anabolism** (building up of the body substances in the constructive phase of metabolism).

The liver manufactures the following important substances:

- **Bile**. Digestive juice important in fat emulsification (the breakdown of large fat globules into smaller particles)
- **Fibrinogen** and **prothrombin**. Coagulants essential for blood clotting

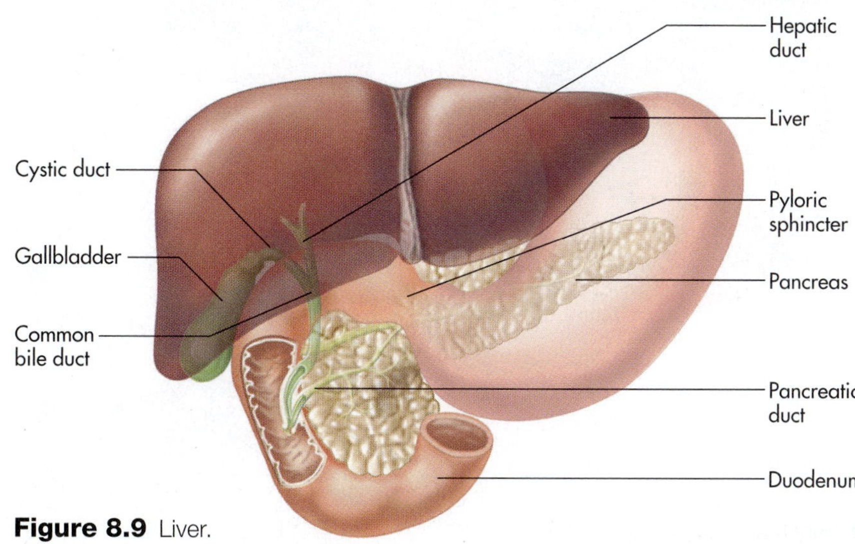

Figure 8.9 Liver.

- **Heparin**. Anticoagulant that helps to prevent the clotting of blood
- **Blood proteins**. Albumin, gamma globulin

Additionally, the liver stores iron and vitamins B_{12}, A, D, E, and K. It also detoxifies many harmful substances (toxins) such as drugs and alcohol.

Gallbladder

The **gallbladder (GB)** is a small pear-shaped sac under the liver. The gallbladder stores bile, which is produced by the liver, and then concentrates it for future use. See Figures 8.1 and 8.10. Bile leaving the gallbladder is 6–10 times more concentrated as that which comes to it from the liver. Concentration is accomplished by removal of water.

Pancreas

The **pancreas** is a large, elongated gland situated behind the stomach and secreting pancreatic juice into the small intestine. See Figures 8.9 and 8.10. The pancreas is 6–9 inches long and contains cells that produce digestive **enzymes**. Other specialized cells in the pancreas secrete the hormones insulin and glucagon directly into the bloodstream. The beta cells of the islets of Langerhans make and release insulin. The alpha cells of the islets of Langerhans synthesize and secrete glucagon.

> **fyi** Newborns produce very little saliva until they are 3 months of age and swallowing is a reflex action. The infant's stomach is small and empties rapidly. The liver of the newborn is often immature, thereby causing **jaundice**. Fat absorption is poor because of a decreased level of bile production.

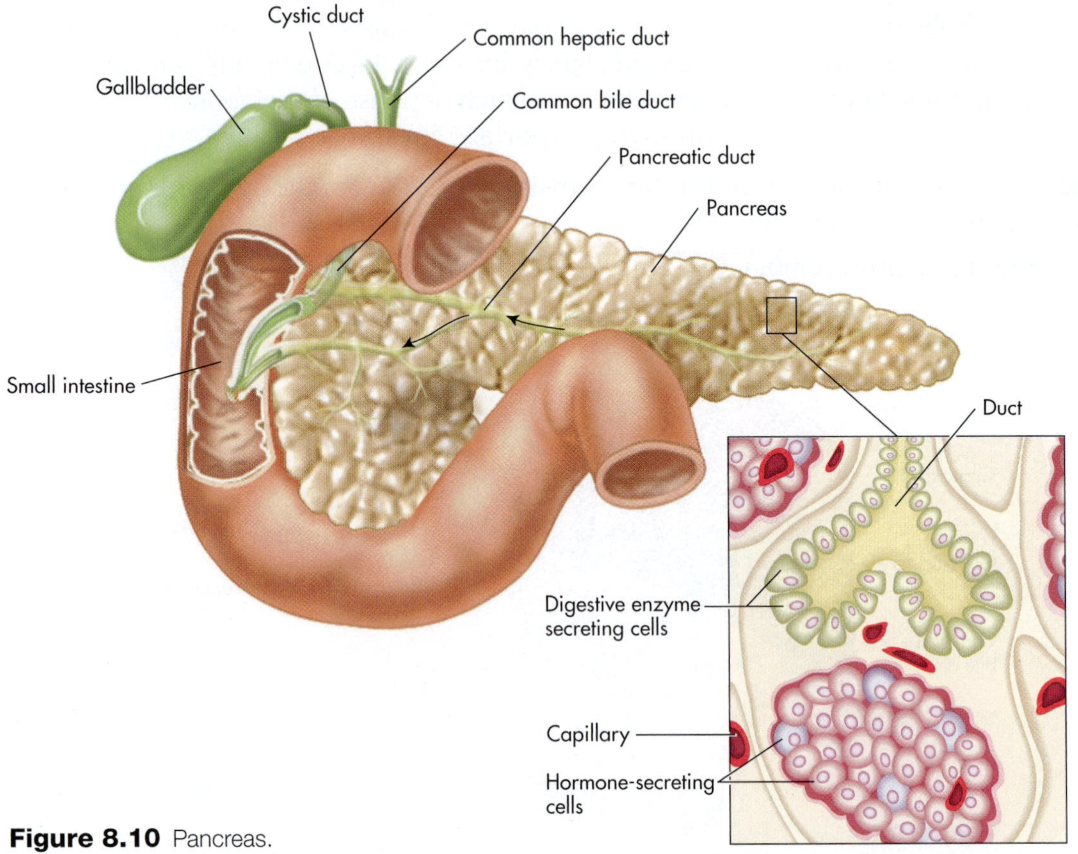

Figure 8.10 Pancreas.

Study and Review I

Anatomy and Physiology

Write your answers to the following questions.

1. Name the primary organs commonly associated with digestion.

   a. ______________________ b. ______________________

   c. ______________________ d. ______________________

   e. ______________________ f. ______________________

2. Name four accessory organs of digestion.

   a. ______________________ b. ______________________

   c. ______________________ d. ______________________

3. State the three main functions of the digestive system.

   a. ______________________ b. ______________________

   c. ______________________

4. Define bolus. ______________________

5. Define peristalsis. ______________________

6. ______________________ and ______________________ convert the food into a semiliquid state.

7. The ______________________ is the first portion of the small intestine.

8. Semiliquid food is called ______________________.

9. The ______________________ transports nutrients to body cells.

10. The large intestine can be divided into four distinct sections called the ______________________, the ______________________, the ______________________, and the ______________________.

11. The ______________________ is the largest glandular organ in the body.

12. State the function of the gallbladder. ______________________

13. Name an important function of the pancreas. ______________________

14. State three functions of the liver.

a. ______________________________ **b.** ______________________________

c. ______________________________

15. Where does digestion and absorption chiefly take place? ______________________________

16. The salivary glands located in and about the mouth are called the ______________________, the ______________________, and the ______________________.

17. Name the two hormones secreted into the bloodstream by the pancreas. ______________________

ANATOMY LABELING

Identify the structures shown below by filling in the blanks.

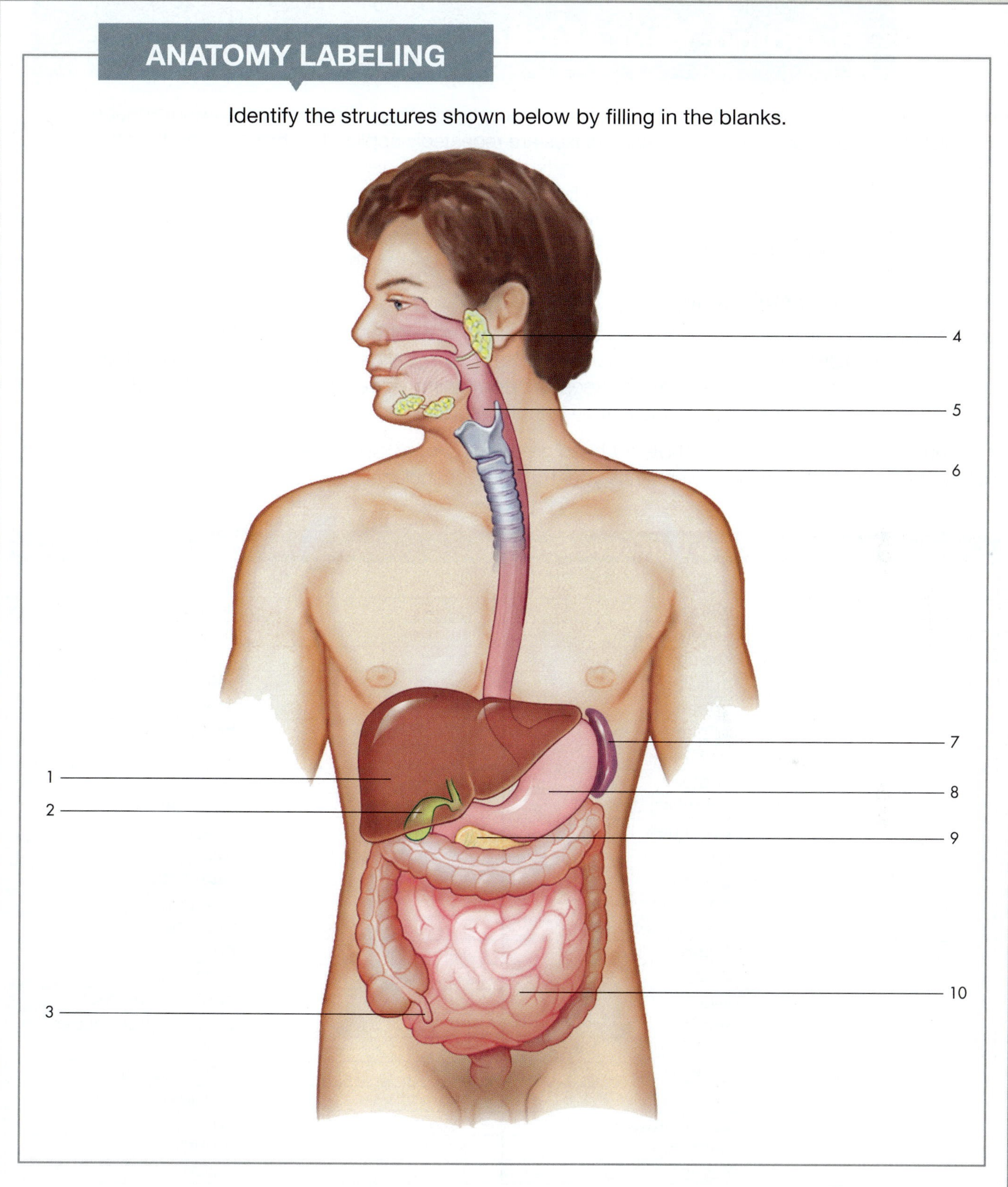

Building Your Medical Vocabulary

This section provides the foundation for learning medical terminology. Review the following alphabetized word list. Note how common prefixes and suffixes are repeatedly applied to word roots and combining forms to create different meanings. The word parts are color-coded: prefixes are yellow, suffixes are blue, roots/combining forms are red. A combining form is a word root plus a vowel. The chart below lists the combining forms for the word roots in this chapter and can help to strengthen your understanding of how medical words are built and spelled.

Remember These Guidelines

1. If the suffix begins with a vowel, drop the combining vowel from the combining form and add the suffix. For example, append/o (*appendix*) + -ectomy (*surgical excision*) becomes appendectomy.
1. If the suffix begins with a consonant, keep the combining vowel and add the suffix to the combining form. For example, herni/o (*hernia*) + -rrhaphy (suture) becomes herniorrhaphy.

You will find that some terms have not been divided into word parts. These are common words or specialized terms that are included to enhance your medical vocabulary.

Combining Forms of the Digestive System

absorpt/o	to take in	**gloss/o**	tongue
aden/o	gland	**glyc/o**	sweet, sugar
aliment/o	nourishment	**halit/o**	breath
amyl/o	starch	**hemat/o**	blood
anabol/o	building up	**hemorrh/o**	vein liable to bleed
append/o	appendix	**hepat/o**	liver
appendic/o	appendix	**herni/o**	hernia
bil/i	gall, bile	**ile/o**	ileum
bucc/o	cheek	**labi/o**	lip
catabol/o	a casting down	**lapar/o**	abdomen
celi/o	abdomen, belly	**lingu/o**	tongue
cheil/o	lip	**odont/o**	tooth
chol/e	gall, bile	**pancreat/o**	pancreas
choledoch/o	common bile duct	**pept/o**	to digest
cirrh/o	orange-yellow	**pharyng/e, pharyng/o**	pharynx
col/o	colon	**pil/o**	hair
colon/o	colon	**prand/i**	meal
cyst/o	bladder	**proct/o**	anus and rectum
dent/o	tooth	**pylor/o**	pylorus, gatekeeper
diverticul/o	diverticula	**rect/o**	rectum
duoden/o	duodenum	**sial/o**	saliva, salivary
enter/o	intestine	**sigmoid/o**	sigmoid
esophage/o, esophag/o	esophagus	**splen/o**	spleen
gastr/o	stomach	**stomat/o**	mouth
gingiv/o	gums	**verm/i**	worm

Medical Word	Word Parts: Part	Word Parts: Meaning	Definition
absorption (ăb-sōrp´ shŭn)	absorpt -ion	to take in process	Process by which nutrient material is transferred from the gastrointestinal tract into the bloodstream or lymph
amylase (ăm´ ĭ-lās)	amyl -ase	starch enzyme	Enzyme that breaks down starch. Ptyalin is a salivary amylase and amylopsin is a pancreatic amylase.
anabolism (ă-năb´ ō-lĭzm)	anabol -ism	a building up condition	Building up of body substances in the constructive phase of metabolism
anorexia (ăn´ ō-rěks´ ĭ-ă)	an- -orexia	lack of appetite	Lack of appetite; decreased desire for food
appendectomy (ăp´ ěn-děk´ tō-mē)	append -ectomy	appendix surgical excision	Surgical excision of the appendix. See Figure 8.11.

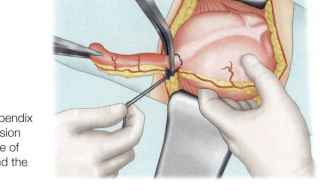

Figure 8.11 Appendectomy. The appendix and cecum are brought through the incision to the surface of the abdomen. The base of the appendix is clamped and ligated, and the appendix is then removed.

Medical Word	Word Parts: Part	Word Parts: Meaning	Definition
appendicitis (ă-pěn˝ dĭ-sī´ tĭs)	appendic -itis	appendix inflammation	Inflammation of the appendix. A point of tenderness in acute appendicitis is known as *McBurney point*, located 1–2 inches above the anterosuperior spine of the ilium on a line between the ilium and the umbilicus. See Figure 8.12.

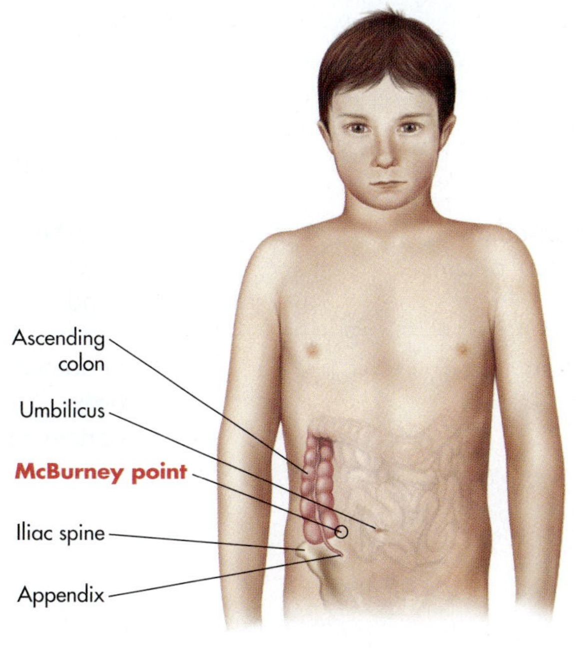

Figure 8.12 McBurney point is the common location of pain in children and adolescents with appendicitis.

Medical Word	Word Parts		Definition
	Part	**Meaning**	
ascites (ă-sī′ tēz)			Significant accumulation of serous fluid in the peritoneal cavity
biliary (bĭl′ ĭ-ār″ ē)	bil/i -ary	gall, bile pertaining to	Pertaining to bile
bilirubin (bĭl″ ĭ-rōō′ bĭn)			Orange-colored bile pigment produced by the separation of hemoglobin into parts that are excreted by the liver cells
black hairy tongue			Condition in which the tongue is covered by hairlike papillae entangled with threads produced by *Aspergillus niger* or *Candida albicans* fungi or by bacteria. This unusual condition could be caused by poor oral hygiene and/or overgrowth of fungi due to antibiotic therapy. See Figure 8.13.

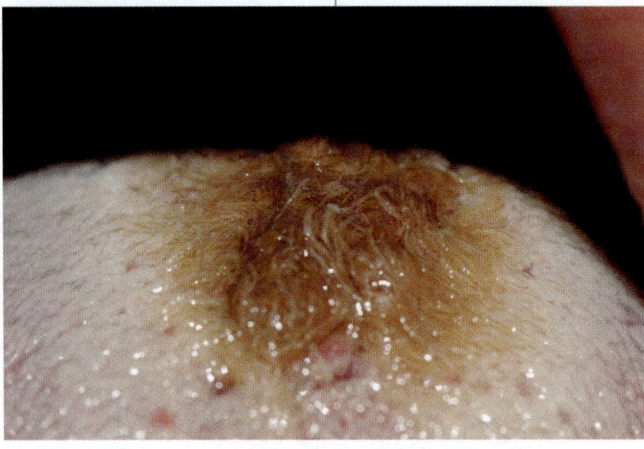

Figure 8.13 Black hairy tongue. (Courtesy of Jason L. Smith, MD)

Medical Word	Part	Meaning	Definition
bowel (bou′ əl)			Intestine; the long tube in the body that stores and then eliminates waste out of the body

insights In ICD-10-CM, *bowel* is listed under disease code K63.9; *functional bowel* is code K59.9, and *psychogenic bowel* is code F45.8. This term is often used to refer to the emptying of the bowel, such as *bowel movement (BM)* or a condition or disease of the bowel.

Medical Word	Part	Meaning	Definition
buccal (bŭk′ ăl)	bucc -al	cheek pertaining to	Literally means *pertaining to the cheek*; relating to the cheek or mouth
catabolism (kă-tăb′ ō-lĭzm)	catabol -ism	a casting down condition	Literally *a casting down*; in metabolism a breaking down of complex substances into more basic elements
celiac (sē′ lĭ-ăk)	celi -ac	abdomen, belly pertaining to	Pertaining to the abdomen

Medical Word	Word Parts		Definition
	Part	Meaning	
cheilosis (kī-lō´ sĭs)	cheil -osis	lip condition	Abnormal condition of the lip as seen in riboflavin and other B-complex deficiencies

RULE REMINDER

The ***o*** has been removed from the combining form because the suffix begins with a vowel.

Medical Word	Part	Meaning	Definition
cholecystectomy (kō″ lē-sĭs-tĕk´ tō-mē)	chol/e cyst -ectomy	gall, bile bladder surgical excision	Surgical excision of the gallbladder. With laparoscopic cholecystectomy, the gallbladder is removed through a small incision near the navel. Gallstones (*cholelithiasis*) are usually present in the removed gallbladder. See Figure 8.14.

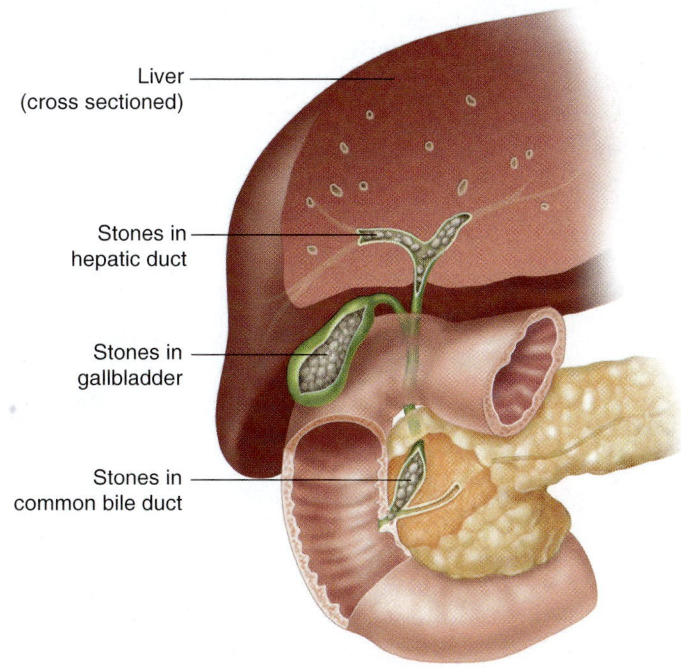

Figure 8.14 Gallbladder with gallstones. Note the stones in the hepatic duct, gallbladder, and common bile duct.

Medical Word	Part	Meaning	Definition
cholecystitis (kō″ lē-sĭs-tī´ tĭs)	chol/e cyst -itis	gall, bile bladder inflammation	Inflammation of the gallbladder
choledochotomy (kō″ lĕd ō-kŏt´ ō-mē)	choledoch/o -tomy	common bile duct incision	Surgical incision of the common bile duct

Medical Word	Word Parts		Definition
	Part	**Meaning**	
cirrhosis (sĭ-rō´ sĭs)	cirrh -osis	orange-yellow condition	Chronic degenerative liver disease characterized by changes in the lobes; parenchymal cells and the lobules are infiltrated with fat. See Figure 8.15.

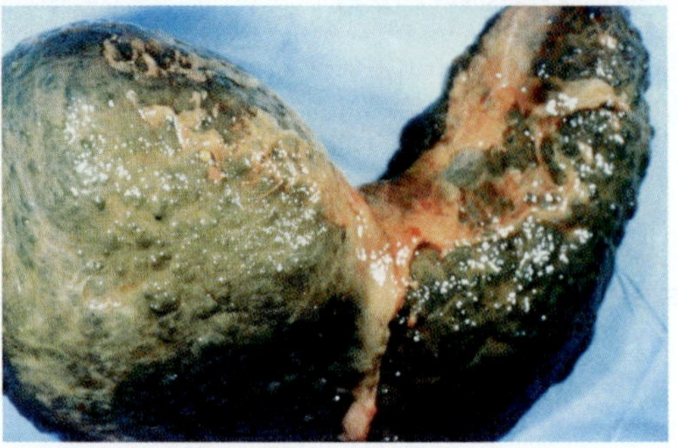

Figure 8.15 The liver in this photograph was from a deceased patient with an advanced state of cirrhosis.

Source: Pearson Education, Inc.

Medical Word	Part	Meaning	Definition
colectomy (kō-lĕk´ tō-mē)	col -ectomy	colon surgical excision	Surgical excision of part of the colon
colon cancer (kō-lŏn kăn´ sĕr)			Malignancy of the colon; sometimes called *colorectal cancer*. See Figure 8.16.

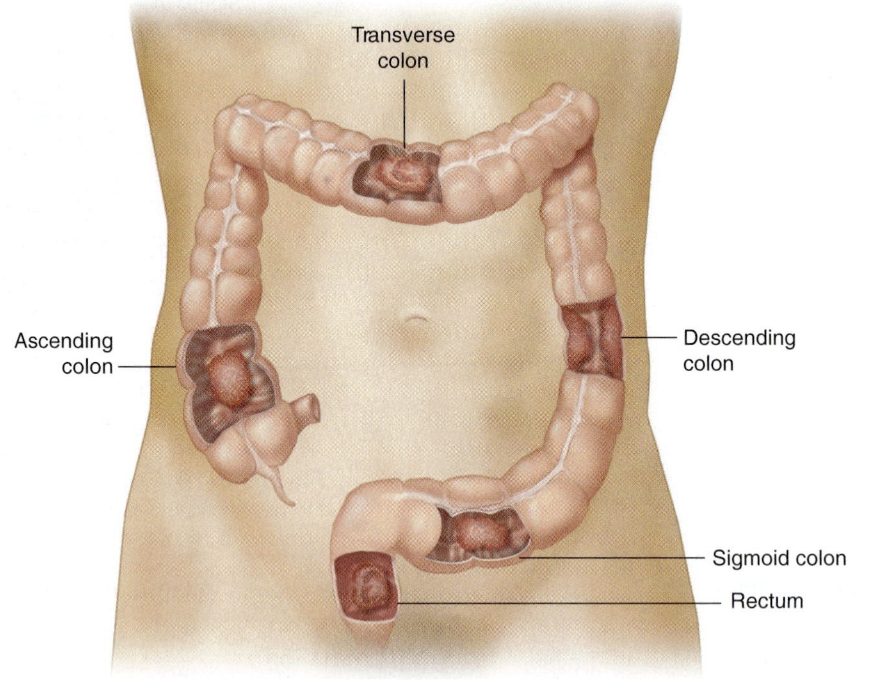

Figure 8.16 Common sites of colorectal cancer.

Medical Word	Part	Meaning	Definition
colonoscope (kō-lŏn´ ō-skōp)	colon/o -scope	colon instrument for examining	Thin, lighted, flexible instrument that is used to view the interior of the colon during a colonoscopy

Medical Word	Word Parts		Definition
	Part	**Meaning**	
colonoscopy (kō-lŏn-ŏs´ kō-pē)	colon/o -scopy	colon visual examination, to view, examine	Visual examination of the colon via a colonoscope. See Figure 8.17.
colostomy (kō-lŏs´ tō-mē)	col/o -stomy	colon new opening	A surgical procedure that brings one end of the large intestine out through an opening (stoma) made in the abdominal wall. Stool moving through the intestine drains through the stoma into a bag attached to the abdomen. A colostomy can be permanent or temporary. The most common types are transverse, descending, and sigmoid, so named due to the site of the disorder and the location of the stoma. See Figure 8.18.

ALERT!

The combining forms **col/o** and **colon/o** mean colon. You can build medical words by using various suffixes such as ***-ectomy***, ***-ic***, ***-scope***, ***-scopy***, and ***-stomy*** to change the meaning of the word.

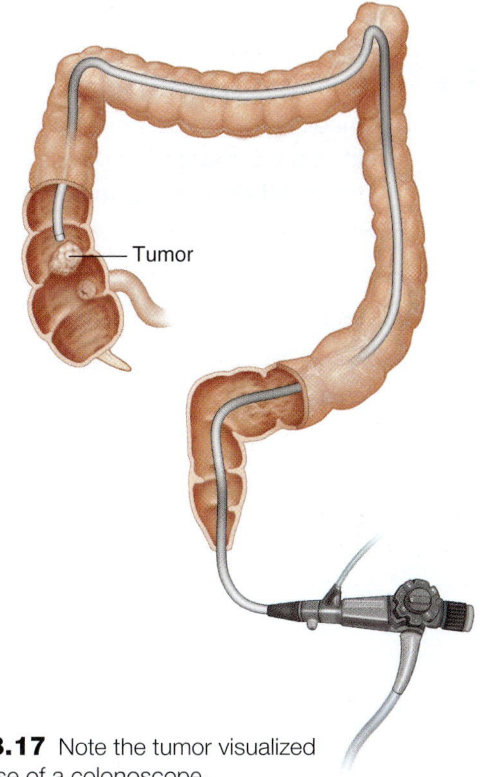

Figure 8.17 Note the tumor visualized with the use of a colonoscope.

RULE REMINDER

This term keeps the combining vowel **o** because the suffix begins with a consonant.

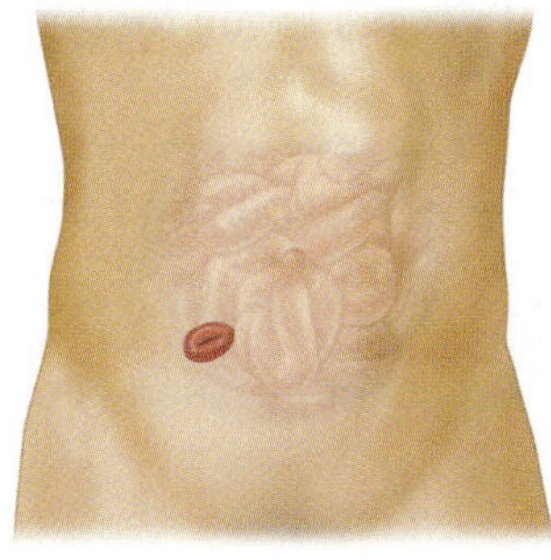
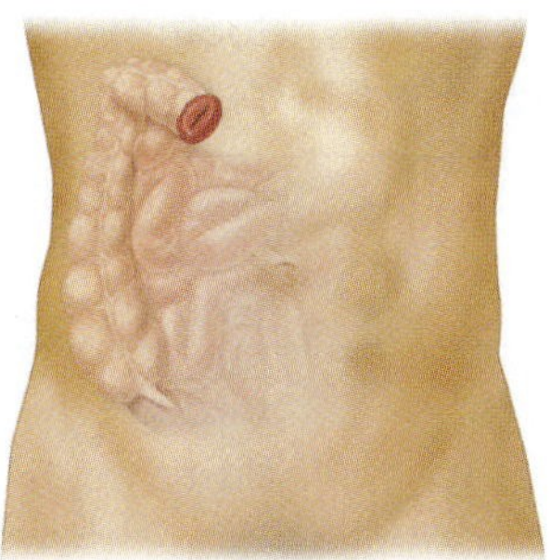
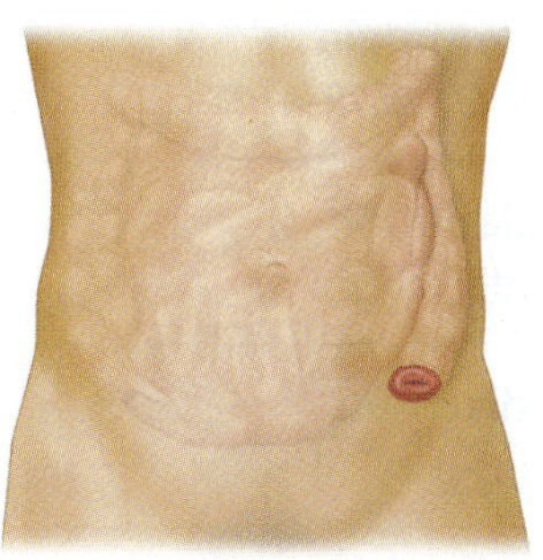

Figure 8.18 Alternate sites that can be used to create a new opening (*-stomy*) in the colon.

Medical Word	Word Parts: Part	Word Parts: Meaning	Definition
constipation (kon″ stĭ-pā′ shŭn)	constipat -ion	to press together process	Infrequent passage of unduly hard and dry feces; *difficult defecation*

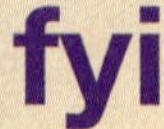

Constipation is a frequent problem among older adults. It is believed that constipation is not a normal age-related change but is caused by low fluid intake, dehydration, lack of dietary fiber, inactivity, medicines, depression, and other health-related conditions. Over time, narcotic medications can slow the bowel and lead to symptoms of constipation, bloating, and nausea. This is known as **opioid-induced constipation (OIC)**.

Medical Word	Word Parts: Part	Word Parts: Meaning	Definition
Crohn disease (krōn)			Chronic autoimmune disease that can affect any part of the gastrointestinal tract but most commonly occurs in the ileum. See Figure 8.19.

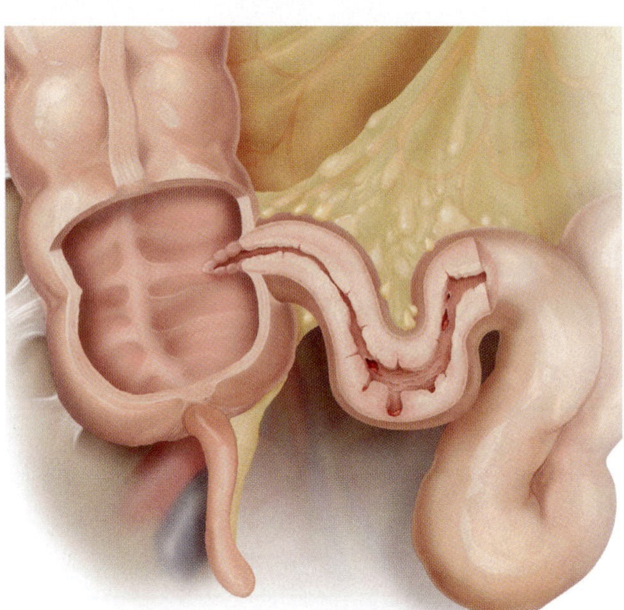

Figure 8.19 Note the thickening of the intestinal wall and the erosion of the inner lining of the ileum, often seen in Crohn disease.

insights In ICD-10-CM, there are combination codes for complications commonly associated with Crohn disease. These combination codes can be found under subcategory K50.0.

Medical Word	Word Parts: Part	Word Parts: Meaning	Definition
dentalgia (dĕn-tăl′ jĭ-ă)	dent -algia	tooth pain, ache	Pain in a tooth; *toothache*
dentition (dĕn-tĭ′ shŭn)			Type, number, and arrangement of teeth in the dental arch
diarrhea (dī-ă-rē′ ă)	dia- -rrhea	through flow	Frequent passage of unformed watery stool

Medical Word	Word Parts		Definition
	Part	Meaning	
diverticulitis (dī″ vĕr-tĭk″ ū-lī′ tĭs)	diverticul -itis	diverticula inflammation	Inflammation of the diverticula (pouches in the walls of an organ) in the colon. Symptoms include pain, fever, chills, cramping, bloating, constipation, and diarrhea. Treatment depends on the severity of the condition. See Figure 8.20.

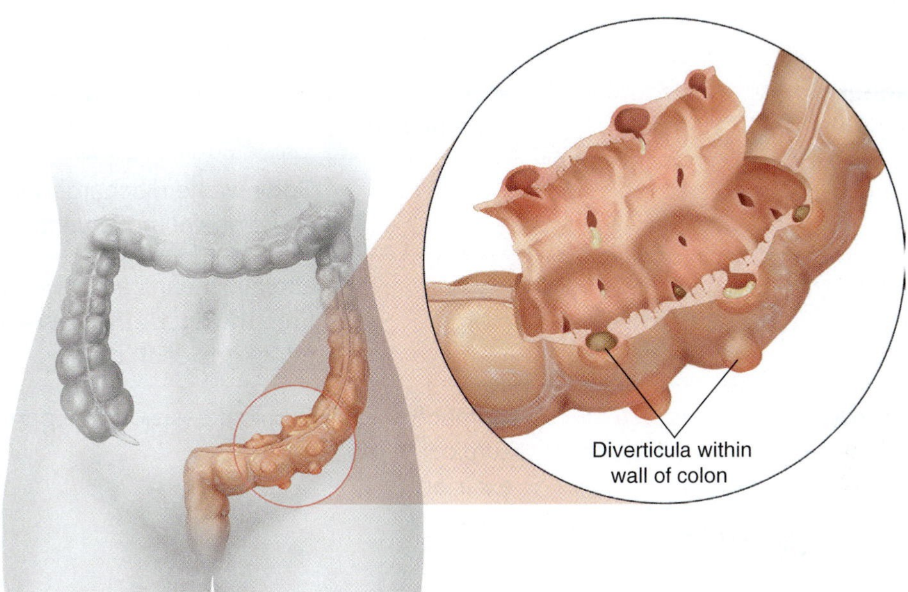

Figure 8.20 Diverticulitis.

Medical Word	Part	Meaning	Definition
duodenal (dū″ ō-dē′ năl)	duoden -al	duodenum pertaining to	Pertaining to the duodenum; the first part of the small intestine
dysentery (dĭs′ ĕn-tĕr″ ē)	dys- enter -y	difficult intestine pertaining to	An intestinal disease characterized by inflammation of the mucous membrane
dyspepsia (dĭs-pĕp′ sĭ-ă)	dys- -pepsia	difficult to digest, digestion	Difficulty in digestion; *indigestion*
dysphagia (dĭs-fā′ jĭ-ă)	dys- -phagia	difficult to eat, to swallow	Difficulty in swallowing
emesis (ĕm′ ĕ-sĭs)	eme -sis	to vomit condition	Vomiting
enteric (ĕn-tĕr′ ĭk)	enter -ic	small intestine pertaining to	Pertaining to the small intestine
enteritis (ĕn″ tĕr-ī′ tĭs)	enter -itis	small intestine inflammation	Inflammation of the small intestine
enzyme (ĕn′ zīm)			Protein substance capable of causing rapid chemical changes in other substances without being changed itself

Medical Word	Word Parts: Part	Word Parts: Meaning	Definition
epigastric (ĕp″ ĭ-găs′ trĭk)	epi- gastr -ic	above stomach pertaining to	Pertaining to the region above the stomach
eructation (ē-rŭk-tā′ shūn)	eructat -ion	a breaking out process	Belching
esophageal (ē-sŏf″ ă-jē′ ăl)	esophage -al	esophagus pertaining to	Pertaining to the esophagus
feces (fē′ sēz)			Body waste discharged from the bowel by way of the anus; *bowel movement (BM)*, *stool*, *excreta*
flatus (flā′ tŭs)			Literally means *a blowing* in Latin; the expelling of gas from the anus. The average person passes 400–1200 mL of gas each day.
gastrectomy (găs-trĕk′ tō-mē)	gastr -ectomy	stomach surgical excision	Surgical excision of a part of or the whole stomach

RULE REMINDER

The ***o*** has been removed from the combining form because the suffix begins with a vowel.

Medical Word	Word Parts: Part	Word Parts: Meaning	Definition
gastric (găs′ trĭk)	gastr -ic	stomach pertaining to	Pertaining to the stomach
gastroenteritis (găs″ trō-ĕn″- tĕr- ī′ tĭs)	gastr/o enter -itis	stomach intestine inflammation	Inflammation of the stomach and intestine
gastroenterologist (găs″trō-ĕn″tĕr-ŏl′ō-jĭst)	gastr/o enter/o -log -ist	stomach intestine study of one who specializes	Physician who specializes in the stomach and intestine
gastroenterology (găs″trō-ĕn″tĕr-ŏl′ō-jē)	gastr/o enter/o -logy	stomach intestine study of	Study of the stomach and intestine
gastroesophageal (găs″ trō ĕ-sŏf″ ă-jē′ al)	gastr/o esophage -al	stomach esophagus pertaining to	Pertaining to the stomach and esophagus

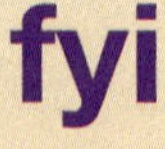

Erosive esophagitis (EE) is a condition in which areas of the esophageal lining are inflamed and ulcerated. The most common cause of erosive esophagitis is chronic acid reflux. **Barrett esophagus (BE)** can also develop as an advanced stage of erosive esophagitis, leading to abnormal changes in the cells of the esophagus, which puts a patient at risk for esophageal cancer.

Medical Word	Word Parts: Part	Word Parts: Meaning	Definition
gastroesophageal reflux disease (GERD) (găs″ trō ĕ-sŏf″ ă-jē′ al rē′ flŭcks)			Condition that occurs when the muscle between the esophagus and the stomach, the lower esophageal sphincter, is weak or relaxes inappropriately, allowing the stomach's contents to back up (*reflux*) into the esophagus. Symptoms include heartburn, belching, and regurgitation of food. See Figure 8.21.

Transient lower esophageal sphincter relaxation

Incompetent lower esophageal sphincter

Increased intragastric pressure

Figure 8.21 Mechanisms of gastroesophageal reflux.

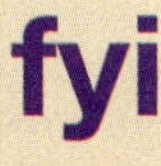

fyi Dietary and lifestyle choices may contribute to GERD. Studies show that cigarette smoking relaxes the lower esophageal sphincter (LES). Obesity and pregnancy can also cause GERD. Some doctors believe a **hiatal hernia** may weaken the lower esophageal sphincter and cause reflux.

Medical Word	Word Parts: Part	Word Parts: Meaning	Definition
gavage (gă-văzh′)			To feed liquid or semiliquid food via a tube (stomach or nasogastric [NG])
gingivitis (jĭn″ jĭ-vī′ tĭs)	gingiv -itis	gums inflammation	Inflammation of the gums
glossectomy (glŏs-ĕk- tō-mē)	gloss -ectomy	tongue excision	Partial or complete surgical excision of the tongue
glycogenesis (glī″ kō-jĕn′ ĕ-sĭs)	glyc/o -genesis	sweet, sugar formation, produce	Formation of glycogen from glucose
halitosis (hăl″ ĭ-tō′ sĭs)	halit -osis	breath condition	Bad breath
hematemesis (hĕm″ ă-tĕm′ ĕ-sĭs)	hemat -emesis	blood vomiting	Vomiting of blood

Medical Word	Word Parts		Definition
	Part	**Meaning**	
hemorrhoid (hĕm´ ō-royd)	hemorrh -oid	vein liable to bleed resemble	Mass of dilated, tortuous veins in the anorectum; can be internal or external. See Figure 8.22.

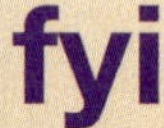

Figure 8.22 Location of internal and external hemorrhoids.

Medical Word	Part	Meaning	Definition
hepatitis (hĕp˝ ă-tī´ tĭs)	hepat -itis	liver inflammation	Inflammation of the liver

fyi

Hepatitis also refers to a group of viral infections that affect the liver. The most common types in the United States are hepatitis A (HAV), hepatitis B (HBV), and hepatitis C (HCV). There are vaccines to prevent hepatitis A and B; however, there is not one for hepatitis C. The common signs and symptoms of hepatitis are malaise, anorexia, hepatomegaly, jaundice, and abdominal pain.

HAV infection is primarily transmitted by the fecal–oral route, by either person-to-person contact or consumption of contaminated food or water. HBV is transmitted by blood transfusion, sexual contact, or the use of contaminated needles or instruments. HCV is most efficiently transmitted through large or repeated percutaneous exposure to infected blood (through the sharing of equipment to inject drugs, needlestick injuries in health care settings, and being born to a mother who is HCV positive).

Hepatitis D (HDV), which can be acute or chronic, is uncommon in the United States. Hepatitis E (HEV) is a serious liver disease that usually results in an acute infection. While rare in the United States, hepatitis E is common in many parts of the world.

Medical Word	Word Parts		Definition
	Part	Meaning	
hernia (hĕr´ nē-ă)			Abnormal protrusion of an organ or a part of an organ through the wall of the body cavity that normally contains it. A *hiatal hernia* occurs when the upper part of the stomach moves up into the chest through a small opening in the diaphragm. An *umbilical hernia* occurs when part of the intestine protrudes through an opening in the abdominal muscles. Umbilical hernias are most common in infants, but they can affect adults as well. In an infant, an umbilical hernia may be especially evident when the infant cries, causing the baby's bellybutton to protrude. An *inguinal hernia* occurs when a loop of intestine enters the inguinal canal, a tubular passage through the lower layers of the abdominal wall. See Figure 8.23.

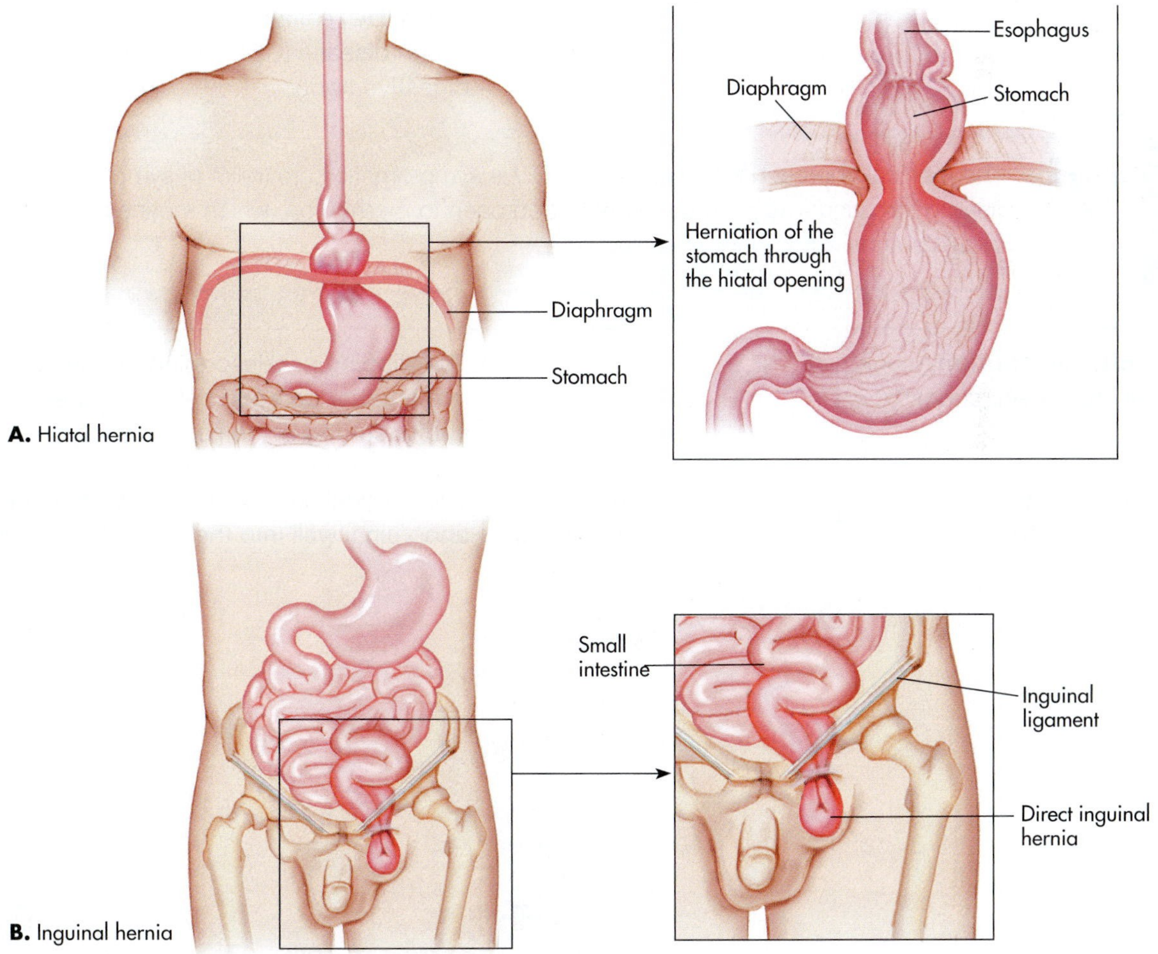

Figure 8.23 Hernias.

insights When coding hernias (K40–K46), ICD-10-CM provides specificity by type, laterality, and with or without obstruction and recurrence.

Medical Word	Word Parts: Part	Word Parts: Meaning	Definition
herniorrhaphy (hĕr″ nē-or′ ă-fē)	herni/o -rrhaphy	hernia suture	Surgical repair of a hernia
hyperemesis (hī″ pĕr-ĕm′ ĕ-sĭs)	hyper- -emesis	excessive, above vomiting	Excessive vomiting
hypogastric (hī″ pō-găs′ trĭk)	hypo- gastr -ic	deficient, below stomach pertaining to	Pertaining to below the stomach
inflammatory bowel disease (IBD)			Broad term that describes conditions with chronic or recurring abnormal immune response and inflammation of the gastrointestinal tract. The two most common inflammatory bowel diseases are ulcerative colitis (UC) (inflammation of the large intestine) and Crohn disease (CD) (inflammation of any portion of the digestive tract).

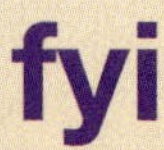

The medical approach for patients with IBD is symptomatic care (relief of symptoms) and mucosal healing following a *step-up* or *stepwise* approach to medication, which means the medical regimen is escalated until a response is achieved.

Medical Word	Word Parts: Part	Word Parts: Meaning	Definition
intussusception (ĭn″ tŭ-sŭ-sĕp′shŭn)			The slipping or telescoping of one part of an intestine into another part just below it; noted chiefly in children and occurring in the ileocecal region
ileostomy (ĭl″ ē-ŏs′ tō-mē)	ile/o -stomy	ileum new opening	The surgical creation of a new opening through the abdominal wall into the ileum. See Figure 8.24.

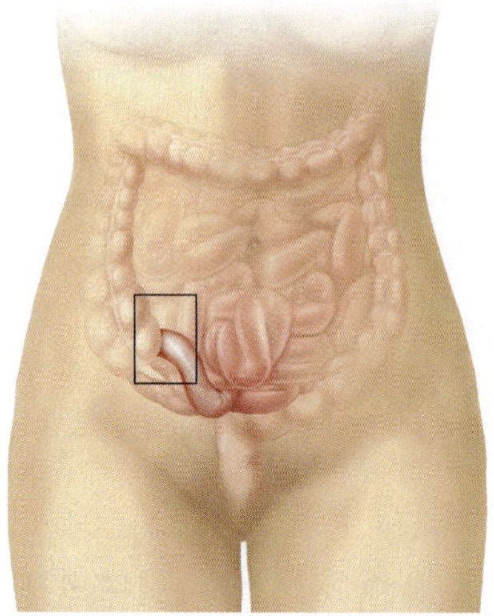

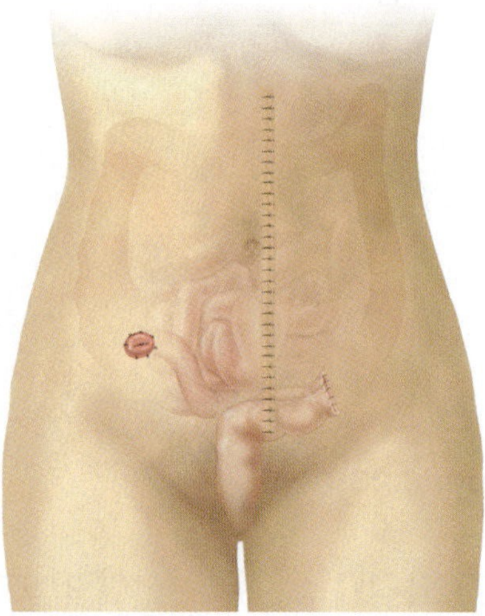

Figure 8.24 Ileostomy. Note that the cecum and colon have been surgically removed.

Medical Word	Word Parts		Definition
	Part	**Meaning**	
irritable bowel syndrome (IBS)			Disorder that affects the muscular contractions of the colon and interferes with its normal functioning; characterized by a group of symptoms, including crampy abdominal pain, bloating, constipation, and diarrhea. *Note:* Inflammatory bowel diseases (IBD) such as ulcerative colitis and Crohn disease should not be confused with IBS. Intestinal inflammation is not a symptom of IBS.
labial (lă´ bĭ-ăl)	labi -al	lip pertaining to	Pertaining to the lip
laparotomy (lăp˝ ăr-ŏt´ ō-mē)	lapar/o -tomy	abdomen incision	Surgical incision into the abdomen
lavage (lă-văzh´)			To wash out a cavity. Gastric lavage is used to remove or dilute gastric contents in cases of acute poisoning or ingestion of a caustic substance. *Vomiting should not be induced*. A closed-system irrigation uses an ordered amount of solution until the desired results are obtained.
laxative (lăk´ să-tĭv)	laxat -ive	to loosen nature of, quality of	Substance that acts to loosen the bowel
lingual (lĭng´ gwal)	lingu -al	tongue pertaining to	Pertaining to the tongue
malabsorption (măl˝ ăb-sōrp´ shŭn)	mal- absorpt -ion	bad to take in process	An inadequate absorption of nutrients from the intestinal tract
mastication (măs˝ tĭ-kā´ shŭn)	masticat -ion	to chew process	Chewing; the physical breaking up of food and mixing with saliva in the mouth
melena (mĕl´ ĕ-nă)			Black, tarry feces (stool) that has a distinctive odor and contains digested blood; usually results from bleeding in the upper GI tract; can be a sign of a peptic ulcer
mesentery (mĕs´ ĕn-tĕr˝ ē)	mes enter -y	middle small intestine pertaining to	Pertaining to the peritoneal fold encircling the small intestine and connecting the intestine to the posterior abdominal wall
nausea (naw´ sē-ă)			Uncomfortable feeling of the inclination to vomit
pancreatitis (păn˝ krē-ă-tī´ tĭs)	pancreat -itis	pancreas inflammation	Inflammation of the pancreas

Medical Word	Word Parts		Definition
	Part	**Meaning**	
paralytic ileus (păr″ ă-lĭt′ ĭk ĭl′ ē-ŭs)	paralyt -ic ile -us	to disable; paralysis pertaining to ileum pertaining to	Paralysis of the intestines that causes distention and symptoms of acute bowel obstruction and prostration
peptic (pĕp′ tĭk)	pept -ic	to digest pertaining to	Pertaining to gastric digestion
peptic ulcer disease (PUD) (pĕp′ tĭk ŭl′ sĕr)	pept -ic	to digest pertaining to	Disease in which an ulcer forms in the mucosal wall of the stomach, the pylorus, the duodenum, or the esophagus. See Figure 8.25.

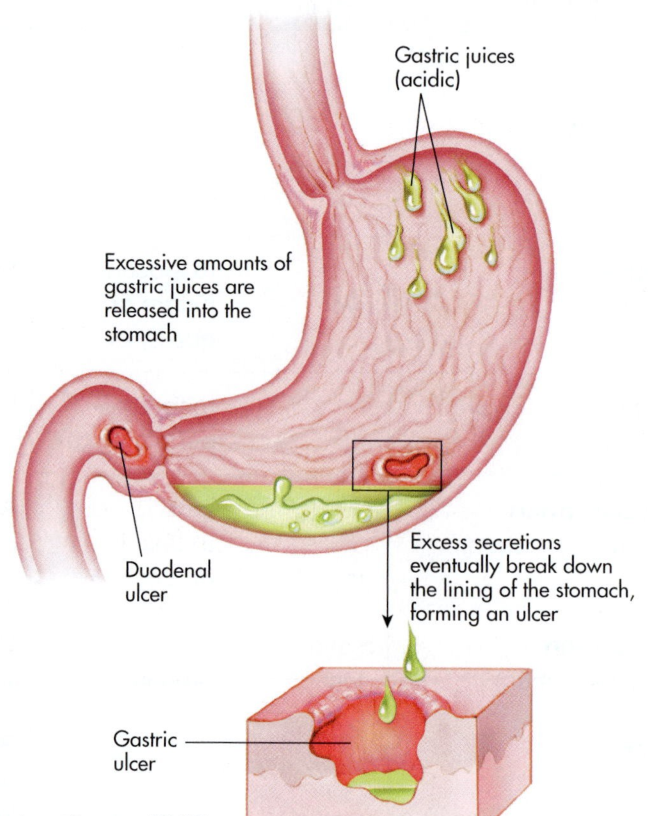

Figure 8.25 Peptic ulcer disease (PUD).

fyi Peptic ulcers are referred to as *gastric*, *duodenal*, or *esophageal*, depending on the location. The erosion of the mucosa that characterizes peptic ulcers is often caused by infection with a bacterium called *Helicobacter pylori (H. pylori)*. Approximately 90% of duodenal ulcers and 80% of peptic ulcers are associated with *Helicobacter pylori*. By killing the bacteria with antibiotics, it is estimated that 90% of the ulcers caused by *H. pylori* can be cured.

Medical Word	Part	Meaning	Definition
periodontal (pĕr″ ē-ō-dŏn′ tăl)	peri- odont -al	around tooth pertaining to	Pertaining to the area around the tooth

Medical Word	Word Parts: Part	Word Parts: Meaning	Definition
periodontal disease			Inflammation and degeneration of the gums and surrounding bone, which frequently causes loss of the teeth
peristalsis (pěr″ ĭ-stăl′ sĭs)	peri- -stalsis	around contraction	Wavelike contraction that occurs involuntarily in hollow tubes of the body, especially the alimentary canal
pharyngeal (făr-ĭn′ jē-ăl)	pharyng/e -al	pharynx pertaining to	Pertaining to the pharynx
pilonidal cyst (pī″ lō-nī′ dăl sĭst)	pil/o nid -al cyst	hair nest pertaining to sac	Closed sac in the crease of the sacrococcygeal region caused by a developmental defect that permits epithelial tissue and hair to be trapped below the skin and cause pain or swelling above the area of the anus or near the tailbone
postprandial (PP) (pōst-prăn′ dĭ-ăl)	post- prand/i -al	after meal pertaining to	Pertaining to after a meal
probiotics			Live microorganisms that, when administered in adequate amounts, confer a health benefit on the digestive system. In the United States, probiotics are available as dietary supplements (including capsules, tablets, and powders) and in dairy foods (such as yogurts with live active cultures).

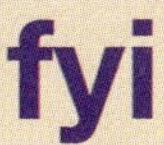

The FDA has not approved any health claims for probiotics; however, they are used for a variety of gastrointestinal conditions such as infectious diarrhea, diarrhea associated with using antibiotics, irritable bowel syndrome, and inflammatory bowel disease.

Medical Word	Word Parts: Part	Word Parts: Meaning	Definition
proctoscope (prŏk′ tō-scōp)	proct/o -scope	anus and rectum instrument for examining	An instrument used in a medical procedure to view the interior of the rectal cavity; a short (10 in or 25 cm long), straight, rigid, hollow metal tube, usually with a small light bulb mounted at the end
pyloric (pī-lōr′ ĭk)	pylor -ic	pylorus, gatekeeper pertaining to	Pertaining to the gatekeeper, the opening between the stomach and the duodenum. In *pyloric stenosis* seen in an infant, the hypertrophied pyloric muscle causes symptoms of projectile vomiting and visible peristalsis.
rectocele (rĕk′ tō-sēl)	rect/o -cele	rectum hernia	Hernia of part of the rectum into the vagina
sialadenitis (sī″ ăl-ăd″ ĕ-nī′ tĭs)	sial aden -itis	saliva gland inflammation	Inflammation of a salivary gland

Medical Word	Word Parts: Part	Word Parts: Meaning	Definition
sigmoidoscope (sĭg-moy´ dō-skōp)	sigmoid/o -scope	sigmoid instrument for examining	An instrument used in a medical procedure to view the interior of the sigmoid colon
splenomegaly (splē˝ nō-mĕg´ ă-lē)	splen/o -megaly	spleen enlargement, large	Enlargement of the spleen
stomatitis (stō˝ mă-tī´ tĭs)	stomat -itis	mouth inflammation	Inflammation of the mouth
sublingual (sŭb-lĭng´ gwăl)	sub- lingu -al	below tongue pertaining to	Pertaining to below the tongue. See Figure 8.26.

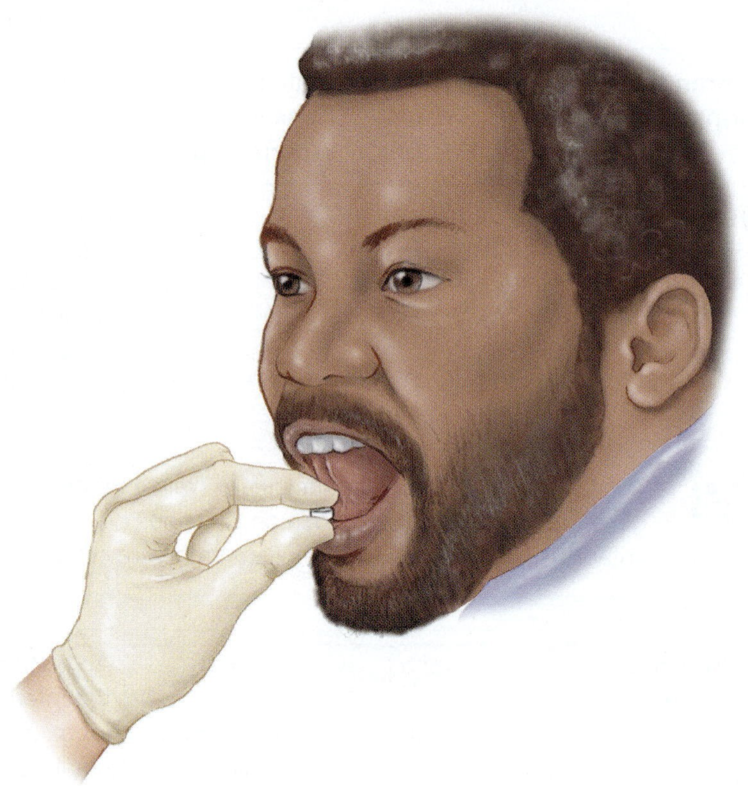

Figure 8.26 Sublingual drug administration.

Medical Word	Word Parts: Part	Word Parts: Meaning	Definition
ulcerative colitis (UC) (ŭl´ sĕr-ă-tĭv kō-lī´ tĭs)			Disease that causes inflammation and ulcers in the lining of the large intestine. The inflammation usually occurs in the rectum and lower part of the colon but can affect the entire colon; also called *colitis* or *proctitis*.
vermiform (vĕr´ mĭ-form)	verm/i -form	worm shape	Shaped like a worm; the vermiform appendix is so named because of its worm-like shape

Medical Word	Word Parts		Definition
	Part	Meaning	
volvulus (vŏl´ vū-lŭs)	volvul -us	to roll pertaining to	Twisting of the bowel on itself that causes an obstruction. See Figure 8.27.

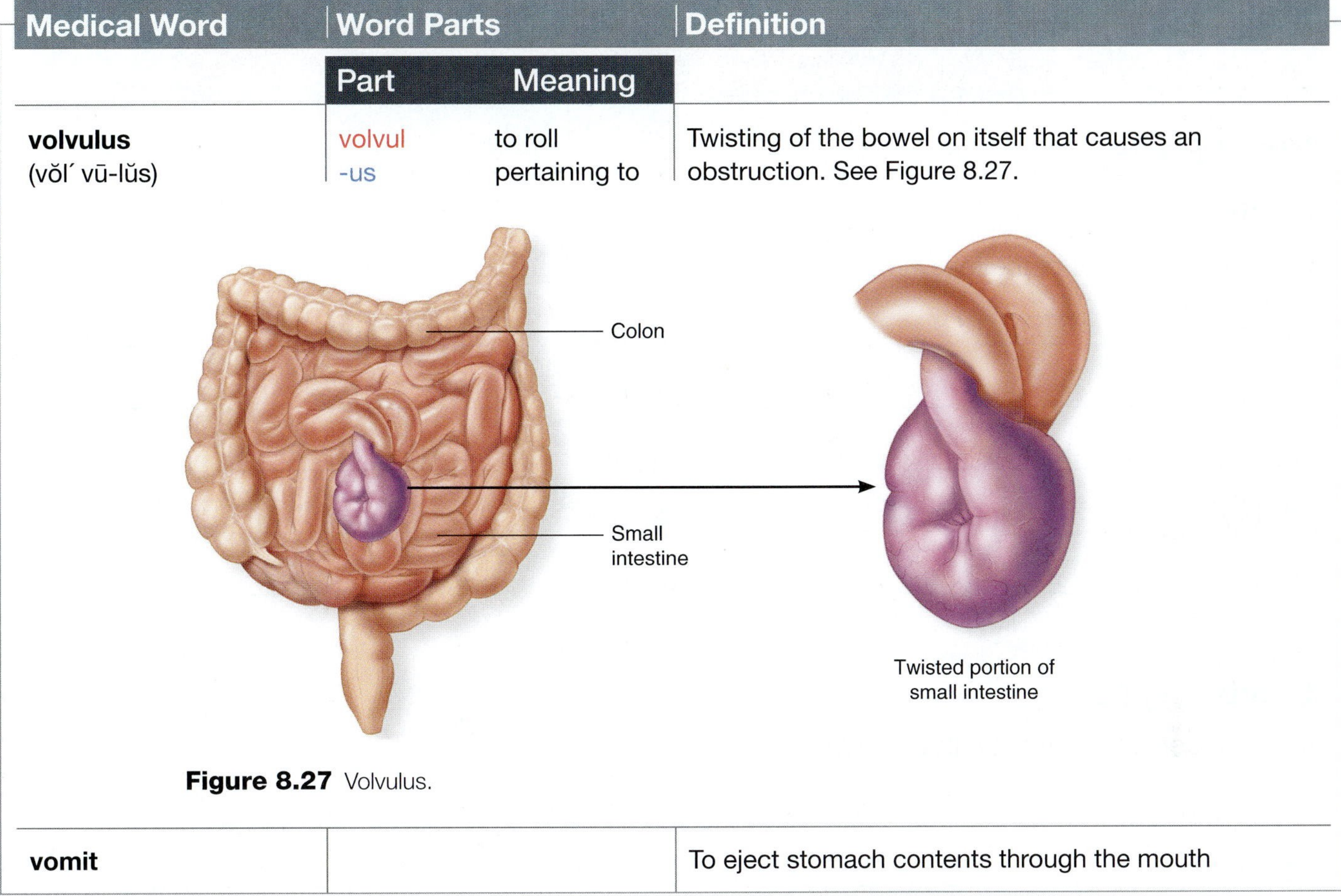

Figure 8.27 Volvulus.

vomit			To eject stomach contents through the mouth

Study and Review II

Word Parts

Prefixes

Give the definitions of the following prefixes.

1. an- ______________________
2. dys- ______________________
3. epi- ______________________
4. hyper- ______________________
5. hypo- ______________________
6. mal- ______________________
7. peri- ______________________
8. post- ______________________
9. dia- ______________________
10. sub- ______________________

Combining Forms

Give the definitions of the following combining forms.

1. amyl/o ______________________
2. append/o ______________________
3. bil/i ______________________
4. bucc/o ______________________
5. celi/o ______________________
6. chol/e ______________________
7. cirrh/o ______________________
8. colon/o ______________________
9. dent/o ______________________
10. enter/o ______________________
11. esophage/o ______________________
12. gastr/o ______________________
13. gingiv/o ______________________
14. gloss/o ______________________
15. hepat/o ______________________
16. ile/o ______________________
17. labi/o ______________________
18. lapar/o ______________________
19. lingu/o ______________________
20. odont/o ______________________
21. prand/i ______________________
22. proct/o ______________________
23. rect/o ______________________
24. stomat/o ______________________

Suffixes

Give the definitions of the following suffixes.

1. -ac	__________	**2.** -al	__________
3. -algia	__________	**4.** -ary	__________
5. -ase	__________	**6.** -cele	__________
7. -oid	__________	**8.** -sis	__________
9. -ectomy	__________	**10.** -emesis	__________
11. -form	__________	**12.** -genesis	__________
13. -ic	__________	**14.** -in	__________
15. -ion	__________	**16.** -ism	__________
17. -ist	__________	**18.** -itis	__________
19. -ive	__________	**20.** -logy	__________
21. -lysis	__________	**22.** -megaly	__________
23. -oma	__________	**24.** -orexia	__________
25. -osis	__________	**26.** -rrhea	__________
27. -pepsia	__________	**28.** -us	__________
29. -phagia	__________	**30.** -scope	__________
31. -scopy	__________	**32.** -stalsis	__________
33. -stomy	__________	**34.** -tomy	__________
35. -y	__________	**36.** -rrhaphy	__________

Identifying Medical Terms

In the spaces provided, write the medical terms for the following meanings.

1. __________ Enzyme that breaks down starch

2. __________ Building up of the body substance in the constructive phase of metabolism

3. __________ Lack of appetite

4. __________ Surgical excision of the appendix

5. __________ Inflammation of the appendix

6. ______________________________ Pertaining to bile

7. ______________________________ Pertaining to the abdomen

8. ______________________________ Difficulty in swallowing

9. ______________________________ Inflammation of the liver

10. ______________________________ Surgical repair of a hernia

11. ______________________________ Pertaining to after meals

12. ______________________________ Enlargement of the spleen

13. ______________________________ An instrument used in a medical procedure to view the interior of the sigmoid colon

Matching

Select the appropriate lettered meaning for each of the following words.

__________ **1.** cirrhosis

__________ **2.** constipation

__________ **3.** diarrhea

__________ **4.** gavage

__________ **5.** hemorrhoid

__________ **6.** hernia

__________ **7.** hyperemesis

__________ **8.** lavage

__________ **9.** pilonidal cyst

__________ **10.** volvulus

a. To wash out a cavity

b. To feed liquid or semiliquid food via a tube

c. Twisting of the bowel on itself that causes an obstruction

d. Frequent passage of unformed watery stool

e. Chronic degenerative liver disease

f. Infrequent passage of unduly hard and dry feces

g. Closed sac in the crease of the sacrococcygeal region

h. Abnormal protrusion of an organ or a part of an organ through the wall of the body cavity that normally contains it

i. Mass of dilated, tortuous veins in the anorectum

j. Excessive vomiting

k. Evacuation of the bowel

Medical Case Snapshots

This learning activity provides an opportunity to relate the medical terminology you are learning to a precise patient case presentation. In the spaces provided, write in your answers.

Case 1

A 54-year-old male was scheduled for a routine visual examination of the colon also known as a ____________. The exam revealed a malignancy of the colon. He was scheduled for a ______________ (a procedure to create a new opening into the colon).

Case 2

A 72-year-old male presents with symptoms of infrequent passage of hard, dry feces. A rectal exam reveals a mass of dilated, tortuous veins in the anorectum. The patient is advised that he has ______________ and ______________. He is to take a laxative to loosen the bowel and is advised to increase his intake of fluids and fiber.

Case 3

A 37-year-old male complains of dull, aching pain in the stomach and back. He has "heartburn and belching." His symptoms suggest peptic ulcer disease, which is often caused by ______________ ______________ (a bacterium). This condition can often be cured with the use of a combination of medications, including ______________ (drugs that kill bacteria).

Drug Highlights

Type of Drug	Description and Examples
antacids	Neutralize hydrochloric acid in the stomach; classified as nonsystemic and systemic.
nonsystemic	EXAMPLES: Amphojel (aluminum hydroxide), Tums (calcium carbonate), Riopan (magaldrate), and Milk of Magnesia (magnesium hydroxide)
systemic	EXAMPLE: sodium bicarbonate
antacid mixtures	Products that combine aluminum (may cause constipation) and/or calcium compounds with magnesium salts (may cause diarrhea). By combining the antacid properties of two single-entity agents, these products provide the antacid action of both yet tend to counter the adverse effects of each other. EXAMPLES: Gaviscon, Gelusil, Maalox Plus, and Mylanta
histamine H_2-receptor antagonists	Inhibit both daytime and nocturnal basal gastric acid secretion and inhibit gastric acid stimulated by food, histamines, caffeine, and insulin used in the treatment of active duodenal ulcer. EXAMPLES: Tagamet (cimetidine), Pepcid (famotidine), Axid (nizatidine), and Zantac (ranitidine)
mucosal protective medications	Medicines that protect the stomach's mucosal lining from acids but do not inhibit the release of acid. EXAMPLES: Carafate (sucralfate) and Cytotec (misoprostol)
gastric acid pump inhibitors (proton-pump inhibitors [PPIs])	Antiulcer agents that suppress gastric acid secretion by specific inhibition of the H + /K + ATPase enzyme at the secretory surface of the gastric parietal cell. Because this enzyme system is regarded as the acid (proton) pump within the gastric mucosa, gastric acid pump inhibitors are so classified because they block the final step of acid production. EXAMPLES: Prilosec (omeprazole), Aciphex (rabeprazole sodium), Prevacid (lansoprazole), Protonix (pantoprazole), and Nexium (esomeprazole magnesium)
other ulcer medications	Treatment regimen for active duodenal ulcers associated with *H. pylori* can involve a two-, three-, or four-drug program. EXAMPLES: A two-drug program—Biaxin (clarithromycin) and Prilosec (omeprazole)—a three-drug program—Flagyl (metronidazole) and either tetracycline or amoxicillin and Pepto-Bismol—and a four-drug program—a proton pump inhibitor plus a single capsule containing bismuth subcitrate potassium, metronidazole, and tetracycline *Note:* For the treatment to be effective, the patient must complete the full treatment program, which usually involves taking the drugs for a total of at least 10-14 days for the two- and three-drug program and 10 days for the four-drug program.

Type of Drug	Description and Examples
agents used for inflammatory bowel disease	Step I – Aminosalicylates (oral, enema, suppository formulations): For treating flare-ups and maintaining remission; more effective in ulcerative colitis (UC) than in Crohn disease (CD) Step IA – Antibiotics: Used sparingly in UC (limited efficacy, increased risk for antibiotic-associated pseudomembranous colitis); in CD, most commonly used for perianal disease, fistulas, intra-abdominal inflammatory masses Step II – Corticosteroids (intravenous, oral, topical, rectal): For acute disease flare-ups only Step III – Immunomodulators: Effective for steroid-sparing action in refractory disease; primary treatment for fistulas and maintenance of remission in patients intolerant of or not responsive to aminosalicylates
laxatives	Used to relieve constipation and to facilitate the passage of feces through the lower gastrointestinal tract. EXAMPLES: Dulcolax (bisacodyl), Milk of Magnesia (magnesium hydroxide), Metamucil (psyllium hydrophilic mucilloid), and Ex-Lax (phenolphthalein)
antidiarrheal agents	Used to treat diarrhea. EXAMPLES: Pepto-Bismol (bismuth subsalicylate), Kaopectate (kaolin mixture with pectin), and Imodium (loperamide HCl)
antiemetics	Prevent or arrest vomiting; also used in the treatment of vertigo, motion sickness, and nausea. EXAMPLES: Dramamine (dimenhydrinate), Phenergan (promethazine HCl), Tigan (trimethobenzamide HCl), and Transderm Scop (scopolamine)
emetics	Used to induce vomiting in people who have taken an overdose of oral drugs or who have ingested certain poisons. An emetic agent should not be given to a person who is unconscious, in shock, or in a semicomatose state. Emetics are also contraindicated in individuals who have ingested strongly caustic substances, such as lye or acid, because their use could result in additional injury to the person's esophagus. EXAMPLE: Ipecac syrup

Diagnostic and Laboratory Tests

Test	Description
alcohol toxicology (ethanol and ethyl) (ăl′ kō-hŏl tŏks″ ĭ-kŏl′ ō-jē)	Test performed on blood serum or plasma to determine levels of alcohol. All 50 states and the District of Columbia have laws defining it as a crime to drive with a blood alcohol concentration (BAC) at or above 0.08%. Increased values indicate alcohol consumption that could lead to cirrhosis of the liver, gastritis, malnutrition, vitamin deficiencies, and other gastrointestinal disorders.
carcinoembryonic antigen (CEA) (kăr″ sĭn-ō-ĕm″ brē-ŏn′ ĭk ăn′ tĭ-jĕn)	Test performed on whole blood or plasma to determine the presence of CEA (antigens originally isolated from colon tumors). Increased values can indicate stomach, intestinal, rectal, and various other cancers and conditions. This test is nonspecific and must be combined with other tests for a final diagnosis. It is being used to monitor the course of cancer therapy.
cholangiography (kō-lăn″ jē-ŏg′ ră-fē)	X-ray examination of the common bile duct, cystic duct, and hepatic ducts in which radiopaque dye is injected and then films are taken. Abnormal results can indicate obstruction, stones, and tumors.
cholecystography (kō″ lē-sĭs-tŏg′ ră-fē)	X-ray examination of the gallbladder in which radiopaque dye is injected and then films are taken. Abnormal results can indicate cholecystitis, cholelithiasis, and tumors.
colonoscopy (kō′ lŏn-ŏs′ kō-pē)	Direct visual examination of the colon via a colonoscope; used to diagnose growths to confirm findings of other tests and to rule out or rule in colon cancer. It can also be used to remove small polyps and to collect tissue samples for analysis. The patient is lightly sedated during the procedure.
comprehensive metabolic panel (CMP)	Includes 14 tests that provide information about the current status of a patient's metabolism, including the health of the kidneys and liver, electrolyte and acid–base balance, and levels of blood glucose and blood proteins. Abnormal results, and especially combinations of abnormal results, can indicate a problem that needs to be addressed.
endoscopic retrograde cholangiopancreatography (ERCP) (ĕn″ dō-skŏp′ ĭk rĕt′ rō-grād kō-lăn″ jē-ō-păn″ krē-ă-tŏg′ ră-fē)	X-ray examination of the biliary and pancreatic ducts by injecting a contrast medium and then films are taken. Abnormal results can indicate fibrosis, biliary or pancreatic cysts, strictures, stones, and chronic pancreatitis.

Test	Description
esophagogastroduodenal endoscopy (ĕ-sŏf″ ă-gō′ găs″ trō-dū″ ō-dē′ năl ĕn-dŏs′kō-pē)	Endoscopic examination of the esophagus, stomach, and small intestine. During the procedure, photographs, biopsy, or brushings may be done.

fyi Upper esophagogastroduodenal endoscopy (also known as *esophagogastroduodenoscopy*) is considered the reference method of diagnosis of peptic ulcer disease. The diagnosis of *H. pylori* can be made by several methods. The biopsy urease test is a colorimetric test based on the ability of *H. pylori* to produce urease; it provides rapid testing at the time of biopsy. Histological identification of organisms is considered the gold standard of diagnostic tests. Culture of biopsy specimens for *H. pylori*, which requires an experienced laboratory, is necessary when antimicrobial susceptibility testing is desired.

Test	Description
fiberoptic colonoscopy (fī″ bĕr-ŏp′ tĭk kō″ lŏn-ŏs′ kō-pē)	Fiberoptic colonoscopy, a direct visual examination of the colon via a flexible colonoscope; used as a diagnostic aid for removal of foreign bodies, polyps, and tissue. The patient is lightly sedated during the procedure.
gamma-glutamyltransferase (GGT) (găm′ ă glōō′ tăm-ĭl-trăns′ fĕr-ās)	Test performed on blood serum to determine the level of GGT (enzyme found in the liver, kidney, prostate, heart, and spleen). Increased values can indicate cirrhosis, liver necrosis, hepatitis, alcoholism, neoplasms, acute pancreatitis, acute myocardial infarction, nephrosis, and acute cholecystitis.
gastric analysis (găs′ trĭk ă-năl′ ĭ-sĭs)	Test performed to determine quality of secretion, amount of free and combined hydrochloric acid (HCl), and absence or presence of blood, bacteria, bile, and fatty acids. Increased level of HCl can indicate peptic ulcer disease, Zollinger–Ellison syndrome (a condition caused by non-insulin-secreting pancreatic tumors, which secrete excess amounts of gastrin), and hypergastrinemia. Decreased level of HCl can indicate stomach cancer, pernicious anemia, and atrophic gastritis.
gastrointestinal (GI) series (găs″ trō-ĭn-tes′ tĭn″ ăl)	Fluoroscopic examination of the esophagus, stomach, and small intestine in which barium is given orally and is observed as it flows through the GI system. Abnormal results can indicate esophageal varices, ulcers, gastric polyps, malabsorption syndrome, hiatal hernias, diverticula, pyloric stenosis, and foreign bodies.
hepatitis panel (hĕp″ ă-tī″ tĭs)	A blood test used to find markers of hepatitis infection. There are different hepatitis panels. Some tests look for proteins (antibodies) that the body makes to fight the infection. Other tests look for antigens or the genetic material (DNA or RNA) of the viruses that cause hepatitis. A common panel checks for: • hepatitis A IgM antibodies (HA Ab-IgM) • hepatitis B surface antigen (HBsAg) • hepatitis B IgM core antibody (HBcAb-IgM) • hepatitis C antibodies (HC Ab)
liver biopsy	Microscopic examination of liver tissue. Abnormal results can indicate cirrhosis, hepatitis, and tumors.

Test	Description
occult blood (ŭ -kŭlt′)	Test performed on feces to determine gastrointestinal bleeding that is not visible. Positive results can indicate gastritis, stomach cancer, peptic ulcer, ulcerative colitis, bowel cancer, bleeding esophageal varices, portal hypertension, pancreatitis, and diverticulitis.
ova and parasites (O&P) (ō′ vă and păr′ ă-sīts)	Test performed on stool to identify ova and parasites. Positive results indicate protozoa infestation.
stool culture	Test performed on stool to identify the presence of organisms.
ultrasonography, gallbladder (ŭl-tră-sŏn-ŏg′ ră-fē)	Test to visualize the gallbladder by using high-frequency sound waves. The echoes are recorded on an oscilloscope and film. Abnormal results can indicate biliary obstruction, cholelithiasis, and acute cholecystitis.
ultrasonography, liver	Test to visualize the liver by using high-frequency sound waves. The echoes are recorded on an oscilloscope and film. Abnormal results can indicate hepatic tumors, cysts, abscess, and cirrhosis.
upper gastrointestinal (UGI) endoscopy (găs′ trō-ĭn-tĕs′ tĭn″ ăl ĕn-dŏs′ kō-pē)	Direct visual examination of the gastric mucosa via a flexible fiberoptic endoscope when gastric neoplasm is suspected. Colored photographs or motion pictures can be taken during the procedure.

Abbreviations

Abbreviation	Meaning
Ba	barium
BAC	blood alcohol concentration
BE	Barrett esophagus
BM	bowel movement
CD	Crohn disease
CEA	carcinoembryonic antigen
CHO	carbohydrate
CMP	comprehensive metabolic panel
EE	erosive esophagitis
ERCP	endoscopic retrograde cholangiopancreatography
GB	gallbladder
GERD	gastroesophageal reflux disease
GGT	gamma-glutamyltransferase
GI	gastrointestinal
HAV	hepatitis A virus
HBIG	hepatitis B immune globulin
HB_sAg	hepatitis B surface antigen
HCl	hydrochloric acid
HCV	hepatitis C virus
HDV	hepatitis D virus
HEV	hepatitis E virus
IBD	inflammatory bowel disease
IBS	irritable bowel syndrome
LES	lower esophageal sphincter
NG	nasogastric (tube)
NH_3	ammonia
O&P	ova and parasites
OIC	opioid-induced constipation
PP	postprandial (after meals)
PPIs	proton-pump inhibitors
PUD	peptic ulcer disease
UC	ulcerative colitis
UGI	upper gastrointestinal

Study and Review III

Building Medical Terms

Using the following word parts, fill in the blanks to build the correct medical terms.

dys-	-al	-itis
bucc	-ectomy	-cele
gingiv	-osis	
lapar/o	-stomy	

Definition	Medical Term
1. Surgical excision of the appendix	append______
2. Literally means pertaining to the cheek	___________al
3. Chronic degenerative liver disease	cirrh ________
4. The creation of a new opening into the colon	colo_________
5. Inflammation of the diverticula in the colon	diverticul_____
6. Difficulty in digestion; indigestion	_______ pepsia
7. Inflammation of the gums	__________itis
8. Surgical incision into the abdomen	________ tomy
9. Pertaining to the tongue	lingu_________
10. Hernia of part of the rectum into the vagina	recto________

Combining Form Challenge

Using the combining forms provided, write the medical term correctly.

absorpt/o	bil/i	gloss/o
append/o	esophage/o	hepat/o

1. Process by which nutrient material is transferred from the gastrointestinal tract into the bloodstream or lymph: ____________ion

2. Surgical excision of the appendix: ____________ectomy

3. Pertaining to bile: ____________ary

4. Pertaining to the esophagus: _____________ al

5. Partial or total surgical excision of the tongue: ______________ectomy

6. Inflammation of the liver: ____________ itis

Select the Right Term

Select the correct answer, and write it on the line provided.

1. Inflammation of the gallbladder is _______________.

   choledochotomy **cholecystitis** **cheilosis** **appendicitis**

2. Significant accumulation of fluid in the peritoneal cavity is ____________.

   ascites **anabolism** **cirrhosis** **celiac**

3. A surgical procedure that brings one end of the large intestine out through an opening (stoma) made in the abdominal wall is called a _____________.

   colonoscopy **colostomy** **colectomy** **cholecystectomy**

4. The term that means pertaining to the stomach and esophagus is _____________.

   gastroenterology **gastroesophageal** **gastoesophaeal** **gastroenteritis**

5. To feed liquid or semiliquid food via a tube is _______________.

   gastric **enteric** **gavage** **deglutition**

6. Chewing; the physical breaking up of food and mixing with saliva is _______.

   malabsorption **mastication** **lavage** **gavage**

Diagnostic and Laboratory Tests

Select the best answer to each multiple-choice question. Circle the letter of your choice.

1. X-ray examination of the common bile duct, cystic duct, and hepatic ducts.
   a. cholangiography **b.** cholecystography
   c. cholangiopancreatography **d.** ultrasonography

2. Direct visual examination of the colon via a flexible colonoscope.
   a. cholangiography **b.** ultrasonography
   c. fiberoptic colonoscopy **d.** cholecystography

3. Fluoroscopic examination of the esophagus, stomach, and small intestine.
   a. colonoscopy **b.** ultrasonography
   c. cholangiography **d.** gastrointestinal series

4. Endoscopic examination of the esophagus, stomach, and small intestine.
   a. cholangiography **b.** gastroduodenoesophagoscopy
   c. esophagogastroduodenoscopy **d.** gastric analysis

5. Test performed to determine the presence of the hepatitis B virus.
   a. occult blood test **b.** stool culture
   c. hepatitis B surface antigen **d.** ova and parasites test

Abbreviations

Place the correct word, phrase, or abbreviation in the space provided.

1. barium ______________________________
2. CHO ______________________________
3. HCV ______________________________
4. hydrochloric acid ______________________________
5. gallbladder ______________________________
6. hepatitis A virus ______________________________
7. NG ______________________________
8. irritable bowel syndrome ______________________________
9. postprandial (after meals) ______________________________
10. proton-pump inhibitors ______________________________

Practical Application

Medical Record Analysis

The Patient Referral Form is an important part of a patient's chart. As part of your learning process and in preparation for a career in a medical environment, you are to assume the role of a medical employee and use the following information—together with your own input—to complete the Patient Referral Form.

PATIENT REFERRAL FORM

Task Edit View Time Scale Options Help Date: 28 September 2017

Patient referred to Seymour Butts, MD, Endoscopy Center, 14 Maddox Drive, Rome, GA 30165, phone number (706) 235-3957, fax (706) 235-8877, for a screening colonoscopy on October 17, 2017, at 8:45 a.m. Advise patient to bring a driver, all current medications, driver's license, and proof of insurance

Referring physician, Angel De'Crohn, MD, Family Practice, 1165 Berry Blvd, Rome, GA 30165, (706) 235-7765, fax (706) 235-6676.

Patient Referral Form

Our practice is affiliated with Mercy Medical Center

Please refer this patient to Mercy Medical Center for any needed surgery or diagnostic procedures so that we can better coordinate this patient's care.

Date: 09/28/17

Patient Name: Ralph J. Starr DOB: 2/24/53 Phone Number 123-456-7890

Appointment Date: ______________________ Time: ______________________

Referred to: ____

____

For:

______________________ Diagnostic Procedure ______________________

______________________ Consultation

______________________ Evaluate and treat, initiating appropriate diagnostic and/or therapeutic services

______________________ Report test results to: ______________________

Reason for referral: ____

Patient Instructions: ____

____

____

Referring Physician's Name: ____________________ Date: ____________________

Phone #: ________________________ Fax #: ________________________

Remit the Record of this Patient's Visit to the Physician Noted Above.

For Office Use Only (appointment made at a time when the patient was not present)

Patient notified of appointment: Date: ____________ Initials: ____________

Unable to contact patient

Attempts to notify: Date/Time/Initials

1. ____

2. ____

3. ____

Comments: ____

Certified Letter Sent: Date: ________________ Initials: ________________

Referral Form Questions

Place the correct answer in the space provided.

1. Write in the Appointment Date: ________________________ Time: ________________________

2. The patient was referred to (write in name of physician, center name, and address):

____

____

____

____

3. The patient was referred for:

_______________________ Diagnostic Procedure

_______________________ Screening Colonoscopy

_______________________ Consultation

_______________________ Evaluate and treat, initiating appropriate diagnostic and/or therapeutic services

_______________________ Report test results to: Angel De'Crohn, MD

4. The Patient Instructions were: ___________________________

5. Write in the name of:

Referring Physician: ___________________________

Date: ______________________________

Phone #: ___________________________

Fax #: _____________________________

Chapter 9

Cardiovascular System

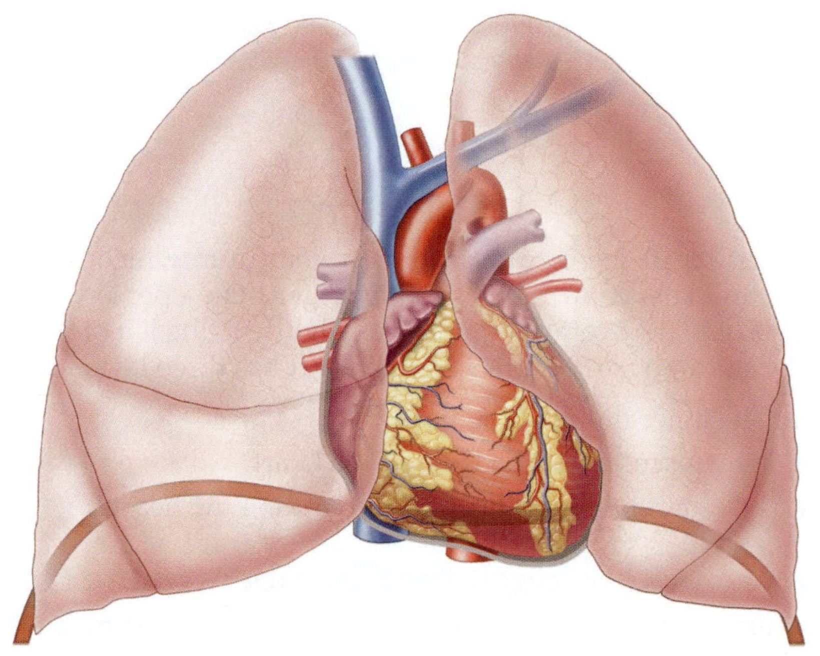

Learning Outcomes

On completion of this chapter, you will be able to:

1. State the description and primary functions of the organs/structures of the cardiovascular system.
2. Explain the circulation of blood through the chambers of the heart.
3. Identify and locate the commonly used sites for taking a pulse.
4. Explain blood pressure.
5. Recognize terminology included in the ICD-10-CM.
6. Analyze, build, spell, and pronounce medical words.
7. Comprehend the drugs highlighted in this chapter.
8. Describe diagnostic and laboratory tests related to the cardiovascular system.
9. Identify and define selected abbreviations.
10. Apply your acquired knowledge of medical terms by successfully completing the *Practical Application* exercise.

Anatomy and Physiology

The cardiovascular (CV) system, also called the *circulatory system*, circulates blood to all parts of the body by the action of the heart. This process provides the body's cells with oxygen and nutritive elements and removes waste materials and carbon dioxide. The heart, a muscular pump, is the central organ of the system. It beats approximately 100,000 times each day, pumping roughly 8,000 liters of blood, enough to fill about 8,500 quart-sized milk cartons. Arteries, veins, and capillaries comprise the network of vessels that transport blood (fluid consisting of blood cells and plasma) throughout the body. Blood flows through the heart, to the lungs, back to the heart, and on to the various body parts. Table 9.1 provides an at-a-glance look at the cardiovascular system. Figure 9.1 shows a schematic overview of the cardiovascular system.

Heart

The **heart** is the center of the cardiovascular system from which the various blood vessels originate and later return. It is slightly larger than a person's fist and weighs approximately 300 g in the average adult. It lies slightly to the left of the midline of the body, behind the sternum (see Figure 9.2). The heart has three layers or linings.

- **Endocardium**. The inner lining of the heart.
- **Myocardium**. The muscular middle layer of the heart.
- **Pericardium**. The outer membranous sac surrounding the heart.

Circulation of Blood through the Chambers of the Heart

The heart is a pump and is divided into the right and left heart by a partition called the **septum**. Each side contains an upper and lower chamber. See Figure 9.3. The **atria**, or upper chambers, are separated by the interatrial septum. The **ventricles**, or lower chambers, are separated by the interventricular septum. The atria receive blood from the various parts of the body. The ventricles pump blood to body parts. Valves control the intake and outflow of blood in the heart chambers. Figure 9.4 shows the functioning of the heart valves and flow of blood through the heart.

Table 9.1 Cardiovascular System at-a-Glance

Organ/Structure	Primary Functions/Description
Heart	The muscular pump that circulates blood through the heart, the lungs (pulmonary circulation), and the rest of the body (systemic circulation)
Arteries	Branching system of vessels that transports blood from the right and left ventricles of the heart to all body parts; transports blood away from the heart
Veins	Vessels that transport blood from peripheral tissues back to the heart
Capillaries	Microscopic blood vessels that connect arterioles with venules; facilitate passage of life-sustaining fluids containing oxygen and nutrients to cell bodies and the removal of accumulated waste and carbon dioxide
Blood	Fluid consisting of formed elements (erythrocytes, thrombocytes, leukocytes) and plasma. It is a specialized bodily fluid that delivers necessary substances to the body's cells (oxygen, foods, salts, hormones) and transports waste products (carbon dioxide, urea, lactic acid) away from those same cells. Blood is circulated around the body through blood vessels by the pumping action of the heart. See Chapter 10, *Blood and Lymphatic System*, for a further discussion of blood.

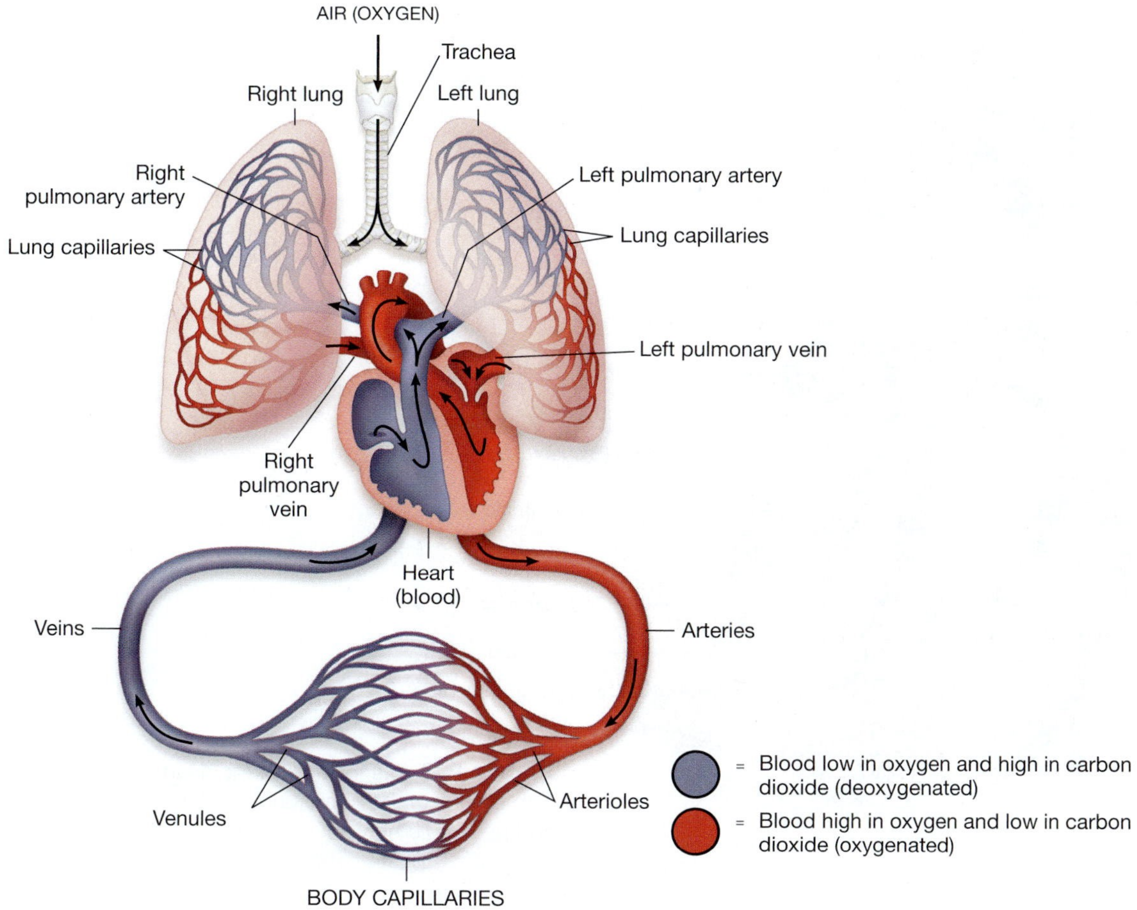

Figure 9.1 Schematic overview of the cardiovascular system.

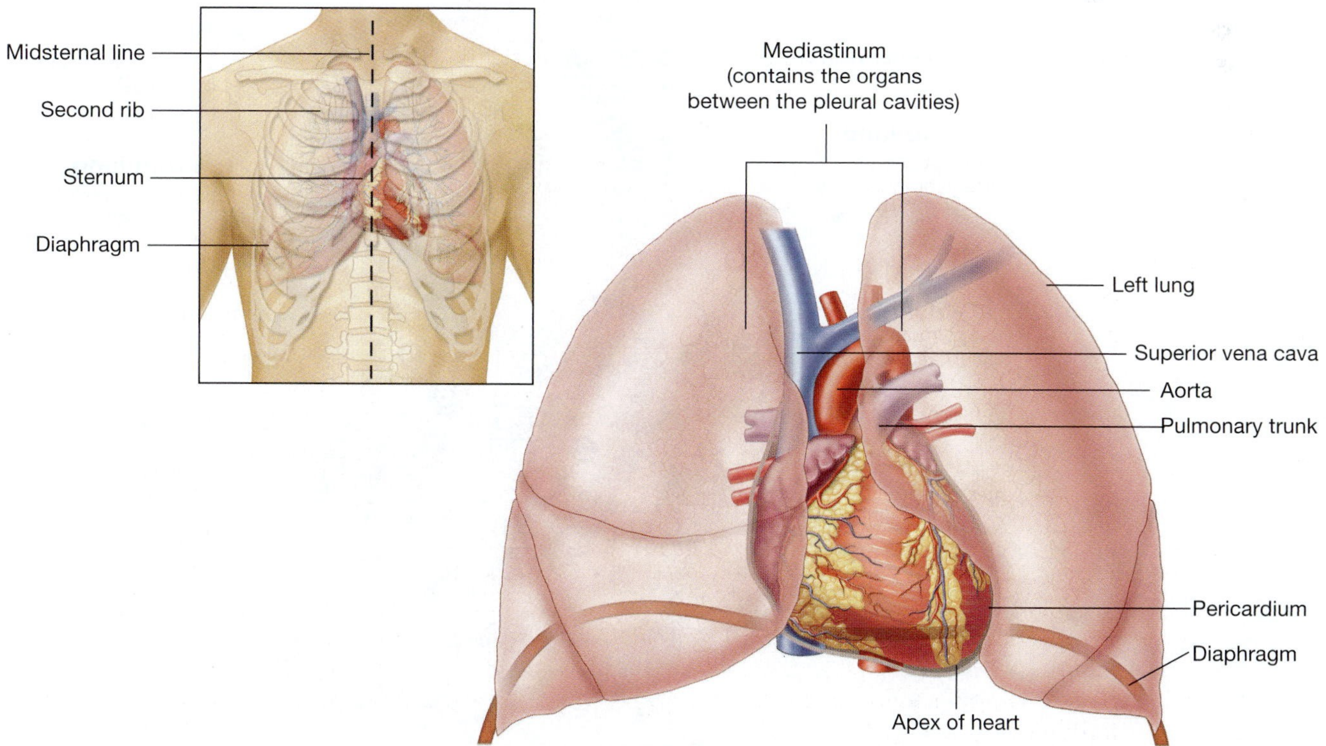

Figure 9.2 Location of the heart in the chest cavity.

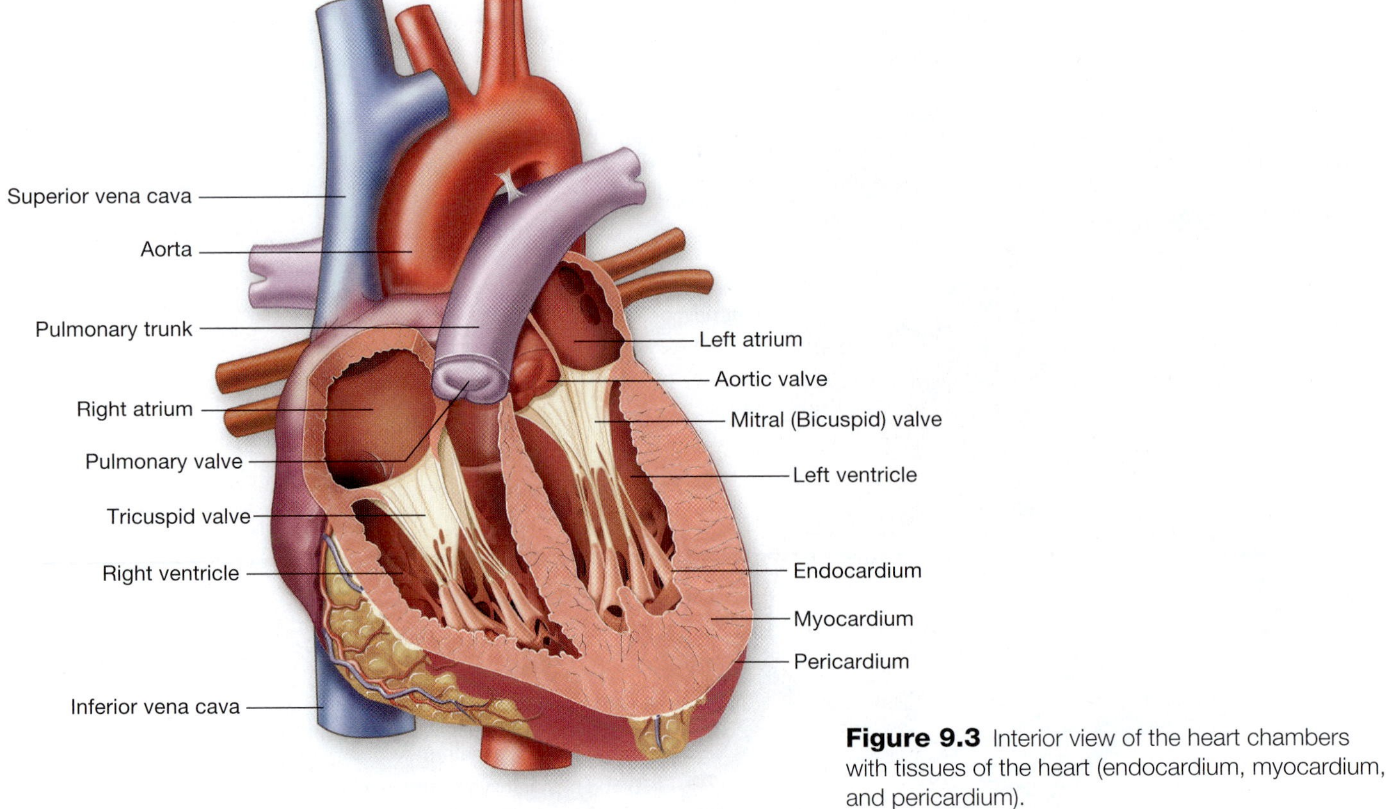

Figure 9.3 Interior view of the heart chambers with tissues of the heart (endocardium, myocardium, and pericardium).

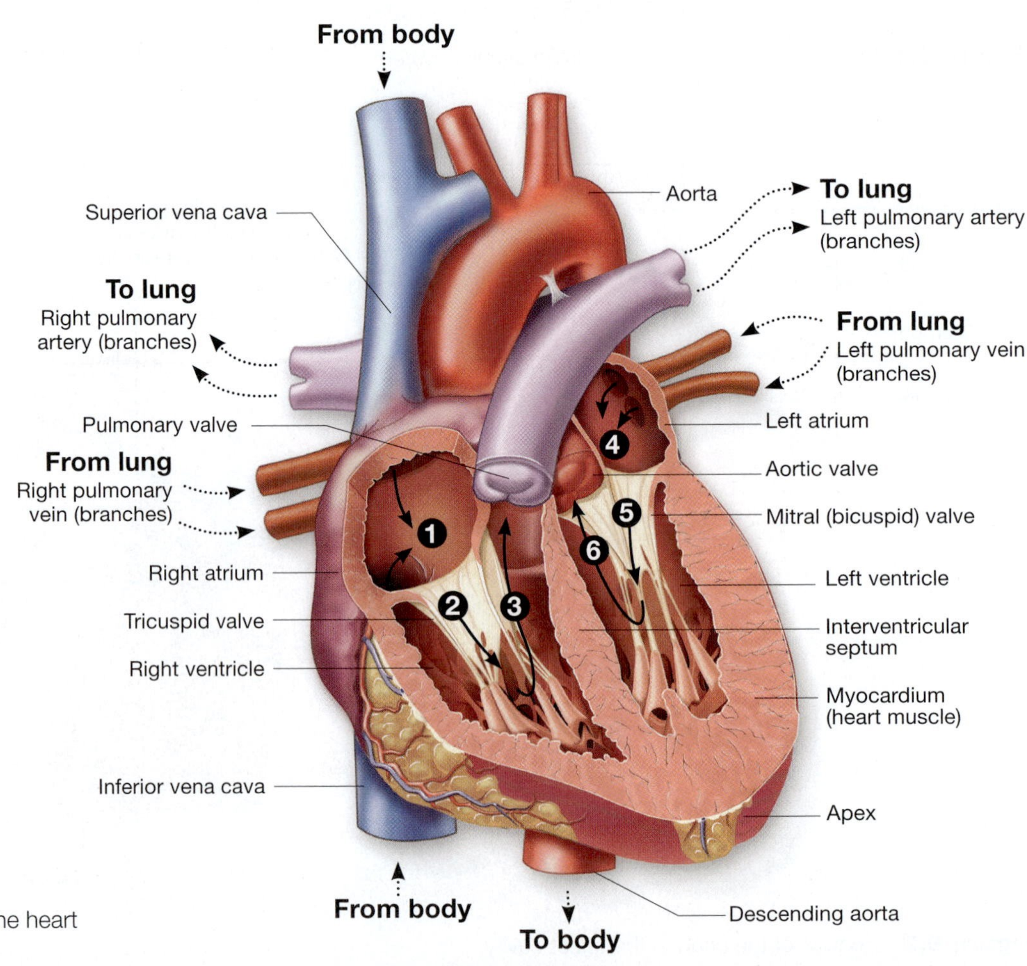

Figure 9.4 The functioning of the heart valves and blood flow.

RIGHT ATRIUM

The right upper portion of the heart is called the **right atrium (RA)**. It is a thin-walled space that receives blood from the upper and lower parts of the body (except the lungs). Two large veins, the superior vena cava and inferior vena cava, bring deoxygenated blood into the right atrium. Deoxygenated blood fills the right atrium before passing through the tricuspid (atrioventricular) valve and into the right ventricle.

RIGHT VENTRICLE

The right lower portion of the heart is called the **right ventricle (RV)**. It receives blood from the right atrium through the tricuspid valve. When filled, the RV contracts. This creates pressure, closing the right atrium and forcing open the pulmonary (semilunar) valve, sending blood into the left and right pulmonary arteries, which carry it to the lungs. The pulmonary artery is the only artery in the body that carries blood deficient in oxygen. In the lungs, the blood gives up wastes and takes on oxygen as it passes through capillary beds into veins. Oxygenated blood leaves the lungs through the left and right pulmonary veins, which carry it to the heart's left atrium. The pulmonary veins are the only veins in the body that carry oxygen-rich (oxygenated) blood. The circulation of blood through the vessels from the heart to the lungs and then back to the heart again is the pulmonary circulation.

LEFT ATRIUM

The left upper portion of the heart is called the **left atrium (LA)**. It receives blood rich in oxygen as it returns from the lungs via the left and right pulmonary veins. As oxygenated blood fills the LA, it creates pressure that forces open the mitral (bicuspid) valve and allows the blood to fill the left ventricle.

LEFT VENTRICLE

The left lower portion of the heart is called the **left ventricle (LV)**. It receives blood from the left atrium through the mitral valve. When filled, the LV contracts. This creates pressure closing the mitral valve and forcing open the aortic valve. The oxygenated blood from the LV flows through the aortic valve and into a large artery known as the **aorta** and from there to all parts of the body (except the lungs) via a branching system of arteries and capillaries.

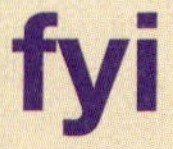

Pediatric cardiologists have recognized more than 50 congenital heart defects. If the left side of the heart is not completely separated from the right side, various septal defects develop. If the four chambers of the heart do not develop normally, complex anomalies form, such as tetralogy of Fallot (TOF), a congenital heart condition involving four defects: pulmonary artery stenosis, ventricular septal defect (VSD), displacement of the aorta to the right, and hypertrophy of the right ventricle.

Heart Valves

The **valves** of the heart are located at the entrance and exit of each ventricle and, as you learned in the preceding section, control the flow of blood within the heart. See Figure 9.5.

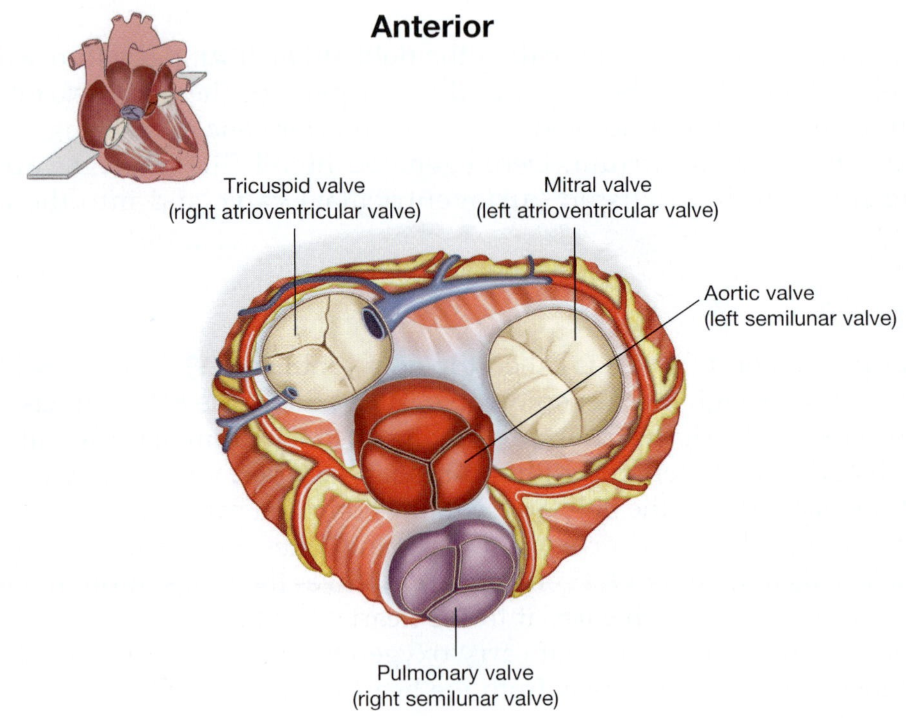

Figure 9.5 Valves of the heart.

TRICUSPID VALVE

The **tricuspid** or **right atrioventricular valve** guards the opening between the right atrium and the right ventricle. In a normal state, the tricuspid valve opens to allow the flow of blood into the ventricle and then closes to prevent any backflow of blood.

PULMONARY (SEMILUNAR) VALVE

The exit point for blood leaving the right ventricle is called the **pulmonary (semilunar) valve**. Located between the right ventricle and the pulmonary artery, it allows blood to flow from the right ventricle through the pulmonary artery to the lungs.

MITRAL (BICUSPID) VALVE

The left atrioventricular valve between the left atrium and the left ventricle is called the **mitral valve (MV)** or **bicuspid valve**. It allows blood to flow to the left ventricle and closes to prevent its return to the left atrium.

AORTIC (SEMILUNAR) VALVE

Blood exits from the left ventricle through the **aortic (semilunar) valve**. Located between the left ventricle and the aorta, it allows blood to flow into the aorta and prevents its backflow to the ventricle.

Vascular System of the Heart

Due to the membranous lining of the heart (endocardium) and the thickness of the myocardium, the heart has its own vascular system to meet its high oxygen demand. The coronary arteries supply the heart with oxygen-rich blood, and the cardiac veins, draining into the coronary sinus, collect the blood (oxygen poor) and return it to the right atrium. See Figure 9.6.

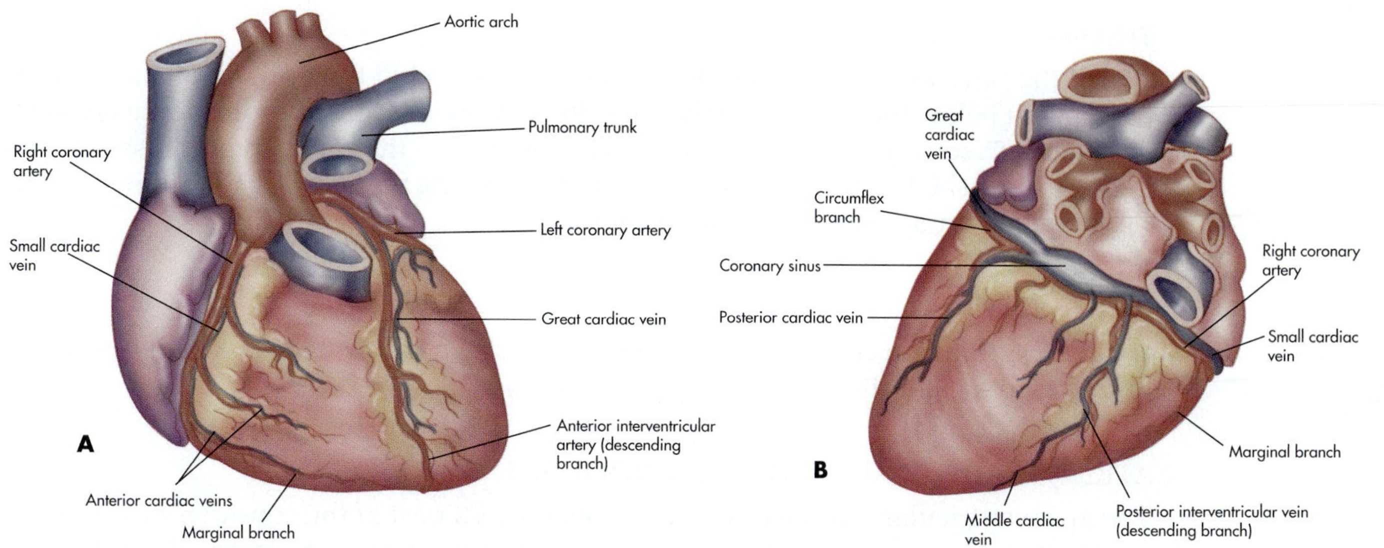

Figure 9.6 Coronary circulation. (A) Coronary vessels portraying the complexity and extent of the coronary circulation. (B) Coronary vessels that supply the posterior surface of the heart.

Conduction System of the Heart

The autonomic nervous system controls the rate and rhythm of the **heartbeat**. It is normally generated by specialized neuromuscular tissue of the heart that is capable of causing cardiac muscle to contract rhythmically. This tissue of the heart comprises the **sinoatrial node**, the **atrioventricular node**, and the **atrioventricular bundle**. See Figure 9.7.

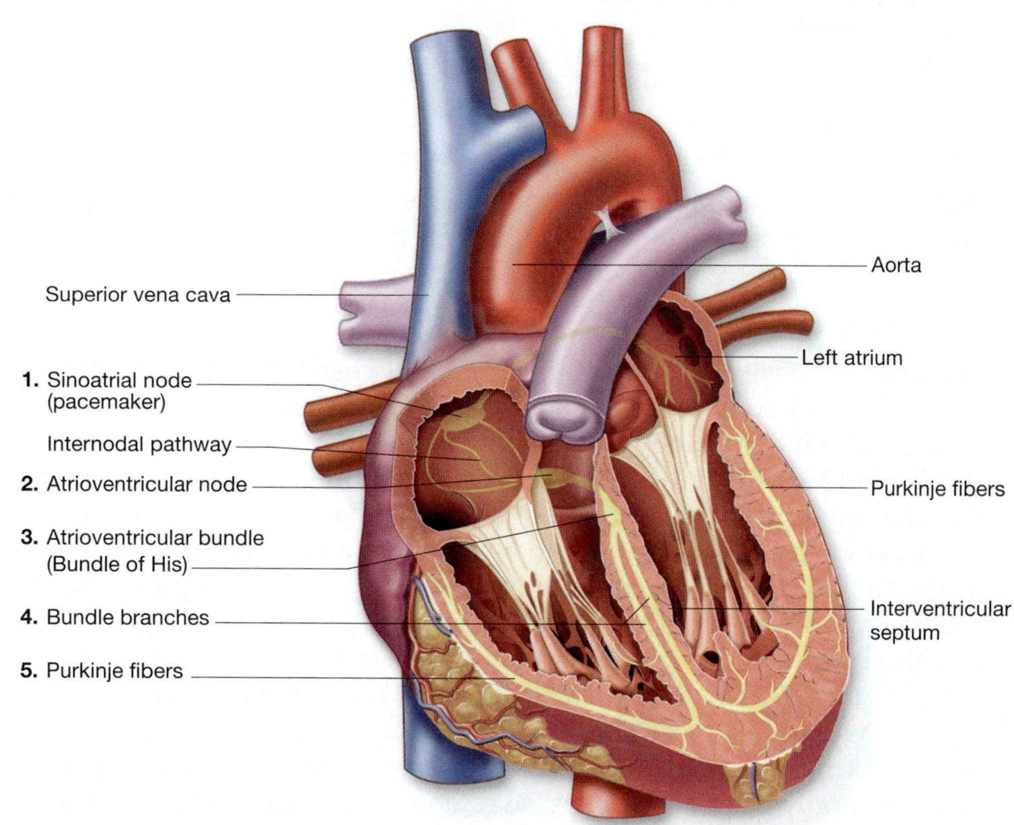

Figure 9.7 Conduction system of the heart.

SINOATRIAL NODE (SA NODE)

Called the *pacemaker* of the heart, the **SA node** is located in the upper wall of the right atrium, just below the opening of the superior vena cava. It consists of a dense network of **Purkinje fibers** (*atypical muscle fibers*) considered to be the source of impulses initiating the heartbeat. Electrical impulses discharged by the SA node are distributed to the right and left atria and cause them to contract.

ATRIOVENTRICULAR NODE (AV NODE)

Located beneath the endocardium of the right atrium, the **AV node** transmits electrical impulses to the bundle of His (*atrioventricular bundle*).

ATRIOVENTRICULAR BUNDLE (BUNDLE OF HIS)

The atrioventricular bundle or **bundle of His** forms a part of the conduction system of the heart. It is a collection of heart muscle cells specialized for electrical conduction that transmits the electrical impulses from the AV node to the point of the apex of the fascicular branches. The bundle of His branches into the two bundle branches that run along the interventricular septum. The bundles give rise to thin filaments known as Purkinje fibers. These fibers distribute the impulse to the ventricular muscle. Together, the bundle branches and **Purkinje network** comprise the ventricular conduction system.

The average adult heartbeat (*pulse*) is between 60 and 90 beats per minute. The rate of the heartbeat can be affected by emotions, smoking, disease, body size, age, stress, the environment, and many other factors.

The heart's electrical activity can be recorded by an **electrocardiogram (ECG, EKG)**, which provides valuable information in diagnosing cardiac abnormalities, such as myocardial damage and arrhythmias (see the section *Diagnostic and Laboratory Tests* and Figure 9.38).

Blood Vessels

There are three main types of blood vessels: arteries, veins, and capillaries. Blood circulates throughout the body through their pathways.

Arteries

The **arteries** constitute a branching system of vessels that transports blood away from the heart to all body parts. See Figure 9.8. In a normal state, arteries are elastic tubes that recoil and carry blood in pulsating waves. All arteries have a pulse, reflecting the rhythmical beating of the heart; however, certain points are commonly used to check the rate, rhythm, and condition of the arterial wall.

A person's pulse can be felt in a place that allows for an artery to be compressed against a bone. The most commonly used sites for taking a pulse are the radial artery, the brachial artery, and the carotid artery. See Table 9.2 and Figure 9.9. The pulse rate can also be measured by using a stethoscope (*auscultation*) and counting the heartbeat for 1 full minute. This is known as the **apical pulse** and is taken over the heart itself. In contrast with other pulse sites, the apical pulse site is unilateral and is located at the apex of the heart or at the fifth intercostal space, just to the left of the midclavicular line. It is commonly used to check pulse rate in infants and children, and when the radial pulse is difficult to palpate (*to feel by touch*).

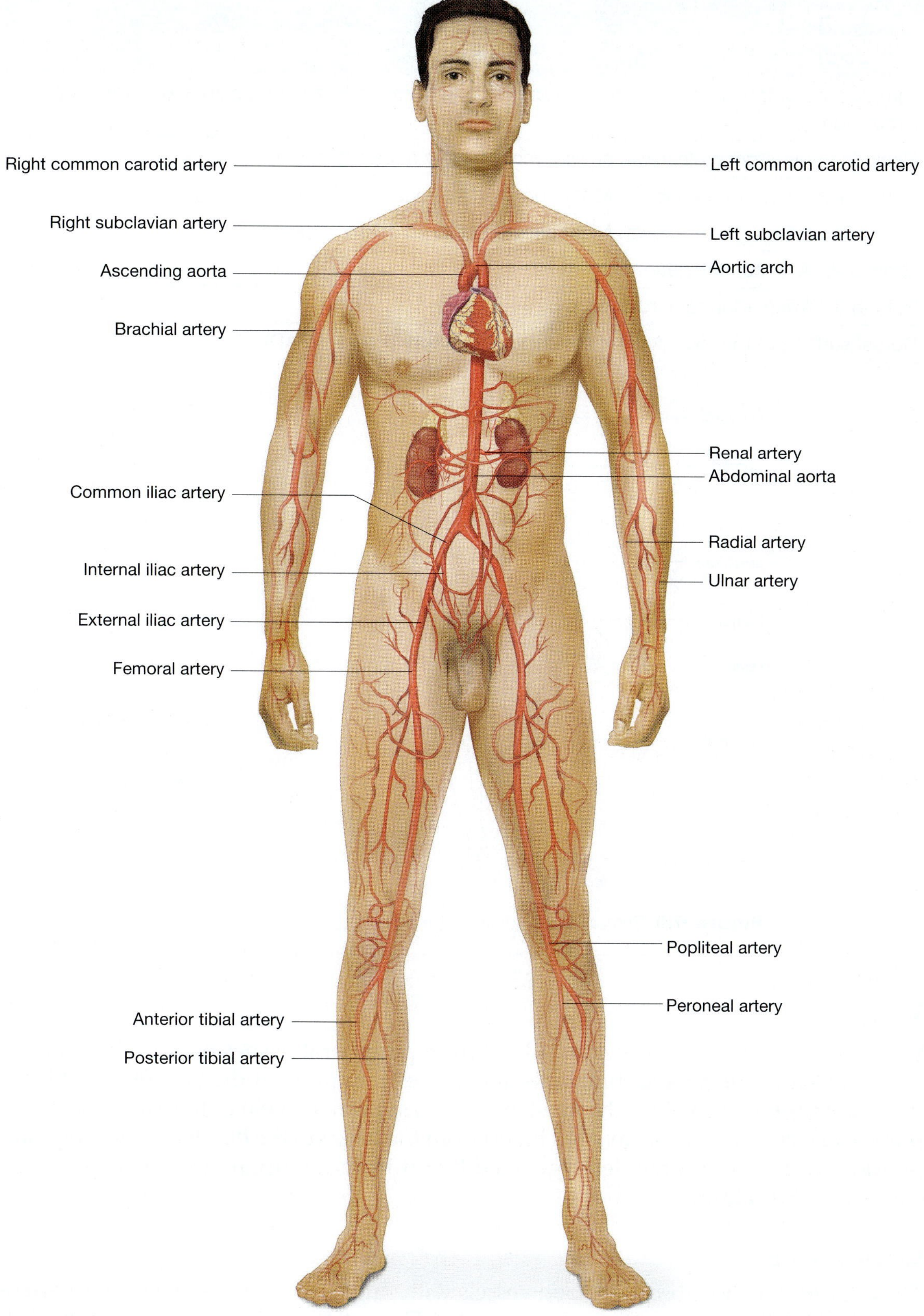

Figure 9.8 Major arteries of the systemic circulation.

Table 9.2 Pulse Checkpoints

Checkpoint	Site/Use
Temporal	Temple area of the head. Used to control bleeding from the head and scalp and to monitor circulation.
Carotid	Neck. In an emergency (*cardiac arrest*), most readily accessible site.
Brachial	Antecubital space of the elbow. Most common site used to check blood pressure.
Radial	Radial (*thumb side*) of the wrist. Most common site for taking a pulse.
Femoral	Groin area. Monitor circulation.
Popliteal	Behind the knee. Monitor circulation.
Dorsalis pedis	Dorsal surface of the foot. Assess for peripheral artery disease (PAD).

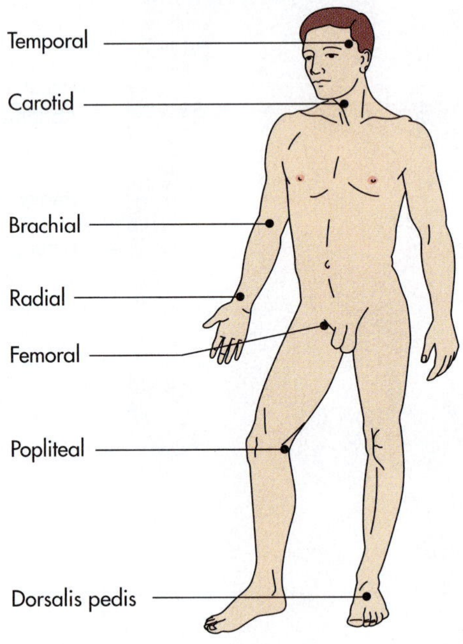

Figure 9.9 Primary pulse points of the body.

Veins

Veins are the vessels that transport blood from peripheral tissues back to the heart. In a normal state, veins have thin walls and valves that prevent the backflow of blood. The great saphenous vein is the most important superficial vein of the lower limb. The pulmonary veins carry oxygenated blood from the lungs to the heart. The superior and inferior venae cavae carry deoxygenated blood from the upper and lower systemic circulation. See Figure 9.10.

Capillaries

The **capillaries** are microscopic blood vessels with single-celled walls that connect **arterioles** (*small arteries*) with **venules** (*small veins*). See Figure 9.11. Blood passing through capillaries gives up the oxygen and nutrients carried to this point by the arteries and picks up waste and carbon dioxide as it enters veins. Veins lead away from the capillaries as tiny vessels and increase in size until they join the superior and inferior venae cavae as they return to the heart. The extremely thin walls of capillaries facilitate passage of oxygen and nutrients to cell bodies and the removal of accumulated waste and carbon dioxide.

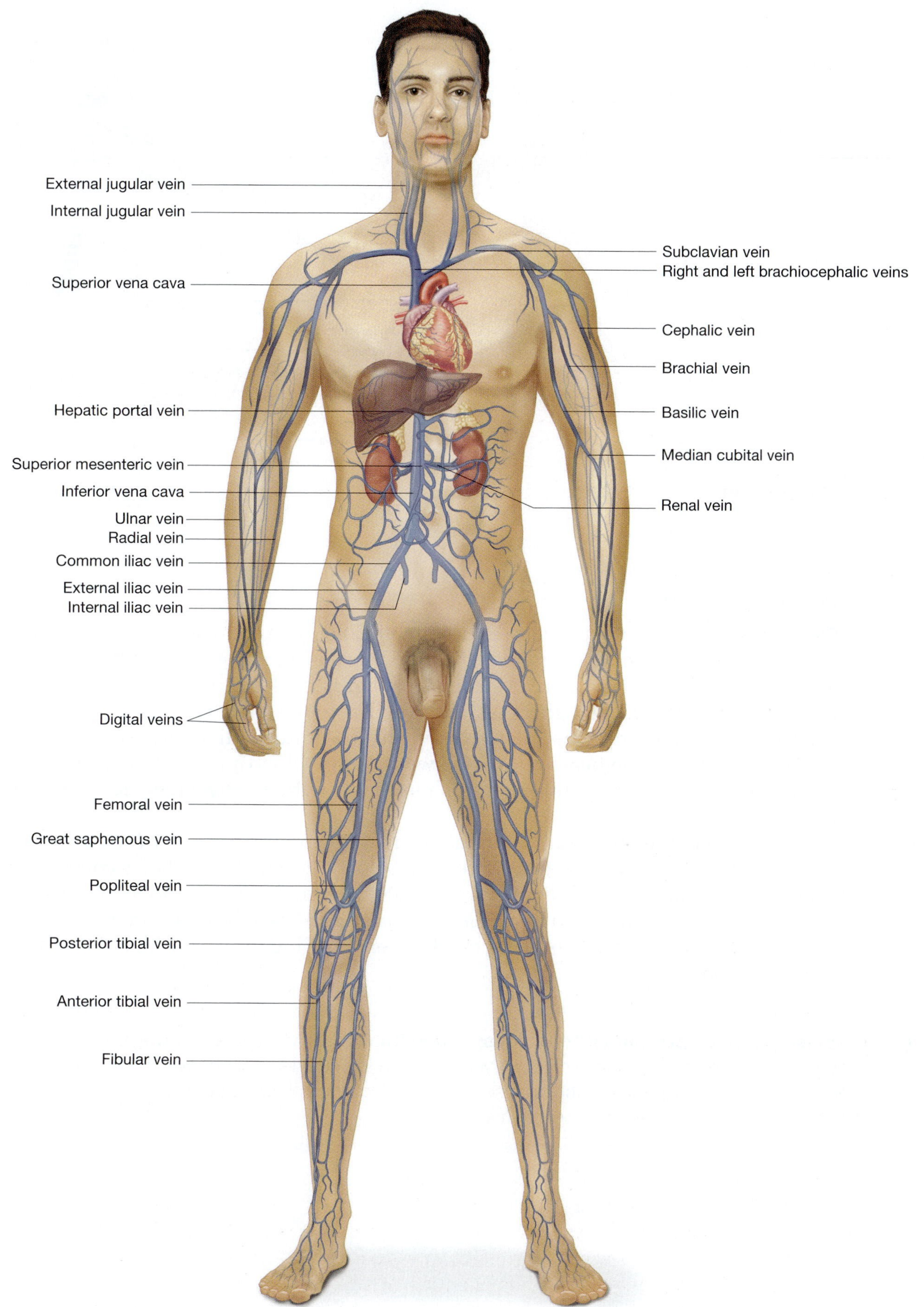

Figure 9.10 Major veins of the systemic circulation.

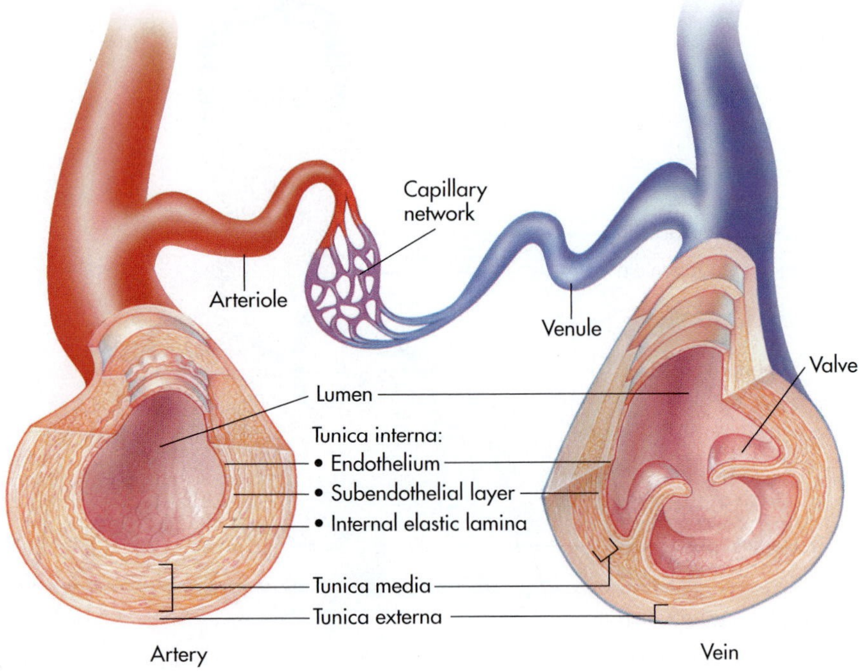

Figure 9.11 Capillaries.

Blood Pressure

Blood pressure (BP) is the pressure exerted by the blood on the walls of the arteries. It results from two forces. One is created by the heart as it pumps blood into the arteries and through the circulatory system. The other is the force of the arteries as they resist the blood flow. The higher (systolic) number represents the pressure while the heart contracts to pump blood to the body. The lower (diastolic) number represents the pressure when the heart relaxes between beats. Blood pressure is reported in millimeters of mercury (mmHg) and is measured with a **sphygmomanometer**. See Figure 9.12.

The systolic pressure is always stated first. For example, 116/74 (116 over 74); systolic = 116, diastolic = 74. Blood pressure below 120 over 80 mmHg is considered optimal for adults. A systolic pressure of 120–139 mmHg or a diastolic pressure of 80–89 mmHg is considered to be *prehypertension* and needs to be monitored on a regular basis. A blood pressure reading of 140 over 90 or higher is considered elevated (hypertension).

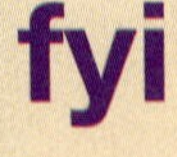

The **pulse (P)**, **blood pressure (BP)**, and **respiration (R)** vary according to a child's age. A newborn's pulse rate is irregular and rapid, varying from 120 to 140 beats/minute. Blood pressure is low and can vary with the size of the cuff used. The average blood pressure at birth is 80/46. The respirations are approximately 35–50 per minute.

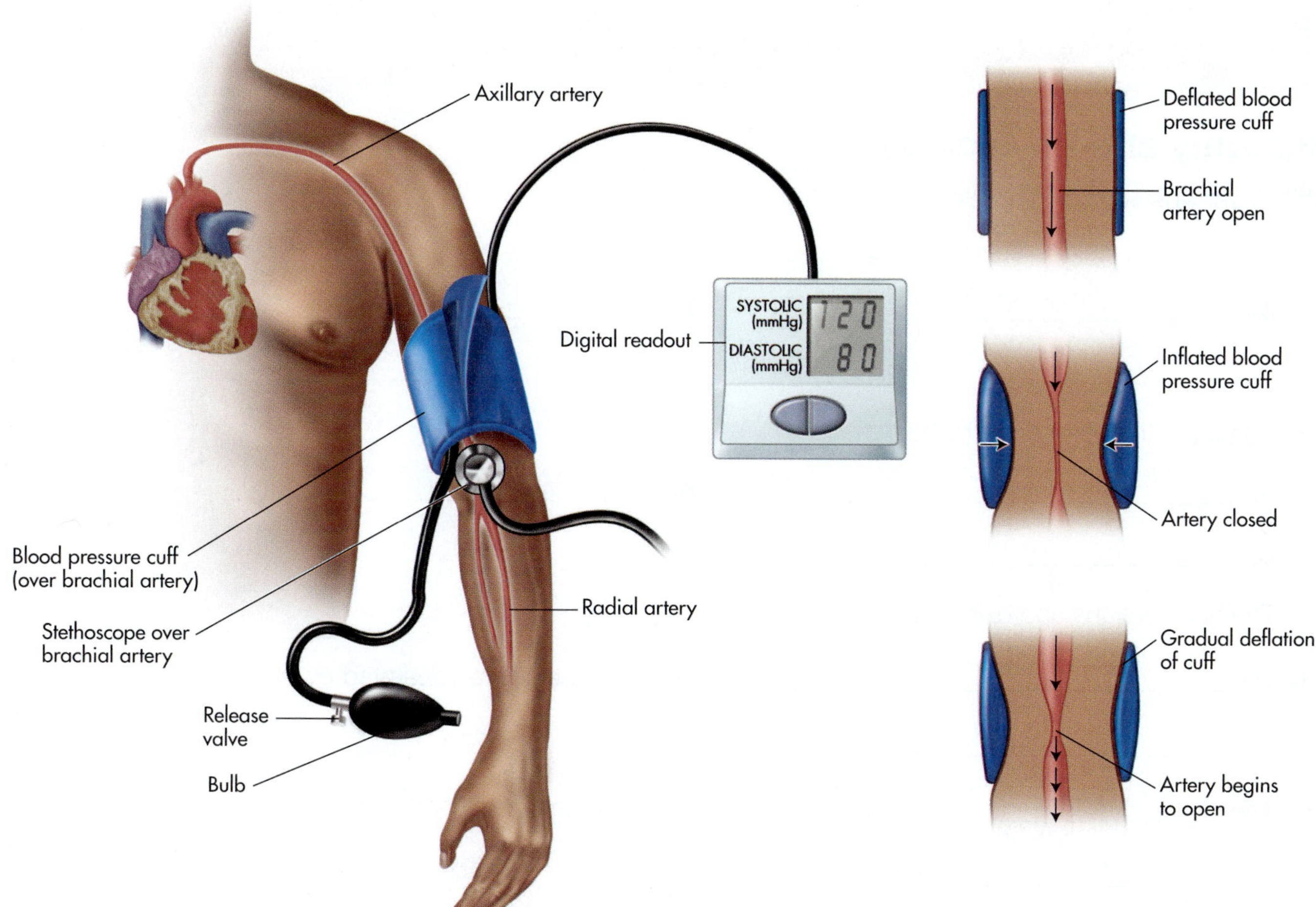

Figure 9.12 Blood pressure measurement.

PULSE PRESSURE

The **pulse pressure** is the difference between the systolic and diastolic readings. This reading indicates the tone of the arterial walls. The normal pulse pressure is found when the systolic pressure is about 40 points higher than the diastolic reading. For example, if the blood pressure is 120/80, the pulse pressure would be 40. A pulse pressure over 50 points or under 30 points is considered abnormal.

Study and Review I

Anatomy and Physiology

Write your answers to the following questions.

1. The cardiovascular system includes:

   a. ______________________ b. ______________________

   c. ______________________ d. ______________________

2. Name the three layers of the heart.

   a. ______________________ b. ______________________

   c. ______________________

3. The heart weighs approximately ________________ grams.

4. The ________________ or upper chambers of the heart are separated by the ________________ septum.

5. The ________________ or lower chambers of the heart are separated by the ________________ septum.

6. A/An ________________ records the heart's electrical activity.

7. The ________________ ________________ ________________ controls the heartbeat.

8. The ________________ ________________ is called the *pacemaker of the heart*.

9. Together, the bundle branches and ________________ comprise the ventricular conduction system.

10. Name the three primary pulse points and state their locations on the body.

    a. ______________________ located ______________________

    b. ______________________ located ______________________

    c. ______________________ located ______________________

11. Define the following terms:

    a. Blood pressure ____

    b. Pulse pressure ____

12. The average adult heart is about the size of a ________________ and normally beats at a pulse rate of ________________ to ________________ beats per minute.

13. A systolic pressure of ________________ to ________________ mmHg or a diastolic pressure of ________________ to ________________ mmHg is considered "prehypertension" and needs to be monitored on a regular basis.

14. State the primary function of arteries. ________________________________

____

____

15. State the primary function of veins. ________________________________

____

____

ANATOMY LABELING

Identify the structures shown below by filling in the blanks.

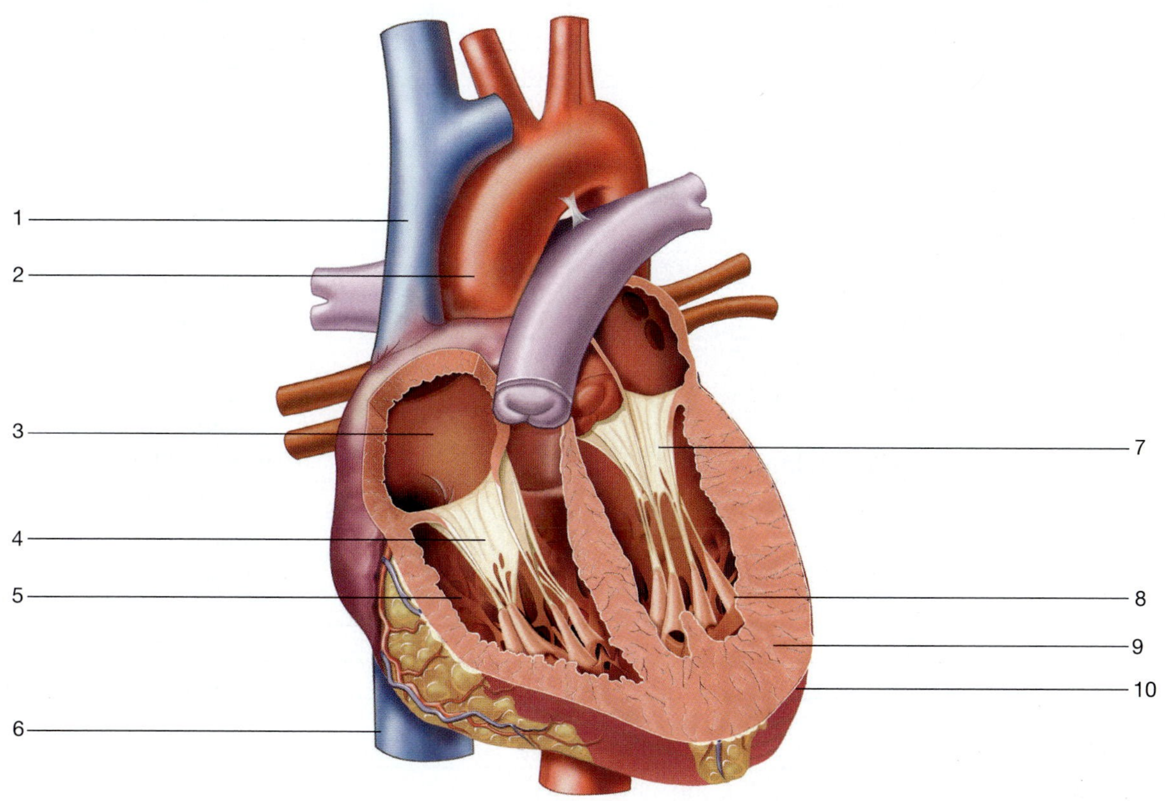

Building Your Medical Vocabulary

This section provides the foundation for learning medical terminology. Review the following alphabetized word list. Note how common prefixes and suffixes are repeatedly applied to word roots and combining forms to create different meanings. The word parts are color-coded: prefixes are yellow, suffixes are blue, roots/combining forms are red. A combining form is a word root plus a vowel. The chart below lists the combining forms for the word roots in this chapter and can help to strengthen your understanding of how medical words are built and spelled.

Remember These Guidelines

1. If the suffix begins with a vowel, drop the combining vowel from the combining form and add the suffix. For example, ather/o (*fatty substance*) + -oma (*tumor*) becomes atheroma.
2. If the suffix begins with a consonant, keep the combining vowel and add the suffix to the combining form. For example, angi/o (*vessel*) + -plasty (*surgical repair*) becomes angioplasty.

You will find that some terms have not been divided into word parts. These are common words or specialized terms that are included to enhance your medical vocabulary.

Combining Forms of the Cardiovascular System			
angi/o	vessel	**mitr/o**	mitral valve
angin/o	to choke	**my/o**	muscle
arteri/o	artery	**occlus/o**	to close up
ather/o	fatty substance, porridge	**ox/i**	oxygen
atri/o	atrium	**oxy**	sour, sharp, acid
auscultat/o	listen to	**palpit/o**	throbbing
cardi/o	heart	**pector/o**	chest
chol/e	bile	**phleb/o**	vein
circulat/o	circular	**pulmon/o**	lung
claudicat/o	to limp	**rrhythm/o**	rhythm
corpor/o	body	**scler/o**	hardening
cyan/o	dark blue	**sept/o**	a partition
dilat/o	to widen	**sin/o**	a curve
dynam/o	power	**sphygm/o**	pulse
ech/o	reflected sound	**sten/o**	narrowing
electr/o	electricity	**steth/o**	chest
embol/o	a throwing in	**thromb/o**	clot of blood
glyc/o	sweet, sugar	**valvul/o**	valve
hem/o	blood	**vas/o**	vessel
infarct/o	infarct (necrosis of an area)	**vascul/o**	small vessel
isch/o	to hold back	**ven/o**	vein
lipid/o	fat	**ventricul/o**	ventricle
lun/o	moon	**vers/o**	turning
man/o	thin		

Medical Word	Word Parts		Definition
	Part	**Meaning**	
anastomosis (ă-năs″ tō-mō´sĭs)	anastom -osis	opening condition	Surgical connection between blood vessels or the joining of one hollow or tubular organ to another
aneurysm (ăn´ ū-rĭzm)			Abnormal widening or ballooning of a portion of an artery due to weakness in the wall of the blood vessel. See Figure 9.13.

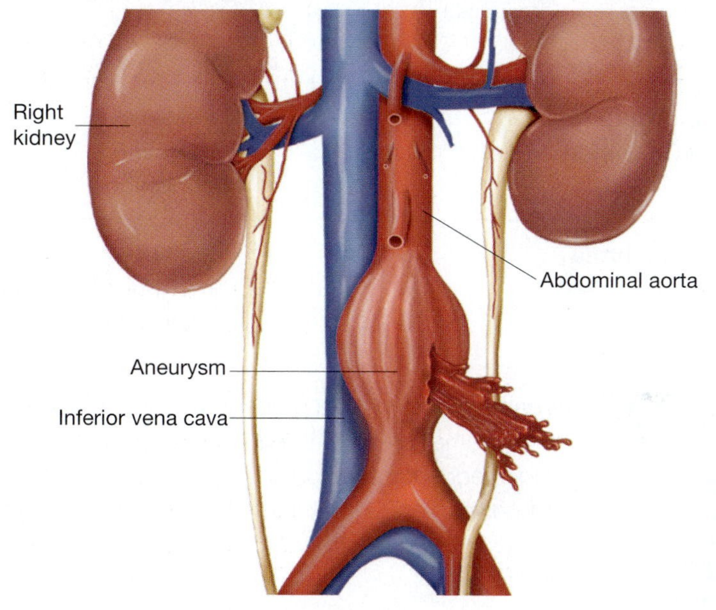

Figure 9.13 Ruptured abdominal aortic aneurysm.

Medical Word	Part	Meaning	Definition
angina pectoris (ăn´ jĭ-nă pĕk´ tōr″ĭs)	angin (a) pector -is	to choke chest pertaining to	Chest pain that occurs when diseased blood vessels restrict blood flow to the heart. It is the most common symptom of coronary artery disease (CAD) and is often referred to as *angina*. The pain can radiate to the neck, jaw, or left arm. It is often described as a crushing, burning, or squeezing sensation. Patients with CAD can present with stable angina pectoris, unstable angina pectoris, or a myocardial infarction (MI), a heart attack.

insights In ICD-10-CM, angina pectoris includes codes I20.0–I20.9. With *stable angina*, the pattern of frequency, intensity, ease of provocation, and duration does not change over a period of several weeks. With *unstable angina*, the pattern of chest pain changes abruptly.

Medical Word	Part	Meaning	Definition
angioma (ăn″ jĭ-ō´ mă)	angi -oma	vessel tumor	Tumor of a blood vessel. See Figure 9.14.

Figure 9.14 Infarction angioma.
(Courtesy of Jason L. Smith, MD)

Medical Word	Word Parts: Part	Word Parts: Meaning	Definition
angioplasty (ăn´ jĭ-ō-plăs˝ tē)	angi/o -plasty	vessel surgical repair	Surgical repair of a blood vessel(s) or a nonsurgical technique for treating diseased arteries by temporarily inflating a tiny balloon inside an artery

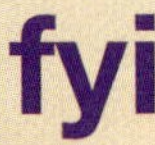

RULE REMINDER

This term keeps the combining vowel ***o*** because the suffix begins with a consonant.

Medical Word	Part	Meaning	Definition
angiostenosis (ăn˝ jĭ-ō-stĕ-nō´ sĭs)	angi/o sten -osis	vessel narrowing condition	Pathological condition of the narrowing of a blood vessel
arrhythmia (ă-rĭth´ mē-ă)	a- rrhythm -ia	lack of rhythm condition	Irregularity or loss of rhythm of the heartbeat; also called *dysrhythmia*. *Note:* The prefix *dys-* means *difficult*.

fyi A *cardiac ablation* is a procedure that can correct heart rhythm problems (arrhythmias). It is used to scar small areas of the heart that may be involved in the arrhythmia. There are two methods. *Radiofrequency ablation* uses heat energy to eliminate the difficult area. *Cryoablation* uses very cold temperatures. During the procedure, small electrodes are placed inside the heart to measure the heart's electrical activity. When the source of the arrhythmia is found, the tissue causing the difficulty is destroyed.

Medical Word	Part	Meaning	Definition
arterial (ăr-tē´ rĭ-ăl)	arter/i -al	artery pertaining to	Pertaining to an artery
arteriosclerosis (ăr-tē˝ rĭ-ō-sklĕ-rō´ sĭs)	arteri/o scler -osis	artery hardening condition	Pathological condition of hardening of arteries. Arteriosclerotic heart disease (ASHD) is hardening of the coronary arteries.

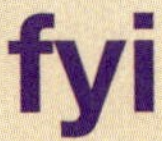

fyi In some older adults, the heart must work harder to pump blood because of hardening of the arteries (*arteriosclerosis*) and a buildup of fatty plaques (cholesterol deposits and triglycerides) in the arterial walls (*atherosclerosis*). Arteries can gradually become stiff and lose their elastic recoil. The aorta and arteries supplying the heart and brain are generally affected first. **Arteriosclerotic heart disease (ASHD)** occurs when the arterial vessels are marked by thickening, hardening, and loss of elasticity in the arterial walls. Reduced blood flow, elevated blood lipids, and defective endothelial repair that can be seen in aging accelerate the course of cardiovascular disease.

Medical Word	Word Parts		Definition
	Part	**Meaning**	
arteritis (ăr″ tĕ-rī′ tĭs)	arter -itis	artery inflammation	Inflammation of an artery. See Figure 9.15.
artificial pacemaker			Electronic device that stimulates impulse initiation within the heart. It is a small, battery-operated device that helps the heart beat in a regular rhythm. See Figure 9.16.

Figure 9.15 Temporal arteritis.
(Courtesy of Jason L. Smith, MD)

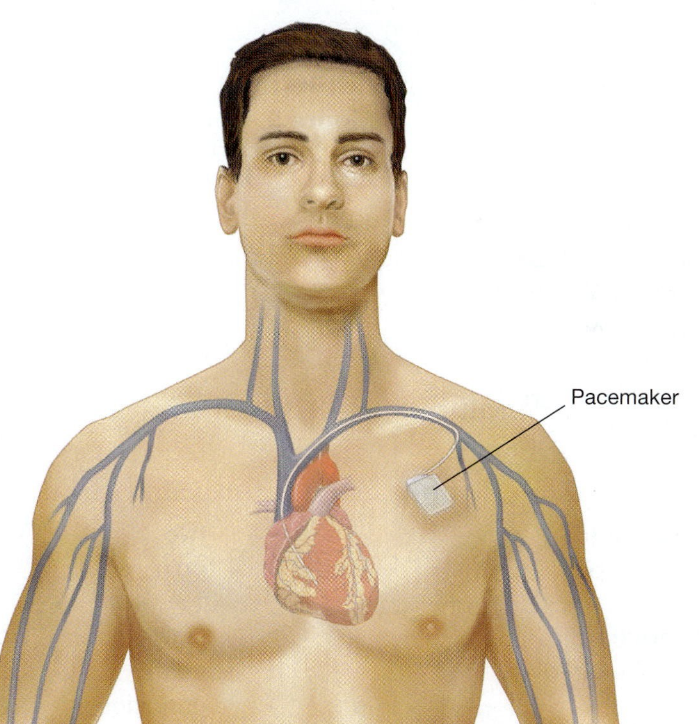

Figure 9.16 A permanent epicardial pacemaker. The pulse generator can be placed in subcutaneous pockets in the subclavian or abdominal regions.

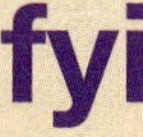

A team of investigators at Children's Hospital Los Angeles and the University of Southern California have developed the first fully implantable *micropacemaker* designed for use in a fetus with complete heart block. The team has done preclinical testing and optimization, as reported in a recent issue of the journal *Heart Rhythm*, and in 2015 the micropacemaker was designated a *humanitarian use device (HUD)** by the U.S. Food and Drug Administration (FDA). The investigators anticipate the first human use of the device in the near future.

* A HUD is a "medical device intended to benefit patients in the treatment or diagnosis of a disease or condition that affects or is manifested in fewer than 4,000 individuals in the United States per year" (From Code of Federal Regulations, Title 21, Chapter 1, Part 814, Subpart A, Section 814.3, U.S. Food and Drug Administration.).

Medical Word	Word Parts		Definition
	Part	**Meaning**	
atheroma (ăth″ ĕr-ō′ mă)	ather -oma	fatty substance, porridge tumor	Tumor of an artery containing a fatty substance
atherosclerosis (ăth″ ĕr-ō-sklĕ-rō′ sĭs)	ather/o scler -osis	fatty substance, porridge hardening condition	Pathological condition of the arteries characterized by the buildup of fatty substances (cholesterol deposits and triglycerides) and hardening of the walls
auscultation (aws″ kŭl-tā′ shŭn)	auscultat -ion	listen to process	Method of physical assessment using a stethoscope to listen to sounds within the chest, abdomen, and other parts of the body. See Figure 9.17.

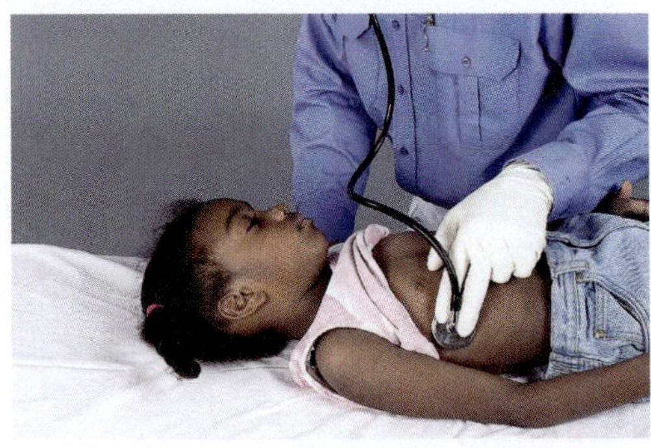

Figure 9.17 During auscultation, sounds can be heard via a stethoscope.

Source: Pearson Education, Inc.

Medical Word	Part	Meaning	Definition
automated external defibrillator (AED) (aw′ tō-māt- ĕd eks-tĕr′ năl dē-fĭb′ rĭ-lā-tor)			Portable automatic device used to restore normal heart rhythm to patients in cardiac arrest. An AED is applied outside the body. It automatically analyzes the patient's heart rhythm and advises the rescuer whether a shock is needed to restore a normal heartbeat. If the patient's heart resumes beating normally, the heart has been defibrillated.
bicuspid (bī-kŭs′ pĭd)	bi- -cuspid	two point	Valve with two cusps; pertaining to the mitral valve
bradycardia (brăd″ ĭ-kăr′ dĭ-ă)	brady- card -ia	slow heart condition	Abnormally slow heartbeat defined as fewer than 60 beats per minute
bruit (brōōt)			Pathological noise; a sound of venous or arterial origin heard on auscultation
cardiac (kăr′ dĭ-ăk)	cardi -ac	heart pertaining to	Pertaining to the heart
cardiac arrest			Loss of effective heart function, which results in cessation of functional circulation. Sudden cardiac arrest (SCA) results in sudden death.

Medical Word	Word Parts: Part	Word Parts: Meaning	Definition
cardiologist (kăr-dē-ŏl′ ō-jĭst)	cardi/o log -ist	heart study of one who specializes	Physician who specializes in the study of the heart
cardiology (kăr″ dē-ŏl′ ō-jē)	cardi/o -logy	heart study of	Literally means *study of the heart*
cardiomegaly (kăr″ dē-ō-mĕg′ ă-lē)	cardi/o -megaly	heart enlargement, large	Enlargement of the heart
cardiomyopathy (CMP) (kăr″ dē-ō-mī-ŏp′ ă-thē)	cardi/o my/o -pathy	heart muscle disease	Disease of the heart muscle that leads to generalized deterioration of the muscle and its pumping ability. It can be caused by multiple factors, including viral infections. See Figure 9.18.

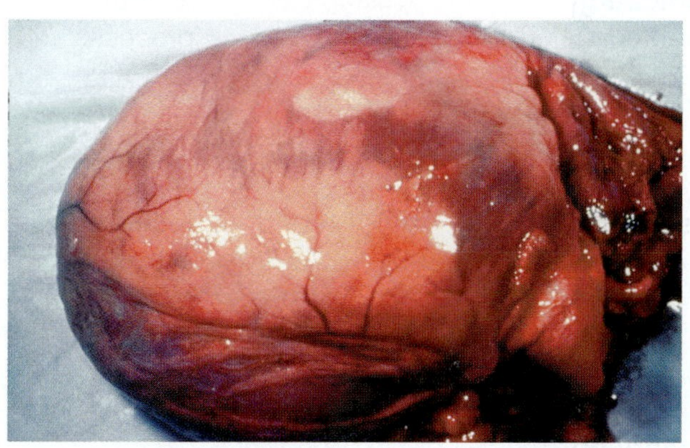

Figure 9.18 An enlarged heart showing the results of cardiomyopathy.

Source: Pearson Education, Inc.

Medical Word	Word Parts: Part	Word Parts: Meaning	Definition
cardiopulmonary (kăr″ dē-ō-pŭl′ mō-nĕr-ē)	cardi/o pulmon -ary	heart lung pertaining to	Pertaining to the heart and lungs (H&L)
cardiotonic (kăr″ dē-ō-tŏn′ ĭk)	cardi/o ton -ic	heart tone pertaining to	A class of medication that is used to increase the tone (pumping strength) of the heart
cardiovascular (CV) (kăr″ dē-ō-văs′ kū-lăr)	cardi/o vascul -ar	heart small vessel pertaining to	Pertaining to the heart and small blood vessels
cardioversion (kăr′ dē-ō-vĕr″ zhŭn)	cardi/o vers -ion	heart turning process	Medical procedure used to treat cardiac arrhythmias. An electrical shock is delivered to the heart to restore its normal rhythm. The electrical energy can be delivered externally through electrodes placed on the chest or directly to the heart by placing paddles on the heart during an open chest surgery.

! ALERT!

The combining form **cardi/o** means *heart.* By adding various suffixes, you can build medical words. How many terms can you build?

Medical Word	Word Parts: Part	Word Parts: Meaning	Definition
cholesterol (chol) (kō-lĕs´ tĕr-ŏl)	chol/e sterol	bile solid (fat)	A normal, soft, waxy substance found among the lipids (fats) in the bloodstream and all body cells. It is the building block of steroid hormones, but it is dangerous when it builds up on arterial walls and can contribute to the risk of coronary heart disease.

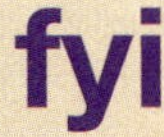

There is evidence that cholesterol can begin clogging the arteries during childhood, leading to atherosclerosis and heart disease later in life. The American Heart Association recommends children and teenagers with high cholesterol take steps to bring it down, as should adults. Ideally, total cholesterol should be below 170 mg/dL in people ages 2–19, and below 200 mg/dL in adults over age 20.

Medical Word	Word Parts: Part	Word Parts: Meaning	Definition
circulation (sĭr″ kū-lā´ shŭn)	circulat -ion	circular process	The moving of the blood in the veins and arteries throughout the body
claudication (klaw-dĭ-kā´ shŭn)	claudicat -ion	to limp process	Literally means *process of lameness or limping*. It is a dull, cramping pain in the hips, thighs, calves, or buttocks caused by an inadequate supply of oxygen to the muscles, due to narrowed arteries. It is one of the symptoms in peripheral artery disease (PAD).
constriction (kən-strĭk´ shŭn)	con- strict -ion	together, with to draw, to bind process	Process of drawing together, as in the narrowing of a vessel
coronary artery bypass graft (CABG) (kŏr´ ō-nă-rē ăr´ tĕr-ē bī´ păs grăft)			Surgical procedure to assist blood flow to the myocardium by using a section of a saphenous vein or internal mammary artery to bypass or reroute blood around an obstructed or occluded coronary artery, thus improving blood flow and oxygen to the heart. See Figure 9.19.

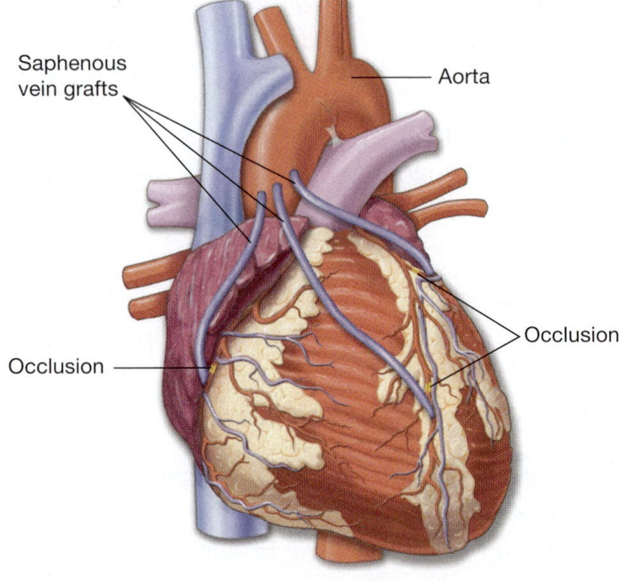

Figure 9.19 A coronary artery bypass graft (CABG) is a procedure to bypass a blocked coronary artery. The procedure involves isolating the blocked coronary artery and grafting a vessel to bypass it. The graft vessel is usually a portion of the saphenous vein of the leg or the internal mammary artery. It is grafted with very fine sutures.

Medical Word	Word Parts		Definition
	Part	Meaning	

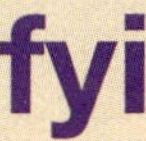

Cardiopulmonary bypass with a pump oxygenator (heart–lung machine) is used for most coronary bypass graft operations. Recently, surgeons have been performing off-pump coronary artery bypass (OPCAB) surgery. In it, the heart continues beating while the bypass graft is sewn in place. In some patients, OPCAB may reduce intraoperative bleeding (and the need for blood transfusion), renal complications, and postoperative neurological deficits (problems after surgery). Increasing blood flow to the heart muscle can relieve chest pain and reduce the risk of heart attack. A patient may undergo several bypass grafts, depending on how many coronary arteries are blocked.

Medical Word	Part	Meaning	Definition
coronary artery disease (CAD)			Most common form of heart disease; it is a progressive disease that increases the risk of myocardial infarction (heart attack) and sudden death. CAD usually results from the buildup of fatty material and plaque in the coronary arteries (atherosclerosis). As the coronary arteries narrow, the flow of blood to the heart can slow or stop. Blockage can occur in one or many coronary arteries. See Figures 9.20 and 9.21.

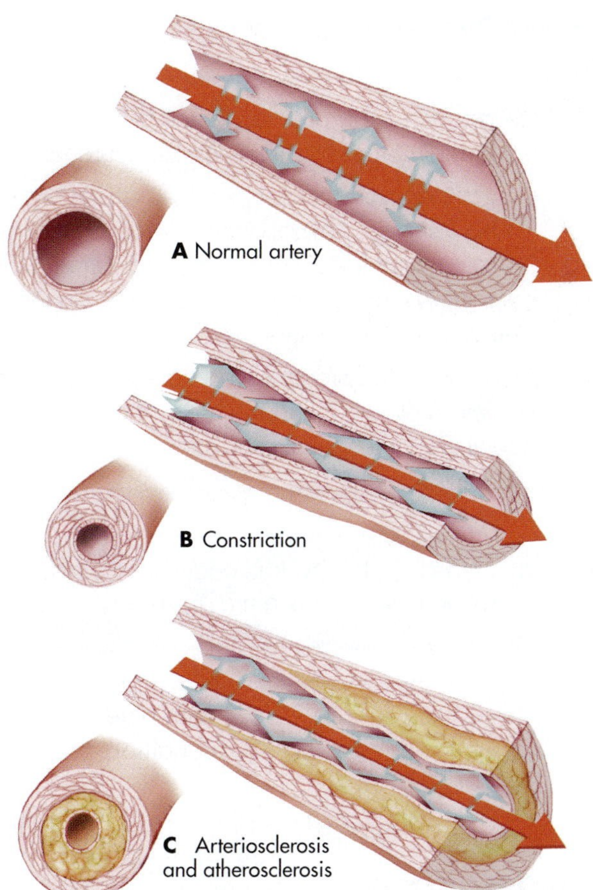

Figure 9.20 Blood vessels: (A) normal artery, (B) constriction, and (C) arteriosclerosis and atherosclerosis.

(*continued*)

Medical Word	Word Parts		Definition
	Part	Meaning	

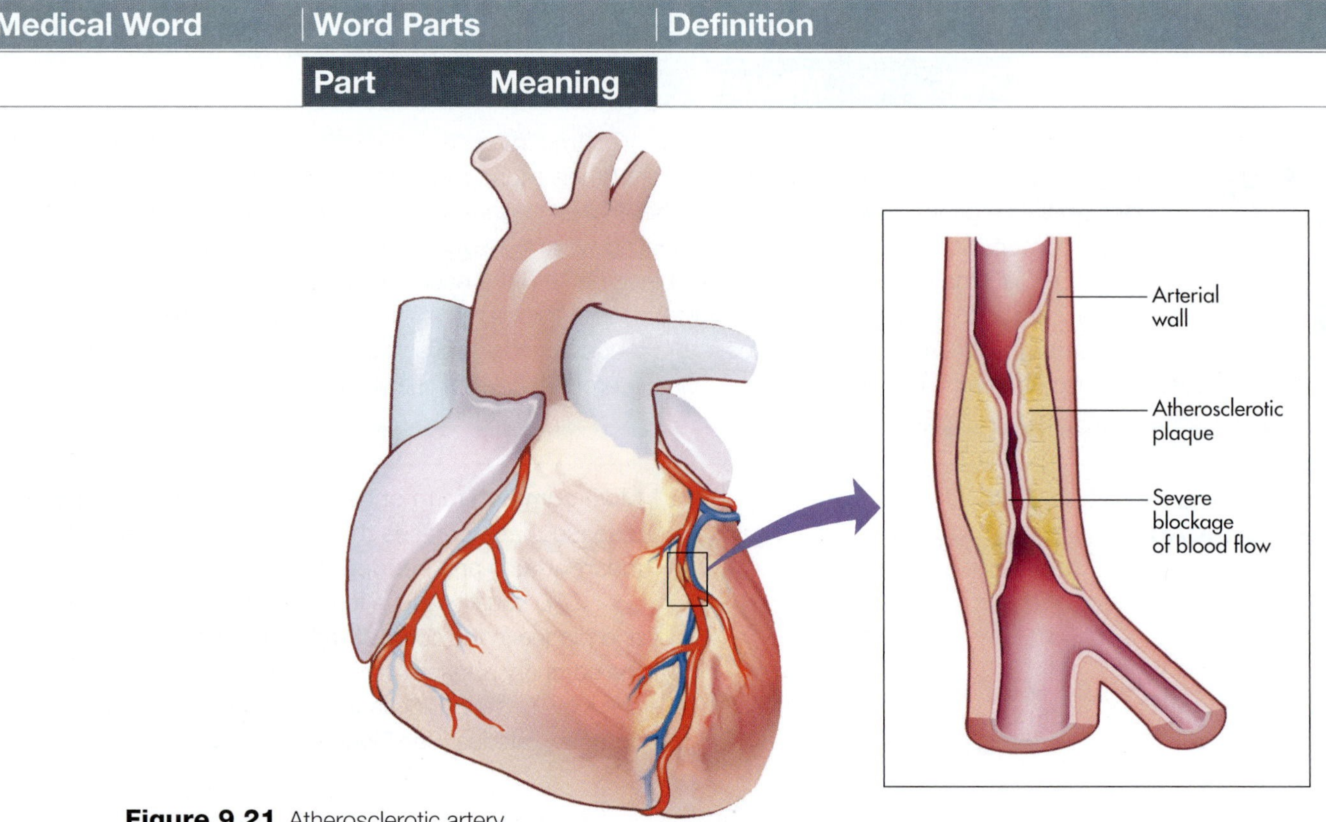

Figure 9.21 Atherosclerotic artery.

fyi *Acute coronary syndrome* is a name given to three types of coronary artery disease that are associated with sudden rupture of plaque inside a coronary artery:

- *Unstable angina* occurs when the pattern of chest pain changes abruptly.
- *Non–ST-segment elevation myocardial infarction (NSTEMI)* (a type of heart attack).
- *ST-segment elevation myocardial infarction (STEMI)* (a type of heart attack). The coronary artery is completely blocked off by a blood clot. Changes can be noted on the ECG as well as in blood levels of key chemical markers.

The type of acute coronary syndrome is determined by the location of the blockage, the length of time blood flow is blocked, and the amount of damage that occurs. These life-threatening conditions require immediate emergency medical care.

insights In the ICD-10-CM, the codes for ST elevation (STEMI) and non-ST elevation (NSTEMI) myocardial infarction are I21–I23.

cyanosis (sī-ă-nō´ sĭs)	cyan -osis	dark blue condition	Abnormal condition of the skin and mucous membranes caused by oxygen deficiency in the blood. The skin, fingernails, and mucous membranes can appear slightly blue or gray.

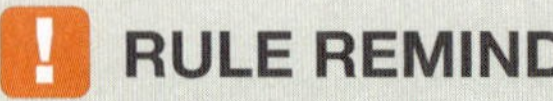

! RULE REMINDER

The ***o*** has been removed from the combining form because the suffix begins with a vowel.

Medical Word	Word Parts		Definition
	Part	**Meaning**	
defibrillator (dē-fĭb´ rĭ-lā˝ tor)			Medical device used to restore a normal heart rhythm by delivering an electric shock; also called a *cardioverter*. See Figure 9.22.

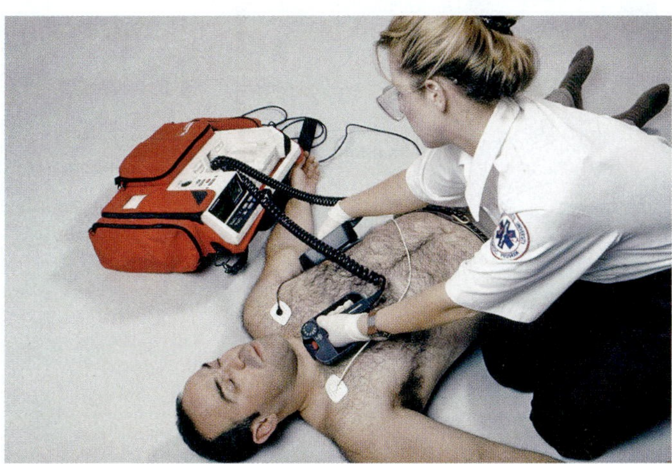

Figure 9.22 Defibrillator (cardioverter).
Source: Pearson Education, Inc.

Medical Word	Part	Meaning	Definition
diastole (dī-ăs´ tō-lē)			Relaxation phase of the heart cycle during which the heart muscle relaxes and the heart chambers fill with blood
dysrhythmia (dĭs-rĭth´ mē-ă)	dys- rhythm -ia	difficult, abnormal rhythm condition	Abnormality of the rhythm or rate of the heartbeat. It is caused by a disturbance of the normal electrical activity within the heart and can be divided into two main groups: *tachycardias* and *bradycardias*. Dysrhythmia is also referred to as an *arrhythmia*.
embolism (ĕm´ bō-lĭzm)	embol -ism	a throwing in condition	Pathological condition caused by obstruction of a blood vessel by foreign substances or a blood clot
endarterectomy (ĕn˝ dăr-tĕr-ĕk´ tō-mē)	end- arter -ectomy	within artery surgical excision	Surgical excision of the inner lining of an artery
endocarditis (ĕn˝ dō-kăr-dī´ tĭs)	endo- card -itis	within heart inflammation	Inflammation of the endocardium (inner lining of the heart), usually involving the heart valves. It typically occurs when microorganisms, especially bacteria from another part of the body such as the gums/teeth, spread through the bloodstream and attach to damaged areas of the heart. Treatments for endocarditis include antibiotics and, in severe cases, surgery. See Figure 9.23.

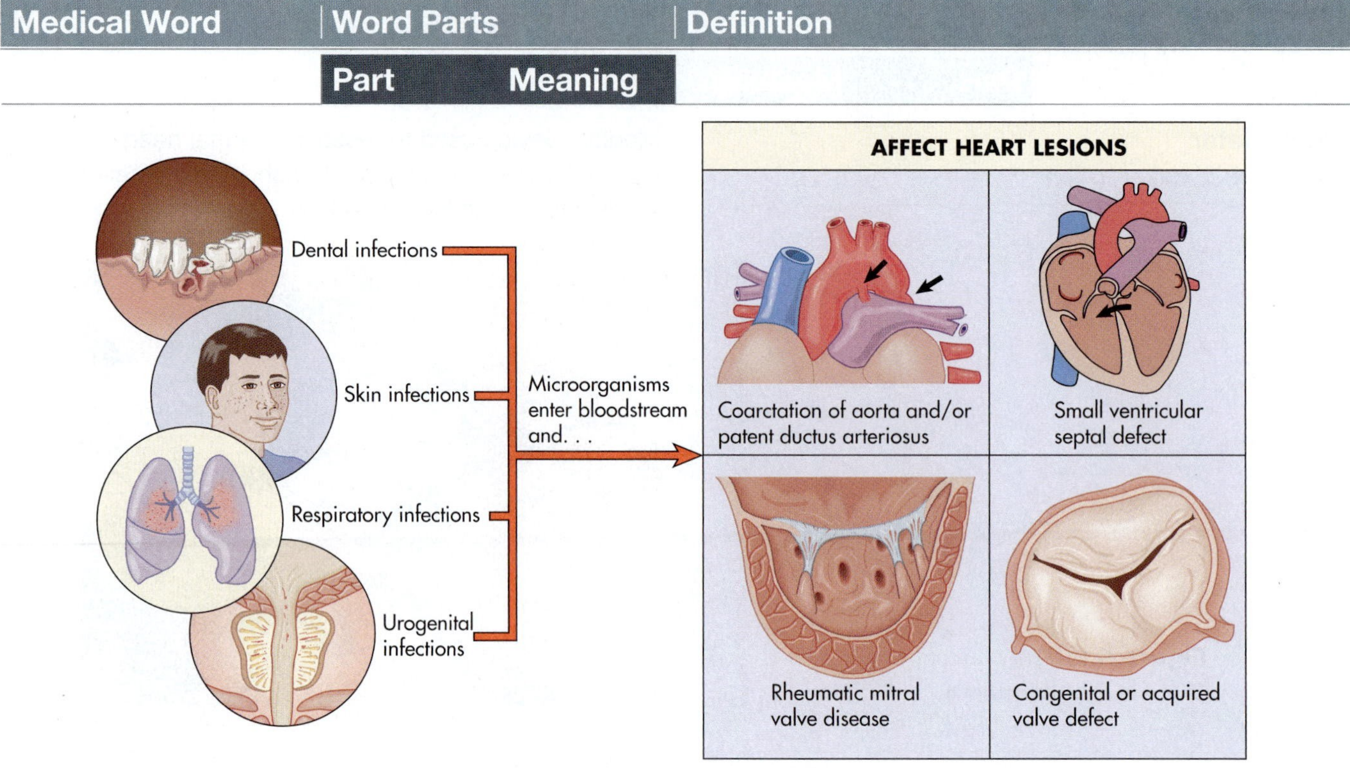

Figure 9.23 How microorganisms enter bloodstream and affect heart lesions, which could result in bacterial endocarditis.

Medical Word	Word Parts: Part	Word Parts: Meaning	Definition
extracorporeal circulation (ECC) (ĕks″ tră-kor-por′ ē-ăl)	extra- corpor -eal circulat -ion	outside body pertaining to circular process	Pertaining to the circulation of the blood outside the body via a heart–lung machine or in hemodialysis
fibrillation (fĭ″ brĭl-ā′ shŭn)	fibrillat -ion	fibrils (small fibers) process	Quivering or spontaneous contraction of individual muscle fibers; an abnormal bioelectric potential occurring in neuropathies and myopathies; disorganized pathological rhythm that can lead to death if not immediately corrected

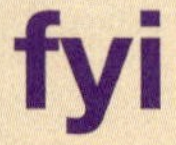

Atrial fibrillation (AF or AFib) is an irregular and often rapid heart rate that can increase the risk of stroke, heart failure, and other heart-related complications. It occurs when rapid, disorganized electrical signals cause the heart's two upper chambers (atria) to *fibrillate* (contract very fast and irregularly). Blood pools in the atria and it is not pumped completely into the heart's two lower chambers (ventricles). As a result, the heart's upper and lower chambers don't work together as they should. Symptoms often include heart palpitations, shortness of breath, and weakness. Episodes of atrial fibrillation can come and go, or one may develop atrial fibrillation that doesn't go away and may require treatment. Although atrial fibrillation itself usually isn't life-threatening, it is a serious medical condition that sometimes requires emergency treatment.

Medical Word	Word Parts		Definition
	Part	Meaning	
flutter			Pathological rapid heart rate that may cause cardiac output (CO) to be decreased. With atrial flutter, the heartbeat is 200–400 beats per minute. With ventricular flutter, the heartbeat is 250 beats or more per minute. On an EKG recording, a flutter will demonstrate a "saw-tooth" appearance.
heart failure (HF)			Pathological condition in which the heart loses its ability to pump blood efficiently. Left-sided heart failure is commonly called *congestive heart failure (CHF)*.

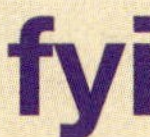

Heart failure (HF) is one of the most common types of cardiovascular disease seen in the older adult. It can involve the heart's left side, right side, or both sides. Left-sided failure leads to a backup of blood, which causes a buildup of fluid in the lungs, or **pulmonary edema**, which causes **dyspnea** and shortness of breath (SOB). Left-sided heart failure is commonly called **congestive heart failure (CHF)**. There are two types of left-sided heart failure. Drug treatments are different for the two types.

- ***Systolic failure*:** *The left ventricle loses its ability to contract normally. The heart can't pump with enough force to push enough blood into circulation.*
- ***Diastolic failure*** *(also called* ***diastolic dysfunction*)**: The left ventricle loses its ability to relax normally (because the muscle has become stiff). The heart can't properly fill with blood during the resting period between each beat.

Right-sided or right-ventricular (RV) heart failure usually occurs as a result of left-sided failure. When the left ventricle fails, increased fluid pressure is, in effect, transferred back through the lungs, ultimately damaging the heart's right side. Right-sided failure is a result of a buildup of blood flowing into the right side of the heart, which can lead to enlargement of the liver, distention of the neck veins, and edema of the ankles. See Figure 9.24 for some signs and symptoms of a patient with heart failure.

Ejection Fraction Heart Failure Measurement

A normal heart pumps a little more than half the heart's blood volume with each beat. **Ejection fraction (EF)** is the percentage of blood that is pumped (ejected) out of the ventricles with each contraction of the heart. It should be measured initially with the first diagnosis of a heart condition, and again as needed, based on changes in the patient's condition. **Left-ventricular ejection fraction (LVEF)** is the measurement of how much blood is being pumped out of the left ventricle of the heart with each contraction. **Right-ventricular ejection fraction (RVEF)** is the measurement of how much blood is being pumped out of the right side of the heart to the lungs for oxygen.

EF Measurement: What It Means	
55–70%	Normal
40–55%	Below normal
Less than 40%	May confirm diagnosis of heart failure
Less than 35%	Patient may be at risk of life-threatening irregular heartbeats

(*continued*)

Medical Word	Word Parts		Definition
	Part	**Meaning**	

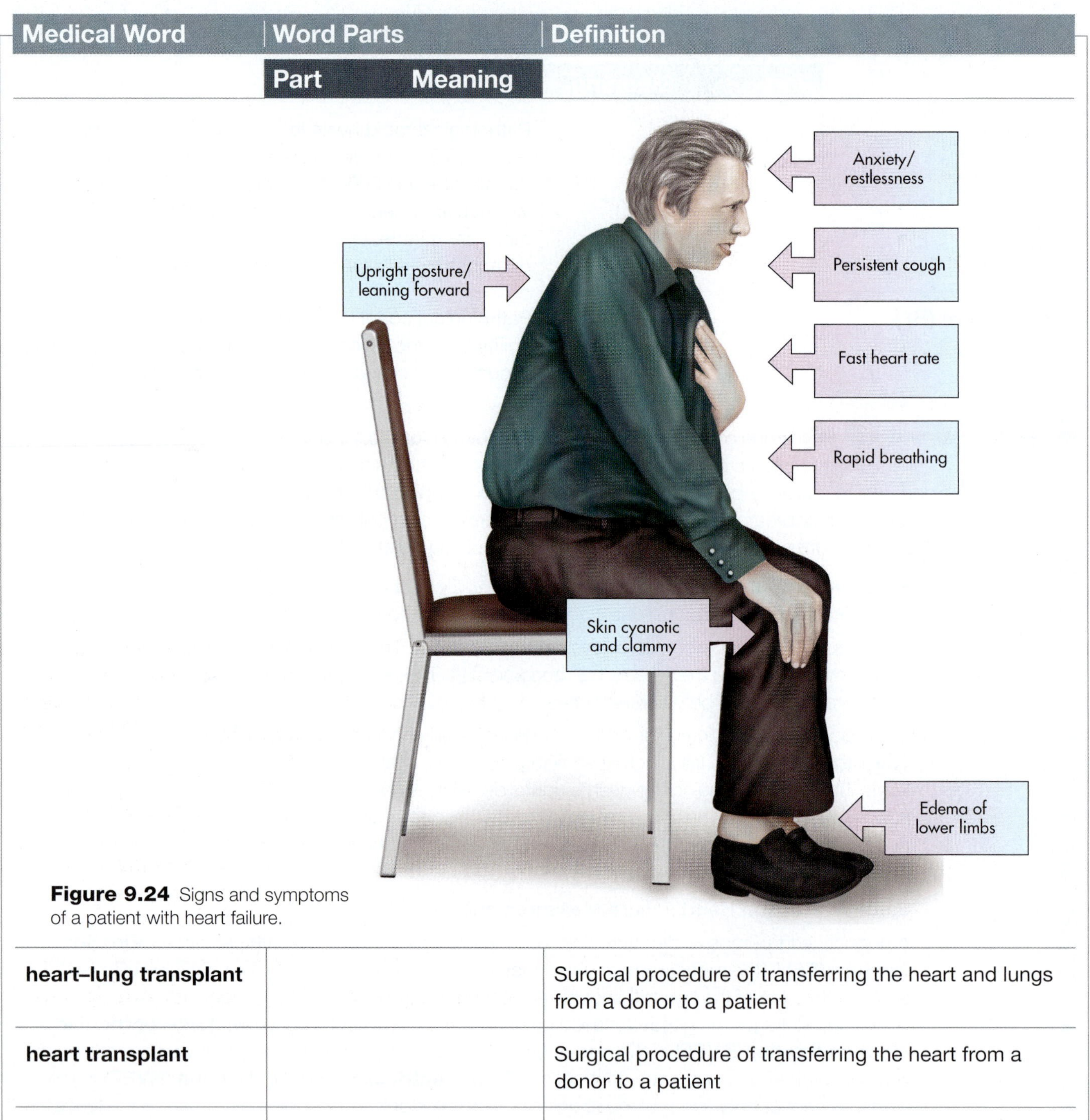

Figure 9.24 Signs and symptoms of a patient with heart failure.

Medical Word	Part	Meaning	Definition
heart–lung transplant			Surgical procedure of transferring the heart and lungs from a donor to a patient
heart transplant			Surgical procedure of transferring the heart from a donor to a patient
hemangioma (hē-măn″ jĭ-ō′ mă)	hem angi -oma	blood vessel tumor	Benign tumor of a blood vessel. See Figures 9.25 and 9.26.

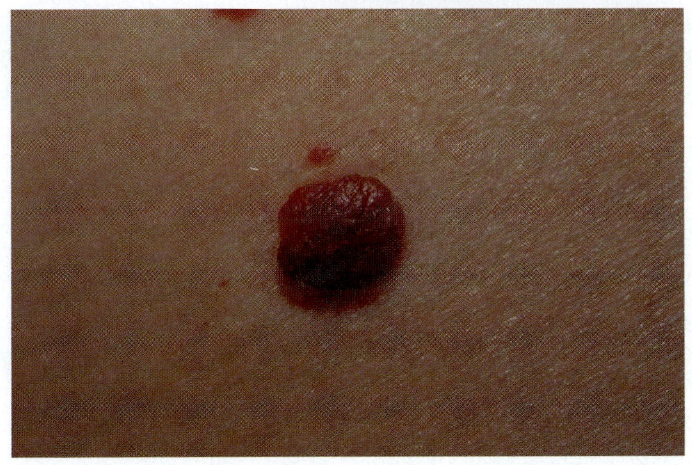
Figure 9.25 Hemangioma. (Courtesy of Jason L. Smith, MD)

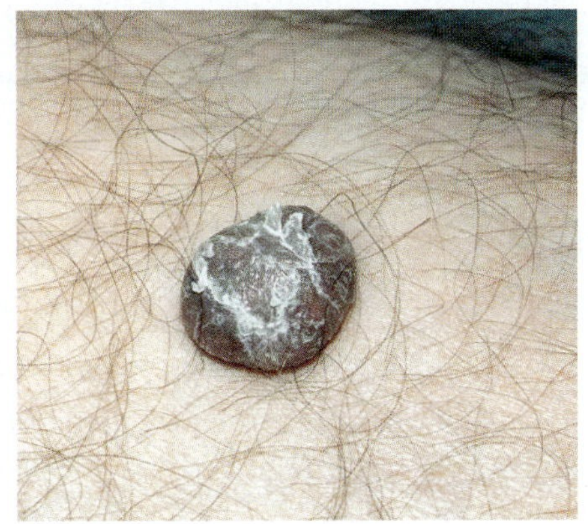
Figure 9.26 Sclerosing hemangioma. (Courtesy of Jason L. Smith, MD)

Medical Word	Word Parts: Part	Word Parts: Meaning	Definition
hemodynamic (hē″ mō-dī-năm′ ĭk)	hem/o dynam -ic	blood power pertaining to	The dynamic study of the heart's function and movement of the blood and pressure
hyperlipidemia (hī″ pĕr-lĭp″ ĭ-dē′ mē-ă)	hyper- lipid -emia	excessive fat blood condition	Abnormal high levels of lipids (fatty substances) in the blood. Lipids include sterols (cholesterol and cholesterol esters), free fatty acids (FFA), triglycerides (glycerol esters of FFA), and phospholipids (phosphoric acid esters of lipid substances).
hypertension (HTN) (hī″ pĕr-tĕn′ shŭn)	hyper- tens -ion	excessive, above pressure process	High blood pressure (HBP) is defined as elevated systolic pressure above 140 or diastolic pressure above 90 with at least two readings on separate office visits. Hypertension often has no symptoms and is frequently called the *silent killer* because, if left untreated, it can lead to kidney failure, stroke, heart attack, peripheral artery disease, and eye damage. Various factors can contribute to developing hypertension, and it is important to know these factors. See Table 9.3.

(*continued*)

Medical Word	Word Parts		Definition
	Part	Meaning	

TABLE 9.3 Factors Contributing to Hypertension

Factors That One Can Control	
Smoking	Avoid the use of tobacco products
Overweight	Maintain a proper weight for age and body size
Lack of exercise	Exercise regularly
Stress	Learn to manage stress
Alcohol	Limit intake of alcohol
Factors That One Cannot Control	
Heredity	Family history of high blood pressure, heart attack, stroke, or diabetes
Race	Incidence of hypertension increases among African Americans
Gender	Chance of developing hypertension increases for males
Age	Likelihood of hypertension increases with age

insights In ICD-10-CM, hypertension codes no longer classify the type of hypertension as benign, malignant, or unspecified. Hypertension is now classified as *essential (primary)* and *secondary*.

Medical Word	Part	Meaning	Definition
hypotension (hī″ pō-tĕn′ shŭn)	hypo- tens -ion	deficient, below pressure process	Low blood pressure
infarction (ĭn-fărk′ shŭn)	infarct -ion	infarct (necrosis of an area) process	Process of development of an infarct, which is death of tissue resulting from obstruction of blood flow
ischemia (ĭs-kē′ mĭ-ă)	isch -emia	to hold back blood condition	Condition in which there is a lack of oxygen due to decreased blood supply to a part of the body caused by constriction or obstruction of a blood vessel

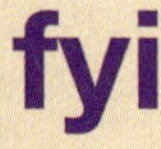

fyi *Ischemic heart disease*, also called *coronary artery disease* or *coronary heart disease*, is a term given to heart problems caused by narrowed coronary arteries. When arteries are narrowed, less blood and oxygen reaches the heart muscle. Ischemia often causes chest pain or discomfort (angina pectoris). *Silent ischemia* is a term given to ischemia without chest pain and a person may experience a heart attack with no prior warning. People who have had previous heart attacks or those with diabetes are especially at risk for developing silent ischemia.

Medical Word	Word Parts		Definition
	Part	**Meaning**	
lipoprotein (lĭp″ ō-prō′ tēn)			Fat (*lipid*) and protein molecules that are bound together. They are classified as **VLDL**—very-low-density lipoproteins; **LDL**—low-density lipoproteins; and **HDL**—high-density lipoproteins. High levels of VLDL and LDL are associated with cholesterol and triglyceride deposits in arteries, which could lead to coronary heart disease, hypertension, and atherosclerosis. See *lipid profile* in the section *Diagnostic and Laboratory Tests*.
mitral stenosis (MS) (mī′ trăl stĕ-nō′sĭs)	mitr -al sten -osis	mitral valve pertaining to narrowing condition	Pathological condition of narrowing of the mitral valve (bicuspid valve) orifice
mitral valve prolapse (MVP) (mī′ trăl vălv prō-lăps′)			Pathological condition that occurs when the leaflets of the mitral valve (bicuspid valve) between the left atrium and left ventricle bulge into the atrium and permit backflow of blood into the atrium. The condition is often associated with progressive mitral regurgitation (blood flows back into the left atrium instead of moving forward into the left ventricle).
murmur (mər′ mər)			An abnormal sound ranging from soft and blowing to loud and booming heard on auscultation of the heart and adjacent large blood vessels. Murmurs range from very faint to very loud. They sometimes sound like a whooshing or swishing noise. Normal heartbeats make a “lub-DUPP” or “lub-DUB” sound. This is the sound of the heart valves closing as blood moves through the heart. Most abnormal murmurs in children are due to congenital heart defects. In adults, abnormal murmurs are most often due to heart valve problems caused by infection, disease, or aging.
myocardial (mī′ ō-kăr′ dĭ-ăl)	my/o cardi -al	muscle heart pertaining to	Pertaining to the heart muscle (myocardium)

Medical Word	Word Parts: Part	Word Parts: Meaning	Definition
myocardial infarction (MI) (mī´ ō-kăr´ dē-ăl ĭn-fărk´ shŭn)	my/o cardi -al infarct -ion	muscle heart pertaining to infarct (necrosis of an area) process	Occurs when a focal area of heart muscle dies or is permanently damaged because of an inadequate supply of oxygen to that area; also known as a *heart attack*. The most common symptom of a heart attack is *angina*, which is chest pain often described as a feeling of crushing, pressure, fullness, heaviness, or aching in the center of the chest. Many times people try to ignore the symptoms or say "it's just indigestion." It is imperative to seek medical help immediately. Calling 911 is almost always the fastest way to get lifesaving treatment.

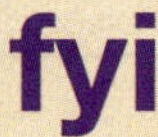

Broken heart syndrome is a term used to describe a type of heart problem that is often brought on by grief or emotional stress. It is a real medical condition with symptoms similar to a heart attack. Traumatic events can trigger the sympathetic nervous system, the "fight-or-flight" mechanism, and the sudden flood of chemicals, including adrenaline, can stun the heart muscle, leaving it temporarily unable to pump properly. Although symptoms may be similar, it is not the same as a heart attack.

Medical Word	Part	Meaning	Definition
myocarditis (mī´ ō-kăr-dī´ tĭs)	my/o card -itis	muscle heart inflammation	Inflammation of the heart muscle that is usually caused by viral, bacterial, or fungal infections that reach the heart
occlusion (ŏ-kloo´ zhŭn)	occlus -ion	to close up process	A blockage in a vessel, canal, or passage of the body
oximetry (ŏk-sĭm´ ĕ-trē)	ox/i -metry	oxygen measurement	Process of measuring the oxygen saturation of blood. A photoelectric medical device (oximeter) measures oxygen saturation of the blood by recording the amount of light transmitted or reflected by deoxygenated versus oxygenated hemoglobin (Hgb). A *pulse oximetry* is a noninvasive method of indicating the arterial oxygen saturation of functional hemoglobin. See Figure 9.27.

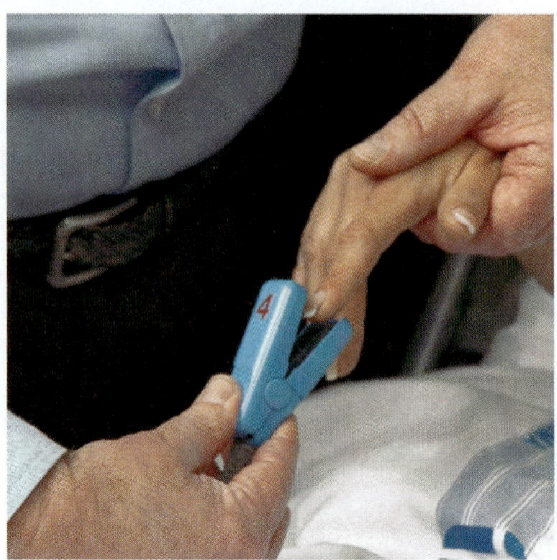

Figure 9.27 Pulse oximetry with the sensor probe applied securely, flush with skin, making sure that both sensor probes are aligned directly opposite each other.

Source: Pearson Education, Inc.

Medical Word	Word Parts		Definition
	Part	**Meaning**	
oxygen (O_2) (ŏk´ sĭ-jĕn)	oxy -gen	sour, sharp, acid formation, produce	Colorless, odorless, tasteless gas essential to respiration in animals
palpitation (păl-pĭ-tā´ shŭn)	palpitat -ion	throbbing process	An abnormal rapid throbbing or fluttering of the heart that is perceptible to the patient and may be felt by the physician during a physical exam
percutaneous transluminal coronary angioplasty (PTCA) (pĕr″ kū-tā´ nē-ŭs trăns-lū´ mĭ-năl kor´ ō-nă-rē ăn´ jĭ-ō-plăs″ tē)			Use of a balloon-tipped catheter to compress fatty plaques against an artery wall. When successful, the plaques remain compressed, which permits more blood to flow through the artery, therefore providing more oxygen to relieve the symptoms of coronary heart disease. See Figure 9.28.

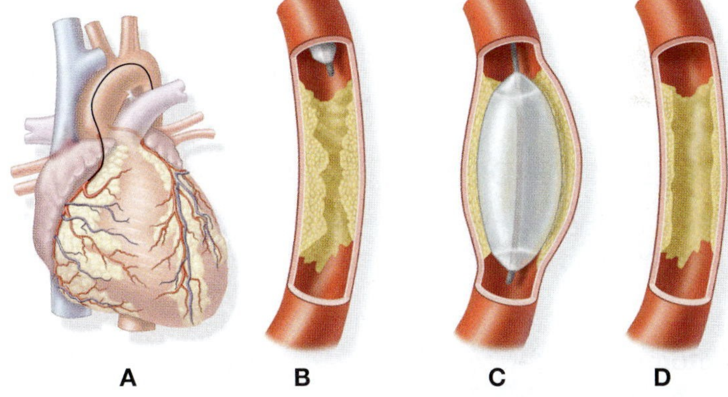

Figure 9.28 Balloon angioplasty. (A) The balloon catheter is threaded into the affected coronary artery. (B) The balloon is positioned across the area of obstruction. (C) The balloon is then inflated, flattening the plaque against the arterial wall. (D) Plaque remains flattened after balloon catheter is removed.

Medical Word	Part	Meaning	Definition
pericardial (pĕr″ ĭ-kăr´ dĭ-ăl)	peri- cardi -al	around heart pertaining to	Pertaining to the pericardium, the sac surrounding the heart
pericardiocentesis (pĕr″ ĭ-kăr″dĭ-ō-sĕn-tē´ sĭs)	peri- cardi/o -centesis	around heart surgical puncture	Surgical procedure to remove fluid from the pericardial sac for therapeutic or diagnostic purposes. See Figure 9.29.

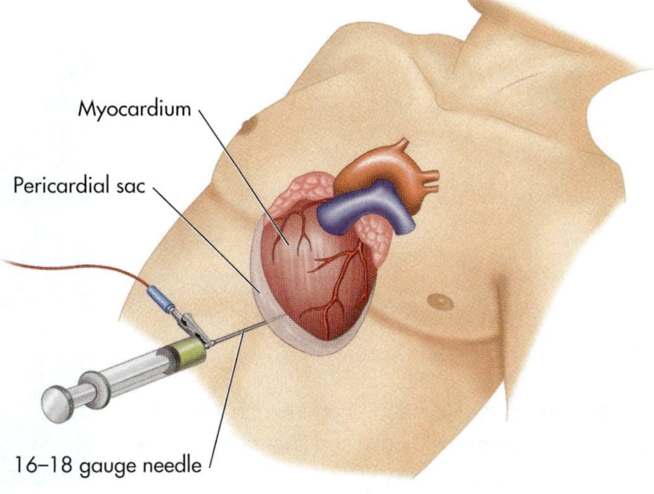

Figure 9.29 Pericardiocentesis.

Medical Word	Word Parts: Part	Word Parts: Meaning	Definition
pericarditis (pĕr″ ĭ-kăr″ dī′ tĭs)	peri- card -itis	around heart inflammation	Inflammation of the pericardium (outer membranous sac surrounding the heart)
peripheral artery disease (PAD) (pər-ĭf′ ər-əl ăr′tĕr-ē)			Pathological condition in which fatty deposits build up in the inner linings of the artery walls. These blockages restrict blood circulation, mainly in arteries leading to the kidneys, stomach, arms, legs, and feet. In its early stages, a common symptom is cramping or fatigue in the legs and buttocks during activity. Such cramping subsides when the person stands still. This is called *intermittent claudication*. If left untreated, PAD can progress to *critical limb ischemia (CLI)*, which occurs when the oxygenated blood being delivered to the leg is not adequate to keep the tissue alive.
phlebitis (flĕ-bī′ tĭs)	phleb -itis	vein inflammation	Literally means *inflammation of a vein*. There will be redness (erythema), swelling (edema), and pain or burning along the length of the affected vein.

RULE REMINDER

The ***o*** has been removed from the combining form because the suffix begins with a vowel.

Medical Word	Word Parts: Part	Word Parts: Meaning	Definition
phlebotomy (flĕ-bŏt′ ō-mē)	phleb/o -tomy	vein incision	Medical term used to describe the puncture of a vein to withdraw blood for analysis
Raynaud phenomenon (rā-nō fĕ-nŏm′ ĕ-nŏn)			Disorder that affects the blood vessels in the fingers and toes; it is characterized by intermittent attacks that cause the blood vessels in the digits to constrict. The cause is believed to be the result of vasospasms that decrease blood supply to the respective regions. Emotional stress and cold are classic triggers of the phenomenon, and discoloration follows a characteristic pattern in time: white, blue, and red. See Figure 9.30.

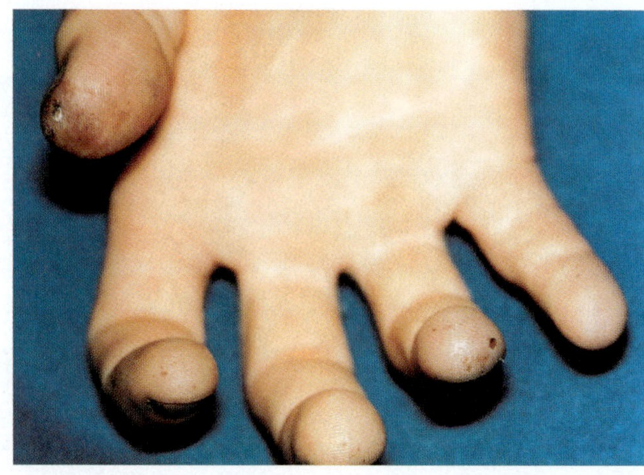

Figure 9.30 Raynaud phenomenon. Note the discoloration in the thumb and fingers.
(Courtesy of Jason L. Smith, MD)

Medical Word	Word Parts: Part	Word Parts: Meaning	Definition
rheumatic heart disease (rōō-măt´ĭk)			Pathological condition in which permanent damage to heart valves is a result of a prior episode of rheumatic fever. The heart valve is damaged by a disease process that generally originates with a strep throat caused by streptococcus A bacteria.
semilunar (sĕm″ ē-lū´ năr)	semi- lun -ar	half moon pertaining to	Valves of the aorta and pulmonary artery; shaped like a crescent (half-moon)
septum (sĕp´ tŭm)	sept -um	a partition tissue, structure	Wall or partition that divides or separates a body space or cavity
shock			A life-threatening condition that occurs when the body is not getting enough blood flow. This can damage multiple organs. Shock requires immediate medical treatment and can get worse very rapidly. In cardiogenic shock, there is failure to maintain the blood supply to the circulatory system and tissues because of inadequate cardiac output. See Figure 9.31.

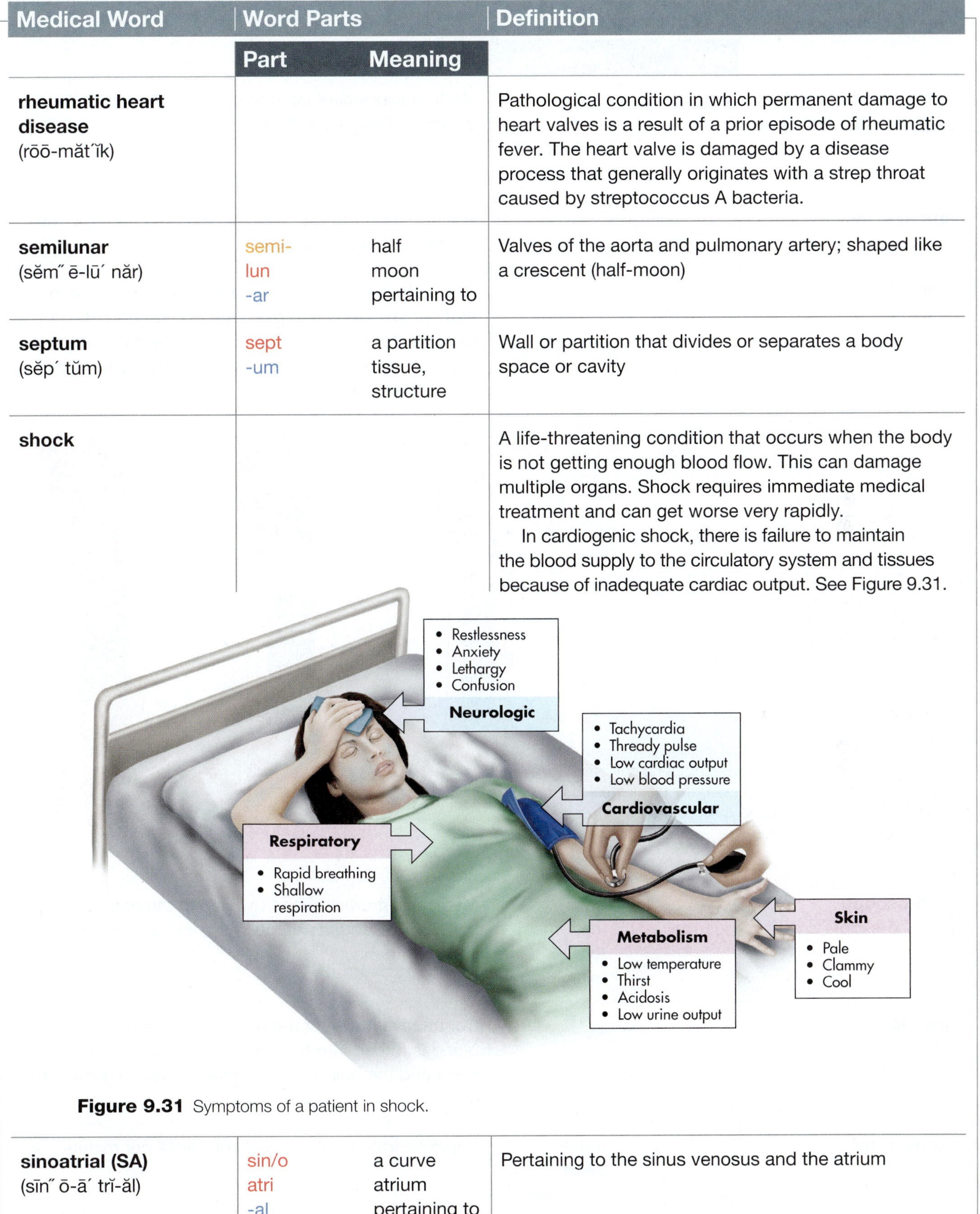

Figure 9.31 Symptoms of a patient in shock.

Medical Word	Word Parts: Part	Word Parts: Meaning	Definition
sinoatrial (SA) (sīn″ ō-ā´ trĭ-ăl)	sin/o atri -al	a curve atrium pertaining to	Pertaining to the sinus venosus and the atrium

Medical Word	Word Parts		Definition
	Part	**Meaning**	
sphygmomanometer (sfĭg″ mō-măn-ŏm′ ĕt-ĕr)	sphygm/o man/o -meter	pulse thin instrument to measure	Medical instrument used to measure the arterial blood pressure. See Figure 9.12.
spider veins			Dilated blood vessels, typically found in the legs, that radiate from a central point
stent			Medical device made of expandable, metal mesh that is placed (by using a balloon catheter) at the site of a narrowing artery. The stent is then expanded and left in place to keep the artery open. See Figure 9.32.

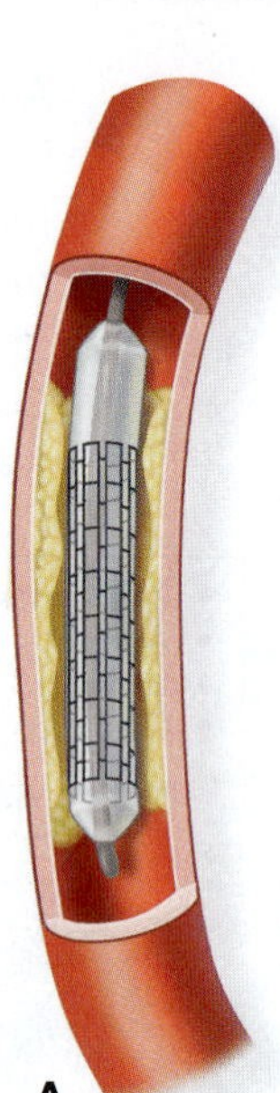

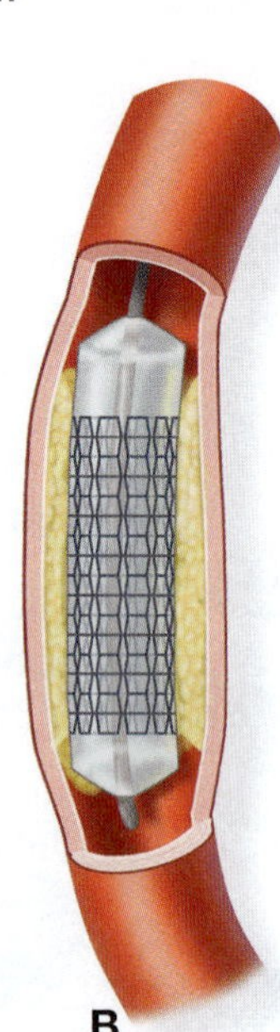

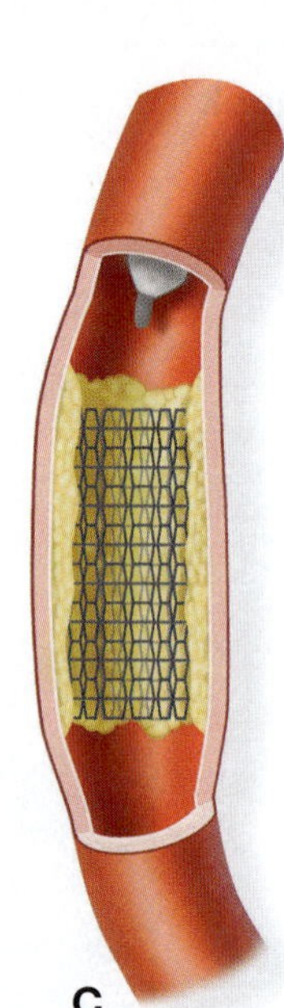

Figure 9.32 Placement of a stent. (A) The stainless steel stent is fitted over a balloon-tipped catheter. (B) The stent is positioned along the blockage and expanded. (C) The balloon is deflated and removed, leaving the stent in place.

Medical Word	Part	Meaning	Definition
stethoscope (stĕth′ ō-skōp)	steth/o -scope	chest instrument for examining	Medical instrument used to listen to the normal and pathological sounds of the heart, lungs, and other internal organs
systole (sĭs′ tō-lē)			Contractive phase of the heart cycle during which blood is forced into the systemic circulation via the aorta and the pulmonary circulation via the pulmonary artery
tachycardia (tăk″ ĭ-kăr′ dĭ-ă)	tachy- card -ia	rapid heart condition	Rapid heartbeat that is over 100 beats per minute

Medical Word	Word Parts		Definition
	Part	**Meaning**	
telangiectasis (tĕl-ăn″ jē-ĕk′ tă-sĭs)	tel angi -ectasis	end vessel dilatation	Vascular lesion formed by dilatation of a group of small blood vessels; can appear as a birthmark or be caused by long-term exposure to the sun. See Figure 9.33.

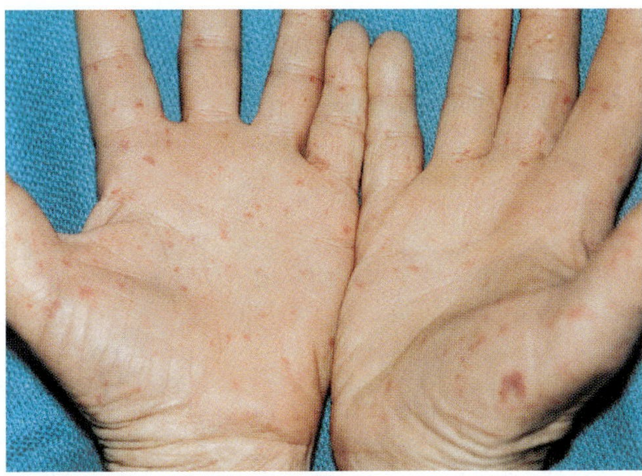

Figure 9.33 Telangiectasis.
(Courtesy of Jason L. Smith, MD)

Medical Word	Part	Meaning	Definition
thrombophlebitis (thrŏm″ bō-flĕ-bī′ tĭs)	thromb/o phleb -itis	clot of blood vein inflammation	Inflammation of a vein associated with the formation of a *thrombus* (blood clot). If the clot breaks off and travels to the lungs, it poses a potentially life-threatening condition called *pulmonary embolism (PE)*. See Figure 9.34.

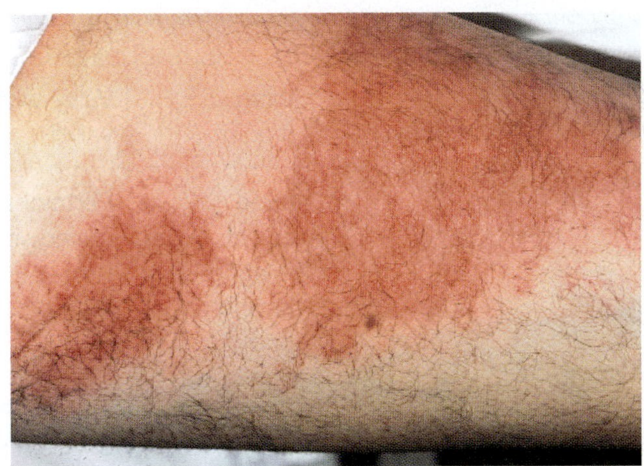

Figure 9.34 Thrombophlebitis.
(Courtesy of Jason L. Smith, MD)

Medical Word	Word Parts		Definition
	Part	**Meaning**	
thrombosis (thrŏm-bō´ sĭs)	thromb -osis	clot of blood condition	A blood clot within the vascular system; *stationary blood clot*. See Figure 9.35.

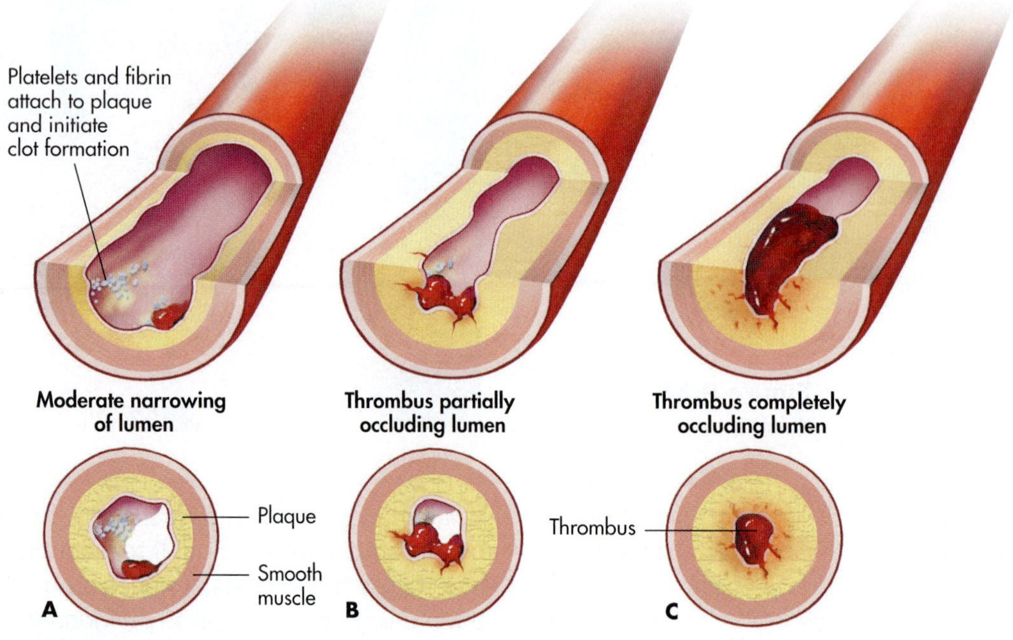

Figure 9.35 Thrombus formation in an atherosclerotic vessel depicting (A) the initial clot formation, and (B) and (C) the varying degrees of occlusion.

Medical Word	Part	Meaning	Definition
tricuspid (trī-kŭs´ pĭd)	tri- -cuspid	three a point	Valve with three cusps; pertaining to the tricuspid valve
triglyceride (trī-glĭs´ ĕr-īd)	tri- glyc -er -ide	three sweet, sugar relating to having a particular quality	Pertaining to an organic compound consisting of three molecules of fatty acids
valve replacement surgery			Surgical replacement of diseased heart valve with an artificial one. There are two types of artificial valves: a mechanical heart valve is made of artificial materials and can usually last a lifetime; a biological heart valve is made from heart valves taken from animals or human cadavers and can wear out over time.
valvuloplasty (văl´ vū-lō-plăs˝ tē)	valvul/o -plasty	valve surgical repair	Surgical repair of a cardiac valve

Medical Word	Word Parts		Definition
	Part	**Meaning**	
varicose veins (văr´ ĭ-kōs)			Swollen, dilated, and knotted veins that usually occur in the lower leg(s). They result from a stagnated or sluggish flow of blood in combination with defective valves and weakened walls of the veins. See Figure 9.36.

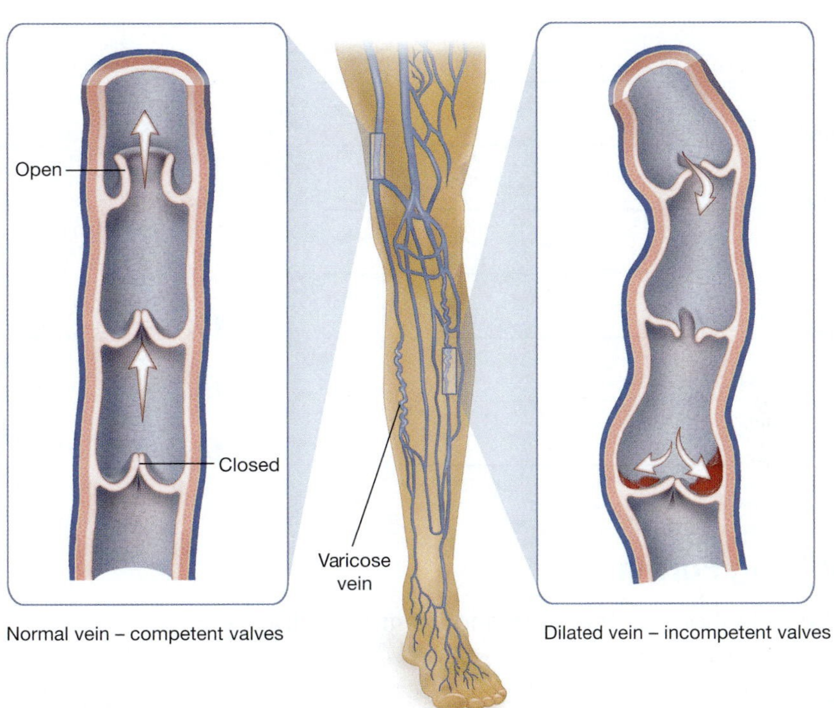

Figure 9.36 Development of varicose veins.

Medical Word	Part	Meaning	Definition
vasoconstrictive (văs″ ō-kŏn-strĭk´ tĭv)	vas/o con- strict -ive	vessel together to draw, to bind nature of, quality of	Causing constriction of the blood vessels
vasodilator (văs″ ō-dī-lā´ tor)	vas/o dilat -or	vessel to widen one who, a doer	Medicine that acts directly on smooth muscle cells within blood vessels to make them widen (dilate)
vasospasm (văs´ ō-spăzm)	vas/o -spasm	vessel contraction, spasm	Spasm of a blood vessel
venipuncture (vĕn´ ĭ-pŭnk″ chūr)			Puncture of a vein for the removal of blood for analysis
ventricular (vĕn-trĭk´ ū-lăr)	ventricul -ar	ventricle pertaining to	Pertaining to a cardiac ventricle

Study and Review II

Word Parts

Prefixes

Give the definitions of the following prefixes.

1. a- ________________
2. bi- ________________
3. brady- ________________
4. con- ________________
5. end- ________________
6. endo- ________________
7. extra- ________________
8. hyper- ________________
9. hypo- ________________
10. peri- ________________
11. dys- ________________
12. semi- ________________
13. tachy- ________________
14. tri- ________________

Combining Forms

Give the definitions of the following combining forms.

1. angi/o ________________
2. arteri/o ________________
3. ather/o ________________
4. cardi/o ________________
5. cyan/o ________________
6. dilat/o ________________
7. ech/o ________________
8. embol/o ________________
9. hem/o ________________
10. isch/o ________________
11. lipid/o ________________
12. lun/o ________________
13. man/o ________________
14. mitr/o ________________
15. occlus/o ________________
16. oxy ________________
17. palpit/o ________________
18. phleb/o ________________
19. scler/o ________________
20. sin/o ________________
21. steth/o ________________
22. thromb/o ________________
23. vas/o ________________
24. ven/o ________________

Suffixes

Give the definitions of the following suffixes.

1. -ac ______________________
2. -al ______________________
3. -ar, -ary ______________________
4. -centesis ______________________
5. -metry ______________________
6. -ectasis ______________________
7. -ectomy ______________________
8. -emia ______________________
9. -er ______________________
10. -gen ______________________
11. -graphy ______________________
12. -ia ______________________
13. -ic ______________________
14. -ide ______________________
15. -ion ______________________
16. -ism ______________________
17. -ist ______________________
18. -itis ______________________
19. -ive ______________________
20. -logy ______________________
21. -malacia ______________________
22. -megaly ______________________
23. -meter ______________________
24. -oma ______________________
25. -or ______________________
26. -osis ______________________
27. -pathy ______________________
28. -plasty ______________________
29. -scope ______________________
30. -spasm ______________________
31. -tomy ______________________
32. -um ______________________

Identifying Medical Terms

In the spaces provided, write the medical terms for the following meanings.

1. ______________________ Tumor of a blood vessel
2. ______________________ Surgical repair of a blood vessel(s)
3. ______________________ Pathological condition of narrowing of a blood vessel
4. ______________________ Irregularity or loss (lack of) rhythm of the heartbeat
5. ______________________ Inflammation of an artery
6. ______________________ Valve with two cusps; pertaining to the mitral valve
7. ______________________ Physician who specializes in the study of the heart

8. ______________________________ Enlargement of the heart

9. ______________________________ Pertaining to the heart and lungs

10. ______________________________ Process of drawing together as in the narrowing of a vessel

11. ______________________________ Condition in which a blood clot obstructs a blood vessel

12. ______________________________ Literally means *inflammation of a vein*

13. ______________________________ Rapid heartbeat

14. ______________________________ Medicine that acts directly on smooth muscle cells within blood vessels to make them widen (dilate)

Matching

Select the appropriate lettered meaning for each of the following words.

____________ **1.** cholesterol

____________ **2.** claudication

____________ **3.** dysrhythmia

____________ **4.** diastole

____________ **5.** fibrillation

____________ **6.** lipoprotein

____________ **7.** cardioversion

____________ **8.** palpitation

____________ **9.** percutaneous transluminal coronary angioplasty

____________ **10.** systole

a. Medical procedure used to treat cardiac arrhythmias

b. Quivering of muscle fiber

c. Fat and protein molecules that are bound together

d. A normal, soft, waxy substance found among the lipids (fats) in the bloodstream and all body cells

e. Literally means *process of lameness, limping*

f. An abnormality of the rhythm or rate of the heartbeat

g. Relaxation phase of the heart cycle

h. Contraction phase of the heart cycle

i. An abnormal rapid throbbing or fluttering of the heart

j. Use of a balloon-tipped catheter to compress fatty plaques against an artery wall

k. Process of being closed

Medical Case Snapshots

This learning activity provides an opportunity to relate the medical terminology you are learning to a precise patient case presentation. In the spaces provided, write in your answers.

Case 1

A 45-year-old male describes experiencing a "squeezing" sensation in his chest during a workout session. This condition, described as _________ _______, occurs when diseased blood vessels restrict blood flow to the heart, causing chest pain that can radiate to the _______ and _______, or to the left arm.

Case 2

A 72-year-old male is diagnosed with arteriosclerotic heart disease (ASHD). Upon _______________ (assessment using a stethoscope to listen to sounds), Dr. Chung hears a bruit or sound of arterial origin. Two conditions often associated with ASHD are _____________ (hardening of the arteries) and _______________ (buildup of fatty substances with subsequent hardening of the arterial walls).

Case 3

The patient is a 62-year-old male experiencing _________ _________ (chest pain). He states that the pain radiates to his neck, jaw, and left arm. An ultrafast CT scan was ordered. After the results of this test were studied, a ____________ _____________ bypass graft (CABG) was discussed with the patient and his wife.

Drug Highlights

Type of Drug	Description and Examples
digitalis drugs	Strengthen the heart muscle, increase the force and velocity of myocardial systolic contraction, slow the heart rate, and decrease conduction velocity through the atrioventricular (AV) node. These drugs are used in the treatment of congestive heart failure, atrial fibrillation, atrial flutter, and paroxysmal atrial tachycardia (PAT). An overdosage of digitalis can cause toxicity. The most common early symptoms of digitalis toxicity are anorexia, nausea, vomiting, and arrhythmias. EXAMPLES: digoxin, Lanoxin (digoxin)
antiarrhythmic agents	Used in the treatment of cardiac arrhythmias (irregular heart rhythms). EXAMPLES: flecainide acetate, Inderal (propranolol HCl), Calan (verapamil), and Cordarone and Pacerone (amiodarone)
vasopressors	Cause contraction of the muscles associated with capillaries and arteries, thereby narrowing the space through which the blood circulates. This narrowing results in an elevation of blood pressure. Vasopressors are useful in the treatment of patients suffering from shock. EXAMPLES: Levophed (norepinephrine bitartrate), dopamine HCl, and metaraminol bitartrate
vasodilators	Cause relaxation of blood vessels and lower blood pressure. Coronary vasodilators are used for the treatment of angina pectoris. EXAMPLES: isosorbide dinitrate and nitroglycerin
antihypertensive agents	Used in the treatment of hypertension. EXAMPLES: Catapres (clonidine HCl), Lopressor (metoprolol tartrate), captopril, and Toprol–XL (metoprolol succinate)
antihyperlipidemic agents	Used to lower abnormally high blood levels of fatty substances (lipids) when other treatment regimens fail. EXAMPLES: Lopid (gemfibrozil), Lipitor (atorvastatin calcium), Pravachol (pravastatin), Zocor (simvastatin), Crestor (rosuvastatin calcium), Vytorin (ezetimibe/simvastatin), Zetia (ezetimibe), niacin, and lovastatin
antiplatelet drugs	Help reduce the occurrence of and death from vascular events such as heart attacks and strokes. *Aspirin* is considered to be the reference standard antiplatelet drug and is recommended by the American Heart Association for use in patients with a wide range of cardiovascular disease. Aspirin helps keep platelets from sticking together to form clots. *Plavix (clopidogrel)* is approved by the Food and Drug Administration for many of the same indications as aspirin. It is recommended for patients for whom aspirin fails to achieve a therapeutic benefit.

Type of Drug	Description and Examples
anticoagulants	Act to prevent blood clots from forming. They are known as "blood thinners" and are used in primary and secondary prevention of deep vein thrombosis (DVT), pulmonary embolism (PE), myocardial infarctions (MI), and cerebrovascular accidents (CVAs; strokes). EXAMPLES: Coumadin (warfarin sodium), heparin, Xarelto (rivaroxaban), and Pradaxa (diabigatran etexilate)
thrombolytic agents	Act to dissolve an existing thrombus when administered soon after its occurrence. They are often referred to as *tissue plasminogen activators* (tPA, TPA) and can reduce the chance of dying after a myocardial infarction by 50%. Unless contraindicated, the drug should be administered within 6 hours of the onset of chest pain. In some hospitals, the time period for administering thrombolytic agents has been extended to 12 and 24 hours. These agents dissolve the clot, reopen the artery, restore blood flow to the heart, and prevent further damage to the myocardium. Bleeding is the most common and potentially serious complication encountered during thrombolytic therapy. Thrombolytic agents are also used in ischemic strokes, deep vein thrombosis, and pulmonary embolism to clear a blocked artery and avoid permanent damage to the perfused tissue. *Note:* Thrombolytic therapy in hemorrhagic strokes is contraindicated because its use would prolong bleeding into the intracranial space and cause further damage. EXAMPLES: streptokinase and Activase (alteplase)

Diagnostic and Laboratory Tests

Test	Description
angiocardiography (ACG) (ăn″ jĭ-ō-kăr″ dĭ-ŏg′ ră-fē)	Video x-ray technique used to follow the passage of blood through the heart and great vessels after an intravenous (IV) injection of a radiopaque contrast substance; used to evaluate patient for cardiovascular (CV) surgery
angiography (ăn″ jē-ŏg′ ră-fē)	A minimally invasive medical test that helps physicians diagnose and treat medical conditions by using x-ray recording (*-graphy*) of a blood vessel after the injection of a radiopaque substance. Used to determine the patency of the blood vessels, organ, or tissue being studied.
cardiac catheterization (CC) (kăr′ dē-ăk kăth″ ĕ-tĕr-ĭ -zā′ shŭn)	Medical procedure used to diagnose heart disorders. A tiny catheter is inserted into an artery in the arm or leg of the patient and is fed through this artery to the heart. Dye is then pumped through the catheter, enabling the physician to locate by x-ray any blockages in the arteries supplying the heart. See Figure 9.37.

(*continued*)

Test	Description
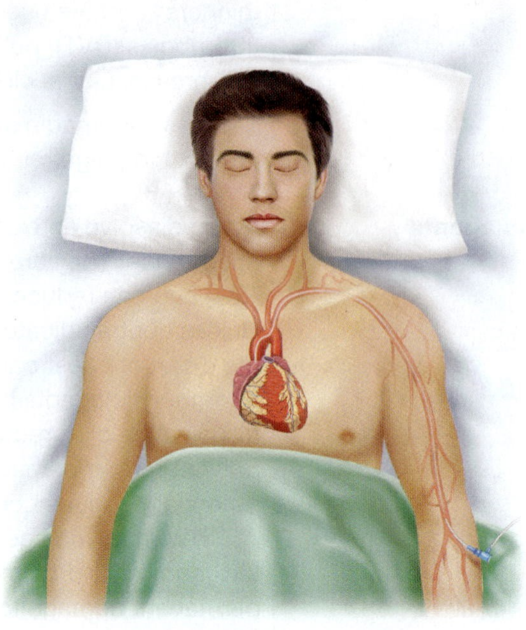 **Figure 9.37** Cardiac catheterization.	
cardiac enzymes (kar´ dē-ăk ĕn´ zīmz)	Blood tests performed to determine cardiac damage in an acute myocardial infarction (AMI). Levels begin to rise 6–10 hours after an AMI and peak at 24–48 hours.
- alanine aminotransferase (ALT)	
- aspartate aminotransferase (AST)	
- creatine kinase (CK)	Used to detect area of damage. Level may be five to eight times normal.
- creatine kinase isoenzymes	Used to indicate area of damage; CK-MB heart muscle, CK-MM skeletal muscle, and CK-BB brain
cardiac muscle protein troponins (kăr´ dē-ăk mŭs´əl prō´tēn trō´ pə-nənz)	Blood tests performed to determine heart muscle injury (microinfarction) not detected by cardiac enzyme tests. Troponin T and troponin I proteins control the interactions between actin and myosin, which contract or squeeze the heart muscle. Normally the level of these cardiac proteins in the blood is very low. It increases substantially within several hours (on average 4–6 hours) of muscle damage, so elevated levels can indicate a heart attack, even a mild one. It peaks at 10–24 hours and can be detected for up to 10–14 days.
cholesterol (chol) (kō-lĕs´ tĕr-ŏl)	Blood test to determine the level of cholesterol in the serum. Elevated levels can indicate an increased risk of coronary heart disease. Any level more than 200 mg/dL is considered too high for heart health.
computed tomography (CT)	Sometimes referred to as a **CAT scan** (computerized axial tomography), this test combines an advanced x-ray scanning system with a powerful minicomputer and has vastly improved imaging quality while making it possible to view parts of the body and abnormalities not previously open to radiography.

Test	Description
echocardiography (ECHO) (ĕk″ ō-kăr″ dē-ŏg′ rah-fē)	Medical procedure using sonographic sound to analyze the size, shape, and movement of structures inside the heart. Usually two echoes are taken: one of the heart at rest and another of the heart under stress. Comparison of the two images helps pinpoint abnormal valves or areas that are not receiving enough blood.
electrocardiogram (ECG, EKG) (ē-lĕk″ trō-kăr′ dē-ō-grăm)	A test that checks for problems with the electrical activity of the heart, an ECG shows the heart's electrical activity recorded as line tracings on paper or displayed on a screen. The spikes and dips in the tracings are called *waves*. A standard electrocardiograph has 12 leads with 10 electrodes placed on the patient's arms, legs, and six positions on the chest, which record electrical activity of different parts of the heart. An ECG provides valuable information in diagnosing cardiac abnormalities, such as myocardial damage and arrhythmias. See Figure 9.38.

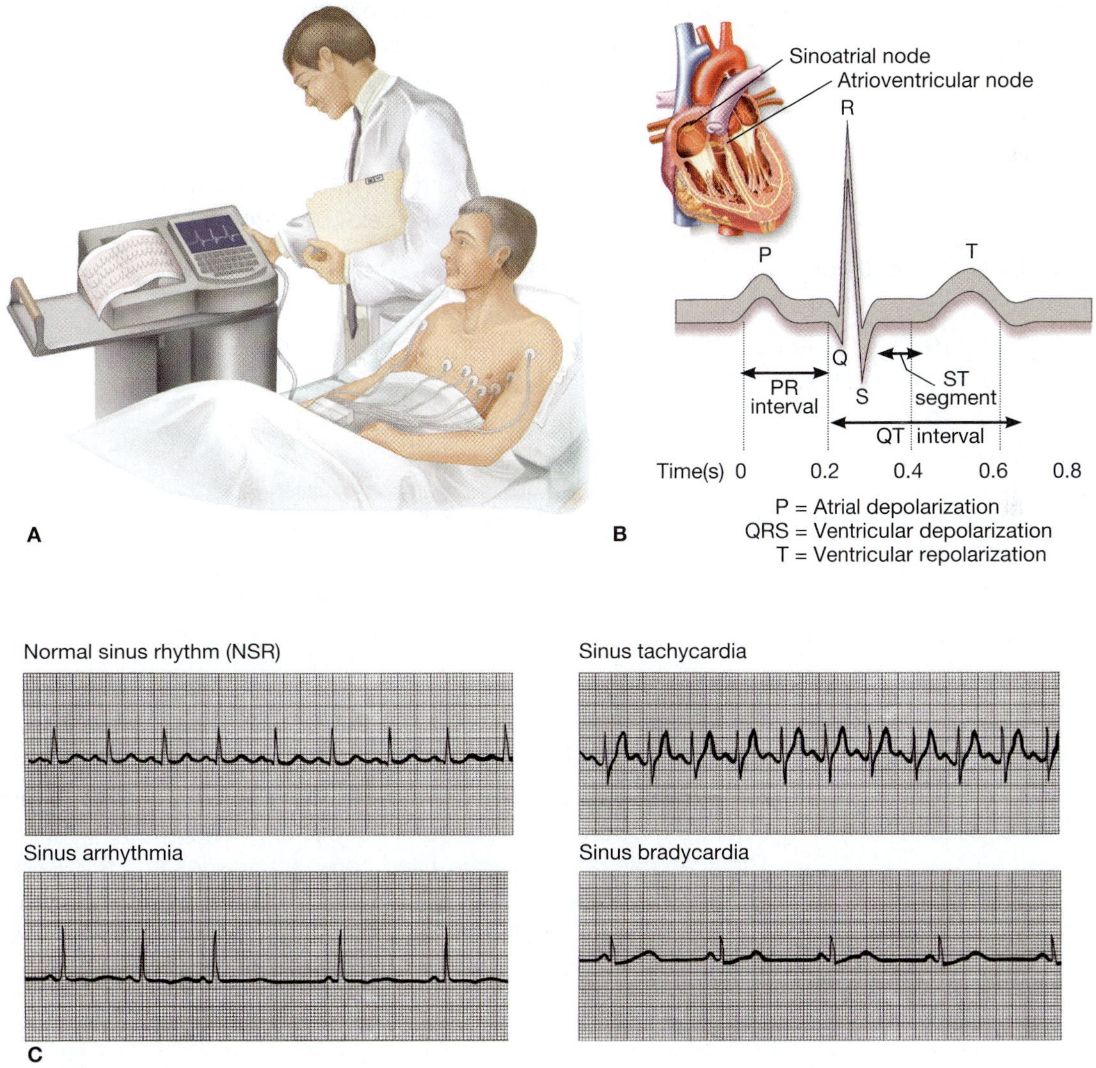

Figure 9.38 Electrocardiography is a commonly used procedure in which the electrical events associated with the beating of the heart are evaluated. (A) Skin electrodes are applied to the chest wall and send electrical signals to a computer that interprets the signals into graph form. (B) Illustration of the electrical events of the heart and a normal ECG/EKG. (C) An electrocardiogram is useful in identifying arrhythmias, as shown here.

Test	Description
electrophysiology study (EPS) (intracardiac) (ĭn″ tră -kăr′ dē-ăk ē-lĕk″ trō-fĭz″ ē-ŏl′ ō-jē)	Invasive cardiac procedure that involves the placement of catheter-guided electrodes within the heart to evaluate and map the electrical conduction of cardiac arrhythmias.
Holter monitor (hōlt′ ər mŏn′ ĭ-tər)	Portable medical device attached to the patient that is used to record a patient's continuous ECG for 24 hours.
lactate dehydrogenase (LD or LDH) (lăk′ tāt dē-hī-drŏj′ ĕ-nās)	Intracellular enzyme present in nearly all metabolizing cells, with the highest concentrations in the heart, skeletal muscles, red blood cells (RBCs), liver, kidney, lung, and brain. When LDH leaks from cardiac cells into the bloodstream, it can be detected and is a good indicator of tissue damage. A high serum level occurs 12–24 hours after cardiac injury.
lipid profile (lĭp′ ĭd)	Series of blood tests including cholesterol, high-density lipoproteins, low-density lipoproteins, and triglycerides. Used to determine levels of lipids and to assess risk factors of coronary heart disease.

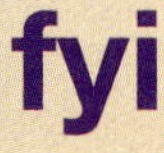

A fasting lipoprotein profile measures the different forms of cholesterol that are circulating in the blood after one avoids eating for 9–12 hours. The evaluations below are for adults.

LDL Cholesterol

below 100	optimal
100–129	near optimal
130–159	borderline high
160–189	high
Above 190	very high

HDL Cholesterol

above 60	optimal
below 40	low for men
below 50	low for women

Total Cholesterol (LDL and HDL)

below 200	optimal
200–239	borderline
above 240	high

Triglycerides

below 150	optimal
150–199	borderline high
above 200	high

Test	Description
magnetic resonance imaging (MRI) (măg-nĕt′ ĭk rĕz′ ō-năns)	Medical imaging technique that uses a magnet that sets the nuclei of atoms in the heart cells vibrating. The oscillating atoms emit radio signals, which are converted by a computer into either still or moving three-dimensional images. The scan can reveal plaque-filled coronary arteries and the layer of fat that envelops most hearts. MRI is also an ideal method for scanning children with congenital heart problems. Patients with pacemakers, stents, or other metal implants cannot have MRI. An MRI scan cannot pick up calcium deposits that could signal narrowed vessels.

Test	Description
positron emission tomography (PET)	Nuclear medicine imaging technique that helps physicians see how the organs and tissues inside the body are functioning. The test involves injecting a very small dose of a radioactive chemical, called a radiotracer, into the vein of the patient's arm. The tracer travels through the body and is absorbed by the organs and tissues being studied. The PET scan detects and records the energy given off by the tracer substance and, with the use of a computer, this energy is converted into three-dimensional pictures. A physician can then look at cross-sectional images of the body organ from any angle in order to detect functional problems. Commonly called a **PET scan**.
stress test	A screening test used in evaluating cardiovascular fitness, also called *exercise test*, *exercise stress test*, or *treadmill test*. The ECG is monitored while the patient is subjected to increasing levels of work using a treadmill or ergometer. It is a common test for diagnosing coronary artery disease, especially in patients who have symptoms of heart disease. The test helps doctors assess blood flow through coronary arteries in response to exercise, usually walking, at varied speeds and for various lengths of time on a treadmill. A stress test can include the use of electrocardiography, echocardiography, and injected radioactive substances.
thallium-201 stress test (thăl′ ē-ŭm)	X-ray study that follows the path of radioactive thallium carried by the blood into the heart muscle. Damaged or dead muscle can be defined, as can the extent of narrowing in an artery.
triglycerides (trī-glĭs′ ĕr-īds)	Blood test to determine the level of triglycerides in the blood. Elevated levels (more than 200 mg/dL) can indicate an increased potential risk of coronary heart disease and diabetes mellitus.
ultrafast CT scan	Ultrafast CT can take multiple images of the heart within the time of a single heartbeat, thus providing much more detail about the heart's function and structures while greatly decreasing the amount of time required for a study. It can detect very small amounts of calcium within the heart and the coronary arteries. This calcium has been shown to indicate that lesions, which can eventually block off one or more coronary arteries and cause chest pain or even a heart attack, are in the beginning stages of formation. Thus, many physicians are using ultrafast CT scanning as a means to diagnose early coronary artery disease in certain people, especially those who have no symptoms of the disease.
ultrasonography (ŭl-tră-sŏn-ŏg′ ră-fē)	Test used to visualize an organ or tissue by using high-frequency sound waves; can be used as a screening test or as a diagnostic tool to determine abnormalities of the aorta, arteries, veins, and the heart.

Abbreviations

Abbreviation	Meaning
ACG	angiocardiography
AED	automated external defibrillator
AF or AFib	atrial fibrillation
AMI	acute myocardial infarction
ASHD	arteriosclerotic heart disease
AST	aspartate aminotransferase
AV	atrioventricular
BP	blood pressure
CABG	coronary artery bypass graft
CAD	coronary artery disease
CC	cardiac catheterization
CHD	coronary heart disease
CHF	congestive heart failure
Chol	cholesterol
CK	creatine kinase
CLI	critical limb ischemia
CMP	cardiomyopathy
CO	cardiac output
CT	computed tomography
CTA	clear to ausculation
CV	cardiovascular
CVA	cerebrovascular accident (stroke)
DVT	deep vein thrombosis
ECC	extracorporeal circulation
ECG, EKG	electrocardiogram
ECHO	echocardiography
EF	ejection fraction
EPS	electrophysiology study (intracardiac)
FDA	Food and Drug Administration
FFA	free fatty acids
HBP	high blood pressure
HDL	high-density lipoprotein
HF	heart failure
Hg	mercury
Hgb	hemoglobin
H&L	heart and lungs
HTN	hypertension
HUD	humanitarian use device
IV	intravenous
LA	left atrium
LD, LDH	lactate dehydrogenase
LDL	low-density lipoprotein
LV	left ventricle
LVEF	left ventricular ejection fraction
MI	myocardial infarction
MRI	magnetic resonance imaging
MS	mitral stenosis
MV	mitral valve
MVP	mitral valve prolapse
NSTEMI	non–ST-segment elevation myocardial infarction
O_2	oxygen
OPCAB	off-pump coronary artery bypass surgery
P	pulse
PAD	peripheral artery disease
PAT	paroxysmal atrial tachycardia
PE	pulmonary embolism
PET	positron emission tomography
PTCA	percutaneous transluminal coronary angioplasty
R	respiration
RA	right atrium
RBCs	red blood cells
RV	right ventricle
RVEF	right ventricular ejection fraction
SA	sinoatrial (node)
SCA	sudden cardiac arrest
SCD	sudden cardiac death
SOB	shortness of breath
STEMI	ST-segment elevation myocardial infarction
TOF	tetralogy of Fallot
tPA, TPA	tissue plasminogen activator
VLDL	very-low-density lipoprotein
VSD	ventricular septal defect

Study and Review III

Building Medical Terms

Using the following word parts, fill in the blanks to build the correct medical terms.

bi-	steth/o	-gen
occlus	veni	-cuspid
sept	-ion	-plasty

Definition	Medical Term
1. Valve with two cusps; pertaining to the mitral valve	_______ cuspid
2. Literally means *process of lameness or limping*	claudicat _____
3. A blockage in a vessel, canal, or passage of the body	__________ ion
4. Colorless, odorless, tasteless gas essential to respiration	oxy _________
5. An abnormal rapid throbbing or fluttering of the heart	palpitat ______
6. Wall or partition that divides a body space or cavity	__________ um
7. Medical instrument used to listen to sounds of the heart	________ scope
8. Valve with three cusps	tri __________
9. Surgical repair of a cardiac valve	valvulo _______
10. Puncture of a vein for the removal of blood for analysis	_____ puncture

Combining Form Challenge

Using the combining forms provided, write the medical term correctly.

angi/o	ather/o	cyan/o
arteri/o	cardi/o	phleb/o

1. Surgical repair of a blood vessel: ________plasty
2. Pertaining to an artery: _______al
3. Tumor of an artery containing a fatty substance: _________oma
4. Enlargement of the heart: ___________megaly
5. The skin, fingernails, and mucous membranes can appear slightly blue: ___________osis
6. Literally means *inflammation of a vein*: ________itis

Select the Right Term

Select the correct answer, and write it on the line provided.

1. Abnormally slow heartbeat defined as less than 60 beats per minute is ______________.

   bruit　　cardioversion　　bradycardia　　tachycardia

2. Abnormal high levels of lipids in the blood is ______________.

   hyperlipidemia　　hyperlipdemia　　hypolipidemia　　hypolipdemia

3. Pertaining to the sac surrounding the heart is ______________.

   pericardial　　pericardiocentesis　　pericarditis　　phlebitis

4. Valves of the aorta and pulmonary artery; shaped like a crescent is ______________.

   sinoatrial　　tricuspid　　bicuspid　　semilunar

5. Pertains to an organic compound consisting of three molecules of fatty acids is ______________.

   tricuspid　　triglyceride　　systole　　triglyeride

6. Condition in which there is a lack of oxygen due to decreased blood supply to a part of the body caused by constriction or obstruction of a blood vessel is ______________.

   infarction　　murmur　　ischemia　　occlusion

Diagnostic and Laboratory Tests

Select the best answer to each multiple-choice question. Circle the letter of your choice.

1. ______________________________ is an intracardiac procedure that maps the electrical conduction of cardiac arrhythmias.
   - **a.** Electrocardiogram
   - **b.** Electrocardiomyogram
   - **c.** Electrophysiology
   - **d.** Cardiac catheterization

2. Blood tests performed to determine cardiac damage in an acute myocardial infarction.
   - **a.** cardiac enzymes
   - **b.** high-density lipoproteins
   - **c.** triglycerides
   - **d.** low-density lipoproteins

3. Method of recording a patient's ECG for 24 hours.
   - **a.** stress test
   - **b.** Holter monitor
   - **c.** ultrasonography
   - **d.** angiography

4. Test used to visualize an organ or tissue by using high-frequency sound waves.
   a. electrophysiology
   b. stress test
   c. ultrasonography
   d. cholesterol

5. X-ray recording of a blood vessel after the injection of a radiopaque contrast medium.
   a. ultrasonography
   b. angiography
   c. stress test
   d. cardiac catheterization

Abbreviations

Place the correct word, phrase, or abbreviation in the space provided.

1. acute myocardial infarction ______________________________
2. atrioventricular ______________________________
3. BP ______________________________
4. CAD ______________________________
5. cardiac catheterization ______________________________
6. ECG, EKG ______________________________
7. HDL ______________________________
8. heart and lungs ______________________________
9. MI ______________________________
10. tPA, TPA ______________________________

Practical Application

Soap: Chart Note Analysis

This exercise will make you aware of the information, abbreviations, and medical terminology typically found in a cardiology patient's chart. Refer to Appendix III, *Abbreviations and Symbols*.

Read the chart note and answer the questions that follow.

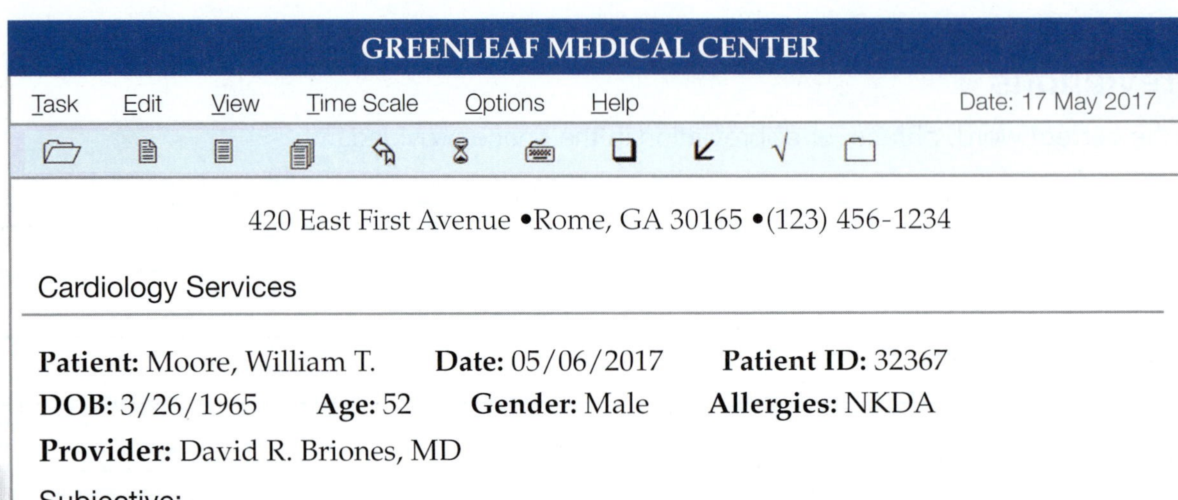

GREENLEAF MEDICAL CENTER

Task Edit View Time Scale Options Help Date: 17 May 2017

420 East First Avenue •Rome, GA 30165 •(123) 456-1234

Cardiology Services

Patient: Moore, William T. **Date:** 05/06/2017 **Patient ID:** 32367
DOB: 3/26/1965 **Age:** 52 **Gender:** Male **Allergies:** NKDA
Provider: David R. Briones, MD

S

Subjective:

Chief Complaint: "Lately I have noticed tightness in my chest during exercise and I feel out of breath. I am real anxious and worried about myself."

52 y/o Caucasian male describes experiencing "tightness" in his chest during a workout session. Noted patient clenching his fist while describing dyspnea (shortness of breath) and how anxious he felt. He denies nausea, vomiting, or radiating pain to his left arm or jaw. The uncomfortable sensation "just went away" after he stopped exercising. He states that he has no prior history of cardiac disease.

O

Objective:

Vital Signs: T: 98.4 F; **P:** 84; **R:** 20; **BP:** 138/90

Ht: 5′ 11″

Wt: 196 lb

General Appearance: Well-developed and muscular. No obvious signs of physical distress noted such as edema, pallor, or diaphoresis. Overall health appears WNL.

Heart: Rate at 84 beats per minute, rhythm regular, no extra sounds, no murmurs.

Lungs: CTA

Abd: Bowel sounds all four quadrants, no masses or tenderness.

MS: Joints and muscles symmetric; no swelling, masses, or deformity; normal spinal curvature. No tenderness to palpation of joints. Full ROM, movement smooth, no crepitant (crackling) sound heard, no tenderness. Muscle strength: able to maintain flexion against resistance and without tenderness.

A

Assessment:

Chest pain (angina pectoris).

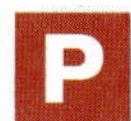

Plan:

1. Schedule patient for an EKG and blood enzyme studies ASAP.
2. Start patient on nitroglycerin (coronary vasodilator) sublingual tablets 0.4 mg prn for chest pain. Instruct patient to seek medical attention immediately if pain is not relieved by nitroglycerin tablets, taken one every 5 minutes over a 15-minute period.
3. To return in 2 weeks for follow-up.
4. Discuss family cardiac history as related to HTN, obesity, diabetes, coronary artery disease, and sudden death of any family member occurring at a young age.
5. Educate patient that angina pectoris occurs due to myocardial ischemia that results when cardiac workload and myocardial oxygen demand exceed the ability of the coronary arteries to supply oxygenated blood. This commonly occurs during exercise or other activity.

Chart Note Questions

Place the correct answer in the space provided.

1. Signs and symptoms of angina pectoris include tightness in the chest, apprehension, and shortness of breath, which is also called ______________________.
2. A complete physical, an EKG, and ______________________ studies are important in determining the diagnosis of angina pectoris.
3. Myocardial ischemia is a result of the body's inability to supply ______________________ blood.
4. EKG is an abbreviation for ______________________.
5. Nitroglycerin is a ______________________ ______________________ used to treat angina pectoris.

Chapter

10 Blood and Lymphatic System

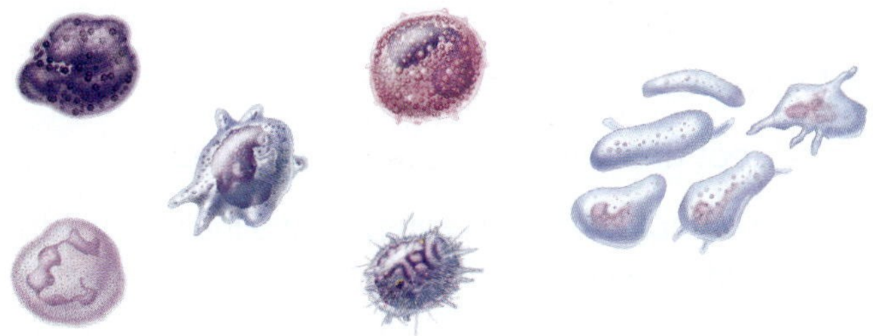

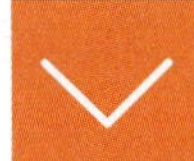

Learning Outcomes

On completion of this chapter, you will be able to:

1. State the description and primary functions of the organs/structures of the blood and lymphatic system.
2. Name the four blood types and their significance in blood typing and blood transfusion.
3. Describe and give the function(s) of the accessory organs of the lymphatic system.
4. Describe the immune system.
5. Explain the immune system's response to foreign substances and the means by which it protects the body.
6. Recognize terminology included in the ICD-10-CM.
7. Analyze, build, spell, and pronounce medical words.
8. Comprehend the drugs highlighted in this chapter.
9. Describe diagnostic and laboratory tests related to blood and the lymphatic system.
10. Identify and define selected abbreviations.
11. Apply your acquired knowledge of medical terms by successfully completing the *Practical Application* exercise.

Anatomy and Physiology

Blood and lymph are two of the body's main fluids and they travel through two separate but interconnected vessel systems. Blood is circulated by the action of the heart, through the circulatory system consisting largely of arteries, veins, and capillaries. Lymph does not actually circulate. It is propelled in one direction, away from its source, through larger lymph vessels, to drain into large veins of the circulatory system located in the upper chest. Numerous valves within the lymph vessels permit one-directional flow, opening and closing as a consequence of pressure caused by the contracting action of muscles on the vessels squeezing the fluid forward.

Table 10.1 provides an at-a-glance look at the blood and lymphatic system.

Blood

Blood is a fluid that circulates through the heart, arteries, veins, and capillaries. It consists of formed elements and plasma, both of which are continuously produced by the body for the purpose of transporting respiratory gases (*oxygen* and *carbon dioxide*), chemical substances (*foods, salts, hormones*), and cells that act to protect the body from foreign substances. The blood volume within an individual depends on body weight. An individual weighing 154 lb (70 kg) has a blood volume of about 5 quarts (qt) or 4.7 liters (L).

Formed Elements

The formed elements in blood are the erythrocytes (red blood cells), thrombocytes (platelets), and leukocytes (white blood cells). See Table 10.2. Formed elements constitute about 45% of the total volume of blood. Together, the plasma and formed elements constitute whole blood. These components can be separated for analysis and clinical purposes. See Figure 10.1.

Table 10.1 Blood and Lymphatic System at-a-Glance

Organ/Structure	Primary Functions/Description
Blood	Fluid consisting of formed elements (erythrocytes, thrombocytes, leukocytes) and plasma. It is a specialized bodily fluid that delivers necessary substances to the body's cells (oxygen, foods, salts, hormones) and transports waste products (carbon dioxide, urea, lactic acid) away from those same cells. Blood is circulated around the body through blood vessels by the pumping action of the heart.
Lymphatic system	Vessel system composed of lymphatic capillaries, lymphatic vessels, lymphatic ducts, and lymph nodes that transport lymph from the tissue to the blood. The three main functions of the lymphatic system are: 1. Transport proteins and fluids, lost by capillary seepage, back to the bloodstream 2. Protect the body against pathogens (microorganisms or substances capable of producing disease) by phagocytosis and immune response 3. Serve as a pathway for the absorption of fats from the small intestine into the bloodstream
Spleen	Major site of erythrocyte (red blood cell) destruction; serves as a reservoir for blood; acts as a filter, removing microorganisms from the blood
Tonsils	Filter bacteria and aid in the formation of white blood cells
Thymus	Plays essential role in the formation of antibodies and the development of the immune response in the newborn; manufactures infection-fighting T cells and helps distinguish normal T cells from those that attack the body's own tissue.

Table 10.2 Types of Blood Cells and Functions

Blood Cell	Function
Erythrocyte (red blood cell)	Transports oxygen and carbon dioxide
Thrombocyte (platelet)	Clots blood
Leukocyte (white blood cell)	Provides body's main defense against invasion of pathogens
Neutrophil	Protects against infection, especially by bacteria; is readily attracted to foreign antigens and destroys them by phagocytosis (engulfing and eating of particulate substances)
Eosinophil	Destroys parasitic organisms; plays a key role in allergic reactions
Basophil	Plays a key role in releasing histamine and other chemicals that act on blood vessels; essential to nonspecific immune response to inflammation
Monocyte	Provides one of the first lines of defense in the inflammatory process, phagocytosis
Lymphocyte	Provides immune capacity to the body
B lymphocyte	Identifies foreign antigens and differentiates into antibody-producing plasma cells
T lymphocyte	Plays essential role in the specific immune response of the body

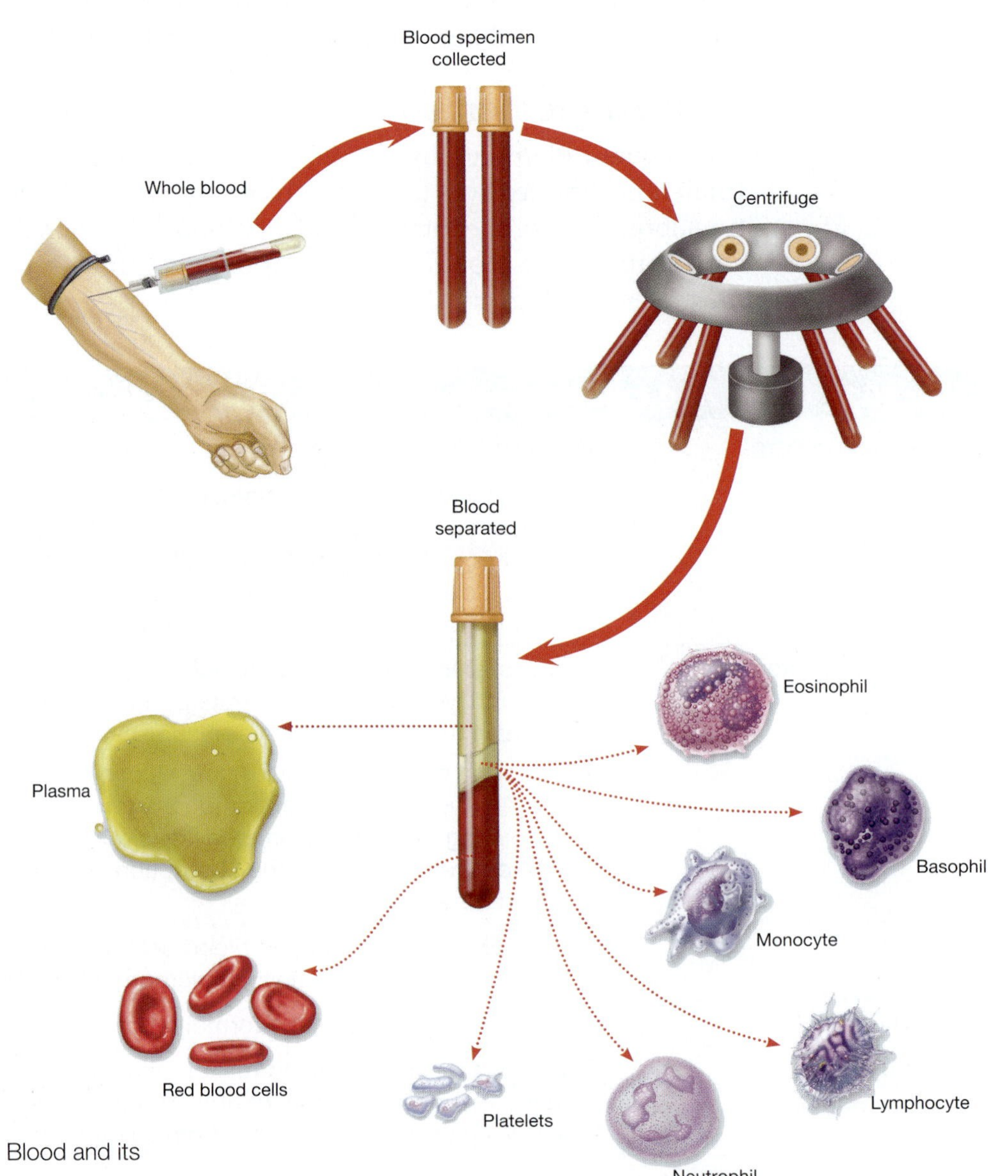

Figure 10.1 Blood and its components.

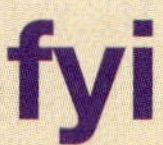

In the embryo, plasma and blood cells are formed about the second week of life. At approximately the fifth week of development, blood formation occurs in the liver and later in the spleen, thymus, lymphatic system, and bone marrow. At 12 weeks, the fetus is 8 cm (3.2 inches) from the crown (or top) of the head to the rump (or bottom) and weighs 45 g (1.6 oz). The fetal **liver** is the chief producer of red blood cells, and the gallbladder secretes **bile**. At 16 weeks, blood vessels are visible through the now-transparent skin. Fetal circulation provides oxygenation and nutrition to the fetus and disposes of carbon dioxide and other waste products.

ERYTHROCYTES

Erythrocytes are commonly called **red blood cells (RBCs)**. Mature RBCs are flexible biconcave disks that lack nuclei. They transport oxygen (most of which is bound to hemoglobin contained in the cell) and carbon dioxide. There are approximately 5 million erythrocytes per cubic millimeter of blood, and they have a lifespan of 80–120 days. Erythrocytes are formed in the red bone marrow. See Figure 10.2.

THROMBOCYTES

Thrombocytes, commonly called *platelets*, are disk-shaped cells about half the size of erythrocytes. See Figure 10.2. They play an important role in the clotting process by releasing *thrombokinase*, which, in the presence of calcium, reacts with *prothrombin* to form *thrombin*. Thrombin (a blood enzyme) converts fibrinogen (a blood protein) into fibrin, an insoluble protein that forms an intricate network of minute threadlike structures called fibrils and causes the blood plasma to coagulate. The blood cells and plasma are enmeshed in the network of fibrils to form the clot.

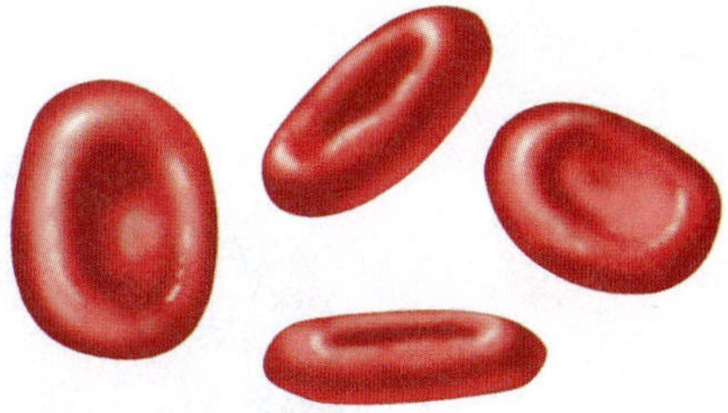

Leukocytes

Basophil

Monocyte

Eosinophil

Neutrophil

Lymphocyte

Platelets

Figure 10.2 Formed elements of blood: erythrocytes, leukocytes (neutrophils, eosinophils, basophils, lymphocytes, and monocytes), and thrombocytes (platelets).

Coagulation is a complex process by which blood forms clots. See Figure 10.3. It is an important part of hemostasis (the cessation of blood loss from a damaged vessel), wherein a damaged blood vessel wall is covered by a platelet and fibrin-containing clot to stop bleeding and begin repair of the damaged vessel. Disorders of coagulation can lead to an increased risk of bleeding (hemorrhage) or clotting (thrombosis).

Coagulation begins almost instantly after an injury to the blood vessel has damaged the endothelium (lining of the vessel). Exposure of the blood to proteins such as tissue factor initiates changes to blood platelets and the plasma protein fibrinogen, a clotting factor. Platelets immediately form a plug at the site of injury; this is called *primary hemostasis*. *Secondary hemostasis* occurs simultaneously: Proteins in the blood plasma, called *coagulation factors* or *clotting factors*, respond in a complex cascade to form fibrin strands, which strengthen the platelet plug. This complex process involves several substances—vitamin K, prothrombin, calcium, thrombin, and fibrinogen—that all aid in forming fibrin.

There are approximately 150,000–400,000 thrombocytes per cubic millimeter of blood. Thrombocytes are fragments of certain giant cells called *megakaryocytes*, which are formed in the red bone marrow.

LEUKOCYTES

Leukocytes, commonly called **white blood cells (WBCs)**, are sphere-shaped cells containing nuclei of varying shapes and sizes. See Figure 10.2. Leukocytes are the body's main defense against the invasion of **pathogens**. In a normal body state, when pathogens enter the tissue, the leukocytes leave the blood vessels through their walls and move in an amoeba-like motion to the area of infection, where they ingest and destroy the invader. There are approximately 8,000 leukocytes per cubic millimeter of blood. The five types of leukocytes are **neutrophils** (neutr/o [*neither*]), **eosinophils** (eos, eosin/o [*rose-colored*]), **basophils** (bas/o [*base*]), **lymphocytes** (lymph/o [*lymph*]), and **monocytes** (mono- [*one*]).

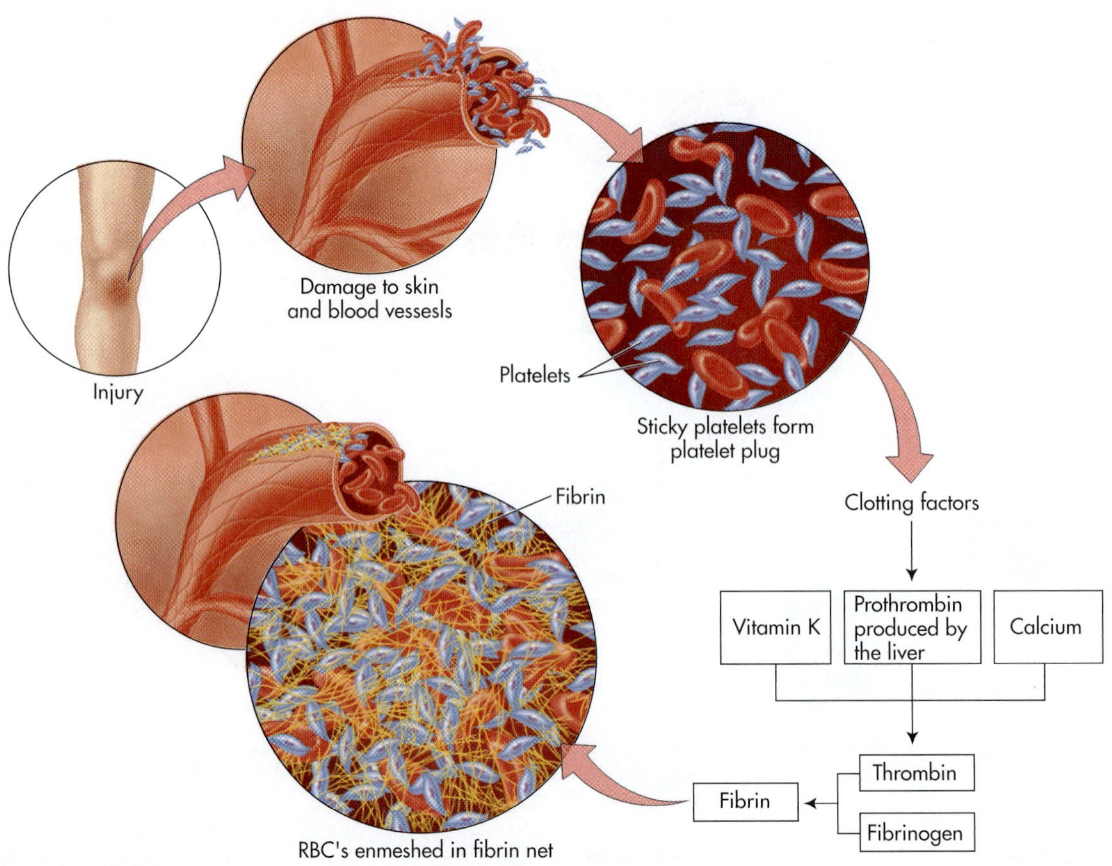

Figure 10.3 The clotting process (coagulation).

Neutrophils, eosinophils, basophils, and monocytes contribute to the body's nonspecific defenses. These immune defenses are activated by a variety of stimuli. Neutrophils aid in the fight of bacterial infection. Lymphocytes are responsible for specific defenses against invading pathogens or foreign proteins. Monocytes are the largest of the leukocytes and fight off bacteria, viruses, and fungi.

Blood Groups

A number of human blood systems are determined by a series of two or more genes closely linked on a single autosomal chromosome. The **ABO** system, which was discovered in 1901 by Karl Landsteiner, is of great significance in blood typing and blood transfusion. The four blood types identified in this system are types A, B, AB, and O. The differences in human blood are due to the presence or absence of certain protein molecules called *antigens* and *antibodies*. The antigens are located on the surface of the red blood cells, and the antibodies are in the blood plasma. Individuals have different types and combinations of these molecules. Individuals in the A group have the A antigen on the surface of their red blood cells and anti-B antibody in the blood plasma; B group has the B antigen and the anti-A antibody; AB group has both A and B antigens and no anti-A or anti-B antibodies; and group O has neither A or B antigens but has both anti-A and anti-B antibodies. Type AB blood is the universal donor of plasma and the universal recipient of cells, and type O is the universal donor of cells only. See Table 10.3.

Rh Factor

The presence of a substance called an **agglutinogen** in the red blood cells is responsible for what is known as the **Rh factor**. It was first discovered in the blood of the rhesus monkey from which the factor gets its name. About 85% of the population have the Rh factor and are called *Rh positive*. The other 15% lack the Rh factor and are designated *Rh negative*. More than 20 genetically determined blood group systems are known today, but the ABO and Rh systems are the most important ones used for blood transfusions.

For a blood transfusion to be safe and successful, ABO and Rh blood groups of the donor and the recipient must be compatible. If they are not, the red blood cells from the donated blood can agglutinate and cause clogging of blood vessels and slow and/or stop the circulation of blood to various parts of the body. The agglutinated red blood cells can also hemolyze (dissolve or be destroyed) and their contents leak out in the body. This can be very dangerous, even life-threatening, to the patient. Before blood can be administered to a patient, a type and crossmatch must be performed. This means mixing the donor cells with the recipient's serum and watching for agglutination. If none occurs, the blood is considered compatible. Even though the blood is checked for compatibility, blood transfusion reactions can still occur and usually involve fever and chills. These reactions typically begin during the first 15 minutes of the transfusion. See Table 10.3 for blood group compatibilities.

Table 10.3 Blood Groups and Compatibilities

Type	Antigen	Plasma Antibody	Percentage/ Population	Compatible Donor Blood Groups	Incompatible Donor Blood Groups
A	A	Anti-B	41%	A, O	B, AB
B	B	Anti-A	10%	B, O	A, AB
AB	Both A and B	No anti-A or anti-B	4%	A, B, AB, O	None
O	No A and B	Both anti-A and anti-B	45%	O	A, B, AB

Plasma

The fluid part of the blood is called **plasma**. Clear and somewhat straw-colored, it comprises about 55% of the total volume of blood and is composed of water (91%) and chemical compounds (9%). Plasma is the fluid part of the circulation medium of blood cells, providing nutritive substances to various body structures and removing waste products of metabolism from body structures. There are four major plasma proteins: **albumin**, **globulin**, **fibrinogen**, and **prothrombin**.

Lymphatic System

The **lymphatic system** is a vessel system apart from, but connected to, the circulatory system. See Figure 10.4. The lymphatic system is composed of *lymphatic capillaries*, *lymphatic vessels*, *lymphatic ducts*, and *lymph nodes*. The system conveys lymph from the tissues to the blood.

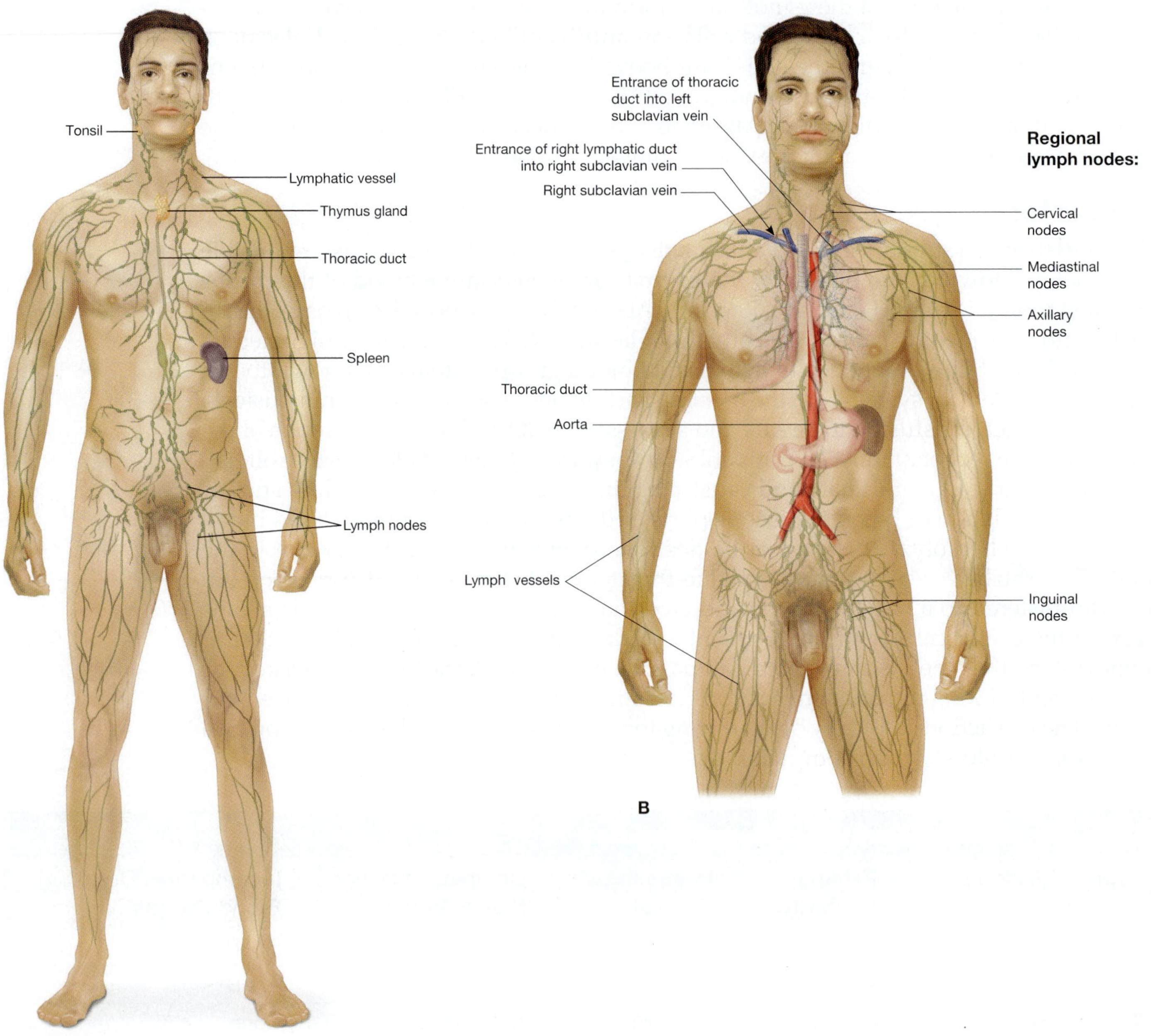

Figure 10.4 Lymphatic system. (A) Lymphatic vessels, major lymph nodes, and lymphatic organs. (B) Areas of lymph node concentration. The direction of lymph flow is toward the heart.

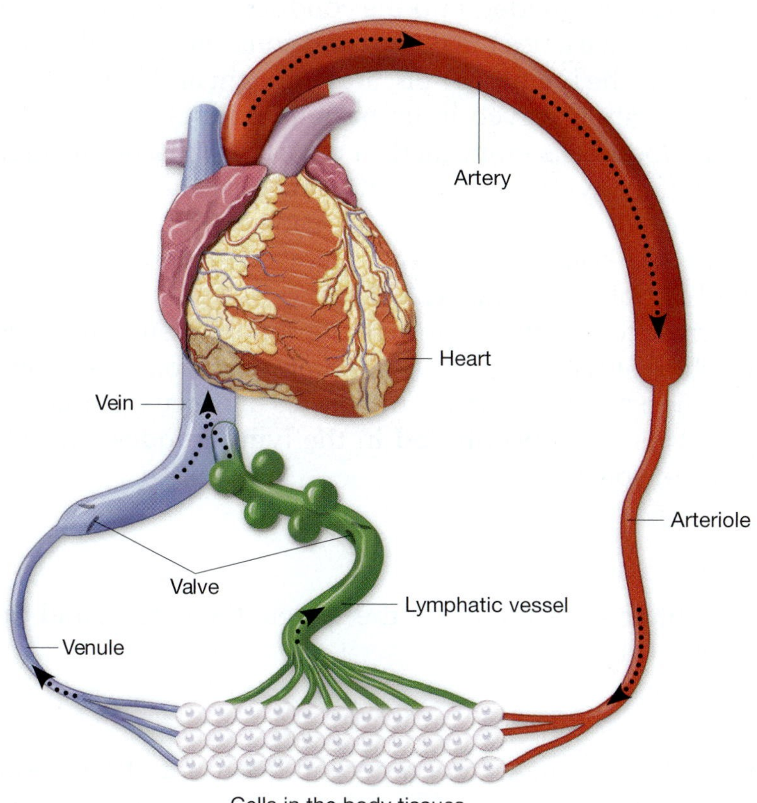

Figure 10.5 Lymphatic vessels pick up excess tissue fluid, purify it in the lymph nodes, and then return it to the circulatory system.

Lymph is a clear, colorless, alkaline fluid (about 95% water) found in the lymphatic vessels. It is fluid derived from body tissues. Lymph contains white blood cells and circulates throughout the lymphatic system, returning to the venous bloodstream through the thoracic duct. See Figure 10.5. The principal component of lymph is fluid from plasma that has seeped out of capillary walls into spaces among the body tissues. Lymph contains proteins (serum albumin, serum globulin, serum fibrinogen), salts, organic substances (urea, creatinine, neutral fats, glucose), and water. Cells present are principally lymphocytes, formed in the lymph nodes and other lymphatic tissues. See Figure 10.6. Lymph from the intestines contains fats and other substances absorbed from the intestines.

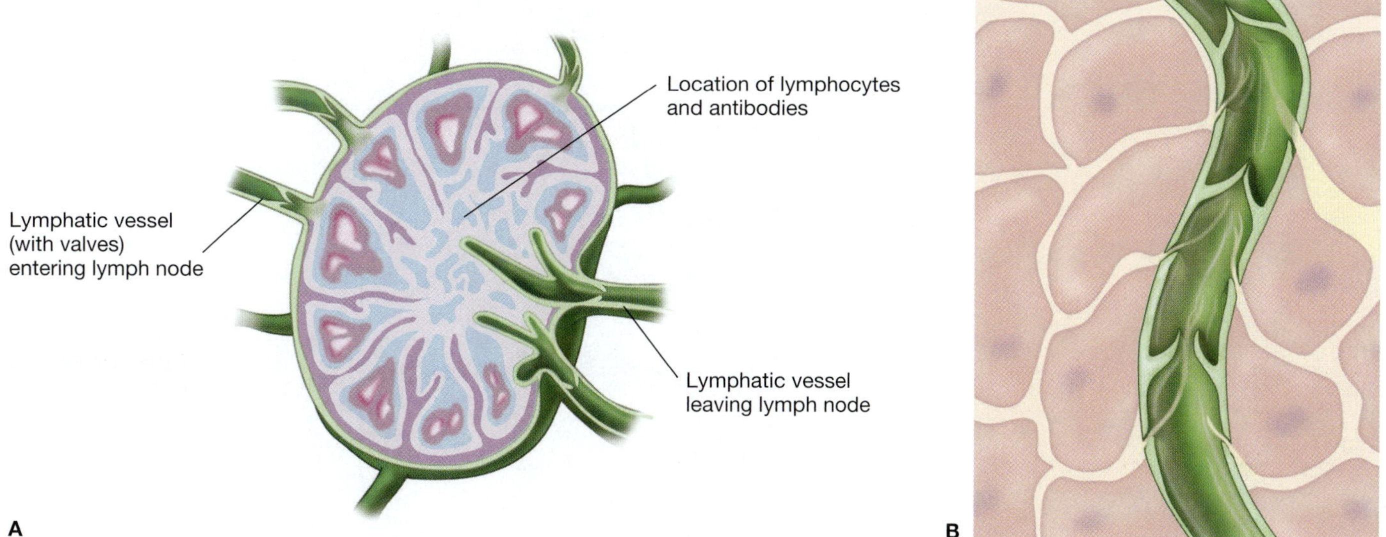

Figure 10.6 (A) Structure of a lymph node. (B) Lymphatic vessel showing valves within tissue cells.

The lymphatic system can be broadly divided into the conducting system and the lymphoid tissue. The conducting system carries the lymph and consists of tubular vessels that include the lymph capillaries, the lymph vessels, and the right and left thoracic ducts. The lymphoid tissue is primarily involved in immune responses and consists of lymphocytes and other white blood cells enmeshed in connective tissue through which the lymph passes. Regions of the lymphoid tissue that are densely packed with lymphocytes are known as *lymphoid follicles*. Lymphoid tissue can either be structurally well organized as lymph nodes or may consist of loosely organized lymphoid follicles known as the mucosa-associated lymphoid tissue (MALT).

The thymus and the bone marrow constitute the primary lymphoid tissues involved in the production and early selection of lymphocytes. Secondary lymphoid tissue provides the environment for the foreign or altered native molecules (antigens) to interact with the lymphocytes. Lymphocytes are concentrated in the lymph nodes, and the lymphoid follicles in the tonsils and spleen.

Accessory Organs

The accessory organs of the lymphatic system include the spleen, the tonsils, and the thymus. See Figure 10.4 and Table 10.1.

Spleen

The **spleen** is a soft, dark red oval body lying in the upper left quadrant of the abdomen. It is the major site of erythrocyte destruction (old erythrocytes over 80–120 days). It serves as a reservoir for blood. The spleen plays an essential role in the immune response and acts as a filter, removing microorganisms from the blood.

Tonsils

The **tonsils** are lymphoid masses located in depressions of the mucous membranes of the face and pharynx. They consist of the *palatine tonsil*, *pharyngeal tonsil (adenoid)*, and the *lingual tonsil*. The tonsils filter bacteria and aid in the formation of white blood cells. See Figure 10.7.

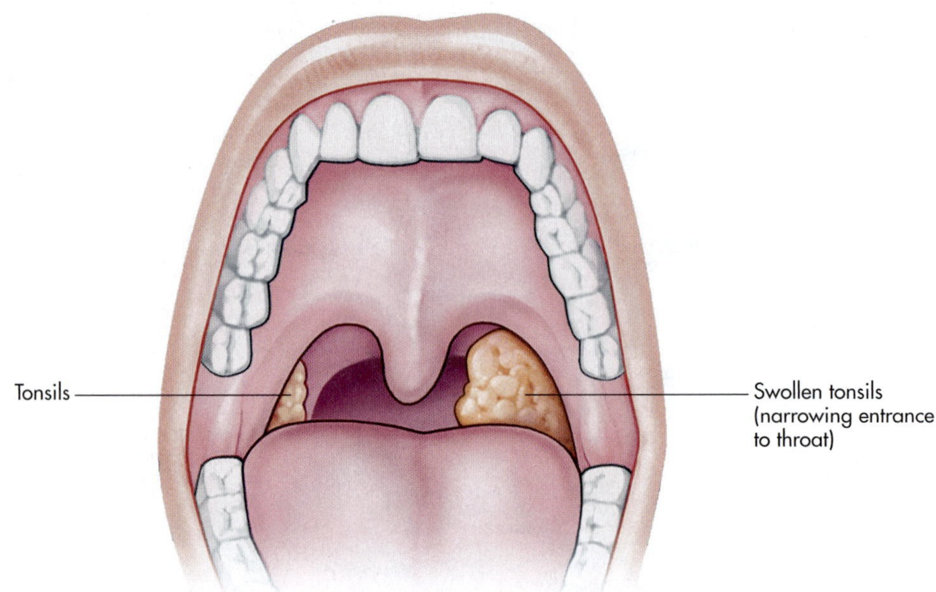

Figure 10.7 Tonsils—normal and enlarged.

Thymus

The **thymus** is considered to be one of the endocrine glands, but because of its function and appearance, it is a part of the lymphoid system. Located in the mediastinal cavity, the thymus plays an essential role in the formation of antibodies and the development of the immune response in the newborn. It manufactures infection-fighting **T cells** and helps distinguish normal T cells from those that attack the body's own tissue. T cells are important in the body's cellular immune response.

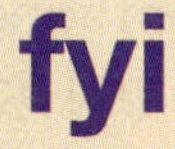

The **thymus gland** plays an important role in the development of the immune response in the newborn. At birth, the average weight of the thymus is 10–15 g. It attains a weight of 28 g (1 oz) at puberty, after which it begins to undergo involution, which replaces the thymus with adipose and connective tissue.

Immune System

The **immune system** is part of the defense mechanism of the body. It consists of the tissues, organs, and physiological processes used by the body to identify and protect against abnormal cells, foreign substances, and foreign tissue cells that may have been transplanted into the body. Many of these tissues and organs are part of the lymphatic system.

Fortunately, the average, healthy human body is equipped with natural defenses that assist it in fighting off disease and cancer. These natural defenses are intact skin, the cleansing action of the body's secretions (such as tears, mucus), white blood cells, body chemicals (such as hormones, enzymes), and antibodies. As long as the immune system is intact and functioning properly, it can defend the body against invading foreign substances and cancer.

Immunity is the state of being immune to or protected from a disease, especially an infectious disease. This state is usually induced by having been exposed to the antigenic marker of an organism that invades the body or by having been immunized with a vaccine capable of stimulating production of specific antibodies. There are several ways that immunity can be described and some of these ways are described here.

Passive immunity is acquired through transfer of antibodies or activated T cells from an immune host, and is short lived, usually lasting only a few months; whereas **active immunity** is induced in the host itself by antigen, and lasts much longer, sometimes lifelong. **Humoral immunity** is the aspect of immunity that is mediated by secreted antibodies, whereas the protection provided by **cell-mediated immunity** involves T lymphocytes alone.

Immune Response

The **immune response** is the reaction of the body to foreign substances and the means by which it protects the body. It is a complex function; the following sections provide an overview of how the immune response works.

The immune response can be described as humoral (pertaining to body fluids) immunity or antibody-mediated immunity and cellular immunity or cell-mediated immunity.

HUMORAL OR ANTIBODY-MEDIATED IMMUNITY

Humoral immunity or **antibody-mediated immunity** involves the production of plasma lymphocytes (B cells) in response to antigen exposure with subsequent formation of antibodies. Humoral immunity is a major defense against bacterial infections. An

antigen is any substance to which the immune system can respond. For example, it may be a foreign substance from the environment such as chemicals, bacteria, viruses, or pollen. If the immune system encounters an antigen that is not found on the body's own cells, it will launch an attack against that antigen.

Antibodies are developed in response to a specific antigen. An antibody is also referred to as an *immunoglobulin;* it is a complex glycoprotein produced by B lymphocytes in response to the presence of an antigen. Antibodies neutralize or destroy antigens in several ways. They can initiate destruction of the antigen by activating the complement system, neutralizing toxins released by bacteria, opsonizing (coating) the antigen, or forming a complex to stimulate phagocytosis, promoting antigen clumping or preventing the antigen from adhering to host cells. See Table 10.4 for the five classes of antibodies: IgG, IgM, IgA, IgE, and IgD.

CELLULAR OR CELL-MEDIATED IMMUNITY

Cellular immunity or cell-mediated immunity involves the production of lymphocytes (T cells) and natural killer (NK) cells that are capable of attacking foreign cells, normal cells infected with viruses, and cancer cells.

Four general phases are associated with the body's immune response to a foreign substance:

1. The first phase recognizes the foreign substance or the invader (enemy).
2. The second phase activates the body's defenses by producing more white blood cells that are designed to seek and destroy the invader(s), especially the macrophages that eat and engulf the foreign substances and lymphocytes, B cells, and T cells. See Table 10.5.
   - T cells of the helper type identify the enemy and rush to the spleen and lymph nodes, where they stimulate the production of other cells to aid in the fight against the foreign substance.
   - T cells of the natural killer (NK) type are large granular lymphocytes that also specialize in killing cells of the body that have been invaded by foreign substances and fighting cells that have turned cancerous.
   - B cells reside in the spleen or lymph nodes and produce antibodies for specific antigens.

Table 10.4 Different Classes of Antibodies

Antibody	Functions
IgG	Crosses placenta to provide passive immunity for the fetus and newborn; opsonizes (coats) microorganisms to enhance phagocytosis; activates *complement system* (a group of proteins in the blood) Components of complement are labeled C1–C9. Complement acts by directly killing organisms; by opsonizing an antigen; and by stimulating inflammation and the B-cell-mediated immune response
IgM	Activates complement; is first antibody produced in response to bacterial and viral infections
IgA	Protects epithelial surfaces; activates complement; is passed to breastfeeding newborn via the colostrum (first milk after birth)
IgE	Responds to allergic reactions and some parasitic infections; triggers mast cells to release histamine, serotonin, kinins, slow-reacting substance of anaphylaxis, and the neutrophil factor, mediators that produce allergic skin reaction, asthma, and hay fever
IgD	Possibly influences B-lymphocyte differentiation

Table 10.5 Functions of Lymphocytes

Type of Cell	Functions
T cells (thymus-dependent)	Provide cellular immunity
B cells (bone marrow–derived)	Provide humoral immunity
NK cells (natural killer)	Attack foreign cells, normal cells infected with viruses, and cancer cells

3. The third phase is the attack phase during which the preceding defenders of the body produce antibodies and/or seek out to kill and/or remove the foreign invader. They do this by phagocytosis in which the macrophages squeeze out between the cells in the capillaries and crawl into the tissue to the site of the infection. Here they surround and eat the foreign substances that caused the infection. Other white blood cells respond to infection by producing antibodies, which are released into the bloodstream and carried to the site of the infection where they surround and immobilize the invaders. Later, the phagocytes can eat both antibody and invader.
4. The fourth phase is the slowdown phase in which the number of defenders returns to normal, following victory over the foreign invader.

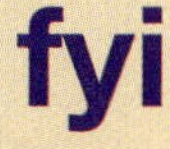

The immune response declines with age, limiting the body's ability to identify and fight foreign substances such as bacteria and viruses. With aging comes the loss of the thymus cortex, which leads to a reduced production of T lymphocytes, including T cells, natural killer cells, and B lymphocytes. Frequency and severity of infections generally increase in older adults because of a decreased ability of the immune system to respond adequately to invading microorganisms.

Study and Review I

Anatomy and Physiology

Write your answers to the following questions.

1. Name the three formed elements of blood.

   a. ______________________ **b.** ______________________

   c. ______________________

2. State the function of erythrocytes. ______________________

   ____

   ____

3. There are approximately ______________________ million erythrocytes per cubic millimeter of blood.

4. The lifespan of an erythrocyte is ____.

5. State the function of leukocytes. ____

6. There are approximately ______________________ thousand leukocytes per cubic millimeter of blood.

7. Name the five types of leukocytes.

   a. ______________________ b. ______________________

   c. ______________________ d. ______________________

   e. ______________________

8. State the function of thrombocytes. ______________________

9. There are approximately ______________________ thrombocytes per cubic millimeter of blood.

10. Name the four blood types.

   a. ______________________ b. ______________________

   c. ______________________ d. ______________________

11. State the three main functions of the lymphatic system.

   a. ____

   b. ____

   c. ____

12. Name the three accessory organs of the lymphatic system.

   a. ____

   b. ____

   c. ____

ANATOMY LABELING

Identify the structures shown below by filling in the blanks.

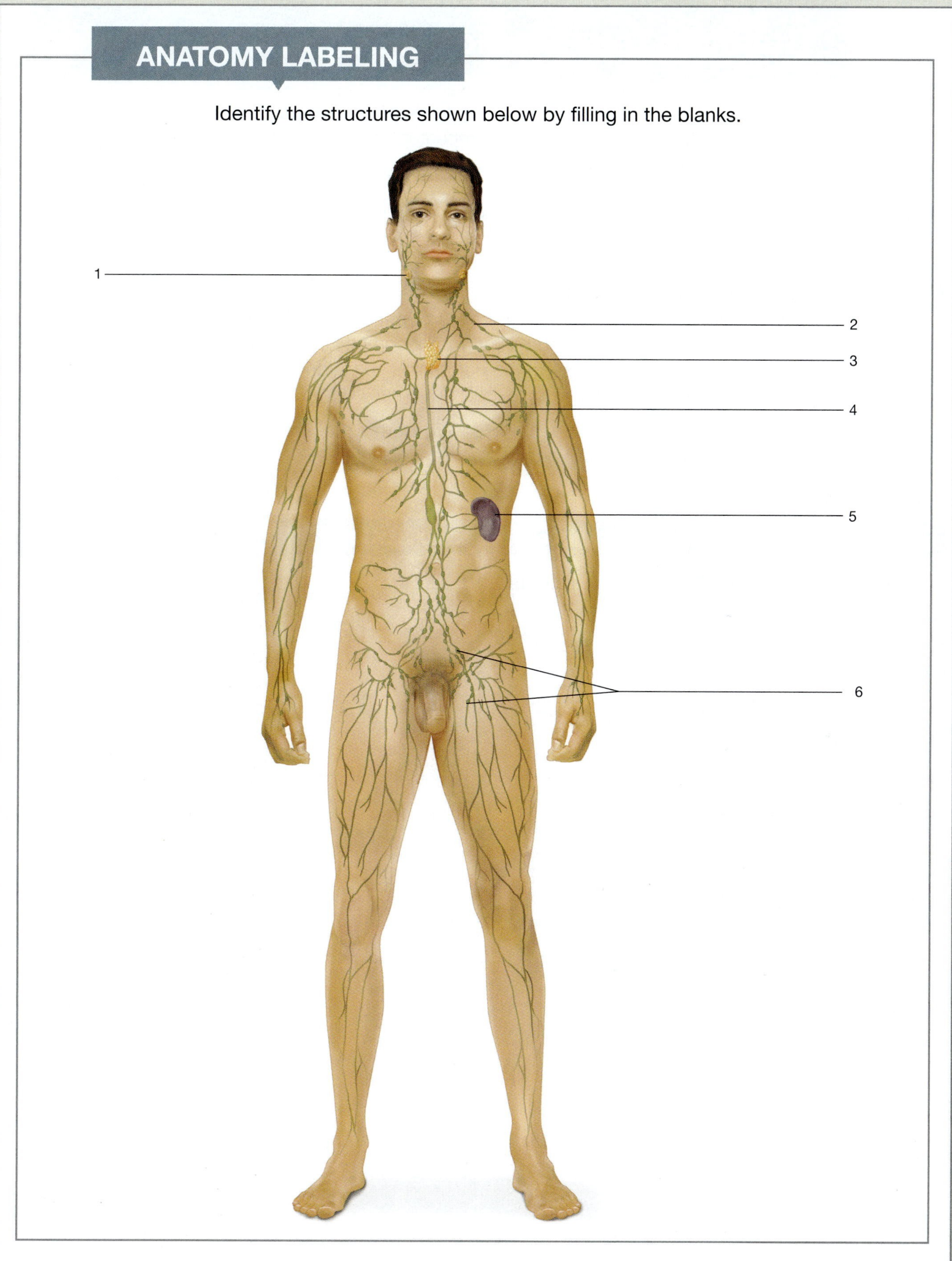

Building Your Medical Vocabulary

This section provides the foundation for learning medical terminology. Review the following alphabetized word list. Note how common prefixes and suffixes are repeatedly applied to word roots and combining forms to create different meanings. The word parts are color-coded: prefixes are yellow, suffixes are blue, roots/combining forms are red. A combining form is a word root plus a vowel. The chart below lists the combining forms for the word roots in this chapter and can help to strengthen your understanding of how medical words are built and spelled.

Remember These Guidelines

1. If the suffix begins with a vowel, drop the combining vowel from the combining form and add the suffix. For example, hemat/o (*blood*) + -oma (*tumor*) becomes hematoma.
2. If the suffix begins with a consonant, keep the combining vowel and add the suffix to the combining form. For example, erythr/o (*red*) + -cyte (*cell*) becomes erythrocyte.

You will find that some terms have not been divided into word parts. These are common words or specialized terms that are included to enhance your medical vocabulary.

Combining Forms of the Blood and Lymphatic System			
aden/o	gland	**hem/o**	blood
agglutin/o	clumping	**immun/o**	immunity
all/o	other	**leuk/o**	white
angi/o	vessel	**lipid/o**	fat
anis/o	unequal	**lymph/o**	lymph
bas/o	base	**macr/o**	large
calc/o	lime, calcium	**neutr/o**	neither
chromat/o	color	**plasm/o**	plasma
coagul/o	clots; to clot	**reticul/o**	net
cyt/o	cell	**septic/o**	putrefying
eosin/o	rose-colored	**ser/o**	whey, serum
erythr/o	red	**sider/o**	iron
fibrin/o	fiber	**splen/o**	spleen
fus/o	to pour	**thromb/o**	clot
globul/o	globe	**thym/o**	thymus
glyc/o	sweet, sugar	**tonsill/o**	tonsil
granul/o	little grain, granular	**vascul/o**	small vessel
hemat/o	blood		

Medical Word	Word Parts		Definition
	Part	Meaning	
acquired immunodeficiency syndrome (AIDS) (ă-kwīrd ĭm″ ū-nō dĕ-f ĭsh′ ĕn-sē)			AIDS is a disease caused by the human immunodeficiency virus (HIV), which is transmitted through sexual contact, exposure to infected blood or blood components, and perinatally from mother to infant. The HIV virus invades the T4 lymphocytes and, as the disease progresses, the body's immune system becomes paralyzed. See Figure 10.8. The patient becomes severely weakened and potentially fatal infections can occur. *Pneumocystis jiroveci* pneumonia (PJP) and Kaposi sarcoma (KS) account for many of the deaths of AIDS patients.

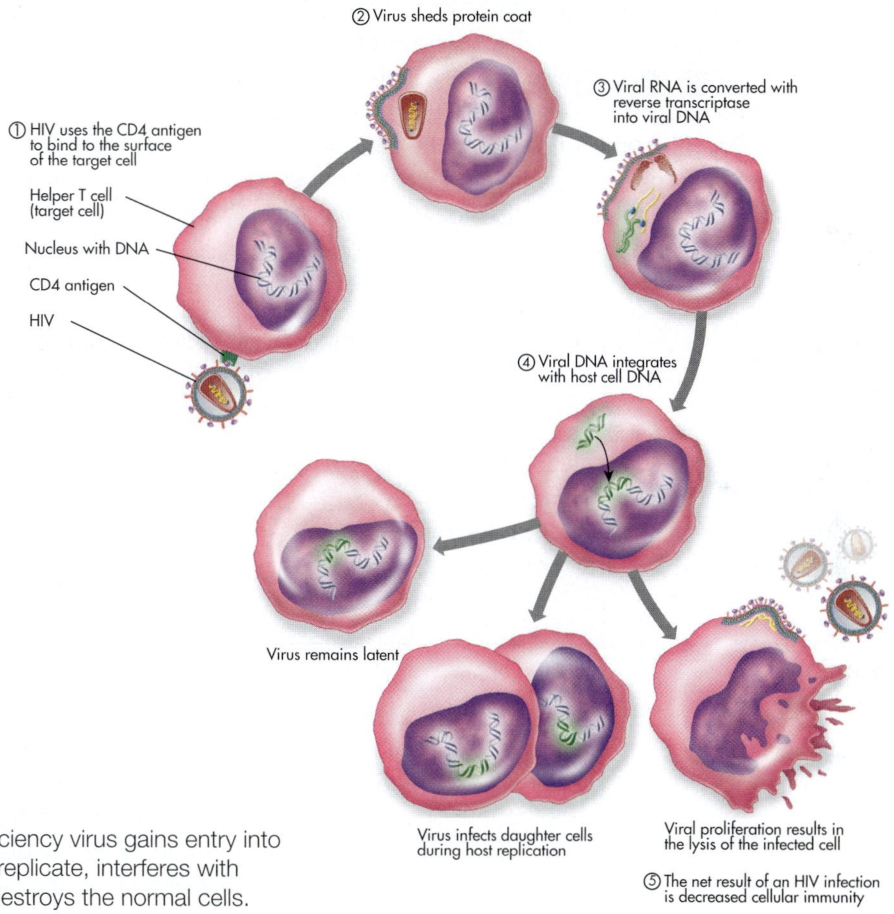

Figure 10.8 Human immunodeficiency virus gains entry into helper T cells, uses the cell DNA to replicate, interferes with normal function of the T cells, and destroys the normal cells.

Medical Word	Word Parts		Definition
	Part	**Meaning**	

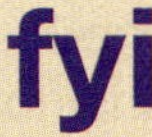

In 2013, people aged 50 and older accounted for 27% of the estimated 26,688 AIDS diagnoses in the United States. Immune function diminishes with age and AIDS infection usually progresses more quickly in older adults.

The main form of treatment of AIDS is with antiviral therapy that suppresses the replication of the HIV virus. This treatment involves a combination of several antiretroviral agents, called *highly active antiretroviral therapy (HAART)*, and has been very effective in reducing the number of HIV particles in the bloodstream (as measured by a blood test called the *viral load*). This can help the immune system recover and improve the T cell count.

The FDA has approved an antiretroviral agent, Truvada (emtricitabine and tenofovir disoproxil fumarate), for *pre-exposure prophylaxis (PrEP)*. The purpose of this drug is to protect uninfected people from HIV. PrEP is not for everyone. The CDC recommends that PrEP be considered for adults who are HIV-negative and at substantial risk for HIV infection through sexual contact or intravenous drug use. People who use PrEP must take the drug every day and return to their healthcare provider every 3 months for a repeat HIV test, prescription refills, and follow-up. In addition, people who take Truvada must be monitored for signs of serious side effects, such as lactic acidosis, liver problems, or worsening of hepatitis B infection. *Truvada does not cure HIV/AIDS.*

agglutination (ă-gloo″ tĭ-nā′ shŭn)	agglutinat -ion	clumping process	Process of clumping together, as of blood cells that are incompatible

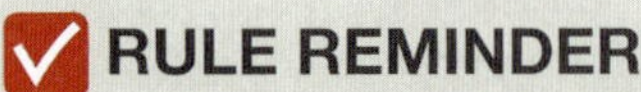

RULE REMINDER

The *o* has been removed from the combining form because the suffix begins with a vowel.

albumin (ăl-bū′ mĭn)			One of a group of simple proteins found in blood plasma and serum
allergy (ăl′ ĕr-jē)	all -ergy	other work	An individual hypersensitivity to a substance that is usually harmless. **Allergic rhinitis** is commonly known as *hay fever*. It is typically caused by the pollens of certain seasonal plants and occurs in people who are allergic to these substances. Symptoms include coughing, headache, sneezing, and itchy nose, mouth, and eyes. See Figure 10.9. This same reaction occurs with allergy to mold, animal dander, dust, and similar inhaled allergens.

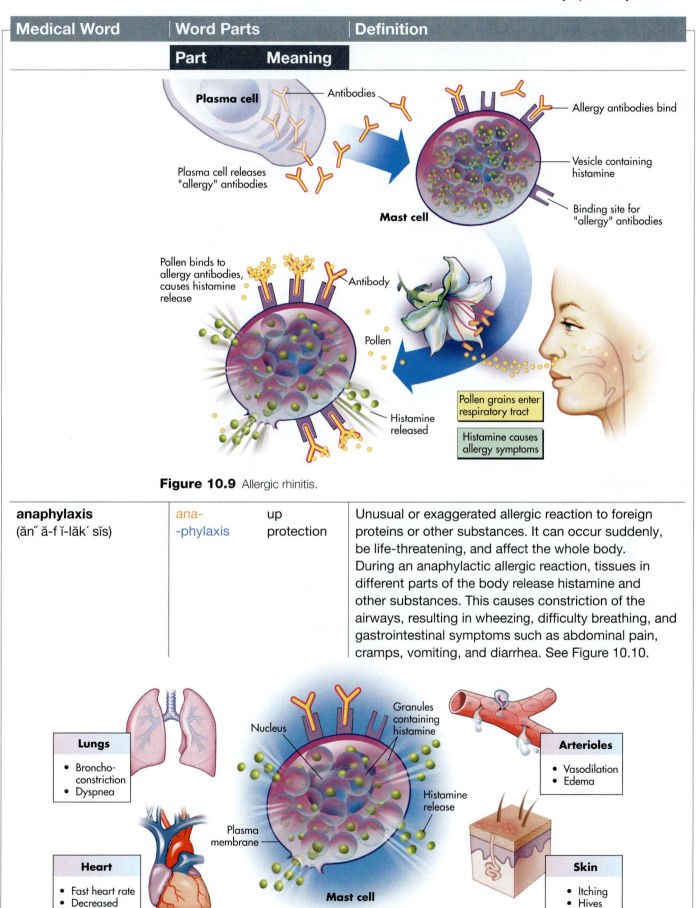

Figure 10.9 Allergic rhinitis.

Medical Word	Word Parts: Part	Word Parts: Meaning	Definition
anaphylaxis (ăn″ ă-f ĭ-lăk′ sĭs)	ana- -phylaxis	up protection	Unusual or exaggerated allergic reaction to foreign proteins or other substances. It can occur suddenly, be life-threatening, and affect the whole body. During an anaphylactic allergic reaction, tissues in different parts of the body release histamine and other substances. This causes constriction of the airways, resulting in wheezing, difficulty breathing, and gastrointestinal symptoms such as abdominal pain, cramps, vomiting, and diarrhea. See Figure 10.10.

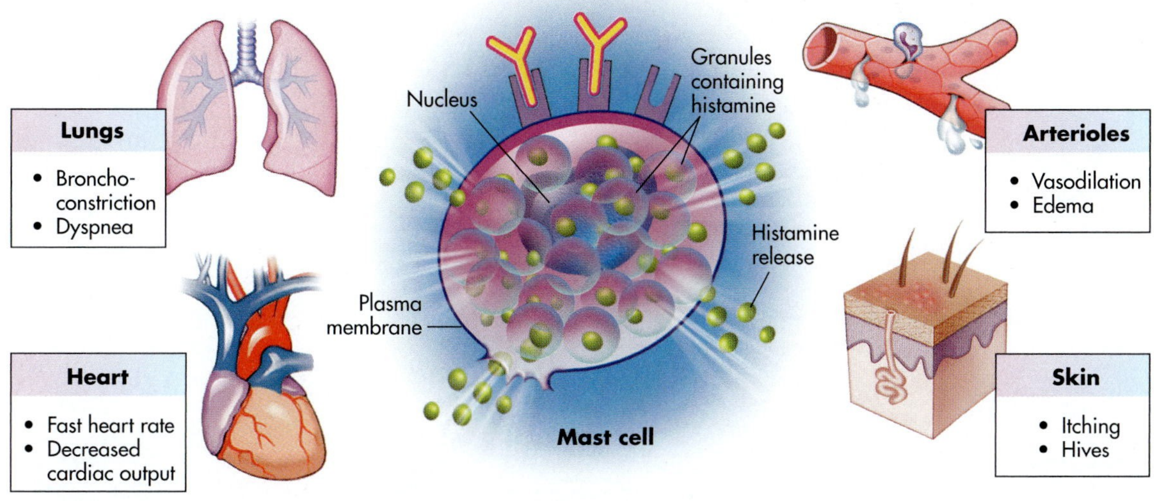

Figure 10.10 Symptoms of anaphylaxis.

Medical Word	Word Parts		Definition
	Part	Meaning	

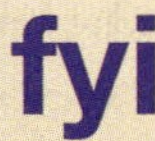

Anaphylaxis is an emergency condition that requires immediate professional medical attention. Shock can occur as a result of lowered blood pressure and blood volume. Hives and angioedema (hives on the lips, eyelids, throat, and/or tongue) often occur, and angioedema could be severe enough to cause obstruction of the airway. Prolonged anaphylaxis can cause heart arrhythmias.

Medical Word	Part	Meaning	Definition
anemia (ă-nē´ mĭ-ă)	an- -emia	lack of blood condition	Literally *a lack of red blood cells*, it is a reduction in the number of circulating red blood cells, the amount of the hemoglobin, or the volume of packed red cells (hematocrit). A normal red blood cell is biconcave with no nuclei and transports oxygen and carbon dioxide. See Figure 10.2. Symptoms of anemia are due to tissue **hypoxia**, or lack of oxygen. General symptoms include pallor, fatigue, dizziness, headaches, decreased exercise tolerance, tachycardia, and shortness of breath (SOB). There are many types of anemia, including hemolytic, pernicious, sickle-cell disease (see Figure 10.11), and thalassemia.

insights In ICD-10-CM, anemias are categorized as:

Nutritional anemias (D50–D53)

- Iron-deficiency anemia (D50)
- Vitamin B_{12}–deficiency anemia (D51)
- Folate-deficiency anemia (D52)
- Other nutritional anemias including megaloblastic anemias, protein-deficiency anemia, and other unspecified anemias (D53)

Anemias due to enzyme disorders (D55–D55.9)

Medical Word	Word Parts		Definition
	Part	Meaning	

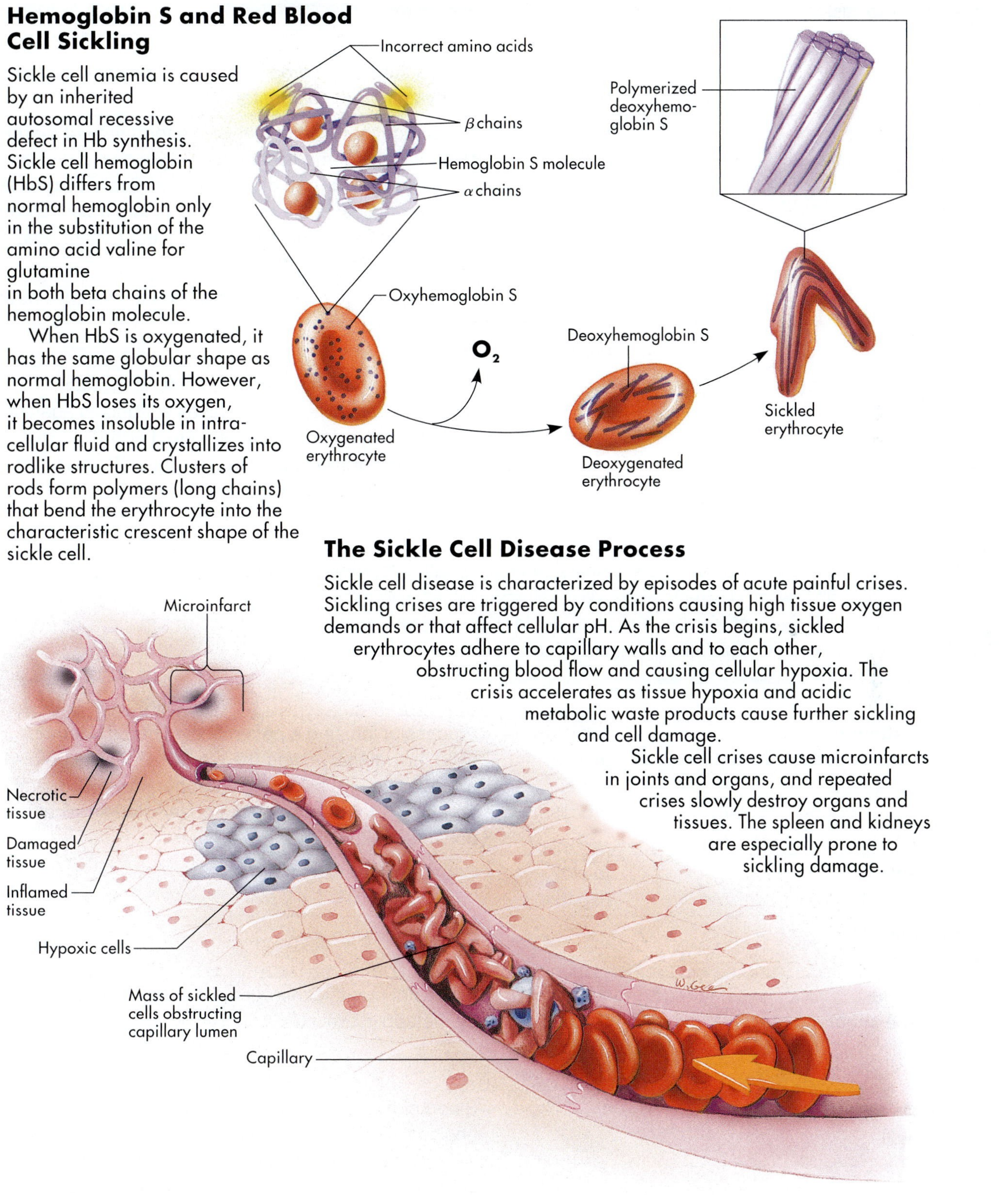
Hemoglobin S and Red Blood Cell Sickling
Sickle cell anemia is caused by an inherited autosomal recessive defect in Hb synthesis. Sickle cell hemoglobin (HbS) differs from normal hemoglobin only in the substitution of the amino acid valine for glutamine in both beta chains of the hemoglobin molecule.
When HbS is oxygenated, it has the same globular shape as normal hemoglobin. However, when HbS loses its oxygen, it becomes insoluble in intracellular fluid and crystallizes into rodlike structures. Clusters of rods form polymers (long chains) that bend the erythrocyte into the characteristic crescent shape of the sickle cell.
Incorrect amino acids
β chains
Hemoglobin S molecule
α chains
Polymerized deoxyhemoglobin S
Oxyhemoglobin S
O2
Deoxyhemoglobin S
Oxygenated erythrocyte
Deoxygenated erythrocyte
Sickled erythrocyte
The Sickle Cell Disease Process
Sickle cell disease is characterized by episodes of acute painful crises. Sickling crises are triggered by conditions causing high tissue oxygen demands or that affect cellular pH. As the crisis begins, sickled erythrocytes adhere to capillary walls and to each other, obstructing blood flow and causing cellular hypoxia. The crisis accelerates as tissue hypoxia and acidic metabolic waste products cause further sickling and cell damage.
Sickle cell crises cause microinfarcts in joints and organs, and repeated crises slowly destroy organs and tissues. The spleen and kidneys are especially prone to sickling damage.
Microinfarct
Necrotic tissue
Damaged tissue
Inflamed tissue
Hypoxic cells
Mass of sickled cells obstructing capillary lumen
Capillary
W. Gee

Figure 10.11 Sickle-cell disease. The clinical manifestations of sickle-cell disease result from pathologic changes to structures and systems throughout the body.

Medical Word	Word Parts		Definition
	Part	**Meaning**	
anisocytosis (ăn-ī″ sō-sī-tō′ sĭs)	anis/o cyt -osis	unequal cell condition	Condition in which the erythrocytes are unequal in size and shape
antibody (ăn′ tĭ-bŏd″ ē)	anti- -body	against body	Protein substance produced in the body in response to an invading foreign substance (antigen)
anticoagulant (ăn″ tĭ-kō-ăg′ ū-lănt)	anti- coagul -ant	against clots forming	Substance that works against the formation of blood clots; a class of medication used in certain patients to prevent blood from clotting; a chemical compound used in medical equipment, such as test tubes, blood transfusion bags, and renal dialysis equipment. See the section *Drug Highlights*.
antigen (ăn′ tĭ-jĕn)	anti- -gen	against formation, produce	Invading foreign substance that induces the formation of antibodies
autoimmune disease (aw″ tō-ĭm-mūn′)			Condition in which the body's immune system becomes defective and produces antibodies against itself. Hemolytic anemia, rheumatoid arthritis, myasthenia gravis, and scleroderma are considered to be autoimmune diseases.

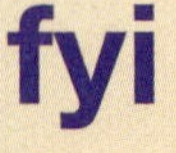

The incidence of autoimmune diseases increases with age, most likely due to a decreased ability of antibodies to differentiate between self and nonself. Failure of the immune response system to recognize mutant, or abnormal, cells could be the reason for the high incidence of cancer associated with increasing age.

Medical Word	Part	Meaning	Definition
autotransfusion (aw″ tō-trăns-fū′ zhŭn)	auto- trans- fus -ion	self across to pour process	Process of infusing a patient's own blood. Methods used include *harvesting* the blood 1–3 weeks before elective surgery; *salvaging* intraoperative blood; and *collecting* blood from trauma or selected surgical patients for infusion within 4 hours.
coagulable (kō-ăg′ ū-lăb-l)	coagul -able	to clot capable	Capable of forming a clot
corpuscle (kŏr′ pŭs-ĕl)			Blood cell
creatinemia (krē″ ă-tĭn-ē′ mĭ-ă)	creatin -emia	flesh, creatine blood condition	Excess of creatine (nitrogenous compound produced by metabolic processes) in the blood
embolus (ĕm′ bō-lŭs)			Blood clot carried in the bloodstream. A mass of undissolved matter present in a blood or lymphatic vessel and brought there by the blood or lymph current. Emboli can be solid, liquid, or gaseous.

Medical Word	Word Parts		Definition
	Part	**Meaning**	
erythroblast (ĕ-rĭth´ rō-blăst)	erythr/o -blast	red immature cell, germ cell	Immature red blood cell that is found only in bone marrow and still contains a nucleus

ALERT!

Check-It-Out! How many words can you build using the combining form **erythr/o**?

Medical Word	Part	Meaning	Definition
erythrocyte (ĕ-rĭth´ rō-sīt)	erythr/o -cyte	red cell	Mature red blood cell, which does not contain a nucleus

RULE REMINDER

This term keeps the combining vowel ***o*** because the suffix begins with a consonant.

Medical Word	Part	Meaning	Definition
erythrocytosis (ĕ-rĭth˝ rō-sī-tō´ sĭs)	erythr/o cyt -osis	red cell condition	Abnormal condition in which there is an increase in production of red blood cells
erythropoiesis (ĕ-rĭth˝ rō-poy-ē´ sĭs)	erythr/o -poiesis	red formation	Formation of red blood cells
erythropoietin (ĕ-rĭth˝ ro-poy´ ĕ´-tĭn)	erythr/o poiet -in	red formation chemical	Hormone that stimulates the production of red blood cells
extravasation (ĕks-tră˝ vă-sā´ shŭn)	extra vas -at(e) -ion	beyond vessel action process	Process by which fluids and/or intravenous (IV) medications can escape from the blood vessel into surrounding tissue
fibrin (fī´ brĭn)	fibr -in	fiber chemical	Insoluble protein formed from fibrinogen by the action of thrombin in the blood-clotting process
fibrinogen (fī-brĭn´ ō-gĕn)	fibrin/o -gen	fiber formation, produce	Blood protein converted to fibrin by the action of thrombin in the blood-clotting process
globulin (glŏb´ ū-lĭn)	globul -in	globe chemical	Plasma protein found in body fluids and cells
granulocyte (grăn´ ū-lō-sīt´)	granul/o -cyte	little grain, granular cell	Granular leukocyte (white blood cell containing granules); a polymorphonuclear white blood cell (includes neutrophils, eosinophils, or basophils)
hematologist (hē˝ mă-tŏl´ ō-jĭst)	hemat/o log -ist	blood study of one who specializes	Literally means *one who specializes in the study of the blood*; physician who specializes in the diagnosis and treatment of blood diseases

Medical Word	Word Parts		Definition
	Part	**Meaning**	
hematology (hē″ mă-tŏl′ ō-jē)	hemat/o -logy	blood study of	Literally means *study of the blood*
hematoma (hē″ mă-tō′ mă)	hemat -oma	blood tumor, mass, fluid collection	Collection of blood that has escaped from a blood vessel into the surrounding tissues; results from trauma or incomplete hemostasis after surgery. See Figure 10.12.

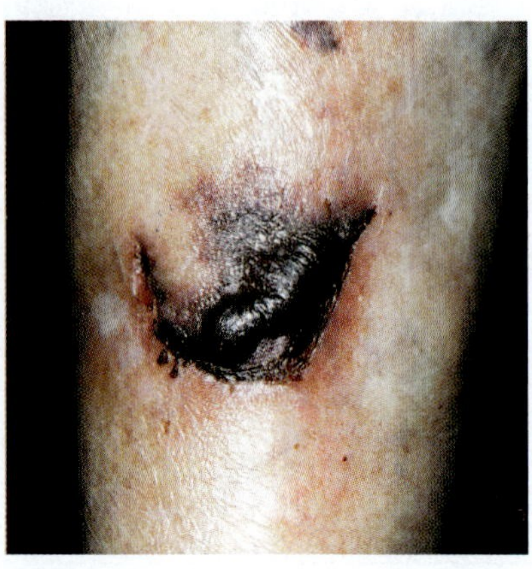

Figure 10.12 Traumatic hematoma.
(Courtesy of Jason L. Smith, MD)

Medical Word	Part	Meaning	Definition
hemochromatosis (hē″ mō-krō″ mă-tō′ sĭs)	hem/o chromat -osis	blood color condition	Genetic disease condition in which iron is not metabolized properly and accumulates in body tissues. The skin has a bronze hue, the liver becomes enlarged, and diabetes and cardiac failure can occur.

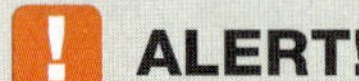

ALERT!

Check-It-Out! How many words can you build using the combining form **hem/o**?

Medical Word	Part	Meaning	Definition
hemoglobin **(Hb, Hgb, HGB)** (hē″ mō-glō′ bĭn)	hem/o -globin	blood globe, protein	Blood protein; the iron-containing pigment of red blood cells that carries oxygen from the lungs to the tissues
hemolysis (hē-mŏl′ ĭ-sĭs)	hem/o -lysis	blood destruction	Destruction of red blood cells
hemophilia (hē″ mō-fĭl′ ĭ-ă)	hem/o -phil -ia	blood attraction condition	Hereditary blood condition characterized by prolonged coagulation and tendency to bleed

Medical Word	Word Parts		Definition
	Part	**Meaning**	
hemorrhage (hĕm´ ĕ-rĭj)	hem/o -rrhage	blood bursting forth	Literally means *bursting forth of blood*; bleeding. See Figure 10.13.
hemostasis (hē´ mō-stā-sĭs)	hem/o -stasis	blood control, stop, stand still	Control or stopping of bleeding. See Figure 10.14.

Figure 10.13 Hemorrhage, vein.
(Courtesy of Jason L. Smith, MD)

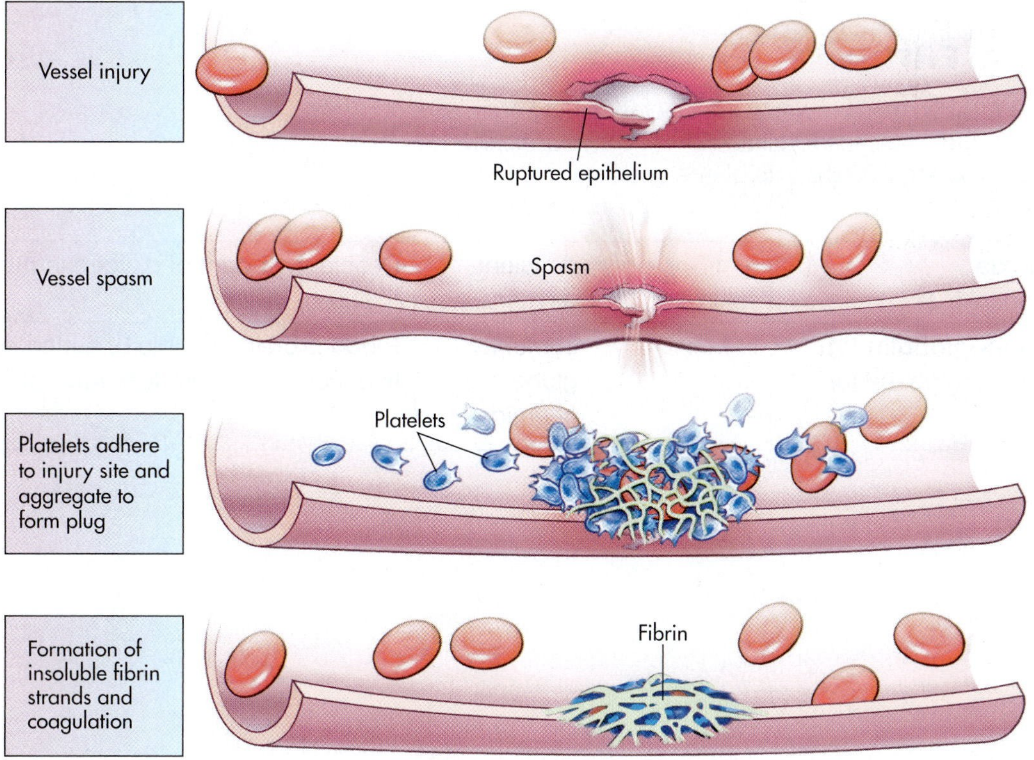

Figure 10.14 Basic steps in hemostasis.

Medical Word	Word Parts		Definition
	Part	**Meaning**	
heparin (hĕp´ ă-rĭn)			Natural substance found in the liver, lungs, and other body tissues that inhibits blood clotting (anticoagulant). As a drug, heparin is used during certain types of surgery and in the treatment of deep vein thrombosis or pulmonary infarction. It can be administered by either subcutaneous or intravenous injection.
hypercalcemia (hī˝ pĕr-kăl-sē´ mĭ-ă)	hyper- calc -emia	excessive lime, calcium blood condition	Pathological condition of excessive amounts of calcium in the blood
hyperglycemia (hī˝ pĕr-glī-sē´ mĭ-ă)	hyper- glyc -emia	excessive sweet, sugar blood condition	Pathological condition of excessive amounts of sugar in the blood
hyperlipidemia (hī˝ pĕr-lĭp-ĭd-ē´ mĭ-ă)	hyper- lipid -emia	excessive fat blood condition	Pathological condition of excessive amounts of lipids (fat) in the blood
hypoglycemia (hī˝ pō-glī-sē´ mĭ-ă)	hypo- glyc -emia	deficient sweet, sugar blood condition	Condition of deficient amounts of sugar in the blood; low blood sugar

ALERT!

It is important to know the difference between **hyper-** *(excessive)* and **hypo-**, **hyp-** *(deficient)*. They are the opposite of one another.

Medical Word	Part	Meaning	Definition
hypoxia (hī˝ pŏks´ ē-ă)	hyp- -oxia	deficient oxygen	Deficient amount of oxygen in the blood, cells, and tissues
immunoglobulin (Ig) (ĭm˝ ū-nō-glŏb´ ū-l ĭn)	immun/o globul -in	immunity globe chemical	Blood protein capable of acting as an antibody. The five major types are IgA, IgD, IgE, IgG, and IgM.

Medical Word	Word Parts: Part	Word Parts: Meaning	Definition
Kaposi sarcoma (KS) (kăp´ ō-sē săr-kō´ mă)			Malignant neoplasm that causes violaceous (violet-colored) vascular lesions and general lymphadenopathy (diseased lymph nodes); it is the most common AIDS-related tumor. See Figure 10.15.

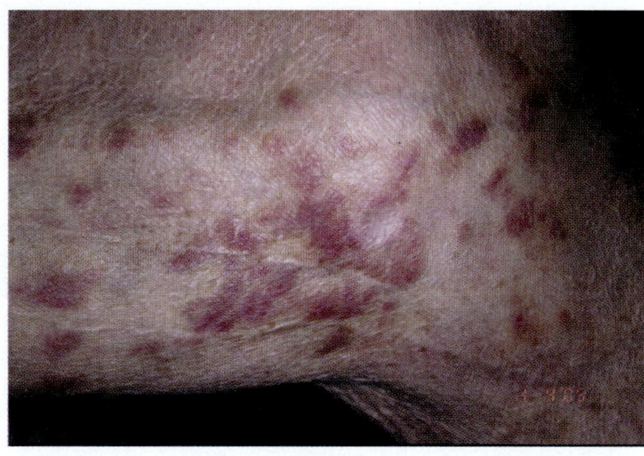

Figure 10.15 Kaposi sarcoma.
(Courtesy of Jason L. Smith, MD)

insights In the ICD-10-CM, the code for Kaposi sarcoma is C46.1. It can also be referred to as *cancer of the soft tissue*. KS of the lymph glands and nodes is coded C46.3.

Medical Word	Word Parts: Part	Word Parts: Meaning	Definition
leukapheresis (loo˝ kă-fĕ-rē´ sĭs)	leuk -apheresis	white removal	Separation of white blood cells from the blood, which are then transfused back into the patient
leukemia (loo-kē´ mē-ă)	leuk -emia	white blood condition	Disease of the blood characterized by overproduction of leukocytes. Common types include chronic lymphocytic leukemia (CLL) and acute lymphocytic leukemia (ALL).

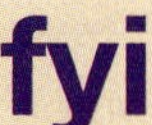

fyi Chronic lymphocytic leukemia (CLL) is a malignancy (cancer) of the white blood cells (lymphocytes) characterized by a slow, progressive increase of these cells in the blood and the bone marrow. Acute lymphocytic leukemia (ALL) is a cancer of the lymph cells. It is characterized by large numbers of immature white blood cells that resemble lymphoblasts. These cells can be found in the blood, the bone marrow, the lymph nodes, the spleen, and other organs.

Medical Word	Word Parts: Part	Word Parts: Meaning	Definition
leukocytopenia (loo˝ kō-sī˝ tō-pē´ nĭ-ă)	leuk/o cyt/o -penia	white cell lack of	Literally means lack of white blood cells
lymphadenitis (lĭm-făd˝ ĕn-ī´ tĭs)	lymph aden -itis	lymph gland inflammation	Inflammation of the lymph glands

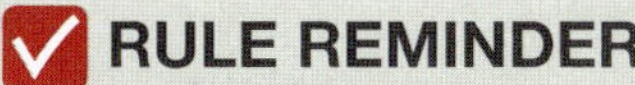

RULE REMINDER

The *o* has been removed from the combining form because the suffix begins with a vowel.

Medical Word	Word Parts: Part	Word Parts: Meaning	Definition
lymphangiitis (lĭm-făn″ jē-ī′ tĭs)	lymph angi -itis	lymph vessel inflammation	Inflammation of lymphatic vessels. See Figure 10.16.

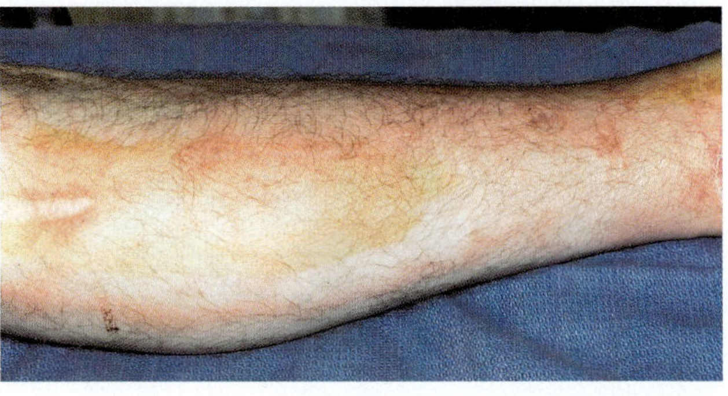

Figure 10.16
Lymphangiitis.
(Courtesy of Jason L. Smith, MD)

Medical Word	Word Parts: Part	Word Parts: Meaning	Definition
lymphedema (lĭmf-ĕ-dē′ mă)	lymph -edema	lymph swelling	Abnormal accumulation of lymph in the interstitial spaces. See Figure 10.17.

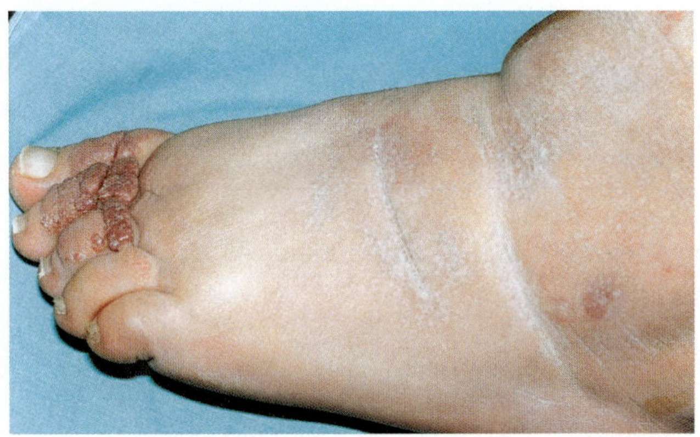

Figure 10.17
Chronic lymphedema.
(Courtesy of Jason L. Smith, MD)

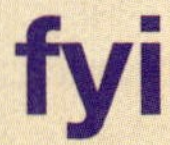

Vascularized lymph node transfer (VLNT) is a microsurgical procedure that involves transferring lymph nodes from the groin to the area under the arm. VLNT may be appropriate for women who have experienced complications during breast cancer surgery. Patients with leg lymphedema may require this procedure at the levels of the knee and groin. Patients with profound soft tissue deformities may require excision (removal) of excess skin and then liposuction of the extremity in a staged fashion.

Medical Word	Word Parts		Definition
	Part	**Meaning**	
lymphoma (lĭm-fō´ mă)	lymph -oma	lymph tumor, mass, fluid collection	Lymphoid neoplasm, usually malignant. See Figures 10.18 and 10.19. Lymphomas are identified as Hodgkin disease or non-Hodgkin lymphomas. Radiation therapy is the primary treatment for early-stage Hodgkin disease.

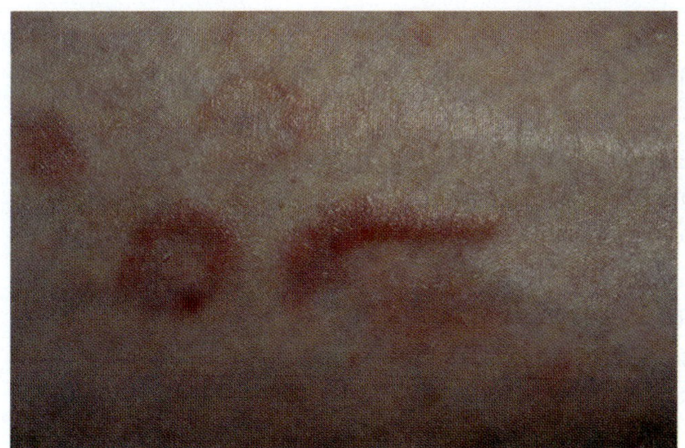

Figure 10.18 Large B cell lymphoma.
(Courtesy of Jason L. Smith, MD)

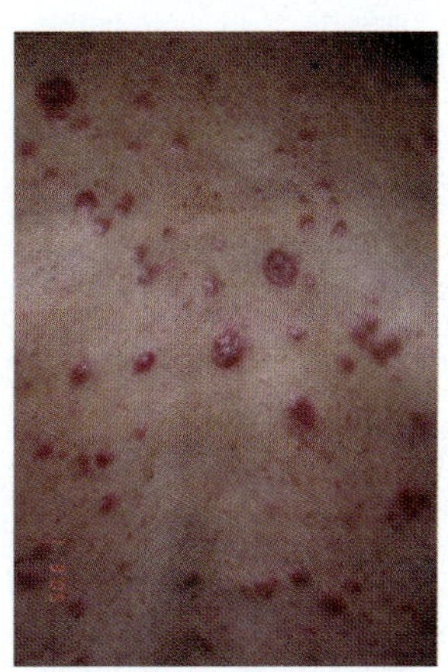

Figure 10.19 Cutaneous T cell lymphoma.
(Courtesy of Jason L. Smith, MD)

Medical Word	Part	Meaning	Definition
lymphostasis (lĭm fŏs´ tă-sĭs)	lymph/o -stasis	lymph control, stop, stand still	Control or stopping of the flow of lymph
macrocytosis (măk˝ rō-sī-tō´ sĭs)	macr/o cyt -osis	large cell condition	Condition in which erythrocytes are larger than normal
mononucleosis (mŏn˝ ō-nū˝ klē-ō´ sĭs)	mono- nucle -osis	one kernel, nucleus condition	Condition of excessive amounts of mononuclear leukocytes in the blood. See Figure 10.20.

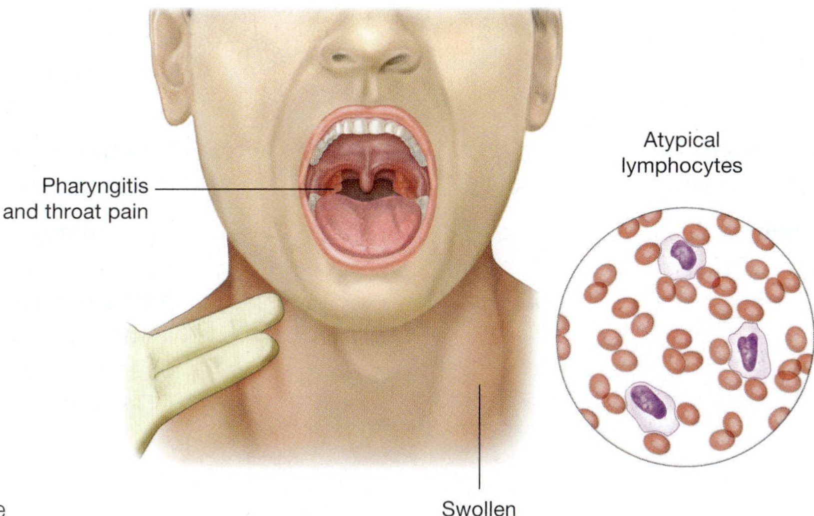

Figure 10.20 Mononucleosis is caused by the Epstein–Barr virus. Symptoms of the infectious disease are swollen palatine tonsils (pharyngitis), swollen cervical lymph nodes (lymphadenopathy), high fever, and a blood sample that shows atypical lymphocytes.

Medical Word	Word Parts		Definition
	Part	**Meaning**	
opportunistic infection (ŏp″ ŏr-too-nĭs′ tĭk)			An infection that occurs more frequently or is more severe in people with weakened immune systems, such as people with HIV or people receiving chemotherapy, than in people with healthy immune systems. AIDS patients are very vulnerable to these types of infections.
pancytopenia (păn″ sī-tō-pē′ nĭ-ă)	pan- cyt/o -penia	all cell lack of	Literally means *lack of the cellular elements of the blood*
phagocytosis (făg″ ō-sī-tō′ sĭs)	phag/o cyt -osis	eat, engulf cell condition	Engulfing and eating of particulate substances such as bacteria, protozoa, cells and cell debris, dust particles, and colloids by phagocytes (leukocytes or macrophages).
plasmapheresis (plăz″ mă-fĕr-ē′ sĭs)	plasm -apheresis	a thing formed, plasma removal	Removal of blood from the body and centrifuging it to separate the plasma from the blood and infusing the cellular elements back into the patient
***Pneumocystis jiroveci* pneumonia (PJP)**			Pneumonia resulting from infection with *Pneumocystis jiroveci*; frequently seen in the immunologically compromised, such as persons with AIDS, steroid-treated individuals, older adults, or premature or debilitated babies during their first 3 months. Patients may be only slightly febrile (or even afebrile), but are likely to be extremely weak, dyspneic, and cyanotic.
polycythemia (pŏl″ ē-sī-thē′ mĭ-ă)	poly- cyt hem -ia	many cell blood condition	Increased number of red blood cells
prothrombin (prō-thrŏm′ bĭn)	pro- thromb -in	before clot chemical	Chemical substance that interacts with calcium salts to produce thrombin
radioimmunoassay (RIA) (rā″ dē-ō-ĭm″ ū-nō-ăs′ā)			Method of determining the concentration of protein-bound hormones in the blood plasma
reticulocyte (rĕ-tĭk′ ū-lō-sīt)	reticul/o -cyte	net cell	Red blood cell containing a network of granules; the last immature stage of a red blood cell
retrovirus (rĕt″ rō-vī′ rŭs)			Virus that contains a unique enzyme called *reverse transcriptase* that allows it to replicate within new host cells. HIV is a retrovirus; once it enters the cell, it can replicate and kill the cells, some lymphocytes directly, and disrupt the functioning of the remaining CD4 cells.

Medical Word	Word Parts		Definition
	Part	Meaning	

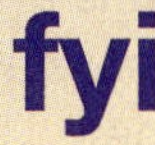

Although the HIV virus can remain inactive in infected cells for years, antibodies are produced to its proteins, a process known as **seroconversion**. These antibodies are usually detectable 6 weeks to 6 months after the initial infection. Helper T or CD4 cells are the primary cells infected by HIV; these cells are involved in cellular immunity and the body's immune response in fighting off infection and disease. The loss of these CD4 cells leads to immunodeficiencies and developing opportunistic infections. A normal CD4 lymphocyte count is 500–1,600 cells/mm^3. It is not uncommon for an HIV-infected person's count to be 180 cells/mm^3.

Medical Word	Part	Meaning	Definition
septicemia (sĕp″ tĭ-sē′ mĭ-ă)	septic -emia	putrefying blood condition	Pathological condition in which bacteria are present in the blood; also known as *sepsis*
seroculture (sē′ rō-kŭl″ chūr)	ser/o -culture	whey, serum cultivation	Bacterial culture of blood
serum (sē′ rŭm)			Blood serum is the clear, thin, and sticky fluid part of the blood that remains after blood clots; any clear watery fluid that has been separated from its more solid elements, such as the exudates from a blister
sideropenia (sĭd″ ĕr-ō-pē′ nĭ-ă)	sider/o -penia	iron lack of	Lack of iron in the blood
splenomegaly (splē″ nō-mĕg′ ă-lē)	splen/o -megaly	spleen enlargement	Abnormal enlargement of the spleen
stem cell			A bone marrow cell that gives rise to different types of blood cells

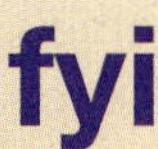

Myelodysplastic syndromes are a group of diseases of the blood and bone marrow in which the bone marrow does not make enough healthy blood cells, thus the blood stem cells do not mature into healthy red blood cells, white blood cells, or platelets. The immature blood cells, called *blasts*, do not function normally and either die in the bone marrow or soon after they enter the blood. This leaves less room for healthy white blood cells, red blood cells, and platelets to form in the bone marrow. When there are fewer blood cells, infection, anemia, or easy bleeding may occur. Myelodysplastic syndromes often do not cause early symptoms and are sometimes found during a routine blood test. Other conditions may cause similar symptoms, such as:

- Shortness of breath
- Weakness or feeling tired
- Having skin that is paler than usual
- Easy bruising or bleeding
- Petechiae (flat, pinpoint spots under the skin caused by bleeding)
- Fever or frequent infections

Medical Word	Word Parts		Definition
	Part	**Meaning**	
thalassemia (thăl-ă-sē´ mĭ-ă)	thalass -emia	sea blood condition	Hereditary anemia occurring in populations bordering the Mediterranean Sea and in Southeast Asia. It is a blood disorder in which the body makes an abnormal form of hemoglobin. The disorder results in large numbers of red blood cells being destroyed, which leads to anemia.

insights In ICD-10-CM, subcategories of thalassemia are coded D56–D56.9 and include:

- Alpha thalassemia
- Beta thalassemia
- Delta-beta thalassemia
- Thalassemia minor
- Hereditary persistence of fetal hemoglobin
- Hemoglobin E-beta thalassemia
- Other thalassemias
- Thalassemia, unspecified

Medical Word	Part	Meaning	Definition
thrombectomy (thrŏm-bĕk´ tō-mē)	thromb -ectomy	clot surgical excision	Surgical excision of a blood clot
thrombin (thrŏm´ bĭn)	thromb -in	clot chemical	Blood enzyme that converts fibrinogen into fibrin
thromboplastin (thrŏm″ bō-plăs´ tĭn)	thromb/o plast -in	clot developing chemical	Essential factor in the production of thrombin and blood clotting
thrombosis (thrŏm-bō´ sĭs)	thromb -osis	clot condition	Formation, development, or existence of a blood clot (thrombus) within the vascular system. In venous thrombosis (thrombophlebitis), a thrombus forms on the wall of a vein, accompanied by inflammation and obstructed blood flow. Thrombi can form in either superficial or deep veins. Deep vein thrombosis (DVT) is generally a complication after hospitalization, surgery, or immobilization. See Figure 10.21.

Medical Word	Word Parts		Definition
	Part	Meaning	

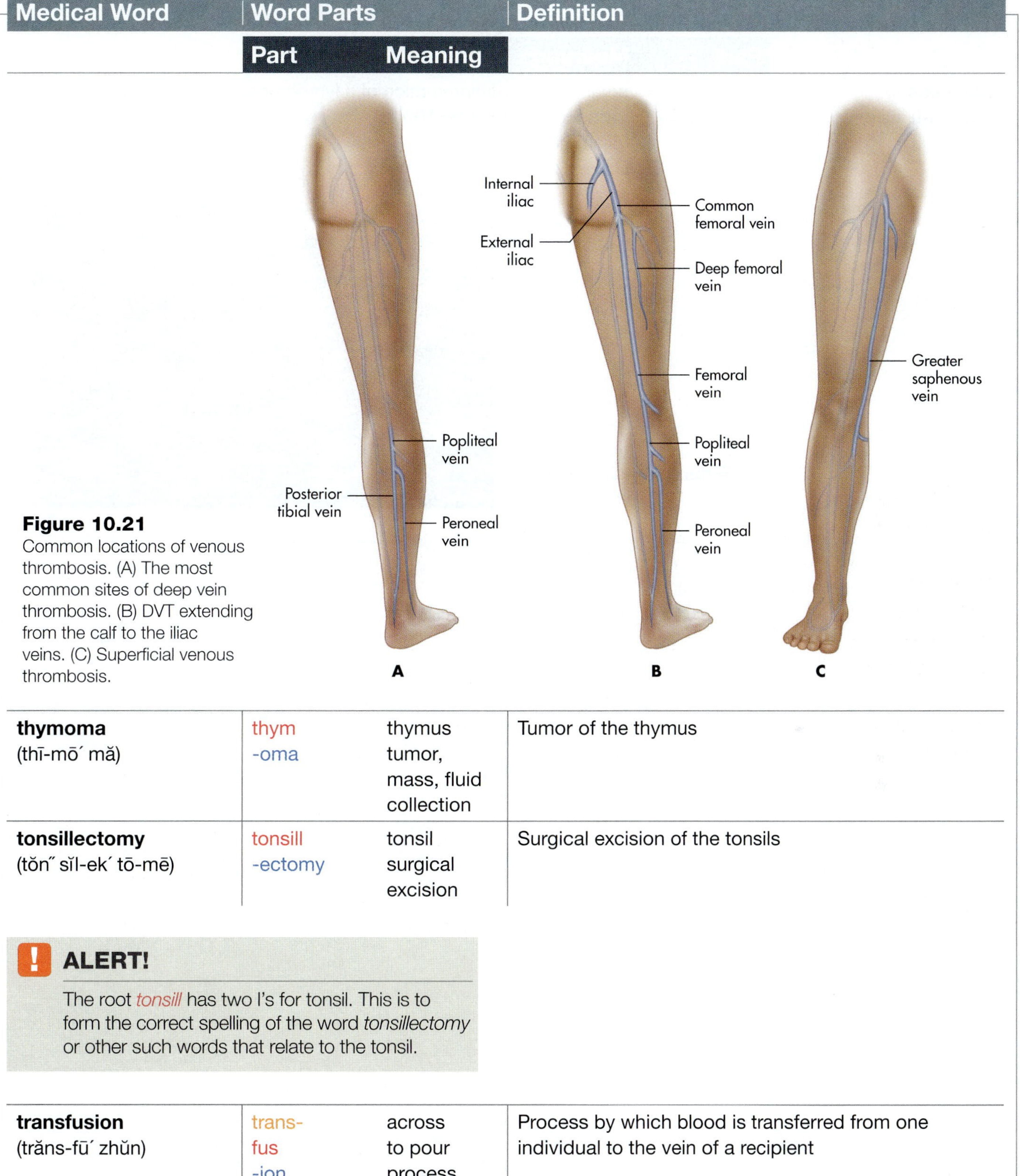

Figure 10.21
Common locations of venous thrombosis. (A) The most common sites of deep vein thrombosis. (B) DVT extending from the calf to the iliac veins. (C) Superficial venous thrombosis.

Medical Word	Part	Meaning	Definition
thymoma (thī-mō´ mă)	thym -oma	thymus tumor, mass, fluid collection	Tumor of the thymus
tonsillectomy (tŏn″ sĭl-ek´ tō-mē)	tonsill -ectomy	tonsil surgical excision	Surgical excision of the tonsils

ALERT!

The root *tonsill* has two l's for tonsil. This is to form the correct spelling of the word *tonsillectomy* or other such words that relate to the tonsil.

Medical Word	Part	Meaning	Definition
transfusion (trăns-fū´ zhŭn)	trans- fus -ion	across to pour process	Process by which blood is transferred from one individual to the vein of a recipient

Medical Word	Word Parts		Definition
	Part	Meaning	
vasculitis (văs″ kū-lī′ tĭs)	vascul -itis	small vessel inflammation	Inflammation of a lymph or blood vessel. See Figure 10.22.

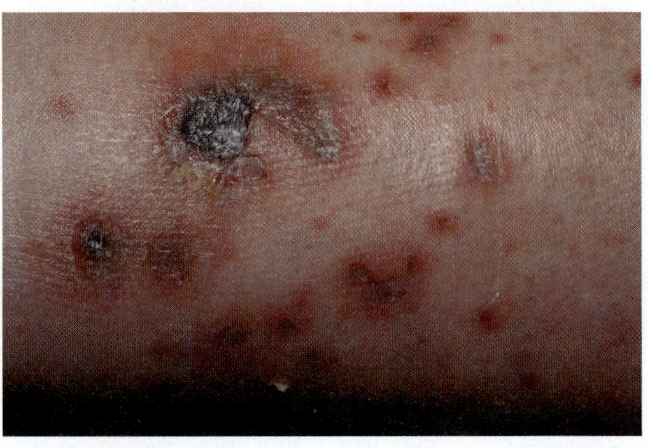

Figure 10.22 Vasculitis.
(Courtesy of Jason L. Smith, MD)

Study and Review II

Word Parts

Prefixes

Give the definitions of the following prefixes.

1. an- ____________________
2. anti- ____________________
3. auto- ____________________
4. ana- ____________________
5. extra- ____________________
6. hyper- ____________________
7. hypo- ____________________
8. mono- ____________________
9. pan- ____________________
10. poly- ____________________
11. pro- ____________________
12. trans- ____________________
13. hyp- ____________________

Combining Forms

Give the definitions of the following combining forms.

1. agglutin/o ____________________
2. angi/o ____________________
3. anis/o ____________________
4. bas/o ____________________
5. chromat/o ____________________
6. coagul/o ____________________
7. cyt/o ____________________
8. eosin/o ____________________
9. erythr/o ____________________
10. glyc/o ____________________
11. hemat/o ____________________
12. hem/o ____________________
13. immun/o ____________________
14. leuk/o ____________________
15. lymph/o ____________________
16. macr/o ____________________
17. neutr/o ____________________
18. plasm/o ____________________
19. septic/o ____________________
20. ser/o ____________________
21. sider/o ____________________
22. splen/o ____________________
23. thym/o ____________________
24. vascul/o ____________________

Suffixes

Give the definitions of the following suffixes.

1. -able ______________________
2. -ant ______________________
3. -apheresis ______________________
4. -blast ______________________
5. -body ______________________
6. -edema ______________________
7. -culture ______________________
8. -cyte ______________________
9. -ectomy ______________________
10. -emia ______________________
11. -ergy ______________________
12. -gen ______________________
13. -phylaxis ______________________
14. -globin ______________________
15. -ic ______________________
16. -in ______________________
17. -ion ______________________
18. -ist ______________________
19. -itis ______________________
20. -logy ______________________
21. -lysis ______________________
22. -megaly ______________________
23. -oma ______________________
24. -osis ______________________
25. -penia ______________________
26. -phil ______________________
27. -poiesis ______________________
28. -rrhage ______________________
29. -stasis ______________________
30. -tomy ______________________
31. -ia ______________________
32. -oxia ______________________

Identifying Medical Terms

In the spaces provided, write the medical terms for the following meanings.

1. ______________________ Process of clumping together, as of blood cells that are incompatible
2. ______________________ An individual hypersensitivity to a substance that is usually harmless
3. ______________________ Protein substance produced in the body in response to an invading foreign substance
4. ______________________ Substance that works against the formation of blood clots
5. ______________________ Invading foreign substance that induces the formation of antibodies
6. ______________________ Process of infusing a patient's own blood
7. ______________________ Capable of forming a clot

8. ______________________ Excess of creatine in the blood

9. ______________________ Blood clot carried in the bloodstream

10. ______________________ Granular leukocyte

11. ______________________ Literally means *one who specializes in the study of the blood*

12. ______________________ Blood protein; the iron-containing pigment of red blood cells

13. ______________________ Pathological condition of excessive amounts of sugar in the blood

14. ______________________ Pathological condition of excessive amounts of lipids (fat) in the blood

15. ______________________ White blood cell

16. ______________________ Control or stopping of the flow of lymph

17. ______________________ Condition of excessive amounts of mononuclear leukocytes in the blood

18. ______________________ Chemical substance that interacts with calcium salts to produce thrombin

19. ______________________ Abnormal enlargement of the spleen

20. ______________________ Clotting cell; blood platelet

Matching

Select the appropriate lettered meaning for each of the following words.

__________ **1.** autotransfusion
__________ **2.** erythrocyte
__________ **3.** erythropoietin
__________ **4.** extravasation
__________ **5.** hemorrhage
__________ **6.** immunoglobulin
__________ **7.** hemochromatosis
__________ **8.** radioimmunoassay
__________ **9.** reticulocyte
__________ **10.** thrombectomy

a. Method of determining the concentration of protein-bound hormones in the blood plasma
b. Genetic disease condition in which iron is not metabolized properly and accumulates in body tissues
c. Blood protein capable of acting as an antibody
d. Mature red blood cell that does not contain a nucleus
e. Hormone that stimulates the production of red blood cells
f. Literally means bursting forth of blood; bleeding
g. Process by which fluids and/or medications escape from the blood vessel into surrounding tissue
h. Process of infusing a patient's own blood
i. Surgical excision of a blood clot
j. Red blood cell containing a network of granules
k. White blood cell

Medical Case Snapshots

This learning activity provides an opportunity to relate the medical terminology you are learning to a precise patient case presentation. In the spaces provided, write in your answers.

Case 1

A 52-year-old female states, "It was months after the death of my husband when I began dating a younger man. We became sexually involved. I am so afraid. Bill has just told me that he is HIV positive and could have AIDS." AIDS is a disease caused by the ______ ____________ virus which invades the ______ lymphocytes.

Case 2

A 15-year-old female complains of being tired, experiencing dizziness, headaches, fast heartbeat, and shortness of breath (_____). A possible diagnosis is anemia. The symptoms of anemia are due to a deficient amount of oxygen in the blood known as ___________. Bloodwork is ordered and the patient is to return in 2 weeks.

Case 3

Two weeks after the initial exam, the 15-year-old female was seen by Dr. Mann. The diagnosis of anemia was confirmed. With anemia special attention is given to the amount of ____________ (or iron-containing pigment of red blood cells) and the percentage of solid components compared to the liquid components of blood called _________. The patient was prescribed an antianemic agent that is used to treat iron-deficiency anemia.

Drug Highlights

Type of Drug	Description and Examples
anticoagulants	Used in inhibiting or preventing a blood clot formation. Hemorrhage can occur at almost any site in patients on anticoagulant therapy. EXAMPLES: heparin sodium, Coumadin (warfarin sodium), and Lovenox (enoxaparin)
hemostatic agents	Used to control bleeding; can be administered systemically or topically. EXAMPLES: Amicar (aminocaproic acid) and vitamin K
antianemic agents (*irons*)	Used to treat iron-deficiency anemia. Oral iron preparations interfere with the absorption of oral tetracycline antibiotics. These products should not be taken within 2 hours of each other. EXAMPLES: Oral iron supplements (ferrous sulfate); prescription IV medications INFeD (iron dextran) and Venofer (iron sucrose)
epoetin alfa (*EPO, Procrit*)	Genetically engineered hemopoietin that stimulates the production of red blood cells. It is a recombinant version of erythropoietin and is indicated for treating anemia in patients with chronic renal failure and HIV-infected patients taking zidovudine.
other agents	Agents used in treating folic-acid deficiency include Folvite (folic acid). Agents used in treating vitamin B_{12}–deficiency include vitamin B_{12} (cyanocobalamin) injection.

Diagnostic and Laboratory Tests

Test	Description
antinuclear antibodies (ANA) (ăn″ tĭ-nū′ klē-ăr ăn′ tĭ-bŏd″ ēs)	Blood test to identify antigen–antibody reactions. ANA antibodies are present in a number of autoimmune diseases (e.g., lupus).
bleeding time	Puncture of the earlobe or forearm to determine the time required for blood to stop flowing. With the Duke method (earlobe), 1–3 minutes is the normal time, and with the Ivy (forearm), 1–9 minutes is the normal time for the flow of blood to cease. Times longer than these can indicate thrombocytopenia, aplastic anemia, leukemia, decreased platelet count, hemophilia, and potential hemorrhage. Anticoagulant drugs delay the bleeding time.
blood typing (ABO groups and Rh factor)	Blood test to determine an individual's blood type (A, B, AB, and O) and Rh factor (can be negative [Rh–] or positive [Rh+]).
bone marrow aspiration (ăs-pĭ-rā′ shŭn)	Removal of bone marrow for examination; can be performed to determine aplastic anemia, leukemia, certain cancers, and polycythemia.

Test	Description
CD4 cell count	Most widely used serum blood test to monitor the progress of AIDS. CD4 count of less than 200/mm^3 confirms AIDS diagnosis. CD4 is a protein on the surface of cells that normally helps the body's immune system fight disease. The HIV attaches itself to the protein to attack white blood cells (WBCs), causing a failure of the patient's defense system.
complete blood count (CBC)	Blood test that includes a hematocrit, hemoglobin, red and white blood cell count, and differential; usually part of a complete physical examination.
enzyme-linked immunosorbent assay (ELISA) (ĕn′ zīm-linkt ĭm″ ū-nō-sŏr′-bĕnt ă-sā)	Most widely used screening test for HIV. The latest generation of ELISA tests is 99.5% sensitive to HIV. Occasionally, the ELISA test will be positive for a patient without symptoms of AIDS from a low-risk group. Because this result is likely to be a false positive, the ELISA must be repeated *on the same sample of the patient's blood*. If the second ELISA is positive, the result should be confirmed by the Western blot test.
erythrocyte sedimentation rate (ESR, sed rate) (ĕ-rĭth′ rō-sīt sĕd″ ĭ-mĕn-tā′ shŭn)	Blood test to determine the rate at which red blood cells settle in a long, narrow tube. The distance the RBCs settle in 1 hour is the rate. Higher or lower rate can indicate certain disease conditions.
hematocrit (Hct, HCT) (hē-măt′ ō-krĭt)	Blood test performed on whole blood to determine the percentage of red blood cells in the total blood volume. The percentage varies with age and gender: men range 40–54%; women 37–47%; children 35–49%; newborns 49–54%.
hemoglobin (Hb, Hgb, HGB) (hē″ mō-glō′ bĭn)	Blood test to determine the amount of iron-containing pigment of the red blood cells.
immunoglobulins (Ig) (ĭm″ ū-nō-glŏb′ ū-lĭns)	Serum blood test to determine the presence of IgA, IgD, IgE, IgG, and/or IgM. Lymphocytes and plasma cells produce immunoglobulins in response to antigen exposure. Increased and/or decreased values can indicate certain disease conditions.
partial thromboplastin time (PTT) (păr′ shāl thrŏm″ bō-plăs′ tĭn)	Test performed on blood plasma to determine how long it takes for fibrin clots to form; used to regulate heparin dosage and to detect clotting disorders.
platelet count (plāt′ lĕt)	Test performed on whole blood to determine the number of thrombocytes present. Increased and/or decreased amounts can indicate certain disease conditions.
prothrombin time (PT) (prō-thrŏm′ bĭn)	Test performed on blood plasma to determine the time needed for oxalated plasma to clot; used to regulate anticoagulant drug therapy and to detect clotting disorders.
red blood count (RBC)	Test performed on whole blood to determine the number of erythrocytes present. Increased and/or decreased amounts can indicate certain disease conditions.

Test	Description
viral load	Blood test that measures the amount of HIV in the blood. Results can range from 50 to more than 1 million copies per milliliter (mL) of blood. Two tests that are used to measure viral load are bDNA and PCR.
Western blot test or immunoblot test (ĭm″ ū-nō-blŏt)	Used as a reference procedure to confirm the diagnosis of AIDS. In Western blot testing, HIV antigen is purified by electrophoresis (large protein molecules are suspended in a gel and separated from one another by running an electric current through the gel). If antibodies to HIV are present, a detectable antigen–antibody response occurs and a positive result is noted.
white blood count (WBC)	Blood test to determine the number of leukocytes present. Increased level indicates infection and/or inflammation and leukemia. Decreased level indicates aplastic anemia, pernicious anemia, and malaria.

Abbreviations

Abbreviation	Meaning
ABO	blood groups
AIDS	acquired immunodeficiency syndrome
ALL	acute lymphocytic leukemia
ANA	antinuclear antibodies
CBC	complete blood count
CLL	chronic lymphocytic leukemia
diff	differential count
DVT	deep vein thrombosis
ELISA	enzyme-linked immunosorbent assay
eos, eosin	eosinophil
ESR, sed rate	erythrocyte sedimentation rate
HAART	highly active antiretroviral therapy
Hb, Hgb, HGB	hemoglobin
Hct, HCT	hematocrit
HIV	human immunodeficiency virus
Ig	immunoglobulin
IV	intravenous
KS	Kaposi sarcoma
lymphs	lymphocytes
MALT	mucosa-associated lymphoid tissue
mL, ml	milliliter
NK	natural killer (cells)
PJP	*Pneumocystis jiroveci* pneumonia
PrEP	pre-exposure prophylaxis
PT	prothrombin time
PTT	partial thromboplastin time
RBC	red blood cell (count)
Rh	Rhesus (factor)
RIA	radioimmunoassay
SOB	shortness of breath
WBC	white blood cell (count)

Study and Review III

Building Medical Terms

Using the following word parts, fill in the blanks to build the correct medical terms.

mono-	sider/o	-culture
erythr/o	thromb	-megaly
hem/o	-in	
lymph	-cyte	

Definition	Medical Term
1. Formation of red blood cells	_______poiesis
2. Plasma protein found in body fluids and cells	globul_______
3. Destruction of red blood cells	_________lysis
4. Red blood cell containing a network of granules	reticulo_______
5. Lymphoid neoplasm, usually malignant	_________oma
6. Red blood cell	_________cyte
7. Bacterial culture of blood	sero________
8. Lack of iron in the blood	________penia
9. Abnormal enlargement of the spleen	spleno_______
10. Formation of a blood clot within the vascular system	_________osis

Combining Form Challenge

Using the combining forms provided, write the medical term correctly.

hem/o	erythr/o	leuk/o
coagul/o	hemat/o	lymph/o

1. Destruction of red blood cells _______ lysis

2. Capable of forming a clot: ______able

3. Immature red blood cell that is found only in bone marrow: ______blast

4. Literally means *study of the blood*: __________ logy

5. Disease of the blood characterized by overproduction of leukocytes: _____ emia

6. Abnormal accumulation of lymph in the interstitial spaces: _______edema

Select the Right Term

Select the correct answer, and write it on the line provided.

1. An individual hypersensitivity to a substance that is usually harmless is _______.

   anaphylaxis **anemia** **AIDS** **allergy**

2. Protein substance produced in the body in response to an invading foreign substance is ___________.

   antigen **antibody** **albumin** **fibrinogen**

3. Hereditary blood disease characterized by prolonged coagulation and tendency to bleed is _______________.

   hemophilia **hemolysis** **hemorrhage** **hemochromatosis**

4. Hereditary anemia occurring in populations bordering the Mediterranean Sea and in Southeast Asia is _______________.

   hemolytic **pernicious** **thalassemia** **sickle cell**

5. Blood clot carried in the bloodstream is _____________.

   thrombus **coagulable** **extravasation** **embolus**

6. Essential factor in the production of thrombin and blood clotting is __________.

   thrombin **thromboplastin** **thrombocyte** **prothrombin**

Diagnostic and Laboratory Tests

Select the best answer to each multiple-choice question. Circle the letter of your choice.

1. Blood test to identify antigen–antibody reactions.
   - **a.** erythrocyte sedimentation rate
   - **b.** hematocrit
   - **c.** immunoglobulins
   - **d.** antinuclear antibodies

2. Blood test that includes a hematocrit, hemoglobin, red and white blood cell count, and differential.
   - **a.** blood typing
   - **b.** sedimentation rate
   - **c.** CBC
   - **d.** Hb, Hgb

3. Blood test performed on whole blood to determine the percentage of red blood cells in the total blood volume.
   - **a.** RBC
   - **b.** WBC
   - **c.** Hct
   - **d.** PTT

4. Blood test to determine the number of leukocytes present.
   - **a.** RBC
   - **b.** WBC
   - **c.** Hct
   - **d.** PTT

5. Puncture of the earlobe or forearm to determine the time required for blood to stop flowing.
   - **a.** bleeding time
   - **b.** platelet count
   - **c.** prothrombin time
   - **d.** PTT

Abbreviations

Place the correct word, phrase, or abbreviation in the space provided.

1. acquired immunodeficiency syndrome ______
2. acute lymphocytic leukemia ______
3. CML ______
4. hemoglobin ______
5. Hct ______
6. human immunodeficiency virus ______
7. PJP ______
8. PT ______
9. RBC ______
10. radioimmunoassay ______

Practical Application

Medical Record Analysis

This exercise contains information, abbreviations, and medical terminology from an actual medical record or case study that has been adapted for this text. The names and any personal information have been created by the author. Read and study each form or case study and then answer the questions that follow. You may refer to Appendix III, *Abbreviations and Symbols*.

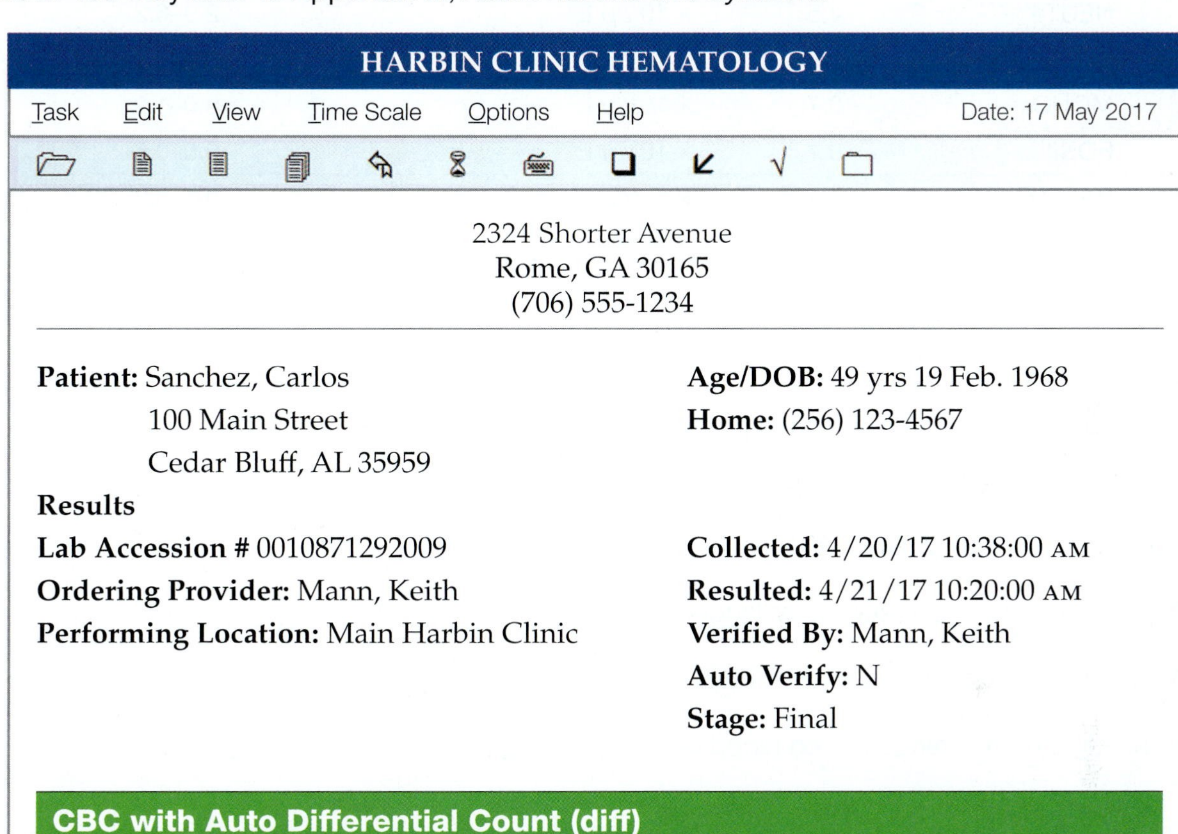

HARBIN CLINIC HEMATOLOGY

Task Edit View Time Scale Options Help Date: 17 May 2017

2324 Shorter Avenue
Rome, GA 30165
(706) 555-1234

Patient: Sanchez, Carlos
100 Main Street
Cedar Bluff, AL 35959

Age/DOB: 49 yrs 19 Feb. 1968
Home: (256) 123-4567

Results

Lab Accession # 0010871292009
Ordering Provider: Mann, Keith
Performing Location: Main Harbin Clinic

Collected: 4/20/17 10:38:00 AM
Resulted: 4/21/17 10:20:00 AM
Verified By: Mann, Keith
Auto Verify: N
Stage: Final

CBC with Auto Differential Count (diff)

Test	Result	Units	Flag	Reference Range
WBC	7.9	$\times 10^3/\mu L$		4.8–10.8
RBC	4.44	$\times 10^3/\mu L$	L	4.6–6.13
HGB	14.4	g/dL		14.1–18.1
HCT	41.9	%	L	43.5–53.7
MCV	94.0	fL		80.0–99.0
MCH	35.4	Pg	H	26.0–34.0
MCHC	34.3	g/dL		33.0–37.0
RDW	12.6	%		11.6–14.8
PLATELETS	248	$\times 10^3/\mu L$		130–400
MPV	8.8	fL		7.4–10.4
NEUT%	56.3	%		37.0–80.0

Test	Result	Units	Flag	Reference Range
LYMPH%	32.4	%		10.0–50.0
MONO%	8.2	%		0.1–10.0
EOS%	1.6	%		0.1–6.0
BASO%	1.5	%		0.0–3.0
NEUT#	4.5	$\times 10^3/\mu L$		2.9–6.2
LYMPH#	2.6	$\times 10^3/\mu L$		0.8–3.9
MONO#	0.7	$\times 10^3/\mu L$		0.0–1.2
EOS#	0.1	$\times 10^3/\mu L$		0.0–0.6
BASO#	0.1	$\times 10^3/\mu L$		0.1–0.3

Medical Record Questions

Place the correct answer in the space provided.

1. What does the abbreviation *CBC* mean? ________________________________
2. What does the abbreviation *diff* mean? ________________________________
3. Which one of the test results was flagged high? ________________________________
4. What is the normal range for white blood cells? ________________________________
5. What is the normal range for red blood cells? ________________________________

Chapter 11

Respiratory System

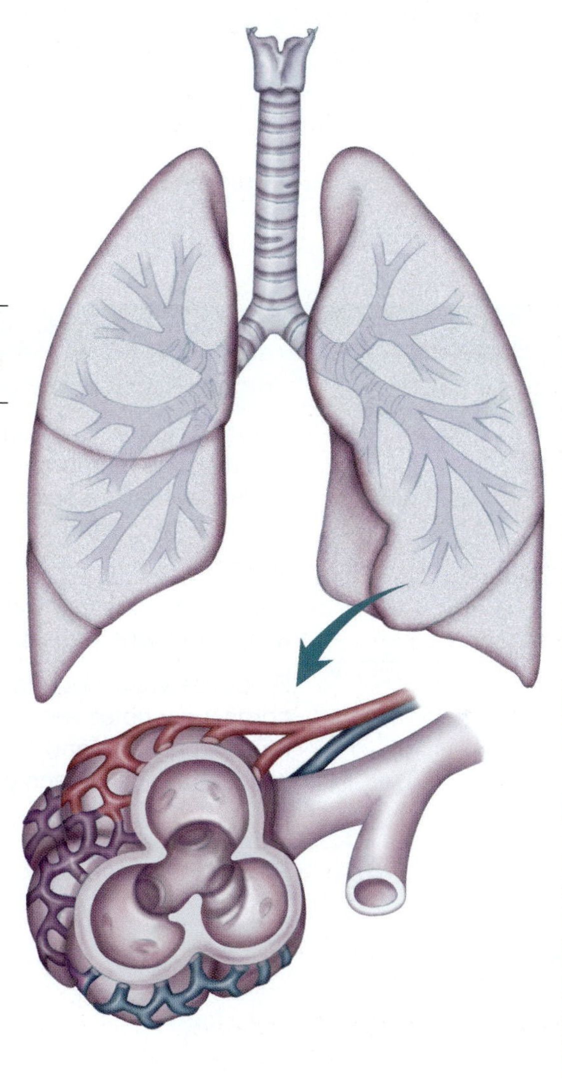

Learning Outcomes

On completion of this chapter, you will be able to:

1. Describe respiration.
2. State the description and primary functions of the organs/structures of the respiratory system.
3. Define terms that physiologists and respiratory specialists use to describe the volume of air exchanged in breathing.
4. Recognize terminology included in the ICD-10-CM.
5. Analyze, build, spell, and pronounce medical words.
6. Comprehend the drugs highlighted in this chapter.
7. Describe diagnostic and laboratory tests related to the respiratory system.
8. Identify and define selected abbreviations.
9. Apply your acquired knowledge of medical terms by successfully completing the *Practical Application* exercise.

Anatomy and Physiology

The respiratory system consists of the nose, pharynx, larynx, trachea, bronchi, and lungs. Its primary function is to *supply* oxygen (O_2) for individual tissue cells to use and to *take away* their gaseous waste product, carbon dioxide (CO_2). See Figure 11.1. This process is accomplished through the act of **respiration (R)**, which consists of external and internal processes. **External respiration** is the process by which the lungs are ventilated and oxygen and carbon dioxide are *exchanged* between the air in the lungs and the blood within capillaries of the alveoli. **Internal respiration** is the process by which oxygen and carbon dioxide are exchanged between the blood in tissue capillaries and the cells of the body. Table 11.1 provides an at-a-glance look at the respiratory system.

Table 11.1 Respiratory System at-a-Glance

Organ(s)/Structure(s)	Primary Functions/Description
Nose	Serves as an air passageway; warms and moistens inhaled air; its cilia and mucous membrane trap dust, pollen, bacteria, and other foreign matter; contains special smell receptor cells (nerve cells), which assist in distinguishing various smells; contributes to phonation and the quality of voice
Pharynx	Serves as a passageway for air and for food; contributes to phonation as a chamber where the sound is able to resonate
Larynx	Produces vocal sounds. High notes are formed by short, tense vocal cords. Low notes are produced by long, relaxed vocal cords. The nose, mouth, pharynx, and bony sinuses aid in phonation and the tone that is produced to give each person a distinctive sound.
Trachea	Provides an open passageway for air to and from the lungs
Bronchi	Provide a passageway for air to and from the lungs

ALERT!

Did you know that *bronchi* is the plural form of bronchus?

Organ(s)/Structure(s)	Primary Functions/Description
Lungs	Bring air into contact with blood so that oxygen and carbon dioxide can be exchanged in the *alveoli*

ALERT!

Did you know that *alveoli* is the plural form of alveolus?

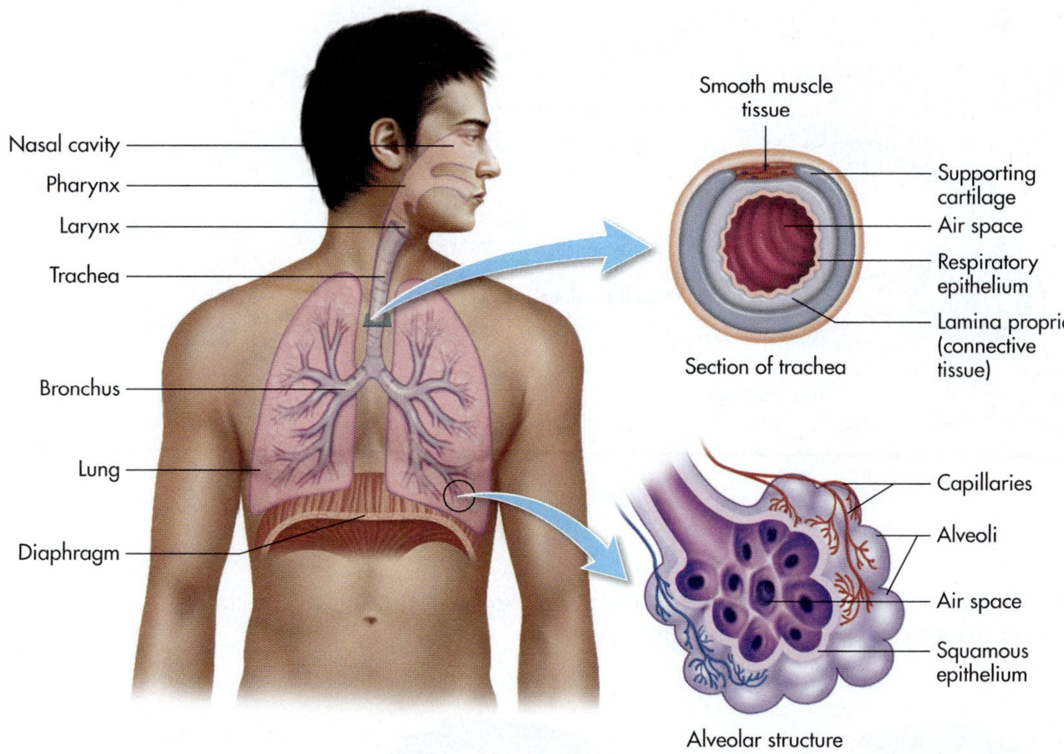

Figure 11.1 The respiratory system: nasal cavity, pharynx, larynx, trachea, bronchus, and lung with expanded views of the trachea and alveolar structure.

Nose

The **nose** consists of an external and internal portion. The *external portion* is a triangle of cartilage and bone that is covered with skin and lined with mucous membrane. The external entrance of the nose is known as the **nostrils** or **anterior nares**. The *internal portion* of the nose is divided into two chambers by a partition, the **septum**, separating it into a right and a left cavity. These cavities are divided into three air passages: the *superior*, *middle*, and *inferior conchae*. These passages lead to the pharynx and are connected with the paranasal sinuses by openings, with the ears by the eustachian tube, and with the region of the eyes by the nasolacrimal ducts. See Figure 11.2.

The nose is lined with mucous membrane and plays an important role in the sense of smell. Smell receptor cells are located in the upper part of the nasal cavity. These cells are special nerve cells that have **cilia** (hairlike processes). The cilia of each cell are sensitive to different chemicals and, when stimulated, create a nerve impulse that is sent to the nerve cells of the olfactory bulb, which lies inside the skull just above the nose. The olfactory nerves carry the nerve impulse from the olfactory bulb directly to the brain, where it is perceived as a smell.

The nasal mucosa produces about 946 mL or 1 qt of mucus per day. Four pairs of paranasal sinuses drain into the nose. These are the *frontal*, *maxillary*, *ethmoidal*, and *sphenoidal* sinuses. See Figure 11.3. The *palatine bones* and *maxillae* separate the nasal cavities from the mouth cavity.

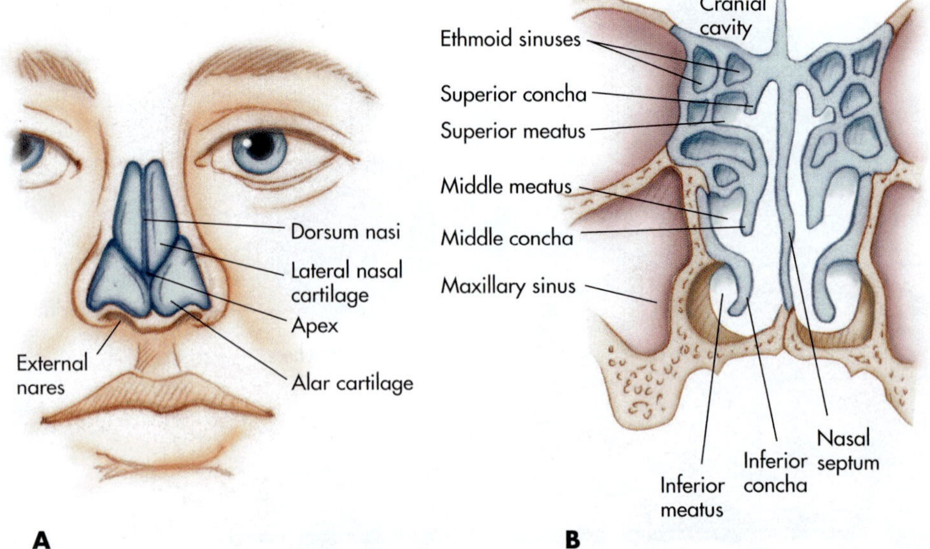

Figure 11.2 Nose and nasal cavity: (A) nasal cartilages and external structure; (B) meatus and positions of the entrance to the ethmoid and maxillary sinuses.

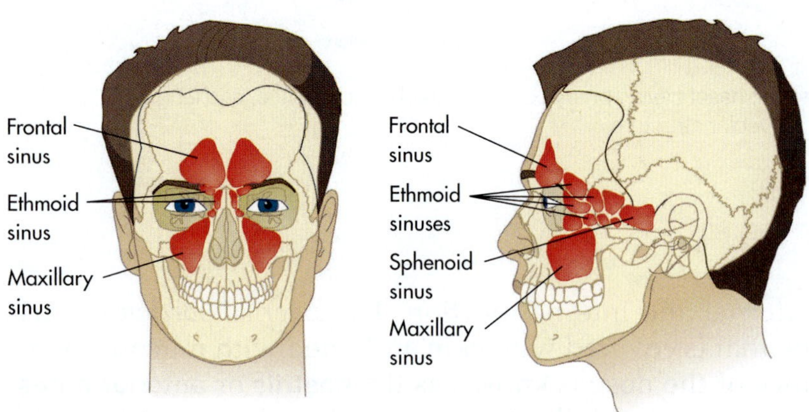

Figure 11.3 Paranasal sinuses.

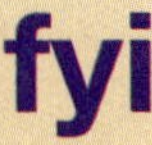

Cleft palate is a condition in which the two plates of the skull that form the hard palate (roof of the mouth) are not completely joined. In most cases, cleft lip, often called harelip, is also present. Cleft palate or lip occurs in about one in 700 infants born in the United States and can range from a small notch in the lip to a groove that runs into the roof of the mouth and nose. This can affect the way the child's face looks. It can also lead to problems with eating, talking, and ear infections. Treatment is usually surgery to close the lip (*cheiloplasty*) and palate (*palatoplasty*). Doctors often do this surgery in several stages. Usually the first surgery is during the baby's first year. With treatment, most children with cleft lip or palate do well.

Pharynx

The **pharynx** is a musculomembranous tube about 5 inches long that extends from the base of the skull, lies anterior to the cervical vertebrae, and becomes continuous with the esophagus. It is divided into three portions: the *nasopharynx* located behind the nose, the *oropharynx* located behind the mouth, and the *laryngopharynx* located behind

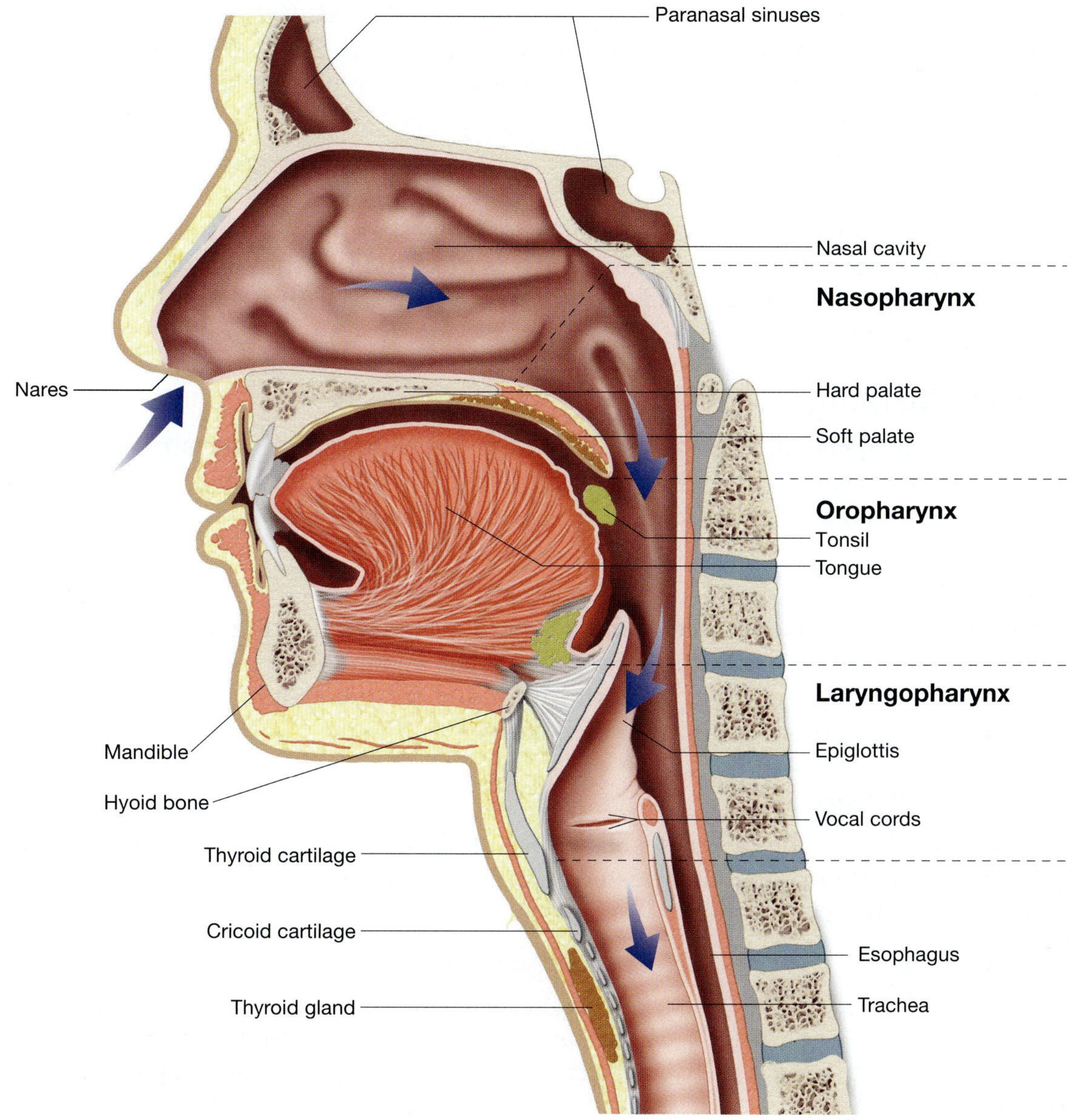

Figure 11.4 Sagittal section of the nasal cavity and pharynx.

the larynx. Seven openings are found in the pharynx: two openings from the eustachian tubes, two openings from the posterior nares into the nasopharynx, the fauces or opening from the mouth into the oropharynx, and the openings from the larynx and the esophagus into the laryngopharynx. See Figure 11.4. Associated with the pharynx are three pairs of lymphoid tissues, which are the **tonsils**. The nasopharynx contains the *adenoids* or *pharyngeal* tonsils. The oropharynx contains the *faucial* or *palatine* tonsils and the *lingual* tonsils. The tonsils are accessory organs of the lymphatic system and aid in filtering bacteria and other foreign substances from the circulating lymph in the head and neck region.

Larynx

The **larynx** or *voice box* is a structure made of muscle and cartilage and lined with mucous membrane. It is the enlarged upper end of the trachea below the root of the tongue and hyoid bone. See Figure 11.1.

The cavity of the larynx contains a pair of *ventricular folds* (false vocal cords) and a pair of vocal folds or true vocal cords. The cavity is divided into three regions: vestibule, ventricle, and entrance to the glottis. The **glottis** is a narrow slit at the opening between the true vocal folds.

Cartilages of the Larynx

The larynx is composed of nine cartilages bound together by muscles and ligaments. The three unpaired cartilages, each of which is described in the following sections, are the *thyroid*, *epiglottis*, and *cricoid*, and the three paired cartilages are the *arytenoid*, *cuneiform*, and *corniculate*.

Thyroid Cartilage

The **thyroid cartilage** is the largest cartilage in the larynx and forms the structure commonly called the *Adam's apple*. This structure is usually larger and more prominent in men than in women and contributes to the deeper male voice.

Epiglottis

The **epiglottis** covers the entrance of the larynx. During swallowing, it acts as a lid to prevent aspiration of food or liquid into the trachea. When the epiglottis fails to cover the entrance to the larynx, food or liquid intended for the esophagus can enter the trachea, causing irritation, coughing, or choking.

Cricoid Cartilage

The **cricoid cartilage** is the lowermost cartilage of the larynx. It is shaped like a signet ring with the broad portion being posterior and the anterior portion forming the arch and resembling the ring's band.

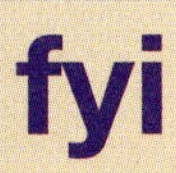

In the older adult, atrophy of the pharynx and larynx muscle can occur, causing a slackening of the vocal cords and a loss of elasticity of the laryngeal muscles and cartilages. These changes can cause a "gravelly," softer voice with a rise in pitch, making communication more difficult, especially if there is impaired hearing.

Trachea

The **trachea** or *windpipe* is a semi-cylindrical cartilaginous tube that is the air passageway extending from the pharynx and larynx to the bronchi. It is about 1 inch wide and 4½ inches (11.4 cm) long. It is composed of smooth muscle that is reinforced at the front and sides by C-shaped rings of cartilage. The mucous membrane lining the trachea contains cilia, which sweep foreign matter out of the passageway. The trachea provides an open passageway for air to and from the lungs. See Figure 11.1.

Bronchi

The **bronchi** are the two main branches of the trachea, which provide the passageway for air to the lungs. The trachea divides into the **right bronchus** and the **left bronchus**. The right bronchus is larger and extends down in a more vertical direction than the left bronchus. When a foreign body is inhaled or aspirated, it more frequently lodges in the right bronchus or enters the right lung. Each bronchus enters the lung at a depression, the **hilum**. The bronchi then subdivide into the bronchial tree composed of smaller bronchi, bronchioles, and alveolar ducts. The bronchial tree terminates in the *alveoli*, which are tiny air sacs supporting a network of capillaries from pulmonary blood vessels. The function of the bronchi is to provide an open passageway for air to and from the lungs. See Figure 11.1.

Lungs

The two **lungs** are conical-shaped spongy organs of respiration. They lie on both sides of the heart within the pleural cavity of the thorax. They occupy a large portion of the thoracic cavity and are enclosed in the **pleura**, a serous membrane composed of several layers. The pleural cavity is a space between the parietal and visceral pleura and contains a serous fluid that lubricates and prevents friction caused by the rubbing together of the two layers. The thoracic cavity is separated from the abdominal cavity by a musculomembranous wall, the **diaphragm**. The central portion of the thoracic cavity, between the lungs, is a space called the **mediastinum**, containing the heart and other structures.

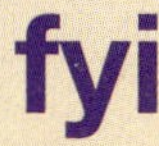

With advancing age, the respiratory system is vulnerable to injuries caused by infections, environmental pollutants, and allergic reactions. The number of cilia declines as one grows older. At the same time, the number of mucus-producing cells may increase, resulting in mucus clogging the airways.

Total lung capacity is relatively constant across the lifespan but vital capacity (volume of air that can be exhaled after a maximal inspiration) decreases because the residual volume increases (amount of air remaining in the lungs after maximal expiration).

The lungs consist of elastic tissue filled with interlacing networks of tubes and sacs that carry air and with blood vessels carrying blood. The broad inferior surface of the lung is the **base**, which rests on the diaphragm, while the **apex**, or pointed upper margin, rises from 2.5 to 5.0 cm above the sternal end of the first rib. The lungs are divided into **lobes**, with the right lung having three lobes and the left lung having two lobes. The left lung is slightly smaller than the right lung and has an indentation, the **cardiac depression**, which allows room for the normal placement of the heart. In an average adult male, the right lung weighs approximately 445 g (1 lb) and the left about 395 g. In an average adult male, the total lung capacity (TLC) is 3.6–9.4 L, whereas in an average adult female it is 2.5–6.9 L. A **lobule** is a primary subdivision of a lobe. In the lungs, it is a physiological unit of the lung consisting of a respiratory bronchiole and its branches (alveolar ducts, alveolar sacs, and alveoli). The lungs contain around 300 million **alveoli**, which are the air cells where the exchange of oxygen and carbon dioxide takes place. The main function of the lungs is to bring air into contact with blood so that oxygen and carbon dioxide can be exchanged in the alveoli. See Figure 11.5.

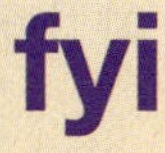

At 12 weeks' gestation, the lungs of the fetus have a definite shape. At 20 weeks, the cellular structure of the alveoli is complete; the fetus is able to suck its thumb and swallow amniotic fluid. At 24 weeks, the nostrils open and respiratory movements occur. At 26–32 weeks, **surfactant** (a substance formed in the lung that regulates the amount of surface tension of the fluid lining the alveoli) is produced. In preterm infants, the lack of surfactant contributes to *neonatal respiratory distress syndrome (NRDS)*, previously called hyaline membrane disease (HMD). It is also called infant respiratory distress syndrome (IRDS) or respiratory distress syndrome (RDS) of the newborn.

During fetal life, gaseous exchange occurs at the placental interface. The lungs do not function until birth.

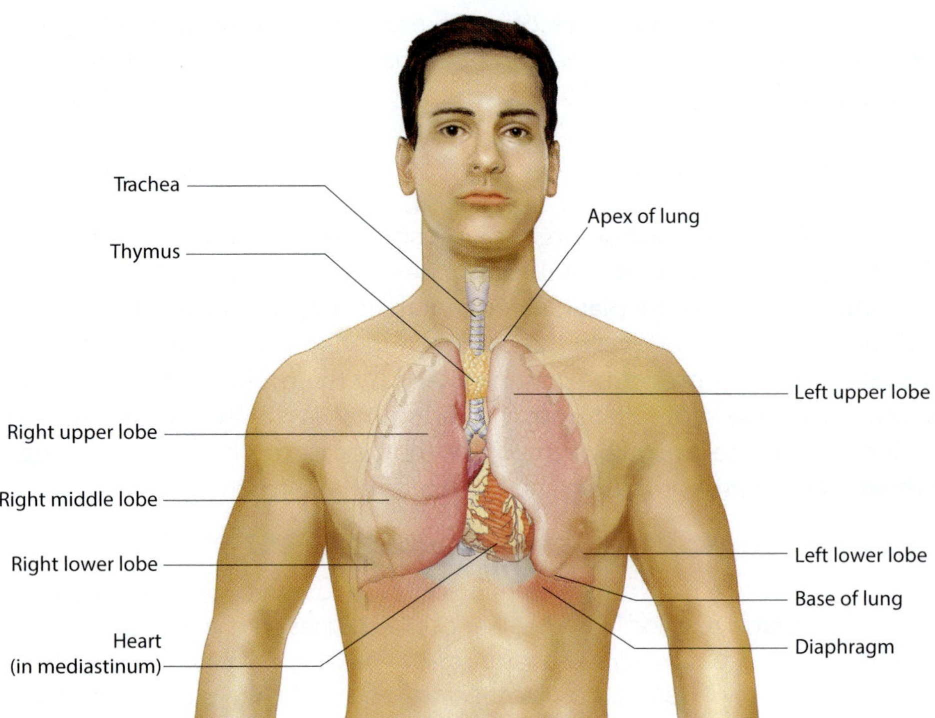

Figure 11.5 Position of the lungs and other thoracic organs.

Respiration

Volume

The following terms are used by physiologists and respiratory specialists to describe the volume of air exchanged in breathing:

Tidal volume (TV). Amount of air in a single inspiration and expiration. In the average adult male, about 500 mL of air enters the respiratory tract during normal quiet breathing.

Expiratory reserve volume (ERV). Amount of air that can be forcibly expired after a normal quiet respiration. This is also called the *supplemental air* and measures approximately 1000–1200 mL.

Inspiratory reserve volume (IRV). Amount of air that can be forcibly inspired over and above a normal inspiration and measures approximately 3000 mL.

Residual volume (RV). Amount of air remaining in the lungs after maximal expiration, about 1500 mL.

Vital capacity (VC). Volume of air that can be exhaled after a maximal inspiration.

Functional residual capacity (FRC). Volume of air that remains in the lungs at the end of a normal expiration.

Total lung capacity (TLC). Maximal volume of air in the lungs after a maximal inspiration.

Vital Function of Respiration

Temperature, pulse, respiration, and **blood pressure** are the vital signs that are essential elements for determining an individual's state of health. A deviation from normal of one or all of the vital signs denotes a state of illness. Evaluation of an individual's response to changes occurring within the body can be measured by taking the vital signs. Through careful analysis of these changes in the vital signs, a physician can determine a diagnosis, a prognosis, and a plan of treatment for the patient. The variations of certain vital signs signify a typical disease process and its stages of development. For example, in a patient who has pneumonia (inflammation of the lungs caused by bacteria, viruses, fungi, or chemical irritants), the temperature can be elevated to 101°F–106°F, and pulse and respiration can increase to almost twice their normal rates. When the temperature falls, the patient will perspire profusely and the pulse and respiration will begin to return to normal rates.

The *medulla oblongata* and the *pons*, two of the structures of the brainstem, regulate and control respiration. The rate, rhythm, and depth of respiration are controlled by nerve impulses from the medulla oblongata and the pons via the spinal cord. See Figure 11.6.

Respiratory Rate

Individuals of different ages breathe at different respiratory rates. The **respiratory rate** is regulated by the respiratory center located in the medulla oblongata. The following are normal resting respiratory rates for some different age groups:

Newborn	30–60 per minute
1–3 years	20–30 per minute
11–14 years	12–20 per minute
Adult	16–20 per minute

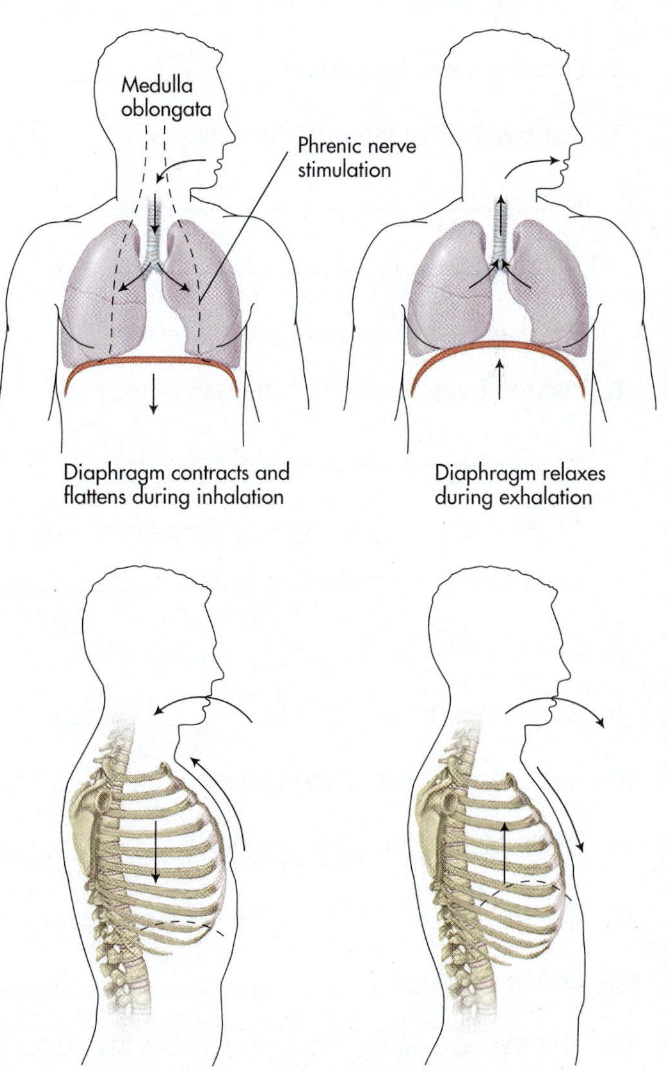
Medulla
oblongata
Phrenic nerve
stimulation
Diaphragm contracts and
flattens during inhalation
Diaphragm relaxes
during exhalation
During inhalation the diaphragm
presses the abdominal organs
forward and downward
During exhalation the diaphragm
rises and recoils to the resting
position

Figure 11.6 The process of respiration.

Study and Review I

Anatomy and Physiology

Write your answers to the following questions.

1. List the organs of the respiratory system.

   a. ______________________ b. ______________________

   c. ______________________ d. ______________________

   e. ______________________ f. ______________________

2. State the primary function of the respiratory system.

   ____

   ____

3. Define external respiration ____

4. Define internal respiration ____

5. List the five functions of the nose.

   a. ______________________ b. ______________________

   c. ______________________ d. ______________________

   e. ______________________

6. List the three functions of the pharynx.

   a. ______________________ b. ______________________

   c. ______________________

7. State the function of the epiglottis ____

8. Define glottis ____

9. State the function of the larynx ____

10. State the function of the trachea ____

11. State the function of the bronchi ____

12. Give a brief description of the lungs ____

13. Define pleura ____

14. The thoracic cavity is separated from the abdominal cavity by a musculomembranous wall commonly known as the ____

15. The central portion of the thoracic cavity between the lungs is a space called the ____________________

16. The right lung has ______________________ lobes and the left lung has ______________________ lobes.

17. The air cells of the lungs are the ____

18. State the main function of the lungs ____

19. The vital signs, which are essential elements for determining an individual's state of health, are ______________________, ______________________, ______________________, and

____

20. Define the following terms:

a. Tidal volume ____

b. Residual volume ____

c. Vital capacity ____

21. The __________________ __________________ and the __________________ of the central nervous system regulate and control respiration.

22. The normal resting respiratory rate for a newborn is ________________ to ________________breaths per minute.

23. The normal resting respiratory rate for an adult is __________________________ to

__________________________ breaths per minute.

ANATOMY LABELING

Identify the structures shown below by filling in the blanks.

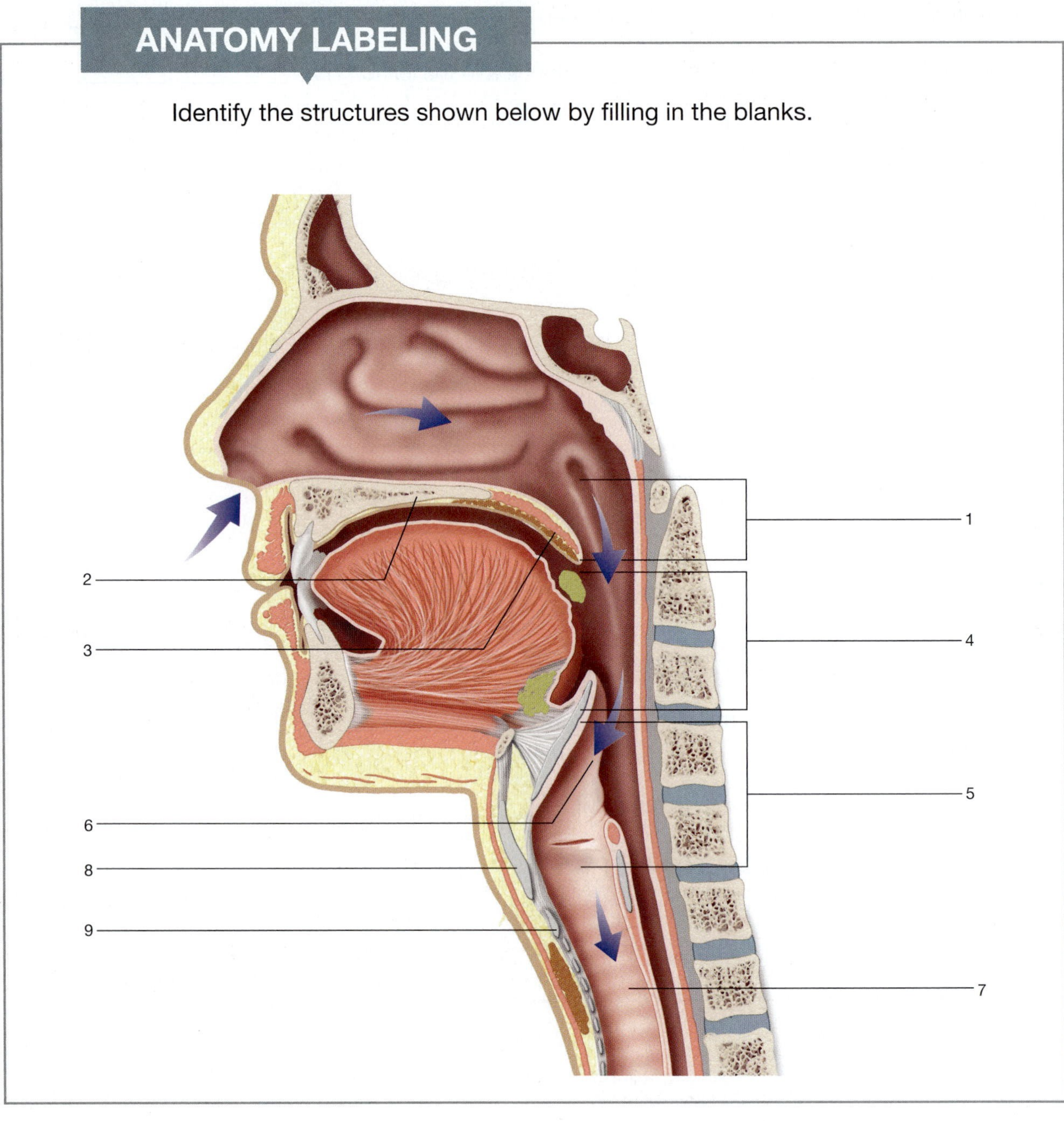

Building Your Medical Vocabulary

This section provides the foundation for learning medical terminology. Review the following alphabetized word list. Note how common prefixes and suffixes are repeatedly applied to word roots and combining forms to create different meanings. The word parts are color-coded: prefixes are yellow, suffixes are blue, roots/combining forms are red. A combining form is a word root plus a vowel. The chart below lists the combining forms for the word roots in this chapter and can help to strengthen your understanding of how medical words are built and spelled.

Remember These Guidelines

1. If the suffix begins with a vowel, drop the combining vowel from the combining form and add the suffix. For example, tubercul/o (*a little swelling*) + -osis (*condition*) becomes tuberculosis.
2. If the suffix begins with a consonant, keep the combining vowel and add the suffix to the combining form. For example, hem/o (*blood*) + -ptysis (*to spit*) becomes hemoptysis.

You will find that some terms have not been divided into word parts. These are common words or specialized terms that are included to enhance your medical vocabulary.

Combining Forms of the Respiratory System			
alveol/o	small, hollow air sac	**ox/o**	oxygen
anthrac/o	coal	**palat/o**	palate
aspirat/o	to draw in	**pector/o**	chest
atel/o	imperfect	**pharyng/o**	pharynx, throat
bronch/o	bronchus	**pleur/o**	pleura
bronchiol/o	bronchiole	**pneum/o**	air
cheil/o	lip	**pneumon/o**	lung
coni/o	dust	**pulmon/o**	lung
cyan/o	dark blue	**py/o**	pus
cyst/o	sac	**respirat/o**	breathing
fibr/o	fiber	**rhin/o**	nose
halat/o	breathe	**rhonch/o**	snore
hem/o	blood	**sarc/o**	flesh
laryng/o	larynx, voice box	**spir/o**	breathe
lob/o	lobe	**theli/o**	nipple
mes/o	middle	**thorac/o**	chest
nas/o	nose	**tonsill/o**	tonsil, almond
olfact/o	smell	**trache/o**	trachea
or/o	mouth	**tubercul/o**	a little swelling
orth/o	straight	**ventilat/o**	to air

Medical Word	Word Parts		Definition
	Part	**Meaning**	
alveolus (ăl-vē´ ō-lŭs)	alveol -us	small, hollow air sac pertaining to	Pertaining to a small air sac in the lungs
anthracosis (ăn″ thră-kō´ sĭs)	anthrac -osis	coal condition	Lung condition caused by inhalation of coal dust and silica; also called *black lung*
apnea (ăp´ nē-ă)	a- -pnea	lack of breathing	Temporary cessation of breathing. **Sleep apnea** is a temporary cessation of breathing during sleep. To be so classified, the apnea must last for at least 10 seconds and occur 30 or more times during a 7-hour period of sleep. Sleep apnea is classified according to the mechanisms involved. **Obstructive apnea** is caused by obstruction to the upper airway. **Central apnea** is marked by absence of respiratory muscle activity.
asphyxia (ăs-fĭk´ sĭ-ă)	a- sphyx -ia	lack of pulse condition	Emergency condition in which there is a depletion of oxygen in the blood with an increase of carbon dioxide in the blood and tissues; symptoms include dyspnea, cyanosis, tachycardia, impairment of senses, and, in extreme cases, convulsions, unconsciousness, and death. Some of the more common causes include drowning, electrical shock, aspiration of vomitus, lodging of a foreign body in the respiratory tract, inhalation of toxic gas or smoke, and poisoning. Artificial ventilation and oxygen should be administered as quickly as possible.
aspiration (ăs″ pĭ-rā´ shŭn)	aspirat -ion	to draw in process	The act of drawing in or out by suction using a device such as a syringe or needle; the process of drawing foreign bodies—such as food, liquid, or other substances—into the nose, throat, or lungs on inspiration

Medical Word	Word Parts		Definition
	Part	Meaning	
asthma (ăz´ mă)			Disease of the bronchi characterized by wheezing, dyspnea, and a feeling of constriction in the chest. See Figure 11.7. Inflammation of the airways causes airflow into and out of the lungs to be restricted. During an asthma attack, the muscles of the bronchial tree constrict and the linings of the air passages swell, reducing airflow and producing the characteristic wheezing sound. See Figure 11.8.

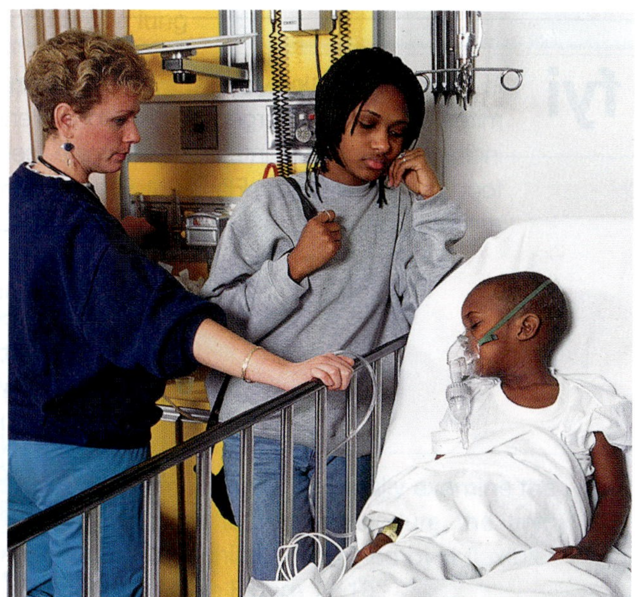

Figure 11.7 Acute exacerbations of asthma can require management in the emergency department. The child is placed in a sitting position to facilitate respiratory effort.

Source: Pearson Education, Inc.

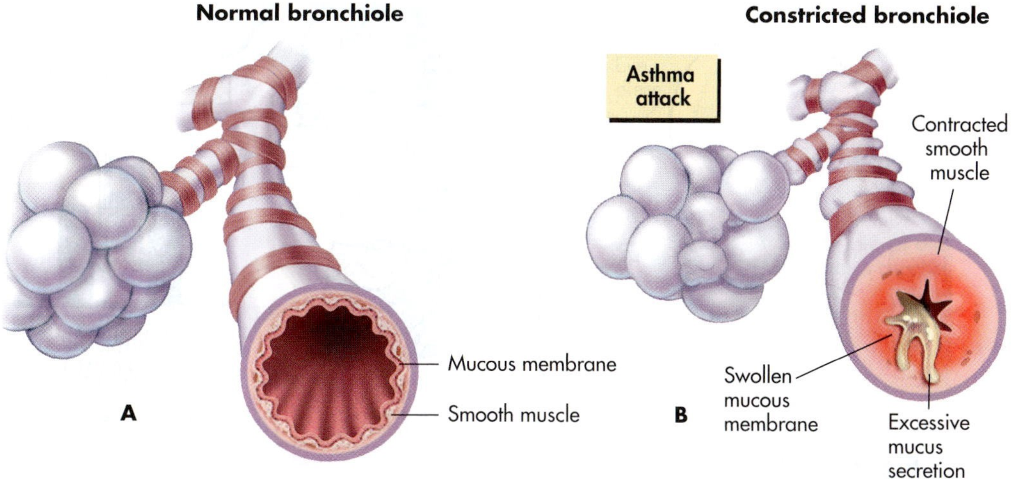

Figure 11.8 Changes in bronchioles during an asthma attack: (A) normal bronchiole and (B) in asthma attack.

Medical Word	Word Parts		Definition
	Part	**Meaning**	

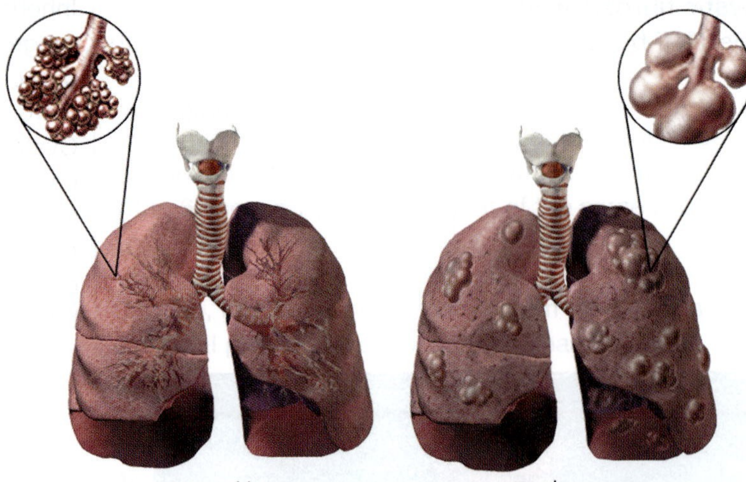

Figure 11.13 Normal lung and one with emphysema.

insights In ICD-10-CM, emphysema includes *panlobular emphysema* (J43.1) and *centrilobular emphysema* (J43.2). Panlobular (pan- [*all*]) emphysema affects all parts of the lobules (alveolar ducts, alveolar sacs, and alveoli). In centrilobular (centri [*center*]) emphysema, destruction begins at the center of the lobule and is associated with cigarette smoking.

Medical Word	Part	Meaning	Definition
empyema (ĕm″ pī-ē′ mă)			Pus in a body cavity, especially the pleural cavity
endotracheal (ET) (ĕn″ dō-trā′ kē-ăl)	endo- trache -al	within trachea pertaining to	Within the trachea. An endotracheal tube is used in general anesthesia, intensive care, and emergency medicine for airway management, mechanical ventilation, and as an alternative route for the administration of medicines when an intravenous (IV) infusion line cannot be established.
epistaxis (ĕp″ ĭ-stăk′ sĭs)	epi- -staxis	upon dripping	Nosebleed; usually results from traumatic or spontaneous rupture of blood vessels in the mucous membranes of the nose
eupnea (ūp-nē′ ă)	eu- -pnea	good, normal breathing	Good or normal breathing
exhalation (ĕks″ hə-lā′ shŭn)	ex- halat -ion	out breathe process	Process of breathing out
expectoration (ĕk-spĕk″ tə rā′ shŭn)	ex- pector(at) -ion	out chest process	Process of coughing up and spitting out material (sputum) from the lungs, bronchi, and trachea

Medical Word	Word Parts		Definition
	Part	**Meaning**	
Heimlich maneuver (hīm´ lĭk mă-nōō´ văr)			Technique for forcing a foreign body (usually a bolus of food) out of the trachea. See Figure 11.14.

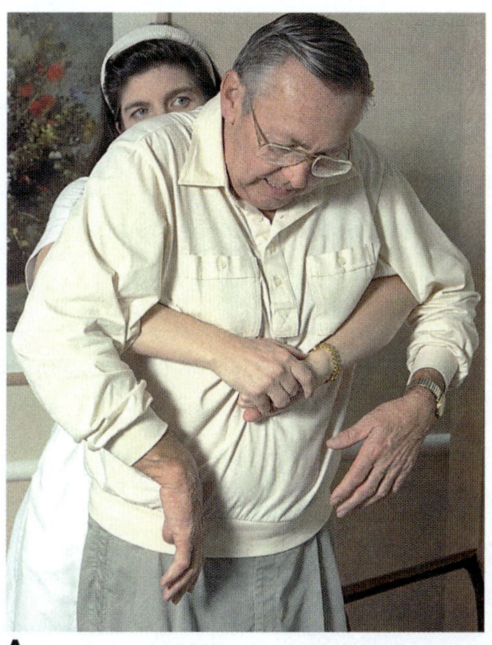

A

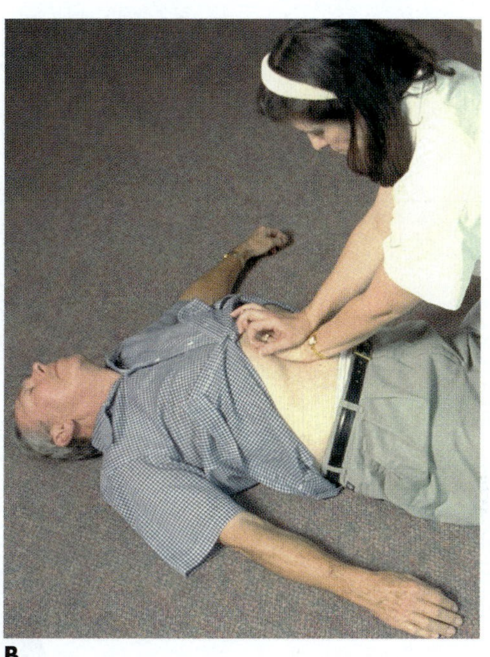

B

Figure 11.14 Administration of abdominal thrusts (the Heimlich maneuver) to (A) a conscious victim and (B) an unconscious victim.

Source: Pearson Education, Inc.

Medical Word	Part	Meaning	Definition
hemoptysis (hē-mŏp´ tĭ-sĭs)	hem/o -ptysis	blood to spit	Spitting up blood

RULE REMINDER

This term keeps the combining vowel ***o*** because the suffix begins with a consonant.

Medical Word	Part	Meaning	Definition
hyperpnea (hī˝ pĕrp-nē´ ă)	hyper- -pnea	excessive breathing	Abnormally deep and rapid breathing
hyperventilation (hī˝ pĕr-vĕn˝ tĭ-lā´ shŭn)	hyper- ventilat -ion	excessive to air process	Process of excessive ventilating, thereby increasing the air in the lungs beyond the normal limit
hypoxia (hī-pŏks´ ĭ-ă)	hyp- ox -ia	below, deficient oxygen condition	Condition of deficient amounts of oxygen in body tissues

Medical Word	Word Parts		Definition
	Part	**Meaning**	
influenza (ĭn″ floo-ĕn′ ză)			Acute, contagious respiratory infection caused by a virus. Onset is usually sudden, and symptoms are fever, chills, headache, myalgia, cough, and sore throat.
inhalation (ĭn″ hă-lā′ shŭn)	in- halat -ion	in breathe process	Process of breathing in
laryngeal (lăr-ĭn′ jĭ-ăl)	laryng -eal	larynx, voice box pertaining to	Pertaining to the larynx (voice box)
laryngitis (lăr″ ĭn-jī′ tĭs)	laryng -itis	larynx, voice box inflammation	Inflammation of the larynx (voice box). See Figure 11.15.

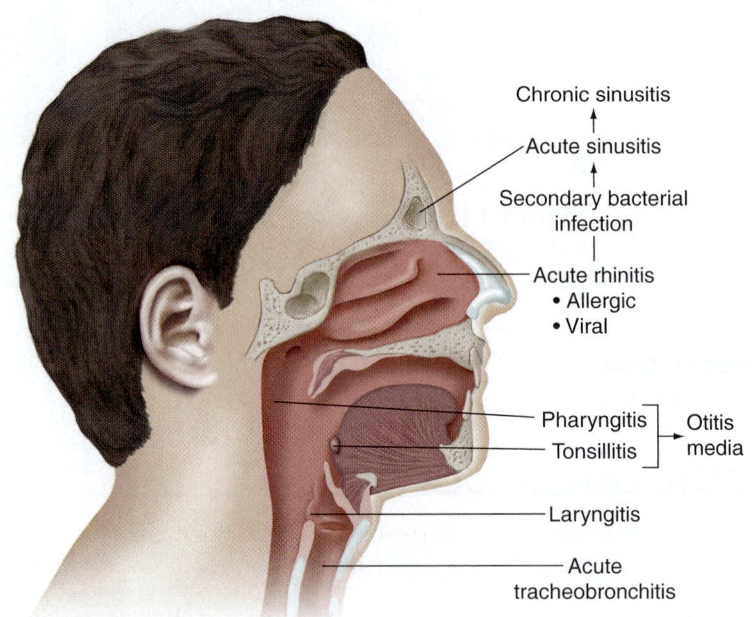

Figure 11.15 Paranasal sinuses are part of the upper respiratory system. From here, infections can spread via the nasopharynx to the middle ear or bronchi. Note locations of laryngitis, pharyngitis, sinusitis, and tonsillitis.

Medical Word	Part	Meaning	Definition
laryngoscope (lăr-ĭn′ gō-skōp)	laryng/o -scope	larynx, voice box instrument for examining	Medical instrument used to visually examine the larynx (voice box). The procedure using a laryngoscope is known as *laryngoscopy*.
Legionnaires disease (lē jə naerz′)			Severe pulmonary pneumonia caused by *Legionella pneumophila*
lobectomy (lō-bĕk′ tō-mē)	lob -ectomy	lobe surgical excision	Surgical excision of a lobe of any organ or gland, such as the lung

Medical Word	Word Parts: Part	Word Parts: Meaning	Definition
mesothelioma (mĕs″ ō-thē″ lĭ-ō′ mă)	mes/o theli -oma	middle nipple tumor	Malignant tumor of mesothelium (serous membrane of the pleura) caused by the inhalation of asbestos
nasopharyngitis (nā″ zō-făr′ ĭn-jī″ tĭs)	nas/o pharyng -itis	nose pharynx, throat inflammation	Inflammation of the nose and pharynx (throat)
olfaction (ŏl-făk′ shŭn)	olfact -ion	smell process	Process of smelling
oropharynx (or″ ō-făr′ ĭnks)	or/o pharynx	mouth pharynx, throat	Central portion of the throat that lies between the soft palate and upper portion of the epiglottis
orthopnea (or″ thŏp′ nē-ă)	orth/o -pnea	straight breathing	Inability to breathe unless in an upright or straight position
palatopharyngoplasty (păl″ ăt-ō-făr″ ĭn′ gō-plăs″ tē)	palat/o pharyng/o -plasty	palate pharynx, throat surgical repair	Type of surgery that relieves snoring and sleep apnea by removing the uvula and the tonsils and reshaping the lining at the back of the throat to enlarge the air passageway
pertussis (pĕr-tŭs′ ĭs)			Acute, infectious disease caused by the bacterium *Bordetella pertussis*; characterized by a peculiar paroxysmal cough ending in a "crowing" or "whooping" sound; also called *whooping cough*
pharyngitis (făr″ ĭn-jī″ tĭs)	pharyng -itis	pharynx, throat inflammation	Inflammation of the pharynx (throat). See Figure 11.15.
pleurisy (ploo′ rĭs-ē)			Inflammation of the pleura caused by injury, infection, or a tumor. The inflamed pleural layers rub against each other every time the lungs expand to breathe in air. This can cause sharp pain with breathing (also called pleuritic chest pain).
pleuritis (ploo-rī″ tĭs)	pleur -itis	pleura inflammation	Inflammation of the pleura
pleurodynia (ploo″ rō-dĭn′ ĭ-ă)	pleur/o -dynia	pleura pain	Pain in the pleura

Medical Word	Word Parts		Definition
	Part	**Meaning**	
pneumoconiosis (nū″ mō-kō″ nĭ-ō′ sĭs)	pneum/o coni -osis	air dust condition	Abnormal condition of the lung caused by the inhalation of dust particles such as coal dust (*anthracosis*), stone dust (*chalicosis*), iron dust (*siderosis*), asbestos (*asbestosis*), and quartz (*silica*) dust (*silicosis*)
pneumonectomy (nū″ mō-nĕk′ tō-mē)	pneumon -ectomy	lung surgical excision	Surgical excision of the left or right lung
pneumonia (nū-mō′ nĭ-ă)	pneumon -ia	lung, air condition	Inflammation of the lung caused by bacteria, viruses, fungi, or chemical irritants. See Figure 11.16.

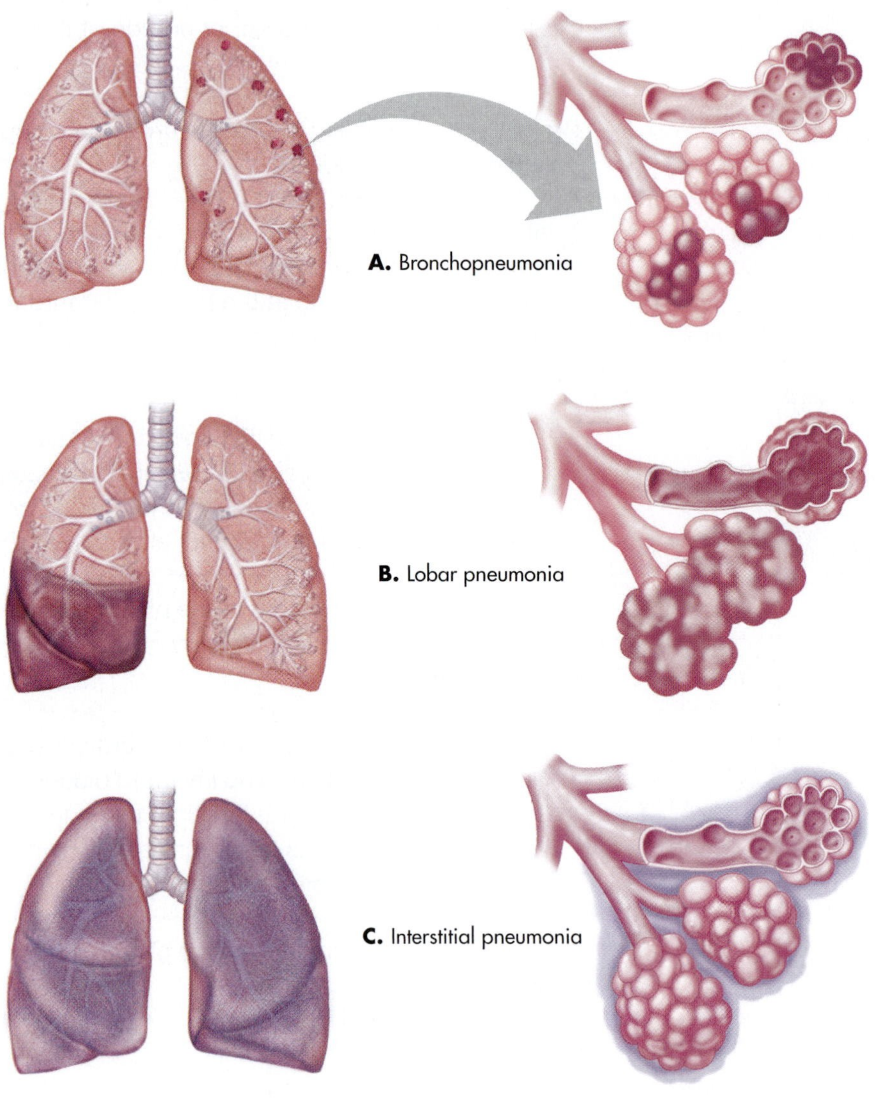

Figure 11.16 (A) Bronchopneumonia with localized pattern. (B) Lobar pneumonia with a diffuse pattern within the lung lobe. (C) Interstitial pneumonia is typically diffuse and bilateral.

(*continued*)

Medical Word	Word Parts: Part	Word Parts: Meaning	Definition

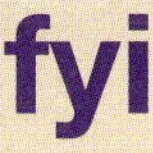

fyi Pneumonia affects 5–10 million people each year in the United States. Symptoms include a cough with greenish mucus or puslike sputum, chills, fever, fatigue, chest pain, and muscle aches. Initial diagnosis is made through auscultation of the chest with a stethoscope. In patients with pneumonia, rales and other abnormal breathing sounds can be heard. Tests that are used to confirm the diagnosis include a chest x-ray and a sputum culture.

Medical Word	Part	Meaning	Definition
pneumonitis (nū″ mō-nī′ tĭs)	pneumon -itis	lung inflammation	Inflammation of the lung
pneumothorax (nū″ mō-thō′ răks)	pneum/o thorax	air chest	A pathological condition in which there is a collection of air between the chest wall and lungs, causing the lung to collapse. It may occur spontaneously or after physical trauma to the chest or as a complication of medical treatment. See Figure 11.17.

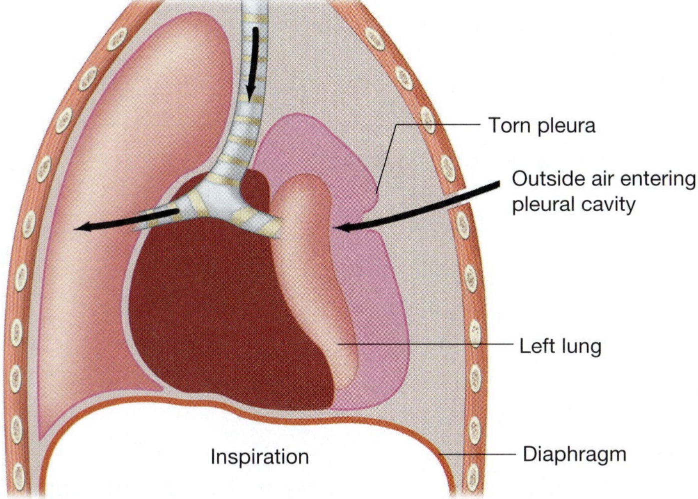

Figure 11.17 Pneumothorax (sucking chest wound).

Medical Word	Part	Meaning	Definition
pulmonologist (pŭl-mō-nŏl′ ō-jĭst)	pulmon/o log -ist	lung study of one who specializes	Physician who specializes in the diagnosis and treatment of pulmonary diseases
pulmonology (pŭl-mō-nŏl′ ō-jē)	pulmon/o -logy	lung study of	The study of pulmonary diseases
pyothorax (pī″ ō-thō′ răks)	py/o thorax	pus chest	Pus in the chest cavity
rale (rāl)			Abnormal sound heard on auscultation of the chest; a crackling, rattling, or bubbling sound

Medical Word	Word Parts		Definition
	Part	**Meaning**	
respirator (rĕs´ pĭ-rā˝ tor)	respirat -or	breathing a doer	Medical device used to assist in breathing; type of machine used for prolonged artificial respiration
respiratory distress syndrome (RDS) (rĕs´ pĭ-ră-tō˝ rē)			Condition that can occur in a premature infant in which the lungs are not matured to the point of manufacturing lecithin, a pulmonary surfactant, resulting in collapse of the alveoli, which leads to cyanosis and hypoxia; previously called *hyaline membrane disease (HMD)*
respiratory syncytial virus (RSV) infection (sĭn-sĭ´ shăl)			Most common cause of bronchiolitis and pneumonia among infants and children under 1 year of age. Illness begins with fever, runny nose, cough, and sometimes wheezing. Most children recover from illness in 8–15 days. It is contagious and spreads through the respiratory secretions of infected persons or contact with contaminated surfaces or objects.
rhinoplasty (rī˝ nō-plăs˝ tē)	rhin/o -plasty	nose surgical repair	Surgical repair of the nose
rhinorrhea (rī˝ nō-rē´ ă)	rhin/o -rrhea	nose flow, discharge	Discharge from the nose

RULE REMINDER

This term keeps the combining vowel ***o*** because the suffix begins with a consonant.

Medical Word	Part	Meaning	Definition
rhinovirus (rī˝ nō-vī˝ rŭs)	rhin/o vir -us	nose virus pertaining to	One of a subgroup of viruses that causes the common cold (*coryza*) in humans
rhonchus (rŏng´ kŭs)	rhonch -us	snore pertaining to	Rale or rattling sound in the throat or bronchial tubes caused by a partial obstruction
sarcoidosis (sar˝ koyd-ō´ sĭs)	sarc -oid -osis	flesh resemble condition	Chronic granulomatous condition that can involve almost any organ system of the body, usually the lungs, causing dyspnea on exertion
severe acute respiratory syndrome (SARS)			Contagious viral respiratory infection that was first described in 2003; serious form of pneumonia resulting in acute respiratory distress and sometimes death
sinusitis (sī˝ nŭs-ī˝ tĭs)	sinus -itis	a curve, hollow inflammation	Inflammation of a sinus. See Figure 11.15.

Medical Word	Word Parts: Part	Word Parts: Meaning	Definition
spirometer (spī-rŏm′ ĕt-ĕr)	spir/o -meter	breathe instrument to measure	Medical instrument used to measure lung volume during inspiration and expiration; in incentive spirometry, a portable spirometer may be used by a patient for deep breathing exercises. See Figure 11.18.
	Figure 11.18 A portable spirometer used by a patient for deep breathing exercises. Source: Pearson Education, Inc.		
sputum (spū′ tŭm)			Substance coughed up from the lungs; can be watery, thick, purulent, clear, or bloody and can contain microorganisms
stridor (strī′ dōr)			High-pitched sound caused by partial obstruction of the air passageway
tachypnea (tăk″ ĭp-nē′ ă)	tachy- -pnea	rapid breathing	Rapid breathing
thoracentesis (thō″ ră-sĕn-tē′ sĭs)	thora -centesis	chest surgical puncture	Surgical puncture of the chest wall for removal of fluid; also called *thoracocentesis*. Can be used in pleurisy to remove excess fluid that has accumulated in the chest cavity. See Figure 11.19.

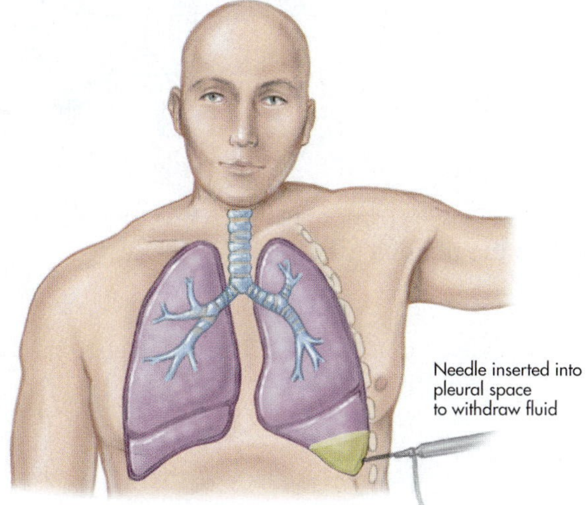

Figure 11.19 Thoracentesis (also called thoracocentesis).

Medical Word	Word Parts		Definition
	Part	**Meaning**	
thoracoplasty (thō´ ră-kō-plăs˝ tē)	thorac/o -plasty	chest surgical repair	Surgical repair of the chest wall
thoracotomy (thō˝ răk-ŏt´ ō-mē)	thorac/o -tomy	chest incision	Incision into the chest wall
tonsillitis (tŏn˝ sĭl-ī´ tĭs)	tonsill -itis	almond, tonsil inflammation	Inflammation of the tonsils. See Figure 11.15.
tracheal (trā´ kē-ăl)	trache -al	trachea, windpipe pertaining to	Pertaining to the trachea (windpipe)
tracheostomy (trā˝ kē-ŏs´ tō-mē)	trache/o -stomy	trachea, windpipe new opening	New opening into the trachea (windpipe). See Figure 11.20.

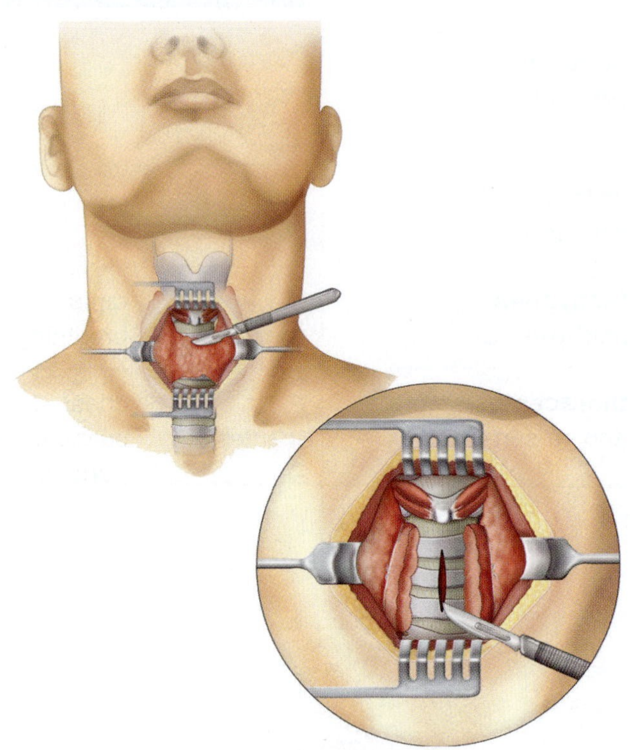

Figure 11.20 Tracheostomy. The surgical creation of a new opening into the trachea.

Medical Word	Part	Meaning	Definition
tracheotomy (trā˝ kē-ŏt´ ō-mē)	trache/o -tomy	trachea, windpipe incision	Incision into the trachea (windpipe)

Medical Word	Word Parts: Part	Word Parts: Meaning	Definition
tuberculosis (TB) (tū-bĕr″ kū-lō′ sĭs)	tubercul -osis	a little swelling condition	Infectious disease caused by the tubercle bacillus, *Mycobacterium tuberculosis*. TB can be diagnosed with a positive sputum culture indicating *Mycobacterium tuberculosis* and a chest x-ray (CXR) revealing lesions in the lung.

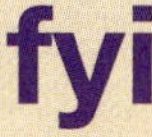

The development of drug-resistant strains of bacteria is one of the most alarming trends in healthcare. The problem is particularly serious with regard to TB bacteria that have developed strains resistant to treatment with one of each of the major tuberculosis medications. Even more dangerous are strains that are resistant to at least two anti-TB drugs, leading to a condition called **multidrug-resistant tuberculosis (MDR TB)**. Although MDR TB can be treated successfully, it is much more difficult to combat than regular tuberculosis and requires long-term therapy—up to 2 years—with drugs that can cause serious side effects.

Medical Word	Word Parts: Part	Word Parts: Meaning	Definition
wheeze (hwēz)			A high-pitched whistling sound caused by constriction of the air passageway associated with an asthma attack or airway obstruction

Study and Review II

Word Parts

Prefixes

Give the definitions of the following prefixes.

1. a- _______________
2. epi- _______________
3. dys- _______________
4. endo- _______________
5. eu- _______________
6. ex- _______________
7. hyp- _______________
8. hyper- _______________
9. in- _______________
10. tachy- _______________

Combining Forms

Give the definitions of the following combining forms.

1. alveol/o _______________
2. anthrac/o _______________
3. atel/o _______________
4. bronch/o _______________
5. coni/o _______________
6. halat/o _______________
7. laryng/o _______________
8. nas/o _______________
9. olfact/o _______________
10. or/o _______________
11. orth/o _______________
12. pector/o _______________
13. pharyng/o _______________
14. pleur/o _______________
15. pneum/o _______________
16. py/o _______________
17. rhin/o _______________
18. rhonch/o _______________
19. spir/o _______________
20. thorac/o _______________
21. tonsill/o _______________
22. trache/o _______________
23. tubercul/o _______________

Suffixes

Give the definitions of the following suffixes.

1. -al ______________________
2. -algia ______________________
3. -centesis ______________________
4. -dynia ______________________
5. -ectasis ______________________
6. -ectomy ______________________
7. -ic ______________________
8. -ia ______________________
9. -ion ______________________
10. -itis ______________________
11. -meter ______________________
12. -osis ______________________
13. -oma ______________________
14. -staxis ______________________
15. -plasty ______________________
16. -or ______________________
17. -pnea ______________________
18. -ptysis ______________________
19. -rrhea ______________________
20. -scope ______________________
21. -stomy ______________________
22. -tomy ______________________
23. -us ______________________

Identifying Medical Terms

In the spaces provided, write the medical terms for the following meanings.

1. ______________________ Pertaining to a small air sac in the lungs
2. ______________________ Chronic dilation of a bronchus or bronchi
3. ______________________ Inflammation of the bronchi
4. ______________________ Condition of difficulty in speaking
5. ______________________ Good or normal breathing
6. ______________________ Spitting up blood
7. ______________________ Process of breathing in
8. ______________________ Inflammation of the larynx
9. ______________________ A collection of air between the chest wall and lungs
10. ______________________ Surgical repair of the nose
11. ______________________ Discharge from the nose
12. ______________________ Inflammation of a sinus

Matching

Select the appropriate lettered meaning for each of the following words.

__________ 1. cough

__________ 2. cystic fibrosis

__________ 3. influenza

__________ 4. inhalation

__________ 5. olfaction

__________ 6. pleurodynia

__________ 7. rhinovirus

__________ 8. sputum

__________ 9. tachypnea

__________ 10. thoracentesis

a. Substance coughed up from the lungs

b. Pain in the pleura

c. Process of smelling

d. One of a subgroup of viruses that causes the common cold in humans

e. Rapid breathing

f. Process of breathing in

g. Surgical puncture of the chest wall for removal of fluid

h. Sudden, forceful expulsion of air from the lungs

i. Inherited disease that affects the pancreas, respiratory system, and sweat glands

j. Slow breathing

k. Acute, contagious respiratory infection caused by a virus

Medical Case Snapshots

This learning activity provides an opportunity to relate the medical terminology you are learning to a precise patient case presentation. In the spaces provided, write in your answers.

Case 1

A 7-year-old male is seen in the emergency room with wheezing, dyspnea, and a feeling of constriction in the chest. He is experiencing an acute exacerbation of ______________. The ER personnel find that he has an inability to breathe unless he is upright. This condition is called ______________ and he is placed in a sitting position. See Figure 11.7.

Case 2

A 58-year-old male presents with ______________ (difficulty in breathing), _________ ___ _________ (abbreviated SOB), fatigue, and wheezing. A smoker for 40 years, he has had bronchitis several times during the past 5 years. With the use of a ______________ (instrument for measuring lung volume), it was determined that he had emphysema or COPD, an abbreviation for ______________ ______________ _______________ ____________.

Case 3

A 28-year-old male returns to the clinic for a follow-up visit after being diagnosed with _____________ (an infectious disease caused by the tubercle bacillus). The lab performs a ___________ culture (to determine the presence of pathogenic microorganisms).

Drug Highlights

Type of Drug	Description and Examples
antihistamines	Act to counter the effects of histamine by blocking histamine 1 (H_1) receptors. They are used to treat allergy symptoms, prevent or control motion sickness, and in combination with cold remedies to decrease mucus secretion and produce bedtime sedation. See Figure 11.21. EXAMPLES: Benadryl (diphenhydramine hcl), Dimetane (brompheniramine maleate), Allegra (fexofenadine), Claritin (loratadine), and Zyrtec (cetirizine)

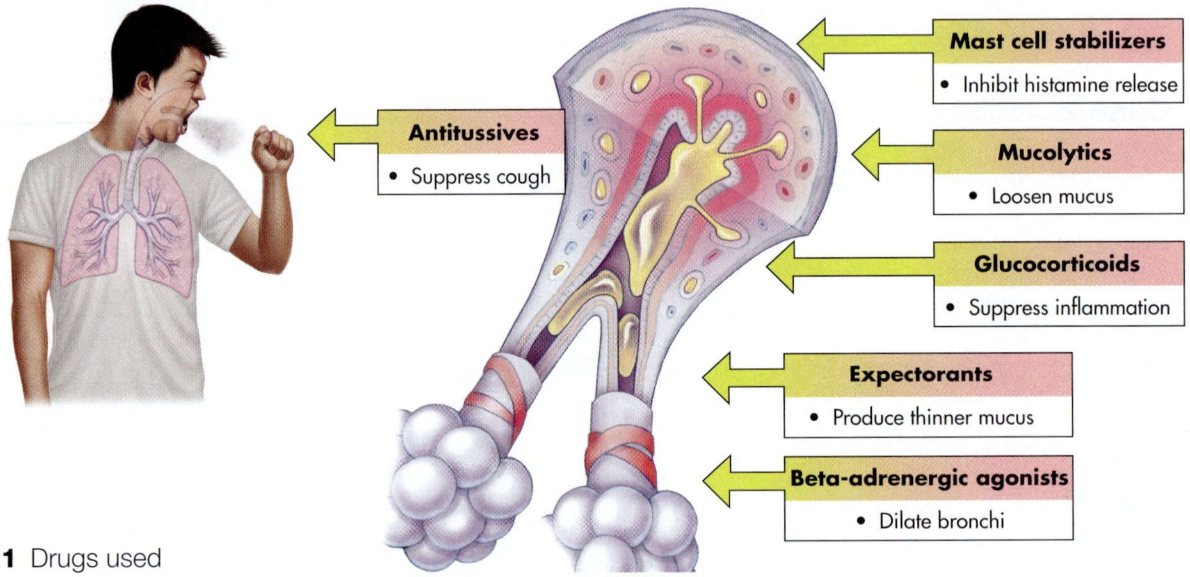

Figure 11.21 Drugs used to treat respiratory disorders.

Type of Drug	Description and Examples
decongestants	These agents are used for the temporary relief of nasal congestion associated with the common cold, hay fever, other upper respiratory allergies, and sinusitis. See Figure 11.21. EXAMPLES: Sudafed (pseudoephedrine HCl) and Afrin (oxymetazoline HCl) *Note:* Sudafed is not available as an over-the-counter drug, and can be obtained only under pharmacy supervision because it contains ingredients that can be used to make the illegal drug methamphetamine, commonly called crystal meth.
antitussives	Can be classified as non-narcotic and narcotic. See Figure 11.21.
non-narcotic agents	Anesthetize the stretch receptors located in the respiratory passages, lungs, and pleura by dampening their activity and thereby reducing the cough reflex at its source. EXAMPLES: Tessalon (benzonatate), diphenhydramine HCl, and Mucinex DM (guaifenesin and dextromethorphan hydrobromide)
narcotic agents	Depress the cough center located in the medulla, thereby raising its threshold for incoming cough impulse. EXAMPLES: codeine and hydrocodone bitartrate

Type of Drug	Description and Examples
expectorants	Promote and facilitate the removal of mucus from the lower respiratory tract. See Figure 11.21. EXAMPLES: Robitussin (guaifenesin) and Mucinex DM (guaifenesin and dextromethorphan hydrobromide)
mucolytics	Break chemical bonds in mucus, thereby lowering its thickness. See Figure 11.21. EXAMPLE: acetylcysteine
bronchodilators	Used to improve pulmonary airflow by dilating air passages. See Figure 11.21. EXAMPLES: Proventil HFA (albuterol sulfate), ephedrine sulfate, aminophylline, Theo-24 (theophylline), and Spiriva (thiotropium)
inhalational glucocorticoids	Used in the treatment of bronchial asthma and in seasonal or perennial allergic conditions when other forms of treatment are not effective. See Figure 11.21. EXAMPLES: Beconase AQ (beclomethasone dipropionate monohydrate), Nasacort AQ (triamcinolone acetonide), Flovent HFA (fluticasone propionate), and flunisolide
antituberculosis agents	Used in the long-term treatment of tuberculosis (9 months to 1 year). They are often used in combination of three or more drugs and the primary drug regimen for active tuberculosis combines the drugs Myambutol (ethambutol HCl), isoniazid, Rifadin, Rimactane (rifampin), pyrazenamide, or Rifater (isoniazid, pyrazinamide, rifampin)

Diagnostic and Laboratory Tests

Test	Description
acid-fast bacilli (AFB) (ăs ĭd-făst″ bă-sĭl′ī)	Test performed on sputum to detect the presence of *Mycobacterium tuberculosis*, an acid-fast bacilli. Positive results indicate tuberculosis.
antistreptolysin O (ASO titer) (ăn″ tĭ-strĕp-tŏl′ ĭ-sĭn)	Test performed on blood serum to detect the presence of streptolysin enzyme O, which is secreted by beta-hemolytic streptococcus. Positive results indicate streptococcal infection.
arterial blood gases (ABGs) (ăr-tē′ rē-ăl)	Test measures the acidity (pH) and the levels of oxygen and carbon dioxide in the blood. This test is used to check how well the lungs are able to move oxygen into the blood and remove carbon dioxide from the blood. Important in determining respiratory acidosis and/or alkalosis and metabolic acidosis and/or alkalosis.
bronchoscopy (brŏng-kŏs′ kō-pē)	Visual examination of the larynx, trachea, and bronchi via a flexible bronchoscope. With the use of biopsy forceps, tissues and secretions can be removed for further analysis.

Test	Description
culture, sputum (spū´ tŭm)	Examination of the sputum to determine the presence of pathogenic microorganisms. Abnormal results can indicate tuberculosis, bronchitis, pneumonia, bronchiectasis, and other infectious respiratory diseases (RDs).
culture, throat	Test that identifies the presence of pathogenic microorganisms in the throat, especially beta-hemolytic streptococci.
laryngoscopy (lăr″ ĭn-gŏs´ kō-pē)	Visual examination of the larynx via a laryngoscope.
pulmonary function test (pŭl´ mō-nĕ-rē)	Series of tests performed to determine the diffusion of oxygen and carbon dioxide across the cell membrane in the lungs, including tidal volume (TV), vital capacity (VC), expiratory reserve volume (ERV), inspiratory capacity (IC), residual volume (RV), forced inspiratory volume (FIV), functional residual capacity (FRC), maximal voluntary ventilation (MVV), total lung capacity (TLC), and flow volume loop (F-V loop). Abnormal results can indicate various respiratory diseases and conditions. See Figure 11.22.

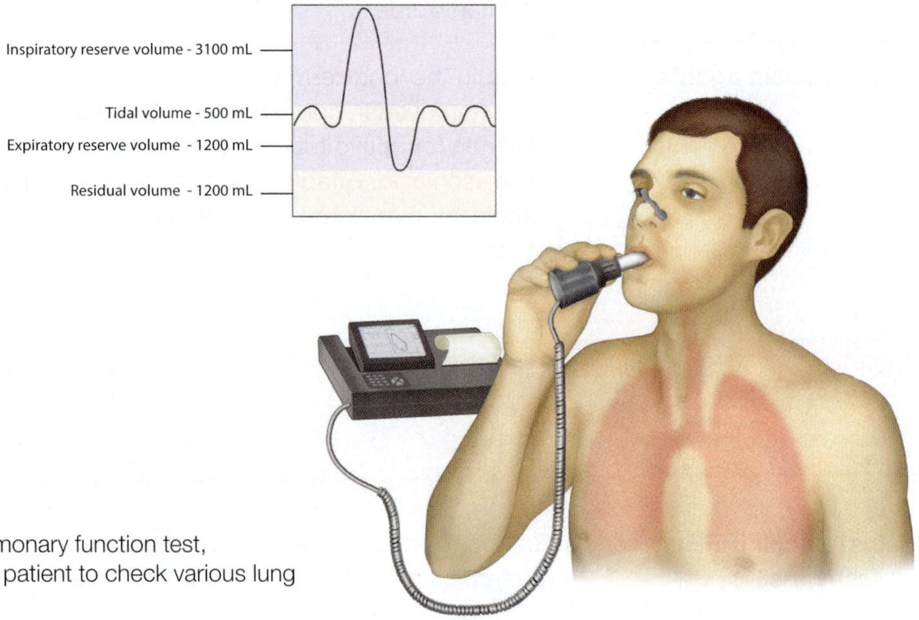

Figure 11.22 As part of a pulmonary function test, a spirometer is being used by the patient to check various lung volume capacities.

Test	Description
rhinoscopy (rī-nŏs´ kō-pē)	Visual examination of the nasal passages.

Abbreviations

Abbreviation	Meaning	Abbreviation	Meaning
ABGs	arterial blood gases	**IRV**	inspiratory reserve volume
AFB	acid-fast bacilli	**IV**	intravenous
ARD	acute respiratory disease	**MDR TB**	multidrug-resistant tuberculosis
ARDS	adult respiratory distress syndrome	**MVV**	maximal voluntary ventilation
ASO	antistreptolysin O	**NRDS**	neonatal respiratory distress syndrome
CF	cystic fibrosis	**O_2**	oxygen
CO_2	carbon dioxide	**R**	respiration
COPD	chronic obstructive pulmonary disease	**RD**	respiratory disease
CXR	chest x-ray	**RDS**	respiratory distress syndrome
DOT	directly observed therapy	**RSV**	respiratory syncytial virus
ERV	expiratory reserve volume	**RV**	residual volume
ET	endotracheal	**SARS**	severe acute respiratory syndrome
FIV	forced inspiratory volume	**SOB**	shortness of breath
FRC	functional residual capacity	**TB**	tuberculosis
F-V loop	flow volume loop	**TLC**	total lung capacity
HMD	hyaline membrane disease	**TV**	tidal volume
IC	inspiratory capacity	**VC**	vital capacity
IRDS	infant respiratory distress syndrome		

Study and Review III

Building Medical Terms

Using the following word parts, fill in the blanks to build the correct medical terms.

dys-	thorac/o	-pnea
pharyng	-ectasis	-ectomy
rhin/o	-staxis	-osis

Definition	Medical Term
1. The collapse of an alveolus, a lobule, or a larger lung unit	atel __________
2. Literally means *difficulty in breathing*	________ pnea
3. Nosebleed	epi _________
4. Abnormally deep and rapid breathing	hyper _______
5. Inflammation of the pharynx	___________ itis
6. Surgical excision of the left or right lung	pneumon ____

(continued)

Definition	Medical Term
7. Surgical repair of the nose	________ plasty
8. Rapid breathing	tachy _______
9. Incision into the chest wall	________ tomy
10. Infectious disease caused by the tubercle bacillus	tubercul _____

Combining Form Challenge

Using the combining forms provided, write the medical term correctly.

anthrac/o	hem/o	olfact/o
bronch/o	laryng/o	orth/o

1. Lung condition caused by inhalation of coal dust and silica: ________osis

2. Medical instrument used to visually examine the bronchi: _______scope

3. Spitting up blood: _______ptysis

4. Medical instrument used to visually examine the larynx: ___________ scope

5. Process of smelling: _________ion

6. Inability to breathe unless in an upright or straight position: ________ pnea

Select the Right Term

Select the correct answer, and write it on the line provided.

1. Disease of the bronchi characterized by wheezing and dyspnea is ________________.

anthracosis **asphyxia** **asthma** **atelectasis**

2. Acute respiratory disease characterized by a barking cough is _________________.

cough **croup** **cystic fibrosis** **dysphonia**

3. Condition of deficient amounts of oxygen in the inspired air is _________________.

eupnea **hyperpnea** **hypoxia** **inhalation**

4. Acute, infectious disease characterized by a cough with a "whooping" sound is __________.

laryngitis **pneumonia** **pharyngitis** **pertussis**

5. Abnormal sound heard on auscultation of the chest; a crackling sound is _____________.

rale **rhonchus** **stridor** **wheeze**

6. One of the subgroup of viruses that causes the common cold is __________________.

syncytial **rhinovirus** **rhinorrhea** **influenza**

Diagnostic and Laboratory Tests

Select the best answer to each multiple-choice question. Circle the letter of your choice.

1. Test performed on sputum to detect the presence of *Mycobacterium tuberculosis*.

a. antistreptolysin O titer
b. acid-fast bacilli
c. pulmonary function test
d. bronchoscopy

2. Visual examination of the nasal passages.

a. bronchoscopy
b. laryngoscopy
c. rhinoscopy
d. rhinoplasty

3. ______________________________ is/are important in determining respiratory acidosis and/or alkalosis and metabolic acidosis and/or alkalosis.

a. Acid-fast bacilli
b. Antistreptolysin O titer
c. Arterial blood gases
d. Pulmonary function test

4. Series of tests to determine the diffusion of oxygen and carbon dioxide across the cell membrane in the lungs.

a. acid-fast bacilli
b. antistreptolysin O titer
c. arterial blood gases
d. pulmonary function test

5. Visual examination of the larynx, trachea, and bronchi via a flexible scope.

a. bronchoscopy
b. laryngoscopy
c. laryngoscope
d. rhinoscopy

Abbreviations

Place the correct word, phrase, or abbreviation in the space provided.

1. acid-fast bacilli ______________________________

2. CF ______________________________

3. chest x-ray ______________________________

4. chronic obstructive pulmonary disease ______________________________

5. ET ______________________________

6. hyaline membrane disease ______________________________

7. respiration ______________________________

8. SARS ______________________________

9. shortness of breath ______________________________

10. TB ______________________________

Chapter

12 Urinary System

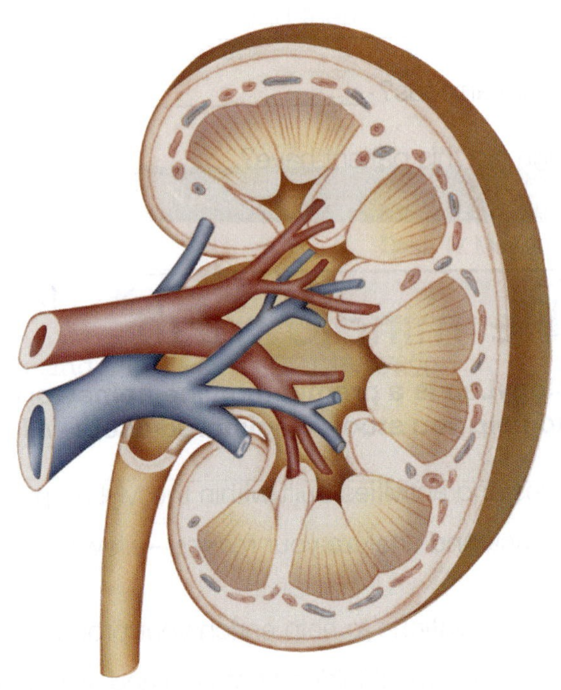

Learning Outcomes

On completion of this chapter, you will be able to:

1. Describe the urinary system and explain its vital function.
2. State the descriptions and primary functions of the organs/structures of the urinary system.
3. Define urinalysis and state its significance.
4. Identify normal and abnormal constituents of urine.
5. Recognize terminology included in the ICD-10-CM.
6. Analyze, build, spell, and pronounce medical words.
7. Comprehend the drugs highlighted in this chapter.
8. Describe diagnostic and laboratory tests related to the urinary system.
9. Identify and define selected abbreviations.
10. Apply your acquired knowledge of medical terms by successfully completing the *Practical Application* exercise.

Anatomy and Physiology

The urinary system consists of two kidneys, two ureters, one bladder, and one urethra (see Figure 12.1). It is also called the excretory, genitourinary (GU), or urogenital (UG) system and is the organ system that produces, stores, and eliminates urine. The vital function of the urinary system is to extract certain wastes from the bloodstream, convert these materials to urine, transport the urine from the kidneys via the ureters to the bladder, and eliminate it (void) at appropriate intervals via the urethra. Through this vital function, homeostasis of body fluids is maintained. Table 12.1 provides an at-a-glance look at the urinary system.

Kidneys

The **kidneys** are purplish-brown, bean-shaped organs located behind the abdominal cavity (*retroperitoneal area*) on either side of the spine between the thoracic vertebrae (T 12) and the lumbar region (Figure 12.2). Each kidney is surrounded by three capsules: the **true capsule**, the **perirenal fat**, and the **renal fascia**. The true capsule is a smooth, fibrous connective membrane that loosely adheres to the surface of the kidney. The perirenal fat is the adipose capsule that embeds each kidney in fatty tissue. The renal fascia is a sheath of fibrous tissue that helps to anchor the kidney to the surrounding structures and helps to maintain its normal position.

External Structure

Each kidney has a *concave* border and a *convex* border. The center of the concave border opens into a notch called the **hilum**. The renal artery and vein, nerves, and lymphatic vessels enter and leave through the hilum. The ureter enters the kidney through the hilum into a saclike collecting area called the *renal pelvis*. See Figure 12.3.

Internal Structure

When a cross-section is made through the kidney, two distinct areas can be seen: the **cortex**, which is the outer layer, and the **medulla** or inner portion (Figure 12.3). The cortex is composed of arteries, veins, convoluted tubules, and glomerular capsules. The medulla is composed of the renal pyramids, conelike masses with papillae projecting into calices of the pelvis.

Microscopic Anatomy

Microscopic examination of the kidney reveals about 1 million **nephrons**, which are the structural and functional units of the organ (Figure 12.3). Each nephron consists of a **renal corpuscle** and **tubule**. The renal corpuscle, also called the *malpighian body*, consists of a **glomerulus**, a network of blood vessels surrounded by the Bowman capsule.

Table 12.1 Urinary System at-a-Glance

Organ/Structure	Primary Functions/Description
Kidneys	Produce urine and help regulate and control body fluids
Ureters	Transport urine from the kidneys to the bladder
Urinary bladder	Serves as a reservoir for urine
Urethra	Passageway of urine to the outside of the body; in the male conveys both urine and semen

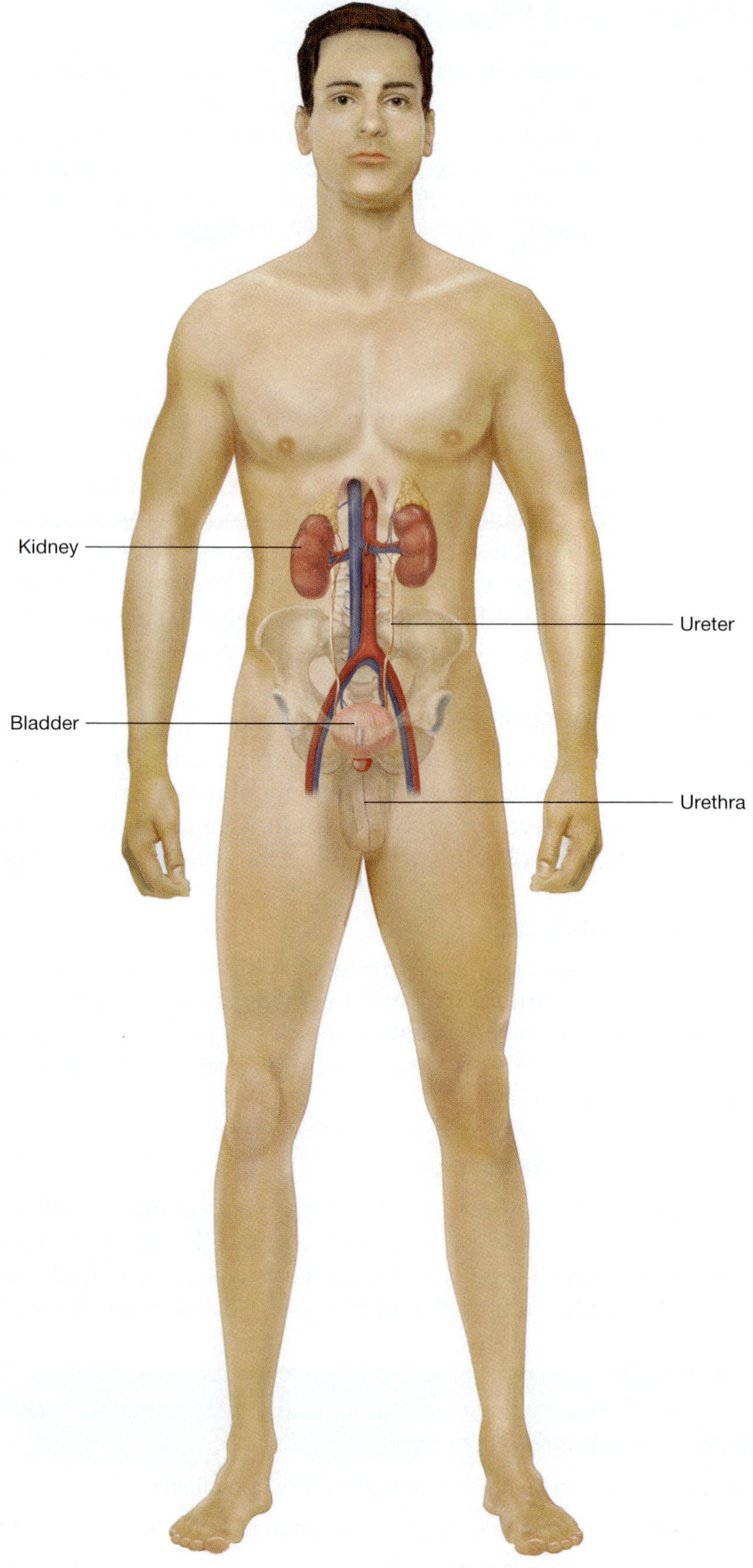

Figure 12.1 The urinary system: kidneys, ureters, bladder, and urethra.

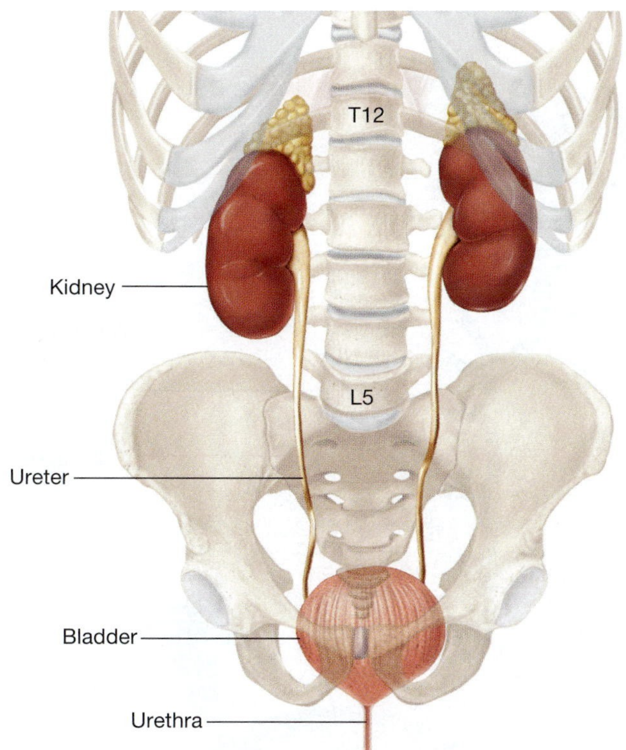

Figure 12.2 Position of the urinary organs.

The **Bowman capsule** is a cup-like sac at the beginning of the tubular component of a nephron in the kidney that performs the first step in the filtration of blood to form urine. Extending from each Bowman capsule is a tubule consisting of the proximal convoluted portion, the loop of Henle, and a distal convoluted portion that opens into a collecting duct.

NEPHRON

The vital function of the *nephron* is to regulate, control, and then remove the waste products of metabolism from the blood plasma. These waste products are urea (chief nitrogenous constituent of urine), uric acid, and creatinine, as well as any excess sodium chloride (NaCl), and potassium ions and ketone bodies. The nephron plays a vital role in the maintenance of normal fluid balance in the body by regulated reabsorption of water and selected electrolytes back into the blood. Approximately 1000–1200 milliliters (mL) of blood flows through the kidney per minute. At a rate of 1000 mL of blood per minute, about 1.5 million mL flows through the kidney in each 24-hour day.

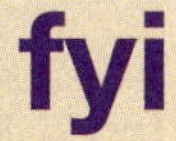

At 10 weeks' gestation, urine forms and enters the bladder of the fetus. At about the third month the fetal kidneys begin to secrete urine. The amount increases gradually as the fetus matures. The newborn's kidneys are immature and lack the ability to concentrate urine. Glomerular filtration and reabsorption are relatively low until the child is 1 or 2 years of age.

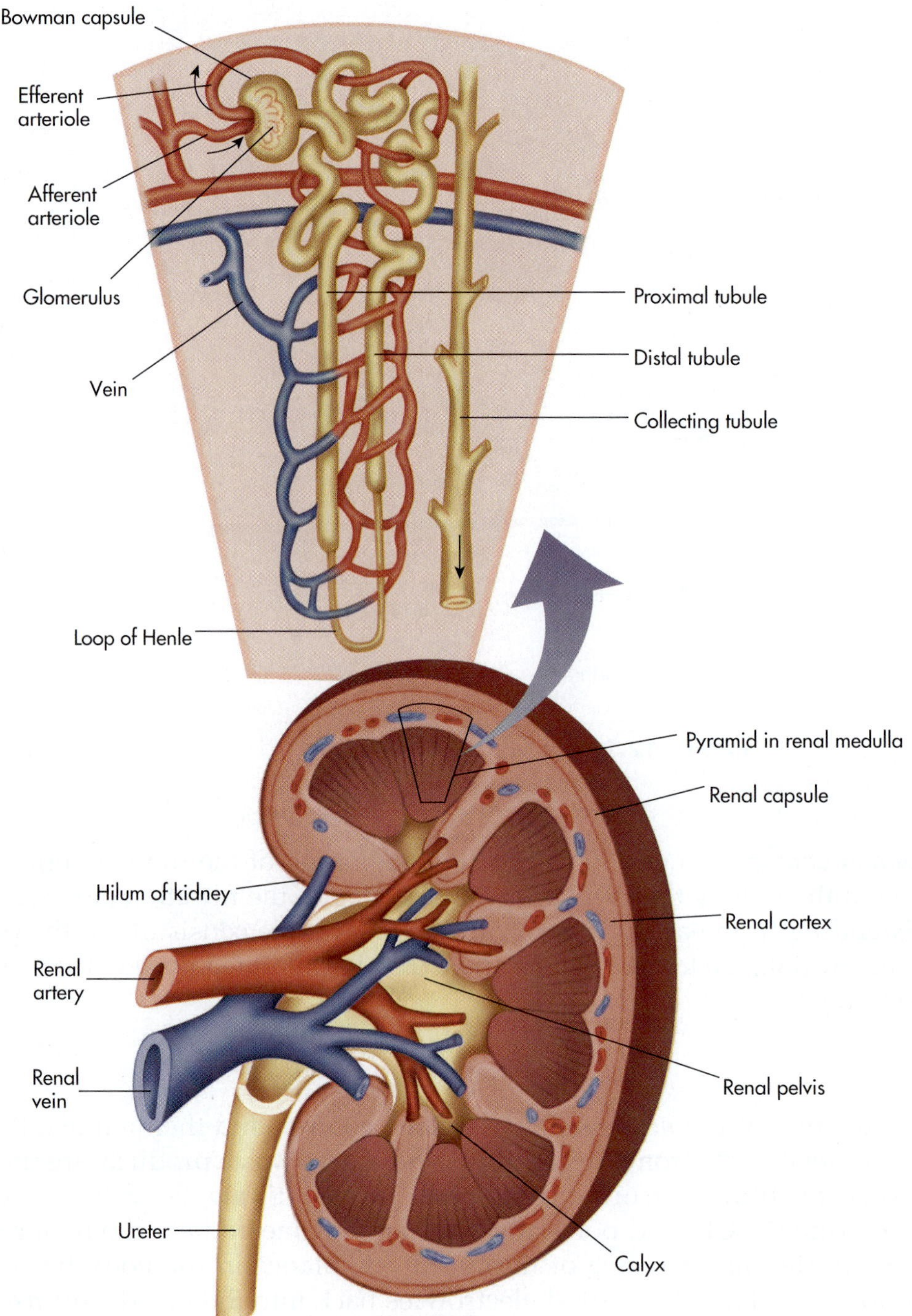

Figure 12.3 Kidney with an expanded view of a nephron.

Ureters

Each kidney has a **ureter**. They are narrow, muscular tubes that drain urine from the kidneys to the bladder (Figure 12.1). They are from 28 to 34 centimeters (cm) long and vary in diameter from 1 millimeter (mm) to 1 cm. The walls of the ureters consist of three layers: an inner coat of mucous membrane, a middle coat of smooth muscle, and an outer coat of fibrous tissue.

Urinary Bladder

The **urinary bladder** (see Figures 12.1 and 12.2) is the muscular, membranous sac that serves as a reservoir for urine. It is located in the anterior portion of the pelvic cavity and consists of a lower portion, the **neck**, which is continuous with the urethra, and an upper portion, the **apex**, which is connected with the umbilicus by the median umbilical ligament. The **trigone** is a small triangular area near the base of the bladder between the openings of the two ureters and the opening of the urethra. The wall of the bladder consists of four layers: an inner layer of epithelium, a muscular coat of smooth muscle, an outer layer composed of longitudinal muscle (*detrusor urinae*), and a fibrous layer. An empty bladder feels firm as the muscular wall becomes thick. As the bladder fills with urine, the muscular wall becomes thinner and distends according to the amount of urine present. Normally, urine is formed continuously and when there is sufficient quantity the need to void occurs.

Urethra

The **urethra** is the musculomembranous tube extending from the bladder to the outside of the body. The external urinary opening is the **urinary meatus**. The male urethra is approximately 20 cm or about 8 inches long and is divided into three sections: *prostatic*, *membranous*, and *penile*. It conveys both urine and semen out of the body. The female urethra is approximately 4 cm or about 1½ inches long. The urinary meatus is situated between the clitoris and the opening of the vagina. The female urethra conveys urine out of the body. See Figure 12.4.

fyi **Urinary tract infections (UTIs)** are common in children. The microorganisms *Escherichia coli*, *Klebsiella*, and *Proteus* cause most urinary tract infections seen in children. The signs and symptoms of a urinary tract infection are age related. Infants can experience fever, weight loss, nausea and vomiting, increased urination (process of voiding urine), foul-smelling urine, persistent diaper rash, and failure to thrive. Older children can have frequent and/or painful urination, abdominal pain, hematuria, fever, chills, and bedwetting episodes in a trained child.

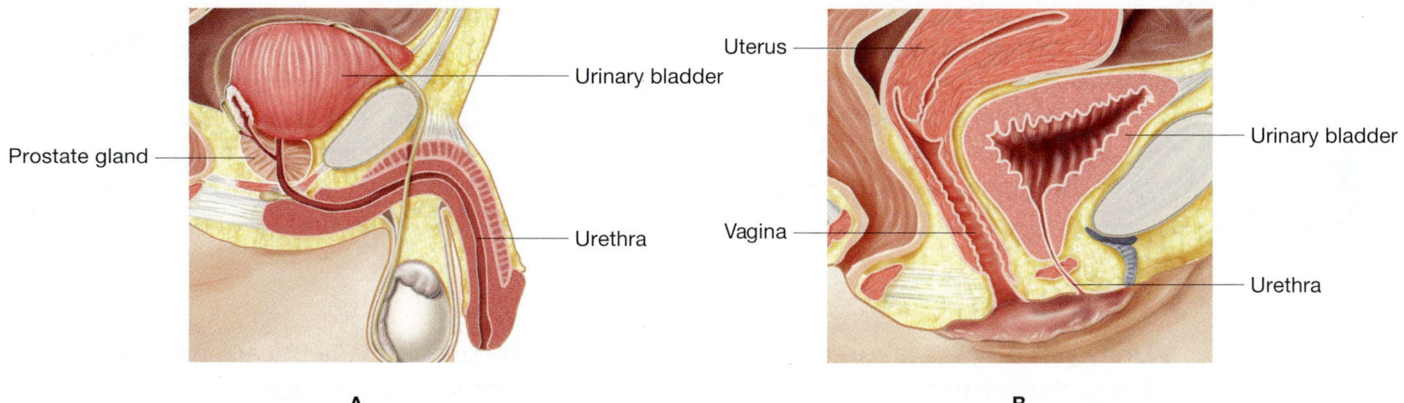

Figure 12.4 (A) The male urethra. (B) The female urethra.

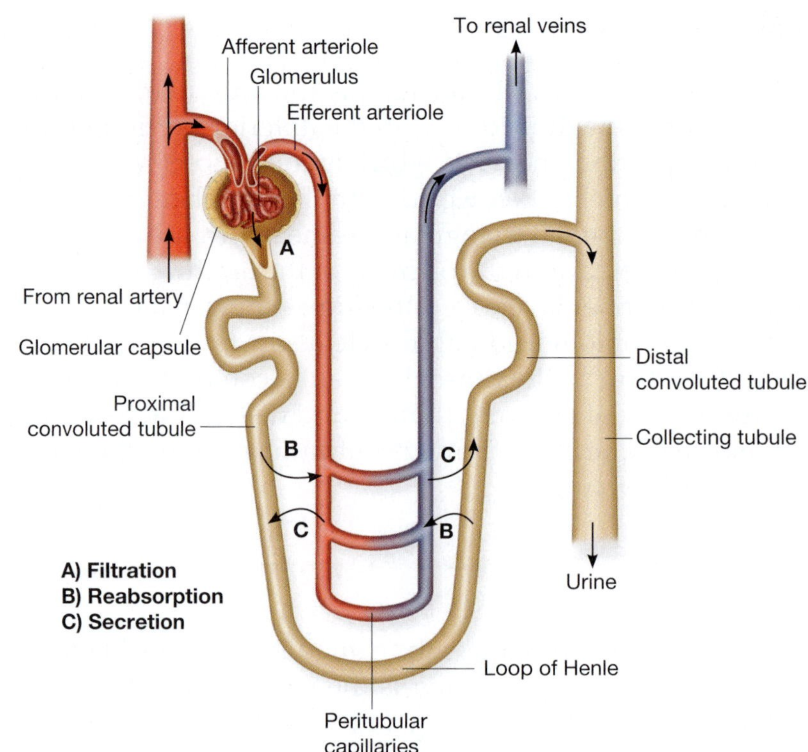

Figure 12.5 Sites of tubular reabsorption and secretion.

Urine

Urine is formed by the process of *filtration* and *reabsorption* in the nephron. It consists of 95% water and 5% solid substances. It is secreted by the kidneys and transported by the ureters to the bladder, where it is stored before being discharged from the body via the urethra. See Figure 12.5.

An average normal adult feels the need to void when the bladder contains around 300–350 mL of urine. An average of 1000–1500 mL of urine is voided daily. Normal urine is clear and yellow to amber in color and has a faintly aromatic odor, a specific gravity of 1.003–1.030, and a slightly acid pH (hydrogen ion concentration).

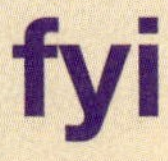

Changes noted in the urinary system of the older adult are loss of muscle tone in the ureters, bladder, and urethra. Bladder capacity can be reduced by half, and the older adult could have to make frequent trips to the bathroom. **Urge incontinence** (or the inability to retain urine voluntarily) is a concern for older adults. There is a leakage of urine due to bladder muscles that contract inappropriately. In men, urge incontinence can be caused by benign prostatic hyperplasia (BPH) or by prostate cancer. In most cases of urge incontinence, no specific cause can be identified. Although urge incontinence may occur in anyone at any age, it is more common in women and older adults.

Urinalysis

Urinalysis (UA) is a laboratory test that evaluates the physical, chemical, and microscopic properties of urine. A freshly voided urine specimen provides for more accurate test results. A urine sample that is left standing for an extended period of time will deteriorate. If the urinalysis cannot be performed on the specimen within 1 hour of the time voided, it should be refrigerated, with the time of collection written on the label of the container. Urine should be collected in a clean, dry, disposable container. When a bacteriological culture is to be done on urine, the specimen is collected by **catheterization**. A urinary catheterization is the process of introducing a catheter through the urethra into the bladder for withdrawal of urine. This is a sterile procedure and performed by individuals trained and skilled in the proper technique.

Urinalysis is a valuable diagnostic tool. Abnormal conditions or diseases can be quickly and easily detected because of the fact that the physical and chemical constituents of normal urine are constant. See Table 12.2.

Table 12.2 Normal and Abnormal Constituents of Urine

Constituent	Normal	Abnormal/Significance
Color	Yellow to amber	Red or reddish—presence of hemoglobin Greenish-brown or black—caused by bile pigments. *The color of urine darkens upon standing.*
Appearance	Clear	Milky—fat globules, pus, bacteria Smoky—blood cells Hazy—refrigeration
Reaction	Between 4.6 and 8.0 pH, with an average of 6.0	High acidity—diabetic acidosis, fever, dehydration Alkaline—urinary tract infection, renal failure
Specific gravity (sp. gr.)	Between 1.003 and 1.030	Low (1.001–1.002)—diabetes insipidus High (over 1.030)—diabetes mellitus, hepatic disease, congestive heart failure
Odor	Faintly aromatic	Fruity sweet—acetone, associated with diabetes mellitus Unpleasant—decomposition of drugs, foods, alcohol
Quantity	Around 1000–1500 mL per day	High—diabetes mellitus, diabetes insipidus, nervousness, diuretics, excessive intake Low—acute nephritis, heart disease, diarrhea, vomiting None—uremia, end-stage renal disease (ESRD)
Protein	Negative	Positive (proteinuria)—renal disease, pyelonephritis
Glucose	Negative	Positive (glycosuria)—diabetes mellitus
Ketones	Negative	Positive (ketonuria)—uncontrolled diabetes mellitus; high-protein, low-carbohydrate diet; starvation
Bilirubin	Negative	Positive (biliuria)—liver disease, biliary obstruction, congestive heart failure
Blood	Negative	Positive (hematuria)—renal disease, trauma
Nitrites	Negative	Positive (nitrituria)—bacteriuria
Urobilinogen	0.1–1.0	Absent—biliary obstruction Reduced—antibiotic therapy Increased—early warning of hepatic or hemolytic disease

Study and Review I

Anatomy and Physiology

Write your answers to the following questions.

1. List the organs of the urinary system.

   a. ______________________ **b.** ______________________

   c. ______________________ **d.** ______________________

2. State the vital function of the urinary system. ______________________

   ____

3. Define hilum. ______________________

4. Define renal pelvis. ______________________

5. The medulla is the ______________________ portion of the kidney.

6. Define nephron. ______________________

7. Each nephron consists of a ______________________ and a ______________________.

8. The renal corpuscle consists of ______________________ and ______________________.

9. Urine is formed by the process of ______________________ and ______________________ in the nephron.

10. An average of ______________________ to ______________________ mL of urine is voided daily.

11. Describe the ureters and state their function. ______________________

    ____

12. Describe the urinary bladder and state its function. ______________________

    ____

13. The external urinary opening is the ______________________.

14. Define urinalysis. ______________________

    ____

15. Give the normal constituents for the physical examination of urine.

a. Color ______________________________

b. Appearance ______________________________

c. Reaction ______________________________

d. Specific gravity ______________________________

e. Odor ______________________________

f. Quantity ______________________________

16. A urine that has a fruity, sweet odor can indicate ______________________________

______________________________.

17. Under chemical examination, the presence of protein in urine is an important sign of ______________________________

______________________________.

ANATOMY LABELING

Identify the structures shown below by filling in the blanks.

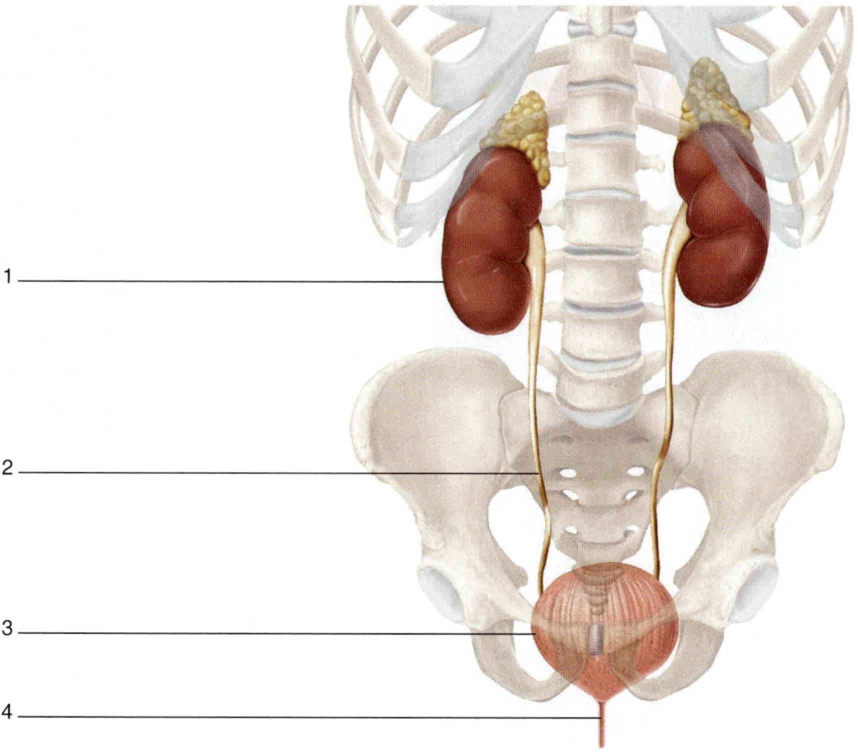

Building Your Medical Vocabulary

This section provides the foundation for learning medical terminology. Review the following alphabetized word list. Note how common prefixes and suffixes are repeatedly applied to word roots and combining forms to create different meanings. The word parts are color-coded: prefixes are yellow, suffixes are blue, roots/combining forms are red. A combining form is a word root plus a vowel. The chart below lists the combining forms for the word roots in this chapter and can help to strengthen your understanding of how medical words are built and spelled.

Remember These Guidelines

1. If the suffix begins with a vowel, drop the combining vowel from the combining form and add the suffix. For example, nephr/o (*kidney*) + -oma (*tumor*) becomes nephroma.
2. If the suffix begins with a consonant, keep the combining vowel and add the suffix to the combining form. For example, cyst/o (*bladder*) + -dynia (*pain*) becomes cystodynia.

You will find that some terms have not been divided into word parts. These are common words or specialized terms that are included to enhance your medical vocabulary.

Combining Forms of the Urinary System			
albumin/o	protein	**micturit/o**	to urinate
bacteri/o	bacteria	**nephr/o**	kidney
calc/i	calcium	**noct/o**	night
corpore/o	body	**perine/o**	perineum
cutane/o	skin	**peritone/o**	peritoneum
cyst/o	bladder	**py/o**	pus
excret/o	sifted out	**pyel/o**	renal pelvis
glomerul/o	glomerulus, little ball	**ren/o**	kidney
glycos/o	glucose, sugar	**scler/o**	hardening
hem/o	blood	**son/o**	sound
hemat/o	blood	**ur/o**	urine, urinate, urination
keton/o	ketone	**ureter/o**	ureter
lith/o	stone	**urethr/o**	urethra
meat/o	passage	**urin/o**	urine

Medical Word	Word Parts		Definition
	Part	**Meaning**	
albuminuria (ăl-bū″ mĭn-oo′ rĭ-ă)	albumin -uria	protein urine	Indicates the presence of serum protein in the urine. Albumin is the major protein in blood plasma. When detected in urine (*albuminuria*), it may indicate a leak in the glomerular membrane, which allows albumin to enter the renal tubule and pass into the urine.
antidiuretic (ăn″ tĭ-dī″ ū-rĕt′ ĭk)	anti- di(a)- uret -ic	against complete, through urine pertaining to	Pertaining to a medication that decreases urine production and secretion
anuria (ăn-ū′ rĭ-ă)	an- -uria	without urine	Literally means *without the formation of urine*; lack of urine production
bacteriuria (băk-tē″ rĭ-ū′ rĭ-ă)	bacteri -uria	bacteria urine	Presence of bacteria in the urine
calciuria (kăl″ sĭ-ū′ rĭ-ă)	calc/i -uria	calcium urine	Presence of calcium in the urine
calculus (kăl′ kū-lŭs)			Pebble; any abnormal concretion (*stone*); plural: calculi. See Figure 12.6.

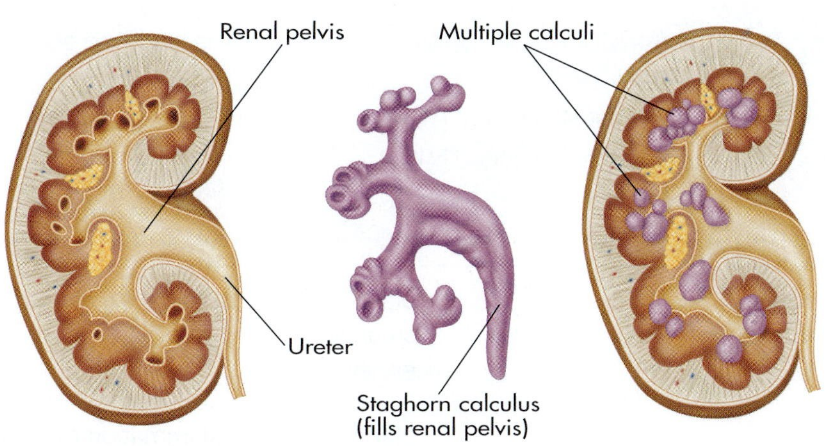

Figure 12.6 Urinary calculi.

Medical Word	Word Parts		Definition
	Part	**Meaning**	
catheter (kăth´ ĕ-tĕr)			Tube of elastic, elastic web, rubber, glass, metal, or plastic that is inserted into a body cavity to remove fluid or to inject fluid. See Figure 12.7.

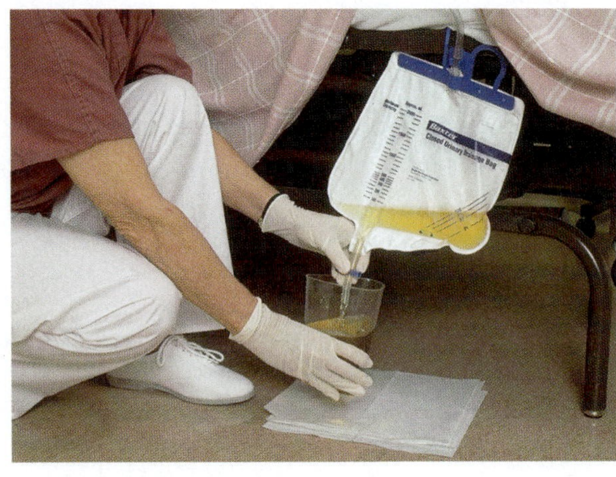

Figure 12.7 Closed urinary drainage system. Urine being measured after it leaves patient's body via catheter.

Source: Pearson Education, Inc.

Medical Word	Part	Meaning	Definition
chronic kidney disease (CKD)			Disease that results from any condition that causes gradual loss of kidney function. When the kidneys are damaged and cannot filter blood as well as healthy kidneys, waste from the blood remains in the body. CKD can lead to kidney failure. Diabetes and high blood pressure are the most common causes of CKD. See *dialysis* and *renal transplantation* for treatment options.

insights In the ICD-10-CM, chronic kidney disease is classified according to its severity and is designated stages 1–5.

- Stage 1 is coded N18.1
- Stage 2 is coded N18.2
- Stage 3 is coded N18.3
- Stage 4 is coded N18.4
- Stage 5 is coded N18.5

Medical Word	Part	Meaning	Definition
cystectomy (sĭs-tĕk´ tō-mē)	cyst -ectomy	bladder surgical excision	Surgical excision of the bladder or part of the bladder
cystitis (sĭs-tī´ tĭs)	cyst -itis	bladder inflammation	Inflammation of the bladder, usually occurring secondarily to ascending urinary tract infections. More than 85% of cases of cystitis are caused by *Escherichia coli*, a bacillus found in the lower gastrointestinal tract.

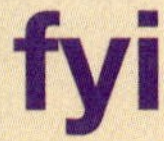

Cystitis is very common and occurs in more than 3 million Americans a year. It frequently affects sexually active women ages 20–50 but can also occur in those who are not sexually active or in young girls and older adults. Females are more prone to cystitis because of their shorter urethra (bacteria do not have to travel as far to enter the bladder) and because of the short distance between the opening of the urethra and the anus.

Interstitial cystitis (IC) is a painful inflammation of the bladder wall. Approximately 1.3 million Americans suffer from this condition and, of those, 90% are women. Symptoms can vary from mild to severe. The cause is unknown, and IC does not respond well to antibiotic therapy.

Medical Word	Word Parts		Definition
	Part	**Meaning**	
cystocele (sĭs′ tō-sēl)	cyst/o -cele	bladder hernia	Hernia of the bladder that protrudes into the vagina

> **RULE REMINDER**
>
> This term keeps the combining vowel ***o*** because the suffix begins with a consonant.

Medical Word	Part	Meaning	Definition
cystogram (sĭs′ tō-grăm)	cyst/o -gram	bladder a mark, record	X-ray record of the bladder

> **ALERT Check-It-Out**
>
> How many words can you build using the root **cyst** and the combining form **cyst/o**?

Medical Word	Part	Meaning	Definition
cystolith (sĭs″ tō-lĭth)	cyst/o -lith	bladder stone	A bladder stone; a vesical calculus
cystoscope (sĭst′ ō-skōp)	cyst/o -scope	bladder instrument for examining	Medical instrument used for visual examination of the bladder
dialysis (dī-ăl′ ĭ-sĭs)	dia- -lysis	complete, through destruction, to separate	Medical procedure to separate waste material from the blood and to maintain fluid, electrolyte, and acid-base balance in impaired kidney function or in the absence of the kidney. The two main types of dialysis, hemodialysis (HD) and peritoneal dialysis (PD), remove wastes from the blood in different ways.
diuresis (dī″ ū-rē′ sĭs)	di(a)- ur -esis	complete, through urinate condition	Pathological condition of increased or excessive flow of urine; occurs in conditions such as diabetes mellitus and diabetes insipidus. Diuretics can also produce diuresis.
dysuria (dĭs-ū′ rĭ-ă)	dys- -uria	difficult, painful urine	Difficult or painful urination
edema (ĕ-dē′ mă)			Pathological condition in which the body tissues contain an accumulation of fluid
enuresis (ĕn″ ū-rē′ sĭs)	en- ur -esis	within urinate condition	Condition of involuntary emission of urine; *bedwetting*

Medical Word	Word Parts: Part	Word Parts: Meaning	Definition
excretory (ěks´ krə-tō-rē)	excretor -y	sifted out pertaining to	Pertaining to the elimination of waste products from the body
extracorporeal shock wave lithotripsy (ESWL) (ěks˝ tră-kor-por´ ē-ăl lĭth´ ō-trip˝ sē)	extra- corpore -al lith/o -tripsy	outside, beyond body pertaining to stone crushing	Process whereby a medical device is used to crush kidney stones (*renal calculi*). The patient is sedated and immersed in a water bath while shock waves pound the stones until they crumble into small pieces. These pieces are generally flushed out with urine. See Figure 12.8.

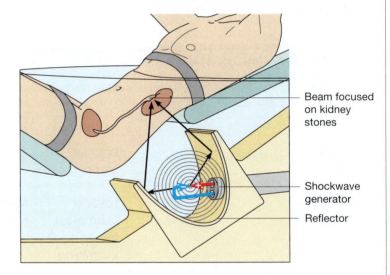

Figure 12.8 Illustration of water immersion lithotripsy procedure. Acoustic shock waves generated by the shock-wave generator travel through soft tissue to shatter the renal stone into fragments, which are then eliminated in the urine.

Medical Word	Word Parts: Part	Word Parts: Meaning	Definition
glomerular (glō-mĕr´ ū-lăr)	glomerul -ar	glomerulus, little ball pertaining to	Literally means *pertaining to the glomerulus*; a network of blood vessels located within the Bowman capsule that permits a greater surface area for filtration. See Figure 12.9.

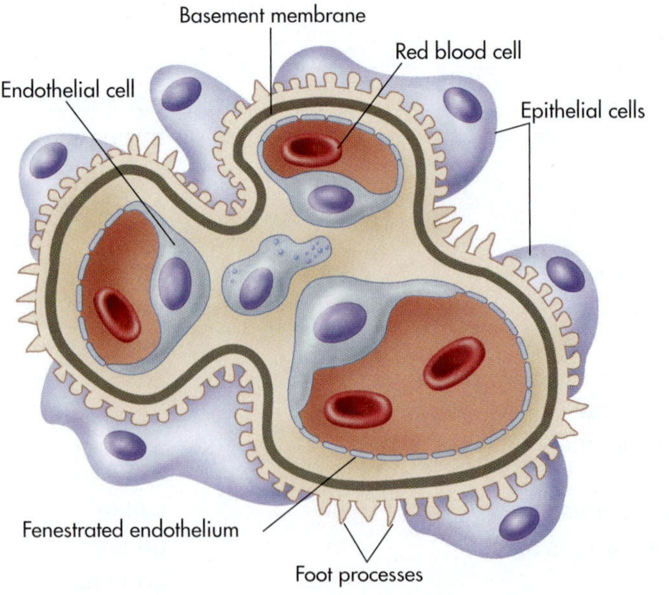

Figure 12.9 Normal glomerulus.

Medical Word	Word Parts: Part	Word Parts: Meaning	Definition
glomerulitis (glō-mĕr″ ū-lī′ tĭs)	glomerul -itis	glomerulus, little ball inflammation	Inflammation of the renal glomeruli
glomerulonephritis (glō-mĕr″ ū-lō-nĕ-frī′ tĭs)	glomerul/o nephr -itis	glomerulus, little ball kidney inflammation	Inflammation of the kidney involving primarily the glomeruli. There are three types: acute glomerulonephritis (AGN), chronic glomerulonephritis (CGN), and subacute glomerulonephritis. See Figure 12.10.

ALERT!

To change glomerul**us** to its singular form, you change **us** to **i** to make glomerul**i**.

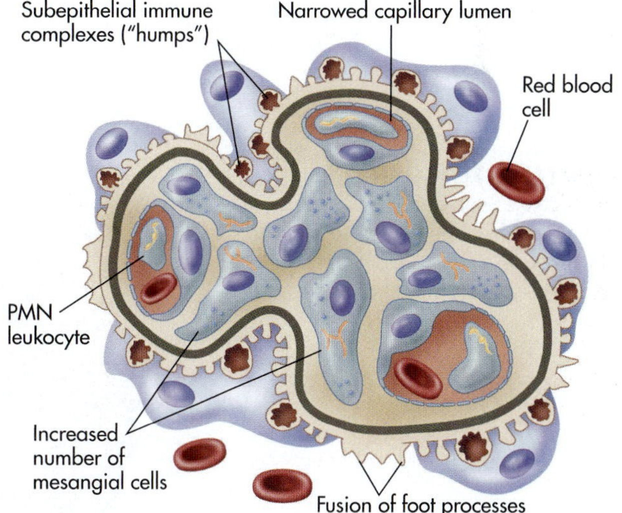

Figure 12.10 Acute glomerulonephritis.

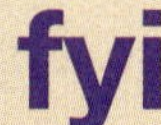

Acute nephritic syndrome (ANS) is a group of symptoms that occur with some disorders that cause glomerulonephritis. It is often caused by an immune response triggered by an infection (causing inflammation) or other disease. The inflammation affects the function of the glomerulus, the part of the kidney that filters blood to make urine and remove waste. As a result, blood and protein appear in the urine and excess fluid builds up in the body. Swelling of the body occurs when the blood loses a protein called albumin, which keeps fluid in the blood vessels. When it is lost, fluid collects in the body tissues. Blood loss from the damaged kidney structures leads to blood in the urine. Acute nephritic syndrome may be related to acute kidney/renal failure and high blood pressure.

Common symptoms of nephritic syndrome include blood in the urine (hematuria); dark, tea-colored, or cloudy urine; decreased urine output (oliguria); lack of urine output; and swelling (edema) of the face, eyes, legs, arms, hands, feet, abdomen, or other areas. See the section *Comparative Analysis of Nephrotic Syndrome and Nephritic Syndrome* later in the chapter.

(*continued*)

Medical Word	Word Parts		Definition
	Part	**Meaning**	

insights In the ICD-10-CM, the code for *acute nephritic syndrome* is N00–N00.9. Included in this classification are *acute glomerular disease*, *acute glomerulonephritis*, and *acute nephritis* (each with a different code number). *Nephrotic syndrome* is N04–N04.9. Included in this classification are *congenital nephrotic syndrome* and *lipoid* (lip [*fat*], -oid [*resemble*]) *nephrosis*.

Medical Word	Part	Meaning	Definition
glycosuria (glī″ kō-soo′ rĭ-ă)	glycos -uria	glucose, sugar urine	Presence of glucose in the urine
hematuria (hē″ mă-tū′ rĭ-ă)	hemat -uria	blood urine	Presence of red blood cells (erythrocytes) in the urine. In microscopic hematuria, the urine appears normal to the naked eye, but examination with a microscope shows a high number of RBCs. Gross hematuria can be seen with the naked eye—the urine is red or the color of cola. If white blood cells are found in addition to red blood cells, then it is a sign of urinary tract infection. See Figure 12.11.

RULE REMINDER

The ***o*** has been removed from the combining form because the suffix begins with a vowel.

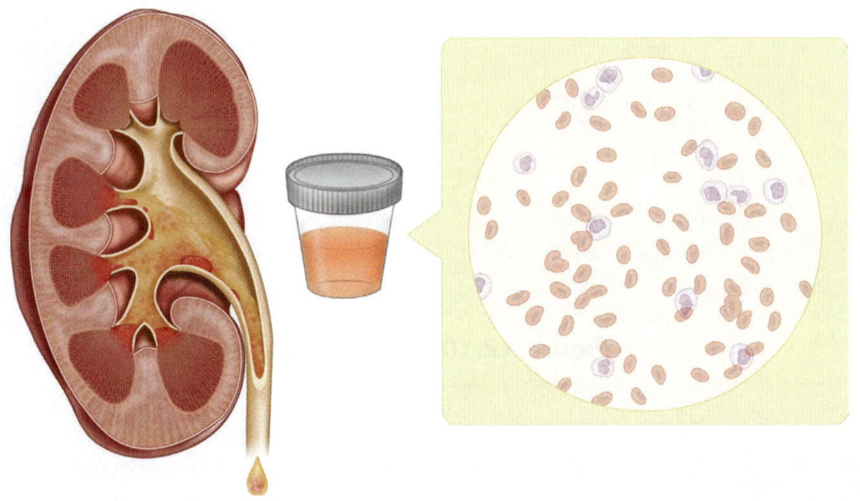

Figure 12.11 Hematuria. Note the color of urine in the specimen container and the microscopic view (in circle) showing red blood cells (red) and white blood cells (purple).

Medical Word	Word Parts		Definition
	Part	**Meaning**	
hemodialysis (HD) (hē″ mō-dī-ăl′ ĭ-sĭs)	hem/o dia- -lysis	blood through, complete separation, loosening, dissolution	Use of an artificial kidney to separate waste from the blood. The blood is circulated through tubes made of semipermeable membranes, and these tubes are continually bathed by solutions that remove waste. See Figure 12.12.

Venous pressure monitor
Air trap
Clean blood returned to patient
Fresh dialyzing solution
Dialyzer
Cellophane membranes
Arterial pressure monitor
Used dialyzing solution
Blood removed for cleaning
Heparin infusion
Blood pump
Inflow pressure monitor

Figure 12.12 Schematic of hemodialysis machine.

Medical Word	Part	Meaning	Definition
hydronephrosis (hī″ drō-nĕf-rō′ sĭs)	hydro- nephr -osis	water kidney condition	Pathological condition in which urine collects in the renal pelvis because of an obstructed outflow, thereby causing distention and damage to the kidney; can be caused by renal calculi, tumor, or hyperplasia of the prostate gland. See Figure 12.13.

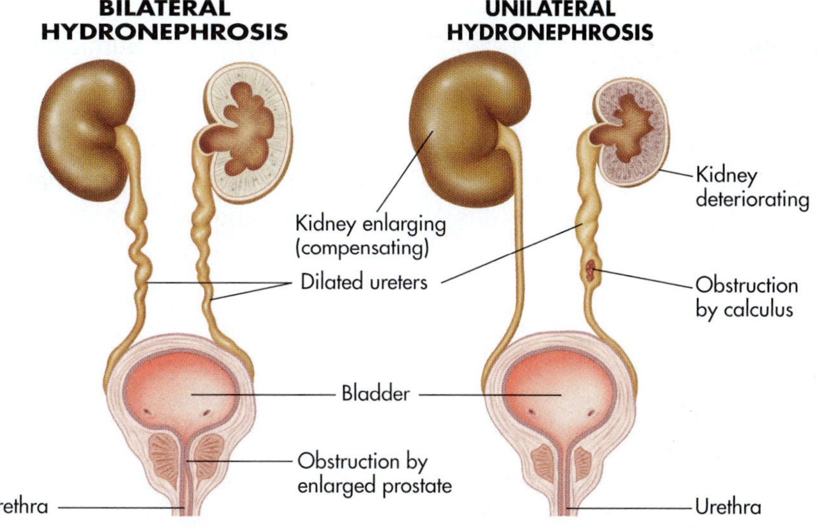

Figure 12.13 Hydronephrosis.

Medical Word	Word Parts		Definition
	Part	**Meaning**	
hypercalciuria (hī″ pĕr-kăl″ sĭ-ū′ rĭ-ă)	hyper- calci -uria	excessive calcium urine	Excessive amount of calcium in the urine
incontinence (ĭn-kən′ tĭn-əns)	in- continence	not to hold	Inability to hold or control urination or defecation
interstitial cystitis (IC) (ĭn″ ter-stĭsh′ al sĭs-tī′ tĭs)			Chronically irritable and painful inflammation of the bladder wall
ketonuria (kē″ tō-nū′ rĭ-ă)	keton -uria	ketone urine	Presence of ketones in the urine resulting from breakdown of fats due to faulty carbohydrate metabolism. It occurs primarily as a complication of diabetes mellitus but can occur in dieting and starvation; also called *ketoacidosis*.
lithotripsy (lĭth′ ō trĭp″ sē)	lith/o -tripsy	stone crushing	Crushing of a kidney stone (Figure 12.8)

RULE REMINDER

This term keeps the combining vowel ***o*** because the suffix begins with a consonant.

Medical Word	Part	Meaning	Definition
meatotomy (mē″ ă-tŏt′ ō-mē)	meat/o -tomy	passage incision	Incision of the urinary meatus to enlarge the opening
meatus (mē-ā′ tŭs)			Opening or passage; the external opening of the urethra
micturition (mĭk′ tū-rĭ″ shŭn)	micturit -ion	to urinate process	Process of urination; to void; emptying the bladder
nephrectomy (nĕ-frĕk′ tō-mē)	nephr -ectomy	kidney surgical excision	Surgical excision of a kidney
nephritis (nĕf-rī′ tĭs)	nephr -itis	kidney inflammation	Inflammation of the kidney

Medical Word	Word Parts		Definition
	Part	**Meaning**	
nephrolithiasis (nĕf˝ rō-lĭth-ī´ ă-sĭs)	nephr/o lith -iasis	kidney stone, calculus condition	Commonly called *kidney stones*; usually deposits of mineral salts, called *calculi*, in the kidney. These stones can pass into the ureter, irritate kidney tissue, and block urine flow. Kidney stones occur when the urine has a high level of minerals (usually calcium) that form stones. See Figure 12.14.

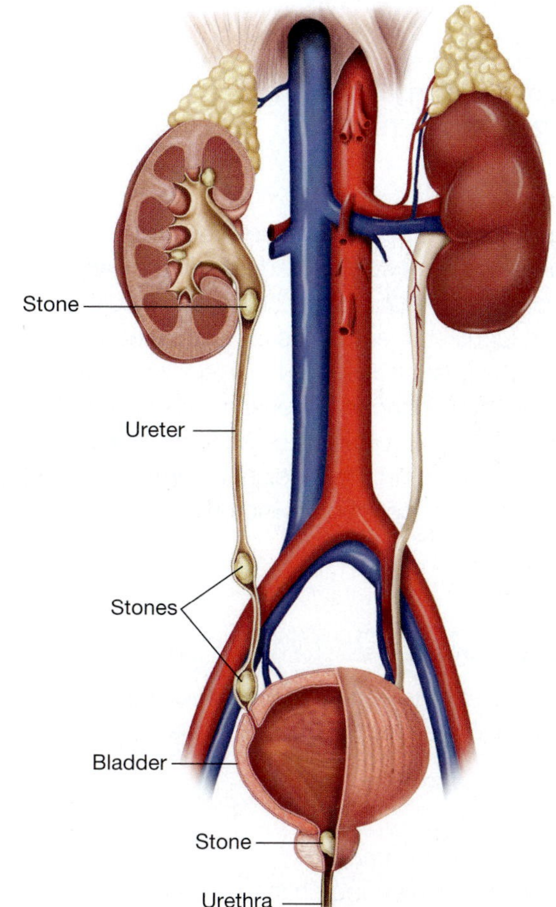

Figure 12.14 Renal calculi (stones) can form in several areas within the urinary tract. When they form in the kidney, they usually arise within the renal pelvis, forming the condition called nephrolithiasis. Stones can also form obstructions in the ureter, bladder, or urethra.

fyi Kidney stones are common and painful disorders of the urinary tract. Men tend to be affected more frequently than women. Most kidney stones pass out of the body without any intervention, but stones that cause lasting symptoms or other complications should be treated. Two treatment techniques used are **extracorporeal shock wave lithotripsy (ESWL)** (see Figure 12.8) or **percutaneous ultrasonic lithotripsy (PUL)** (see Figure 12.15).

Usually, the first symptom of a kidney stone is extreme pain, which begins suddenly when a stone moves in the urinary tract, causing irritation or blockage. A sharp, cramping pain in the back and side in the area of the kidney or in the lower abdomen is felt; nausea and vomiting may occur. If the stone is too large to pass easily, pain continues and blood may appear in the urine.

Medical Word	Part	Meaning	Definition
nephrology (nĕ-frŏl´ ō-jē)	nephr/o -logy	kidney study of	Literally means *study of the kidney*; study of kidney function as well as diagnosis and treatment of renal diseases

Medical Word	Word Parts		Definition
	Part	**Meaning**	
nephroma (nĕ-frō´ mă)	nephr -oma	kidney tumor	Kidney tumor
nephron (nĕf´ rŏn)			Basic structural and functional unit of the kidney
nephropathy (nĕ-frŏp´ ă-thē)	nephr/o -pathy	kidney disease	Pathological disease of the kidney
nephrosclerosis (nĕf″ rō-sklĕ-rō´ sĭs)	nephr/o scler -osis	kidney hardening condition	Condition of hardening of the kidney

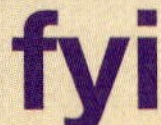

Nephrotic syndrome, also known as **nephrosis**, is a group of symptoms that includes protein in the urine (proteinuria), low blood protein levels (hypoalbuminemia), and swelling (edema). It may affect anyone regardless of age, gender, or race. Some of the causes are nephropathy and systemic diseases such as untreated/uncontrolled hypertension, diabetes, and lupus erythematosus (an autoimmune disease in which the body's immune system mistakenly attacks healthy tissue). Nephrotic syndrome can be termed *primary*, specific to the kidneys, or can be termed *secondary*, a renal manifestation of a systemic disease. In all cases, damage to the glomeruli is an essential feature, leading to the release of too much protein into the urine. Swelling (edema) in the face and around the eyes; in the arms and legs, especially the feet and ankles; and in the abdominal area is the most common symptom.

Comparative Analysis of Nephrotic Syndrome and Nephritic Syndrome

Nephrotic Syndrome	Nephritic Syndrome
Damage to the glomeruli caused by a variety of diseases or injury	Immune response triggered by infection causing inflammation and affecting the function of the glomerulus*
Hypoalbuminemia (low blood protein levels) Loss of protein 3.5 g/day*	Hypertension
Protein in urine (proteinuria)	Protein in urine (proteinuria) Granular casts in urine (tube-shaped proteins) Sediments appear in urine (pyuria)
Frothy urine	Oliguria (scanty amount of urine)
Swelling (edema)	Swelling (edema)
↑ Lipids (hyperlipidemia)	↑WBC (white blood cells—sign of infection)
↓ Antithrombin III (potential formation of deep vein thrombosis)	↑RBC (red blood cells—hematuria)
*In nephr**o**tic syndrome, loss of protein is the distinguishing sign.	*In nephr**i**tic syndrome, the immune response and hematuria are the distinguishing signs.

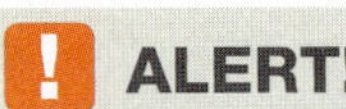

ALERT!

Nephrotic syndrome or nephritic syndrome? Pay close attention to the spelling. One letter does make a difference.

Medical Word	Word Parts		Definition
	Part	**Meaning**	
nocturia (nŏk-tū´ rĭ-ă)	noct -uria	night urine	Urination during the night
oliguria (ŏl-ĭg-ū´ rĭ-ă)	olig- -uria	scanty urine	Scanty, decreased amount of urine. The decreased production of urine may be a sign of dehydration, renal failure, hypovolemic shock, multiple organ dysfunction syndrome, or urinary obstruction/urinary retention. It can be contrasted with anuria, which represents a more complete suppression of urination.
percutaneous ultrasonic lithotripsy (PUL) (pĕr˝ kū-tā´ nē-ŭs) ŭl-tră-sŏn´ ĭk lĭth´ ō-trĭp˝ sē)	per- cutane -ous ultra- son -ic lith/o -tripsy	through skin pertaining to beyond sound pertaining to stone crushing	Crushing of a kidney stone by using ultrasound. This is an invasive surgical procedure performed by using a nephroscope or fluoroscopy. See Figure 12.15.

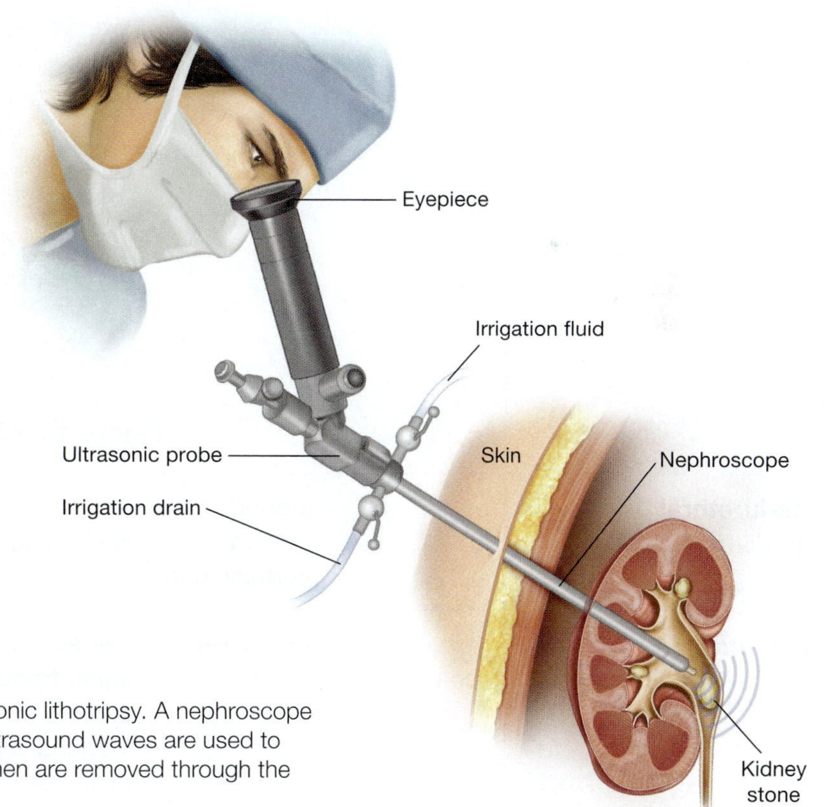

Figure 12.15 Percutaneous ultrasonic lithotripsy. A nephroscope is inserted into the renal pelvis, and ultrasound waves are used to fragment the stones. The fragments then are removed through the nephroscope.

Medical Word	Word Parts		Definition
	Part	**Meaning**	
peritoneal dialysis (PD) (pĕr″ ĭ-tō-nē′ ăl dī-ăl′ ĭ-sĭs)	peritone -al dia- -lysis	peritoneum pertaining to complete, through to separate	Separation of waste from the blood by using a peritoneal catheter and dialysis. Fluid is introduced into the peritoneal cavity, and wastes from the blood pass into this fluid. The fluid and waste are then removed from the body. Types of peritoneal dialysis are IPD—intermittent and CAPD—continuous ambulatory. See Figure 12.16.
periurethral (pĕr″ ĭ-ū-rē′ thrăl)	peri- urethr -al	around urethra pertaining to	Literally means *pertaining to around the urethra*; the immediate area surrounding the urethra
polyuria (pŏl″ ē-ū′ rĭ-ă)	poly- -uria	excessive urine	Literally means *excessive secretion and discharge of urine*; frequent urination; occurs in diabetes mellitus, chronic nephritis, and nephrosclerosis, and can be induced with diuretics and following excessive intake of liquids
pyelitis (pī″ ĕ-lī′ tĭs)	pyel -itis	renal pelvis inflammation	Inflammation of the renal pelvis
pyelolithotomy (pī″ ĕ-lō-lĭth-ŏt′ ō-mē)	pyel/o lith/o -tomy	renal pelvis stone incision	Surgical incision into the renal pelvis for removal of a stone

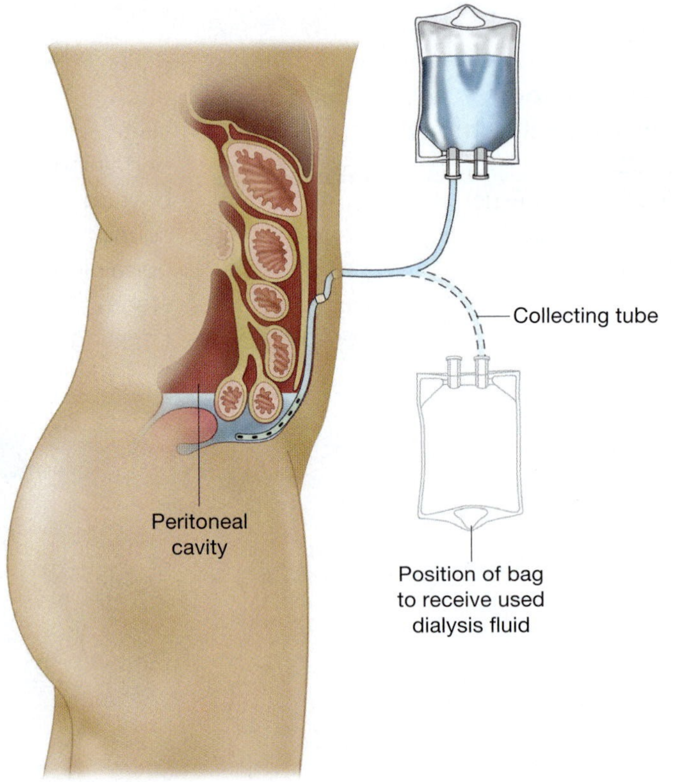

Figure 12.16 Peritoneal dialysis.

Medical Word	Word Parts		Definition
	Part	**Meaning**	
pyelonephritis (pī″ ĕ-lō-nĕ-frī′ tĭs)	pyel/o nephr -itis	renal pelvis kidney inflammation	Inflammation of the kidney and renal pelvis. It is usually caused by bacteria entering the kidneys from the bladder. *Escherichia coli* is a bacillus that is normally found in the large intestine. These infections usually spread from the lower urinary tract via the urethra, to the ureters, and then, into the renal pelvis. See Figure 12.17. From the lymph From the blood (descending) Renal pelvis From the urine (ascending) Ureter **Figure 12.17** Routes of infection for pyelonephritis.
pyuria (pī-ū′ rĭ-ă)	py -uria	pus urine	Pus or white blood cells in the urine; caused by infection (most commonly bacterial) or response to an inflammatory process in the body
renal (rē′ năl)	ren -al	kidney pertaining to	Pertaining to the kidney
renal colic (kŏl′ ĭk)			Sharp, severe pain in the lower back over the kidney, radiating forward into the groin. It usually accompanies forcible dilation of a ureter, followed by spasm as a stone is lodged or passed through it.
renal failure			Pathological failure of the kidney to function; also referred to as *kidney failure*

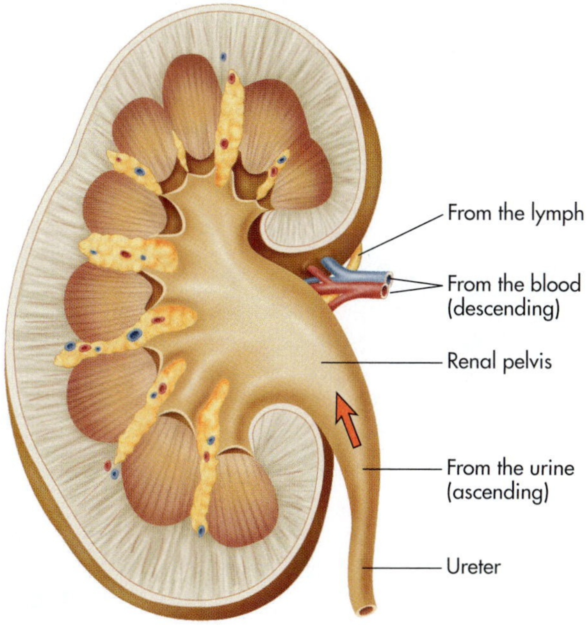

insights In the ICD-10-CM, renal failure (N18.6–N18.9) may be listed as *end-stage renal disease*, *chronic kidney disease requiring dialysis*, *chronic kidney disease unspecified*, *renal disease*, *renal insufficiency*, or *uremia*.

Medical Word	Word Parts		Definition
	Part	**Meaning**	
renal transplantation			The organ transplant of a healthy donor kidney into a patient with end-stage renal disease. The transplanted kidney takes over the work of the two kidneys that failed, so dialysis is no longer needed. Also called *kidney transplantation*. See Figure 12.18.

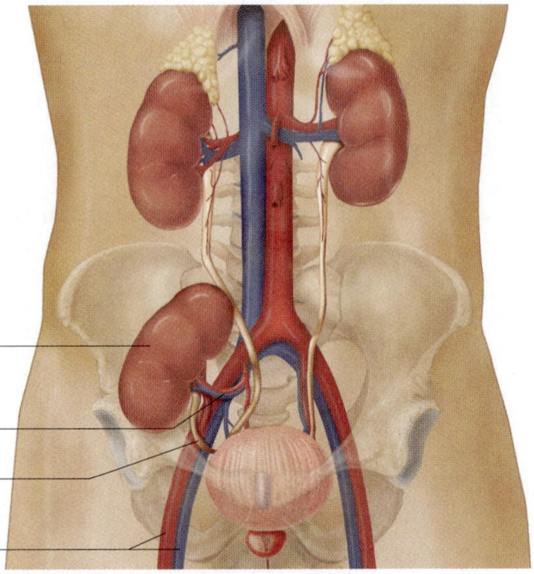

Figure 12.18 Placement of transplanted kidney.

Medical Word	Part	Meaning	Definition
renin (rĕn´ ĭn)			An enzyme produced by the kidney that stimulates vasoconstriction and secretion of aldosterone. The blood renin level is elevated in some types of hypertension.
sediment (sĕd´ ĭ-mĕnt)			Substance that settles at the bottom of a liquid; a precipitate; can be produced by centrifuging urine or other body fluids
sterile (stĕr´ ĭl)			State of being free from living microorganisms; *aseptic*
uremia (ū-rē´ mĭ-ă)	ur -emia	urine blood condition	Excess of urea, creatinine, and other nitrogenous end products of protein and amino acid metabolism accumulated in the blood; also referred to as *azotemia*. In current usage, it refers to the syndrome associated with end-stage renal failure.
ureteroplasty (ū-rē´ tĕr-ō-plăs˝ tē)	ureter/o -plasty	ureter surgical repair	Surgical repair of the ureter

Medical Word	Word Parts		Definition
	Part	**Meaning**	
ureterostomy (ū-rē″ tĕr-ŏs´ tō-mē)	ureter/o -stomy	ureter new opening	Surgical creation of a new opening into the ureter to provide an alternate route for drainage of urine. Example: cutaneous ureter is the surgical implantation of the ureter into the skin.
urethral stricture (ū-rē´ thrăl strĭk´ chŭr)	urethr -al strict -ure	urethra pertaining to to tighten, contraction process	Narrowing or constriction of the urethra
urethroperineal (ū-rē″ thrō-pĕr″ ĭ-nē´ ăl)	urethr/o perine -al	urethra perineum pertaining to	Pertaining to the urethra and perineum

ALERT!

Note the difference between the combining forms **ureter/o** and **urethr/o**. The *ureters* are tubes that lead from the kidney to the bladder and the *urethra* is a tube that leads from the bladder to the outside of the body. What a difference a few letters make!

Medical Word	Part	Meaning	Definition
urgency			Sudden need to void, urinate
urinometer (ū″ rĭ-nŏm´ ĕ-tĕr)	urin/o -meter	urine instrument to measure	Medical instrument used to measure the specific gravity of urine. See Figure 12.19.

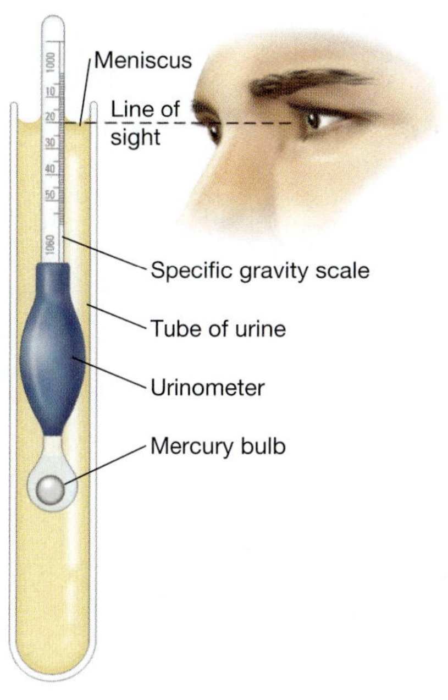

Figure 12.19 Urinometer. In this procedure, a urine sample and urinometer are placed within a tube, and the liquid level is compared to the scale. The procedure provides information on the concentration of solids within a urine sample.

Medical Word	Word Parts		Definition
	Part	**Meaning**	
urobilin (ū″ rō-bī′ lĭn)	ur/o bil -in	urination bile chemical	Brown pigment formed by the oxidation of urobilinogen; may be formed in the urine after exposure to air
urochrome (ū′ rō-krōm)			Pigment that gives urine the normal yellow color
urologist (ū-rŏl′ ō-jĭst)	ur/o log -ist	urination study of one who specializes	Physician who specializes in the study of the urinary system
urology (ū-rŏl′ ō-jē)	ur/o -logy	urination study of	Study of the urinary system

Study and Review II

Word Parts

Prefixes

Give the definitions of the following prefixes.

1. an- ______________________
2. anti- ______________________
3. dia- ______________________
4. dys- ______________________
5. en- ______________________
6. hydro- ______________________
7. extra- ______________________
8. in- ______________________
9. olig- ______________________
10. per- ______________________
11. ultra- ______________________
12. poly- ______________________

Combining Forms

Give the definitions of the following combining forms.

1. albumin/o ______________________
2. bacter/i ______________________
3. calc/i ______________________
4. corpore/o ______________________
5. cyst/o ______________________
6. excret/o ______________________
7. glomerul/o ______________________
8. glycos/o ______________________
9. hemat/o ______________________
10. keton/o ______________________
11. lith/o ______________________
12. meat/o ______________________
13. micturit/o ______________________
14. nephr/o ______________________
15. noct/o ______________________
16. perine/o ______________________
17. peritone/o ______________________
18. pyel/o ______________________
19. ren/o ______________________
20. son/o ______________________
21. ur/o ______________________
22. ureter/o ______________________
23. urethr/o ______________________
24. urin/o ______________________

Suffixes

Give the definitions of the following suffixes.

1. -al ______________________
2. -ar ______________________
3. -cele ______________________
4. -dynia ______________________
5. -y ______________________
6. -ous ______________________
7. -ectomy ______________________
8. -emia ______________________
9. -gram ______________________
10. -ic ______________________
11. -in ______________________
12. -ion ______________________
13. -ist ______________________
14. -itis ______________________
15. -lith ______________________
16. -logy ______________________
17. -lysis ______________________
18. -tripsy ______________________
19. -ure ______________________
20. -meter ______________________
21. -oma ______________________
22. -osis ______________________
23. -pathy ______________________
24. -plasty ______________________
25. -scope ______________________
26. -esis ______________________
27. -stomy ______________________
28. -tomy ______________________
29. -uria ______________________

Identifying Medical Terms

In the spaces provided, write the medical terms for the following meanings.

1. ______________________ Pertaining to a medication that decreases urine production and secretion
2. ______________________ Surgical excision of the bladder or part of the bladder
3. ______________________ Inflammation of the bladder
4. ______________________ Difficult or painful urination
5. ______________________ Inflammation of the renal glomeruli
6. ______________________ Excessive amount of calcium in the urine
7. ______________________ Process of voiding urine
8. ______________________ Kidney stones

9. ______________________ Pertaining to around the urethra

10. ______________________ Pus in the urine

11. ______________________ Surgical repair of the ureter

12. ______________________ Analysis of urine

13. ______________________ Physician who specializes in the study of the urinary system

Matching

Select the appropriate lettered meaning for each of the following words.

______ **1.** ESWL

______ **2.** hemodialysis

______ **3.** lithotripsy

______ **4.** peritoneal dialysis

______ **5.** renal colic

______ **6.** urethral stricture

______ **7.** urgency

______ **8.** urination

______ **9.** urochrome

______ **10.** urinometer

a. Sharp, severe pain in the lower back over the kidney radiating forward into the groin caused by a stone in a ureter

b. Crushing of a kidney stone

c. Process of voiding urine

d. Medical device used to crush kidney stones

e. Use of an artificial kidney to separate waste from the blood

f. Separation of waste from the blood by using a peritoneal catheter and dialysis

g. Narrowing or constriction of the urethra

h. Pigment that gives urine its normal yellow color

i. Medical instrument used to measure the specific gravity of urine

j. Sudden need to void, urinate

k. Analysis of urine

Medical Case Snapshots

This learning activity provides an opportunity to relate the medical terminology you are learning to a precise patient case presentation. In the spaces provided, write in your answers.

Case 1

A 10-year-old girl is referred to an urologist. She complained that "It hurts me every time I have to go to the bathroom and I go a lot at night." The medical term ______________ (means painful urination) and the term ______________ (means urination during the night). The clean-catch urine specimen appeared smoky and had an unpleasant odor. Under microscopic examination, the urine was found to contain red blood cells. This condition is called ______________.

Case 2

The physician ordered a complete UA, an abbreviation for ________________. The results show: *color* (reddish), which indicated the presence of ______________; *reaction* 9.0 pH (alkaline urine), which is indicative of ______________ ______________ ______________; and *nitrites positive*, indicating ________________ (presence of bacteria in the urine). The diagnosis of ______________ (inflammation of the bladder) was confirmed.

Case 3

A 30-year-old male is seen in the ER. He complains of sharp, severe pain in the lower back, over the kidney, radiating forward into his groin. Because of the patient's symptoms, the physician wants to evaluate him for ______________ (commonly called kidney stones). Two treatment techniques that can be used are: ESWL, which stands for ______________ ______________ ______________ lithotripsy, and PUL, or percutaneous ______________ lithotripsy. See Figures 12.8 and 12.15.

Drug Highlights

Type of Drug	Description and Examples
diuretics	Decrease in reabsorption of sodium chloride by the kidneys, thereby increasing the amount of salt and water excreted in the urine. This action reduces the amount of fluid retained in the body and prevents edema. Diuretics are classified according to site and mechanism of action. The following are different types of diuretics.
thiazide	Appear to act by inhibiting sodium and chloride reabsorption in the early portion of the distal tubule. EXAMPLES: Diuril (chlorothiazide), hydrochlorothiazide, and indapamide
loop	Act by inhibiting the reabsorption of sodium and chloride in the ascending loop of Henle. EXAMPLES: bumetanide and Lasix (furosemide)
potassium sparing	Act by inhibiting the exchange of sodium for potassium in the distal tubule; inhibits potassium excretion. EXAMPLES: Aldactone (spironolactone) and Dyrenium (triamterene)
osmotic	Capable of being filtered by the glomerulus but have a limited capability of being reabsorbed into the bloodstream. EXAMPLE: Osmitrol (mannitol)
carbonic anhydrase inhibitor	Act to increase the excretion of bicarbonate (HCO_3) ion, which carries out sodium (Na), water (H_2O), and potassium (K). EXAMPLE: Diamox (acetazolamide)
urinary tract antibacterials	Sulfonamides are generally the drugs of choice for treating acute, uncomplicated urinary tract infections, especially those caused by *Escherichia coli* and *Proteus mirabilis* bacterial strains. They exert a bacteriostatic effect against a wide range of gram-positive and gram-negative microorganisms. EXAMPLES: sulfadiazine, Bactrim, and Septra, which are mixtures of trimethoprim and sulfamethoxazole
urinary tract antiseptics	May inhibit the growth of microorganisms by bactericidal, bacteriostatic, anti-infective, and/or antibacterial action. EXAMPLES: Furadantin and Macrodantin (nitrofurantoin), methenamine hippurate, and Cipro (ciprofloxacin HCl)

Type of Drug	Description and Examples
other drugs	Treat disorders of the lower urinary tract by either stimulating or inhibiting smooth muscle activity, thereby improving urinary bladder functions. These functions are the storage of urine and its subsequent excretion from the body. EXAMPLES: flavoxate HCl and Urecholine (bethanechol chloride)
Rimso-50 (dimethyl sulfoxide)	Used in the treatment of interstitial cystitis.
flavoxate HCl	Reduces dysuria, nocturia, and urinary frequency.
Tofranil (imipramine HCl)	Treats nocturnal enuresis in children.
Ditropan XL (oxybutynin chloride)	Relaxes the muscles in the bladder, thereby decreasing the occurrence of wetting accidents.
Detrol (tolterodine tartrate)	Helps control involuntary contractions of the bladder muscle.

Diagnostic and Laboratory Tests

Test	Description
blood urea nitrogen (BUN) (ū-rē´ ă nī´ trō-jĕn)	Blood test to determine the amount of urea excreted by the kidneys. Abnormal results indicate renal dysfunction.
creatinine (krē-ăt´ ĭ-nēn)	Blood test to determine the amount of creatinine present and to determine the glomerular filtration rate (GFR). Abnormal results indicate renal dysfunction.

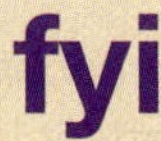

Kidney function is measured by how well the kidneys clean the blood. The glomerular filtration rate (GFR) tests how well the kidneys are working. The main factor in estimating the GFR is determining the level of *creatinine* in the blood. When kidneys are functioning, they remove creatinine from the blood. As kidney function slows, blood levels of creatinine rise. This test is also used to determine the patient's stage of kidney disease.

GFR Classification of Chronic Kidney Disease

Stage	Description	GFR
3	Moderately decreasing GFR	30–59 mL/min
4	Severely decreasing GFR	15–29 mL/min
5	Kidney failure	<15 mL/min

Note: Normal GFR is >60 mL/min

Test	Description
creatinine clearance (krē-ăt´ ĭ-nēn)	Urine test to determine the glomerular filtration rate (GFR). Abnormal results indicate renal dysfunction.

Test	Description
culture, urine	Urine test to determine the presence of microorganisms. Abnormal results indicate urinary tract infection.
cystoscopy (cysto) (sĭs-tŏs´ kŭ-pē)	Visual examination of the bladder and urethra via a lighted cystoscope. Abnormal results can indicate the presence of renal calculi, a tumor, prostatic hyperplasia, and/or bleeding.
intravenous pyelography (pyelogram) (IVP) (ĭn-tră-vē´ nŭs pī˝ ĕ-lŏg´ ră-fē)	Test to visualize the kidneys, ureters, and bladder. A radiopaque substance is intravenously injected, and x-rays are taken. Abnormal results can indicate renal calculi, kidney or bladder tumors, and kidney disease.
kidney, ureter, bladder (KUB)	With the patient supine, a flat-plate x-ray is taken of the abdomen to indicate the size and position of the kidneys, ureters, and bladder
renal biopsy	Removal of tissue from the kidney. Abnormal results can indicate kidney cancer, kidney transplant rejection, and glomerulonephritis.
retrograde pyelography (RP) (rĕt´rō-grād)	X-ray recording of the kidneys, ureters, and bladder following the injection of a contrast medium backward through a urinary catheter into the ureters and the calyces of the pelvis of the kidneys. Useful in locating urinary stones and obstructions. See Figure 12.20. 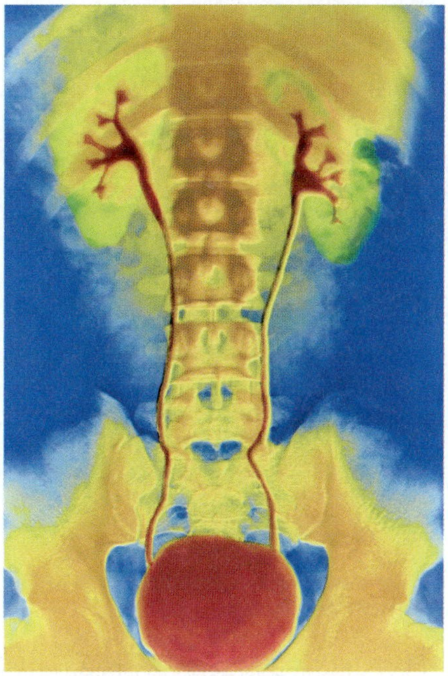 **Figure 12.20** Retrograde pyelography (RP). Note the contrasting of the renal calyces, ureters, and bladder following an injection of a contrast medium. (Courtesy of CNRI/Science Source)
ultrasonography, kidneys (ŭl-tră-sŏn-ŏg´ ră-fē)	Use of high-frequency sound waves to visualize the kidneys. The sound waves (echoes) are recorded on an oscilloscope and film. Abnormal results can indicate kidney tumors, cysts, abscess, and kidney disease.

Abbreviations

Abbreviation	Meaning	Abbreviation	Meaning
AGN	acute glomerulonephritis	**H_2O**	water
ANS	acute nephritic syndrome	**IC**	interstitial cystitis
BPH	benign prostatic hyperplasia	**IPD**	intermittent peritoneal dialysis
BUN	blood urea nitrogen	**IVP**	intravenous pyelogram
CAPD	continuous ambulatory peritoneal dialysis	**K**	potassium
CGN	chronic glomerulonephritis	**KUB**	kidney, ureter, bladder
CKD	chronic kidney disease	**mL**	milliliter
CLIA	clinical laboratory improvement amendments	**mm**	millimeter
cm	centimeter	**Na**	sodium
cysto	cystoscopy	**NaCl**	sodium chloride
ESRD	end-stage renal disease	**PD**	peritoneal dialysis
ESWL	extracorporeal shock wave lithotripsy	**pH**	hydrogen ion concentration
GFR	glomerular filtration rate	**PUL**	percutaneous ultrasonic lithotripsy
GU	genitourinary	**RP**	retrograde pyelography
HCO_3	bicarbonate	**sp. gr.**	specific gravity
HD	hemodialysis	**UA**	urinalysis
		UG	urogenital
		UTI	urinary tract infection

Study and Review III

Building Medical Terms

Using the following word parts, fill in the blanks to build the correct medical terms.

olig-	meat/o	-ion
cyst/o	nephr/o	-uria
continence	ren	

Definition	Medical Term
1. Indicates the presence of serum protein in the urine	albumin______
2. X-ray record of the bladder	________gram
3. Inability to hold or control urination or defecation	in__________
4. Incision of the urinary meatus to enlarge the opening	________tomy
5. Process of urination	micturit______
6. Kidney stones	_______lithiasis

Definition	Medical Term
7. Scanty, decreased amount of urine	_________uria
8. Literally means excessive secretion and discharge of urine	poly_________
9. Pertaining to the kidney	___________al
10. Process of voiding urine	urinat_______

Combining Form Challenge

Using the combining forms provided, write the medical term correctly.

cyst/o	lith/o	noct/o
glycos/o	nephr/o	ureter/o

1. Hernia of the bladder that protrudes into the vagina: ___________ cele
2. Presence of glucose in the urine: ___________ uria
3. Crushing of a kidney stone: ___________ tripsy
4. Kidney tumor: ___________ oma
5. Urination during the night: ___________ uria
6. Disease of the ureter: ___________ pathy

Select the Right Term

Select the correct answer, and write it on the line provided.

1. Presence of calcium in the urine.

   anuria **calciuria** **calculus** **calcuria**

2. Pathological condition in which the body tissues contain an accumulation of fluid is ____________.

   excretory **diuresis** **enuresis** **edema**

3. Presence of red blood cells in the urine is ___________.

   glycosuria **hematuria** **calciuria** **ketonuria**

4. Condition of hardening of the kidney is _________.

   nephology **nephrectomy** **nephritis** **nephrosclerosis**

5. Inflammation of the kidney and renal pelvis is ____________.

   pyelitis **pyelolithotomy** **pyelonephritis** **pyelcystitis**

6. Sharp, severe pain in the lower back over the kidney is ____________.

   renal failure **renal colic** **rennin** **stricture**

Diagnostic and Laboratory Tests

Select the best answer to each multiple-choice question. Circle the letter of your choice.

1. Urine test to determine the glomerular filtration rate.

a. BUN
b. creatinine
c. creatinine clearance
d. KUB

2. Urine test to determine the presence of microorganisms.

a. BUN
b. creatinine
c. urine culture
d. KUB

3. Test to visualize the kidneys, ureters, and bladder. A radiopaque substance is used and x-rays are taken.

a. cystoscopy
b. intravenous pyelography
c. KUB
d. renal biopsy

4. Use of high-frequency sound waves to visualize the kidneys.

a. retrograde pyelography
b. intravenous pyelography
c. ultrasonography
d. cystoscopy

5. Flat-plate x-ray of the abdomen to indicate the size and position of the kidneys, ureters, and bladder.

a. cystoscopy
b. KUB
c. BUN
d. retrograde pyelography

Abbreviations

Place the correct word, phrase, or abbreviation in the space provided.

1. acute glomerulonephritis ______________________________

2. BUN ______________________________

3. chronic kidney disease ______________________________

4. cysto ______________________________

5. GU ______________________________

6. HD ______________________________

7. intravenous pyelogram ______________________________

8. PD ______________________________

9. pH ______________________________

10. urinalysis ______________________________

Practical Application

Medical Record Analysis

This exercise contains information, abbreviations, and medical terminology from an actual medical record or case study that has been adapted for this text. The names and any personal information are made up by the author. Read and study each form or case study and then answer the questions that follow. You may refer to Appendix III, *Abbreviations and Symbols*.

Note: Congress passed the Clinical Laboratory Improvement Amendments (CLIA) in 1988, establishing quality standards for all laboratory testing to ensure the accuracy, reliability, and timeliness of patient test results regardless of where the test was performed.

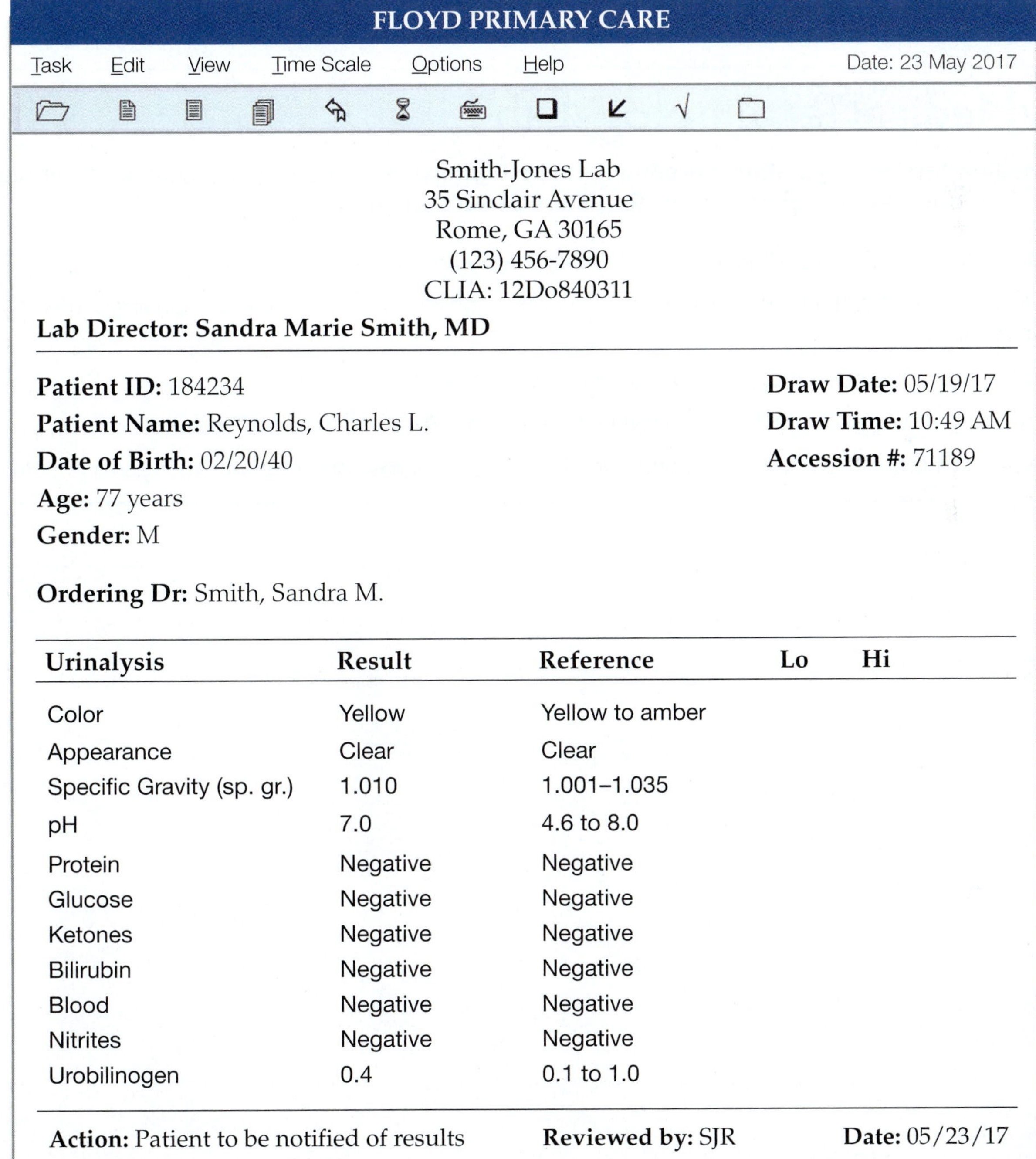

FLOYD PRIMARY CARE

Task Edit View Time Scale Options Help   Date: 23 May 2017

Smith-Jones Lab
35 Sinclair Avenue
Rome, GA 30165
(123) 456-7890
CLIA: 12Do840311

Lab Director: Sandra Marie Smith, MD

Patient ID: 184234
Patient Name: Reynolds, Charles L.
Date of Birth: 02/20/40
Age: 77 years
Gender: M

Draw Date: 05/19/17
Draw Time: 10:49 AM
Accession #: 71189

Ordering Dr: Smith, Sandra M.

Urinalysis	Result	Reference	Lo	Hi
Color	Yellow	Yellow to amber		
Appearance	Clear	Clear		
Specific Gravity (sp. gr.)	1.010	1.001–1.035		
pH	7.0	4.6 to 8.0		
Protein	Negative	Negative		
Glucose	Negative	Negative		
Ketones	Negative	Negative		
Bilirubin	Negative	Negative		
Blood	Negative	Negative		
Nitrites	Negative	Negative		
Urobilinogen	0.4	0.1 to 1.0		

Action: Patient to be notified of results   **Reviewed by:** SJR   **Date:** 05/23/17

Medical Record Questions

Place the correct answer in the space provided.

1. What is the normal color of urine? ______________________
2. Define specific gravity and give the normal sp. gr. of urine. ______________________
3. This patient's pH was 7.0. Is this higher or lower than the average pH? ______________________
4. This patient's report indicated a urobilinogen of 0.4. Is this within normal range? ______________________
5. What would an increased amount of urobilinogen indicate? ______________________

Chapter 13

Endocrine System

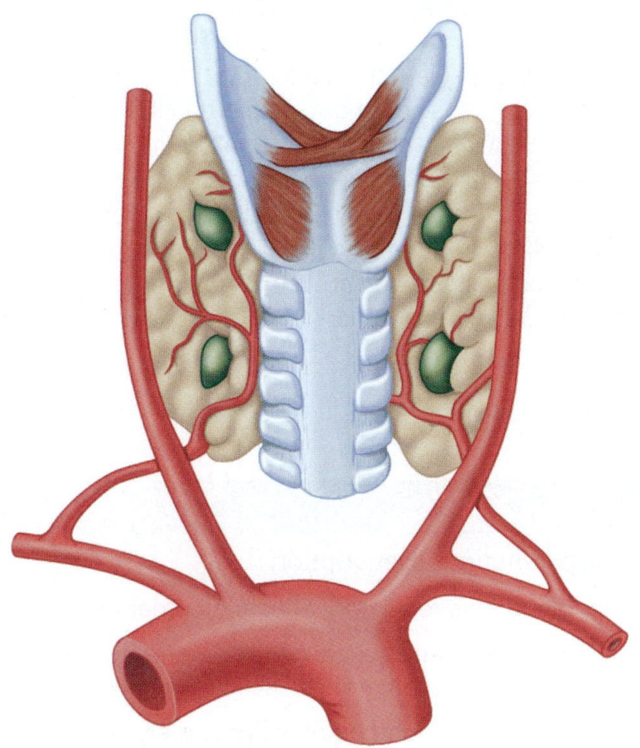

Learning Outcomes

On completion of this chapter, you will be able to:

1. Describe the vital function of the endocrine system.
2. State the description and primary functions of the organs/structures of the endocrine system.
3. Identify the various hormones secreted by the endocrine glands and their hormonal function.
4. Recognize terminology included in the ICD-10-CM.
5. Analyze, build, spell, and pronounce medical words.
6. Comprehend the drugs highlighted in this chapter.
7. Describe diagnostic and laboratory tests related to the endocrine system.
8. Identify and define selected abbreviations.
9. Apply your acquired knowledge of medical terms by successfully completing the *Practical Application* exercise.

Anatomy and Physiology

The endocrine system is made up of glands, each of which secretes a type of hormone into the bloodstream. The glands of the endocrine system and the hormones they release influence almost every cell, organ, and function of the body. Although the endocrine glands are the body's main hormone producers, some other organs such as the brain, heart, lungs, liver, skin, thymus, and the gastrointestinal mucosa, as well as the placenta during pregnancy, produce and release hormones. The primary glands of the endocrine system are the pituitary, pineal, thyroid, parathyroid, pancreas (islets of Langerhans), adrenals, ovaries in the female, and testes in the male.

The vital function of the endocrine system involves the production and regulation of chemical substances called *hormones*. A hormone is a chemical transmitter that is released in small amounts and transported via the bloodstream to a target organ or other cells. The word *hormone* is derived from the Greek language and means *to excite* or *to urge on*. As the body's chemical messengers, hormones transfer information and instructions from one set of cells to another. They regulate growth, development, mood, tissue function, homeostasis, metabolism, and sexual function in the male and female. Table 13.1 provides an at-a-glance look at the endocrine system. Figure 13.1 shows the primary glands of the endocrine system.

Table 13.1 Endocrine System at-a-Glance

Gland	Primary Functions/Description
Pituitary (hypophysis)	Master gland; has regulatory effects on other endocrine glands
Anterior lobe (adenohypophysis)	Influences growth and sexual development, thyroid function, adrenocortical function; regulates skin pigmentation
Posterior lobe (neurohypophysis)	Stimulates the reabsorption of water and elevates blood pressure; stimulates the uterus to contract during labor, delivery, and parturition; stimulates the release of milk during suckling
Pineal	Helps regulate the release of gonadotropin and controls body pigmentation
Thyroid	Plays vital role in metabolism; regulates the body's metabolic processes; influences bone and calcium metabolism; helps maintain plasma calcium homeostasis
Parathyroid	Maintains normal serum calcium level; plays a role in the metabolism of phosphorus
Pancreas (islets of Langerhans)	Regulates blood glucose levels; plays a vital role in metabolism of carbohydrates, proteins, and fats
Adrenals (suprarenals)	
Adrenal cortex	Regulates carbohydrate metabolism, anti-inflammatory effect; helps body cope during stress; regulates electrolyte and water balance; promotes development of male characteristics
Adrenal medulla	Synthesizes, secretes, and stores catecholamines (sympathomimetic hormones: dopamine, epinephrine, norepinephrine)
Ovaries	Promote growth, development, and maintenance of female sex organs
Testes	Promote growth, development, and maintenance of male sex organs

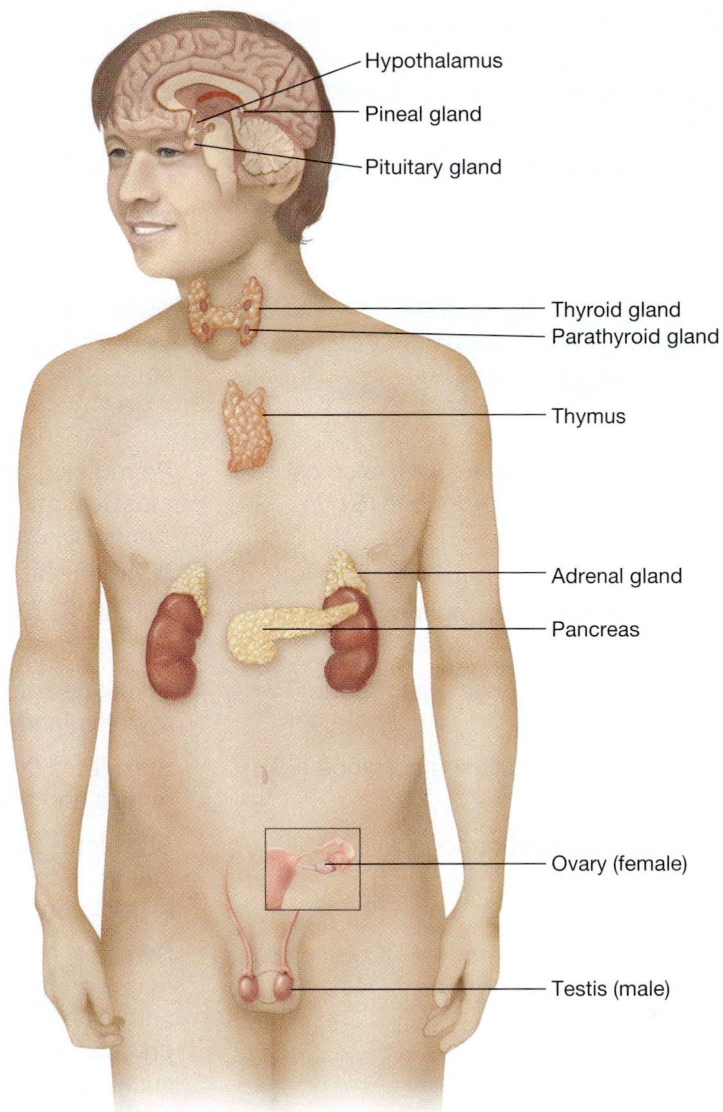

Figure 13.1 Glands of the endocrine system.

Hyposecretion or hypersecretion of specific hormones of the endocrine system cause or are associated with many pathological conditions. Too much or too little of any hormone can be harmful to the body. Controlling the production of or replacing specific hormones can treat many hormonal disorders and/or conditions.

The endocrine system and the nervous system work closely together to help maintain homeostasis (a state of equilibrium that is maintained within the body's internal environment). The **hypothalamus**, a collection of specialized cells that are located in the lower central part of the brain, is the primary link between the endocrine and nervous system (see Figure 13.1). Nerve cells in the hypothalamus control the pituitary gland by producing chemicals that either stimulate or suppress hormone secretions from the pituitary. The hypothalamus synthesizes and secretes releasing hormones such as thyrotropin-releasing hormone (TRH) and gonadotropin-releasing hormone (GnRH) and releasing factors such as corticotropin-releasing factor (CRF), growth hormone–releasing factor (GHRF), prolactin-releasing factor (PRF), and melanocyte-stimulating hormone–releasing factor (MRF). The hypothalamus also synthesizes and secretes release-inhibiting hormones such as growth hormone release-inhibiting hormone. It also produces release-inhibiting factors such as prolactin release-inhibiting factor (PIF) and melanocyte-stimulating hormone release-inhibiting factor (MIF). The hypothalamus also exerts direct nervous control over the adrenal medulla and controls the secretion of the hormones epinephrine and norepinephrine. See Table 13.2 for an overview of the endocrine glands, hormones, and hormonal functions.

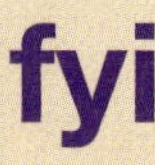

Most of the structures and glands of the endocrine system develop in the fetus during the first 3 months of pregnancy. The endocrine system of the newborn is supplemented by hormones that cross the placental barrier. Both male and female newborns may have swelling of the breast and genitalia from maternal hormones.

Table 13.2 Summary of the Endocrine Glands, Hormones, and Hormonal Functions

Endocrine Glands	Hormones	Hormonal Functions
Pituitary gland		
Anterior lobe	Growth hormone (GH) (also called *somatotropin hormone [STH]*)	Promotes growth and development of bones, muscles, and other organs; enhances protein synthesis, decreases the use of glucose, and promotes fat destruction (lipolysis)
	Adrenocorticotropin hormone (ACTH)	Stimulates growth and development of the adrenal cortex
	Thyroid-stimulating hormone (TSH)	Stimulates growth and development of the thyroid gland
	Follicle-stimulating hormone (FSH)	Stimulates the growth of ovarian follicles in the female and sperm in the male
	Luteinizing hormone (LH)	Stimulates the development of the corpus luteum in the female and the production of testosterone in the male
	Prolactin hormone (PRL) (also called *lactogenic hormone [LTH]*)	Stimulates the development and growth of the mammary glands; important in the initiation and maintenance of milk production during pregnancy. Following childbirth, the act of suckling provides the stimulus for prolactin synthesis and release. When suckling ceases, prolactin secretion slows and milk production decreases and then stops.
	Melanocyte-stimulating hormone (MSH)	Regulates skin pigmentation and promotes the deposit of melanin in the skin after exposure to sunlight
Posterior lobe	Antidiuretic hormone (ADH) (also called *vasopressin [VP]*)	Stimulates the reabsorption of water by the renal tubules and has a pressor (stimulating) effect that elevates the blood pressure
	Oxytocin	Stimulates the uterus to contract during labor, delivery, and parturition; stimulates the release of milk during suckling
Pineal gland	Melatonin	Helps regulate the release of gonadotropin and influences the body's internal clock
	Serotonin	Stimulates neurotransmitter, vasoconstrictor, and smooth muscle; acts to inhibit gastric secretion

(*continued*)

Table 13.2 Summary of the Endocrine Glands, Hormones, and Hormonal Functions (*continued*)

Endocrine Glands	Hormones	Hormonal Functions
Thyroid gland	Thyroxine (T_4)	Maintains and regulates the basal metabolic rate (BMR); influences growth and development, both physical and mental, and the metabolism of fats, proteins, carbohydrates, water, vitamins, and minerals; can be synthetically produced or extracted from animal thyroid glands in crystalline form to be used in the treatment of thyroid dysfunction, especially cretinism, myxedema, and Hashimoto disease
	Triiodothyronine (T_3)	Influences the basal metabolic rate and is more biologically active than thyroxine
	Calcitonin	Influences bone and calcium metabolism and helps maintain plasma calcium homeostasis; also known as thyrocalcitonin
Parathyroid glands	Parathyroid hormone (PTH) (also called *parathormone*)	Plays a role in maintenance of a normal serum calcium level and in the metabolism of phosphorus
Pancreas		
Islets of Langerhans	Glucagon	Facilitates the breakdown of glycogen to glucose
	Insulin	Plays a role in maintenance of normal blood sugar. It promotes the entry of glucose into the cells, thereby lowering the blood glucose (BG) level.
	Somatostatin	Suppresses the release of glucagon and insulin
Adrenal glands		
Cortex	Cortisol	Regulates carbohydrate, protein, and fat metabolism; needed for gluconeogenesis; increases blood sugar level; provides anti-inflammatory effect; helps body cope during times of stress
	Corticosterone	Essential for normal use of carbohydrates, the absorption of glucose, and gluconeogenesis; also influences potassium (K) and sodium (Na) metabolism
	Aldosterone	Essential in regulating electrolyte and water balance by promoting sodium and chloride reabsorption and potassium excretion
	Testosterone	Influences development of male secondary sex characteristics
	Androsterone	Influences development of male secondary sex characteristics
Medulla	Dopamine	Dilates systemic arteries, elevates systolic blood pressure, increases cardiac output, increases urinary output
	Epinephrine (also called *adrenaline*)	Acts as vasoconstrictor, vasopressor, cardiac stimulant, antispasmodic, and sympathomimetic
	Norepinephrine (also called *noradrenaline*)	Acts as vasoconstrictor, vasopressor, and neurotransmitter

(*continued*)

Table 13.2 Summary of the Endocrine Glands, Hormones, and Hormonal Functions (*continued*)

Endocrine Glands	Hormones	Hormonal Functions
Ovaries	Estrogens (estradiol, estrone, and estriol)	Essential for the growth, development, and maintenance of female sex organs and secondary sex characteristics; promote the development of the mammary glands; play a vital role in a woman's emotional well-being and sexual drive
	Progesterone	Prepares the uterus for pregnancy
Testes	Testosterone	Essential for normal growth and development of the male accessory sex organs; plays a vital role in the erection process of the penis and thus is necessary for the sexual act, *copulation* (sexual intercourse)
Thymus gland	Thymosin	Promotes the maturation process of T lymphocytes
	Thymopoietin	Influences the production of lymphocyte precursors and aids in their process of becoming T lymphocytes
Gastrointestinal mucosa	Gastrin	Stimulates gastric acid secretion
	Secretin	Stimulates pancreatic juice, bile, and intestinal secretion
	Cholecystokinin	Causes contraction and emptying of the gallbladder and secretion of pancreatic enzymes
	Enterogastrone	Regulates gastric secretions

Pituitary Gland (Hypophysis)

The **pituitary gland** is a small gray gland located at the base of the brain (Figure 13.1). It lies or rests in a shallow depression of the sphenoid bone known as the *sella turcica*. It is attached by the infundibulum stalk to the hypothalamus. The pituitary is approximately 1 centimeter (cm) in diameter and weighs approximately 0.6 gram (g). It is divided into the anterior lobe (*adenohypophysis*) and the posterior lobe (*neurohypophysis*). The pituitary is also called the **master gland** of the body because of its regulatory effects on the other endocrine glands.

Anterior Lobe

The *adenohypophysis* or **anterior lobe** secretes several hormones that are essential for the growth and development of bones, muscles, other organs, sex glands, the thyroid gland, and the adrenal cortex. The hormones secreted by the anterior lobe and their functions are described in Table 13.2 and shown in Figure 13.2.

Posterior Lobe

The *neurohypophysis* or **posterior lobe** stores and secretes two important hormones that are synthesized in the hypothalamus. The hormones secreted by the posterior lobe and their functions are described in Table 13.2 and shown in Figure 13.2.

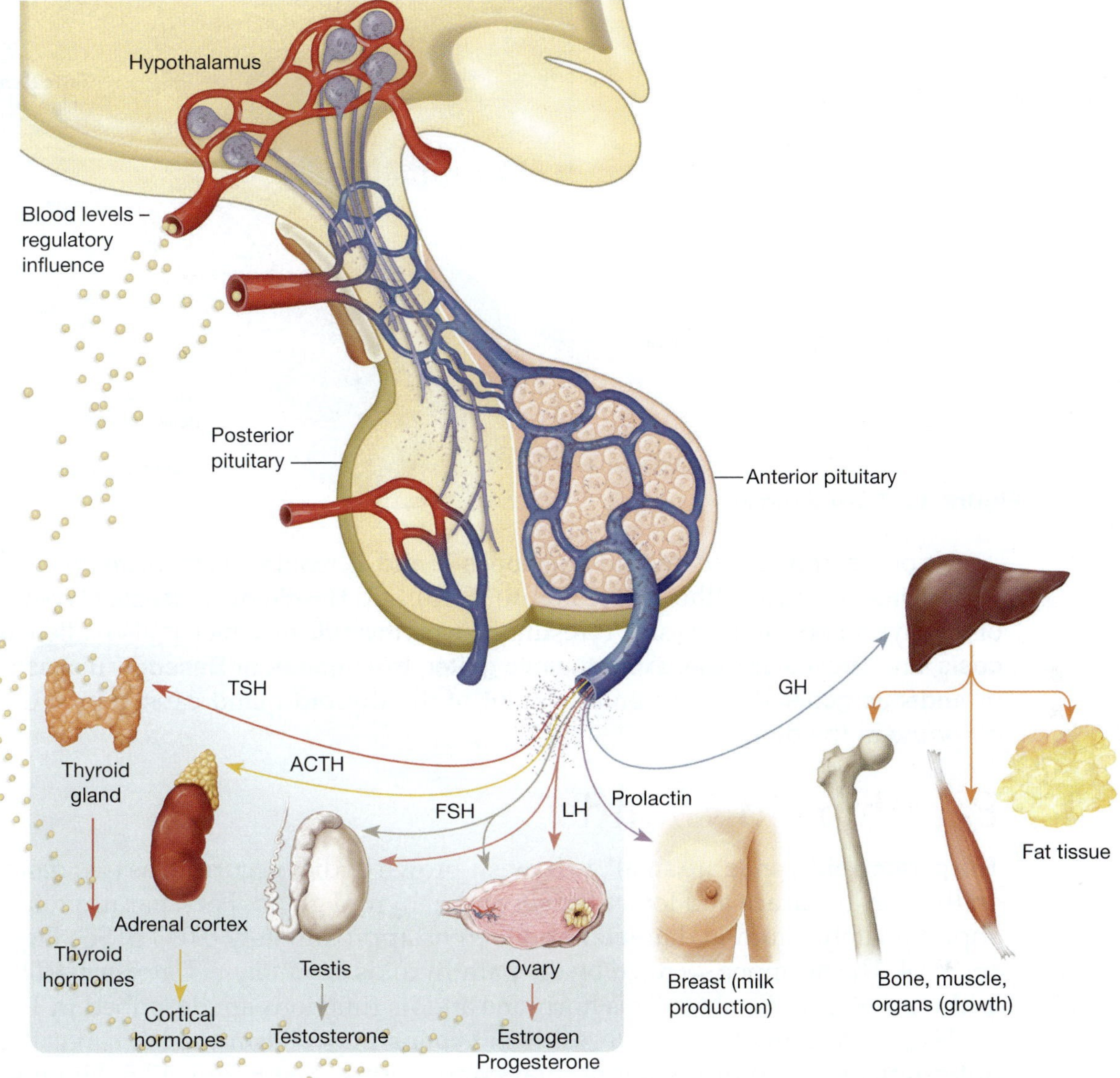

Figure 13.2 The pituitary gland with examples of the pituitary hormones it secretes, showing their target cells, tissues, and/or organs.

Pineal Gland

The **pineal gland** is a small, pine cone–shaped gland located near the posterior end of the corpus callosum. It is less than 1 cm in diameter and weighs approximately 0.1 g (see Figure 13.1). The pineal gland secretes **melatonin** and **serotonin**. Melatonin is a hormone that can be released at night to help regulate the release of gonadotropin. Serotonin is a hormone that is a neurotransmitter, vasoconstrictor, and smooth muscle stimulant and acts to inhibit gastric secretion.

Thyroid Gland

The **thyroid gland** is a large, bilobed gland located in the neck. It is anterior to the trachea and just below the thyroid cartilage. The thyroid is approximately 5 cm long and 3 cm wide and weighs approximately 30 g. See Figures 13.1 and 13.3. It plays a vital role in metabolism and regulates the body's metabolic processes. The hormones secreted by the thyroid gland and their functions are described in Table 13.2.

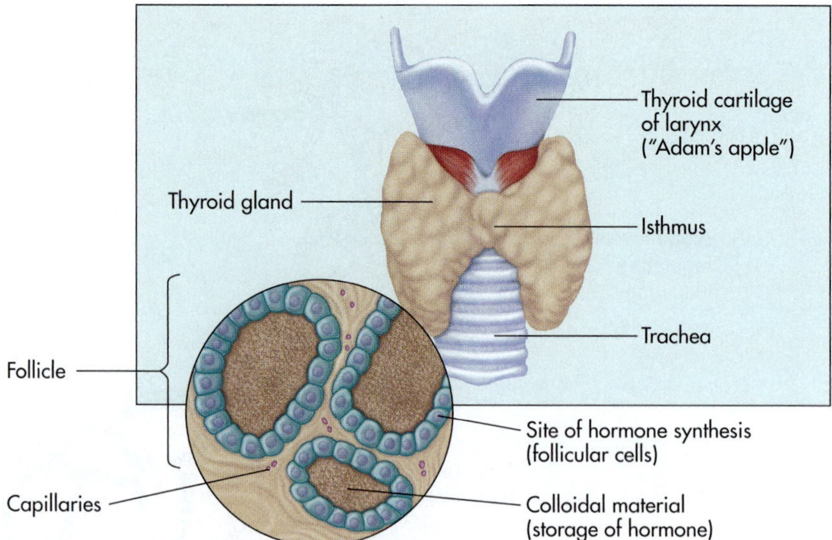

Figure 13.3 Thyroid gland.

Hyposecretion of the thyroid hormones T_3 and T_4 results in **cretinism** during infancy, **myxedema** during adulthood (see Figure 13.15), and **Hashimoto disease.** Hypersecretion of the thyroid hormones T_3 and T_4 results in **hyperthyroidism**, which is also called **thyrotoxicosis**, and **Graves disease**, **exophthalmic goiter**, **toxic goiter**, or **Basedow disease.** Simple or **endemic goiter** shows an enlargement of the thyroid gland caused by a deficiency of iodine in the diet.

Parathyroid Glands

The **parathyroid glands** are small, yellowish-brown bodies occurring as two pairs located on the dorsal surface and lower aspect of the thyroid gland. Each parathyroid gland is approximately 6 mm in diameter and weighs approximately 0.033 g. See Figures 13.1 and 13.4. The hormone secreted by the parathyroids is *parathyroid hormone (PTH)*, which is also called *parathormone*. This hormone and its functions are described in Table 13.2.

Hyposecretion of PTH can result in **hypoparathyroidism**, which can cause **tetany** (intermittent cramp or tonic muscular contractions). See Figure 13.5. Hypersecretion of PTH can result in **hyperparathyroidism**, which can cause **osteoporosis**, **kidney stones**, and **hypercalcemia**.

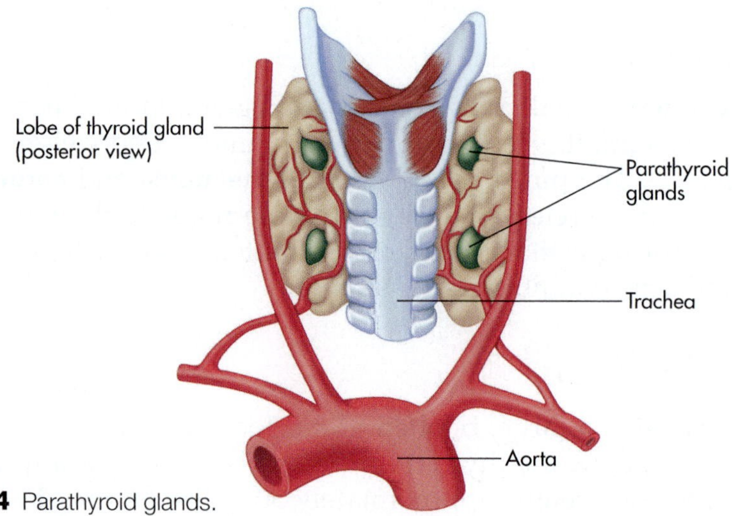

Figure 13.4 Parathyroid glands.

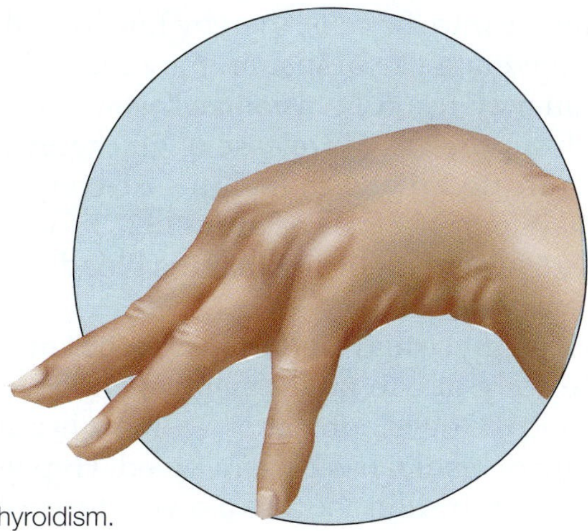

Figure 13.5 Tetany of the hand in hypoparathyroidism.

Pancreas (Islets of Langerhans)

The **islets of Langerhans** are small clusters of cells located within the pancreas. See Figures 13.1 and 13.6. They are composed of three major types of cells: **alpha**, **beta**, and **delta**. The alpha cells secrete the hormone glucagon, which facilitates the breakdown of glycogen to glucose, thereby elevating blood sugar.

The beta cells secrete the hormone insulin (see Figure 13.6), which is essential for the maintenance of normal blood sugar (fasting: 70–99 mg/dL). Insulin is essential to life. It acts to regulate the metabolism of glucose and the process necessary for the intermediary metabolism of carbohydrates, fats, and proteins. It promotes the entry

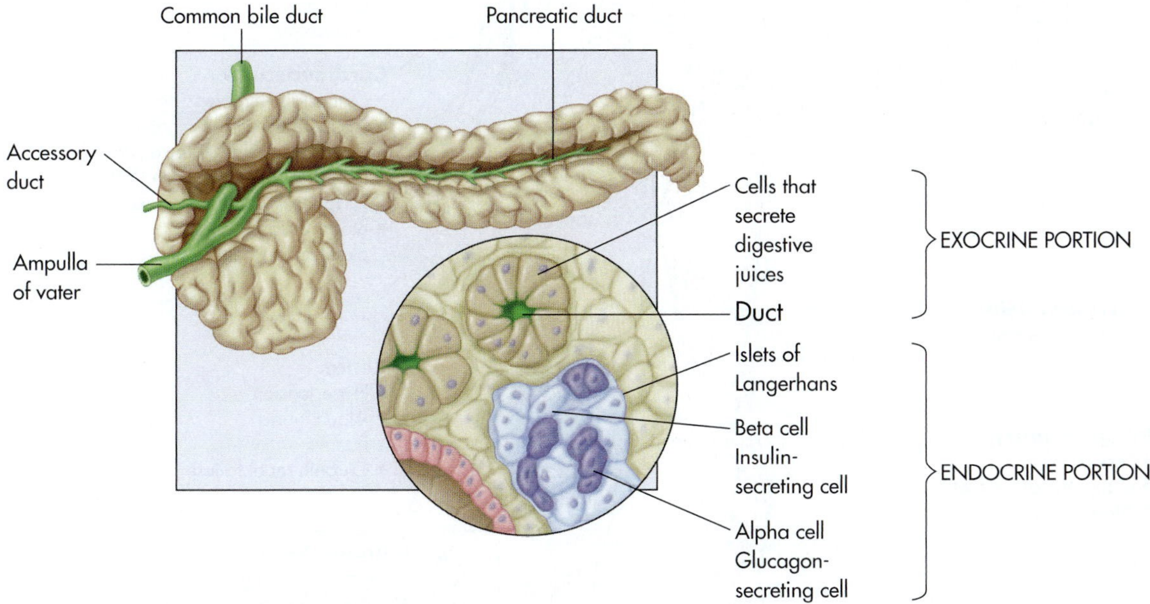

Figure 13.6 Pancreas—an endocrine and exocrine gland. The inset shows the islets of Langerhans. The alpha cells secrete glucagon, which raises the blood glucose level. The beta cells secrete insulin, which lowers the blood glucose level.

of glucose into the cells, thereby lowering the blood glucose (BG) level. Hyposecretion or inadequate use of insulin may result in **diabetes mellitus (DM)**. Hypersecretion of insulin may result in **hyperinsulinism**. The delta cells secrete a hormone, *somatostatin*, which suppresses the release of glucagon and insulin.

Untreated diabetes mellitus or complications of diabetes can result in various multisystem effects. See Figure 13.7. Progressive complications include **hyperglycemia** (excessive amount of sugar in the blood) and **hypoglycemia** (deficient amount of sugar in the blood).

Hyperglycemia can lead to **diabetic ketoacidosis** (accumulation of ketones and acids in the body due to faulty metabolism of carbohydrates and the improper burning of fats) and the development of a coma when the blood sugar is too high or an insufficient amount of insulin has been received. Hypoglycemia occurs when too much insulin has been taken. Insulin shock is a severe form of hypoglycemia and requires an immediate dose of glucose. Convulsions, coma, and death can occur if the patient is not treated.

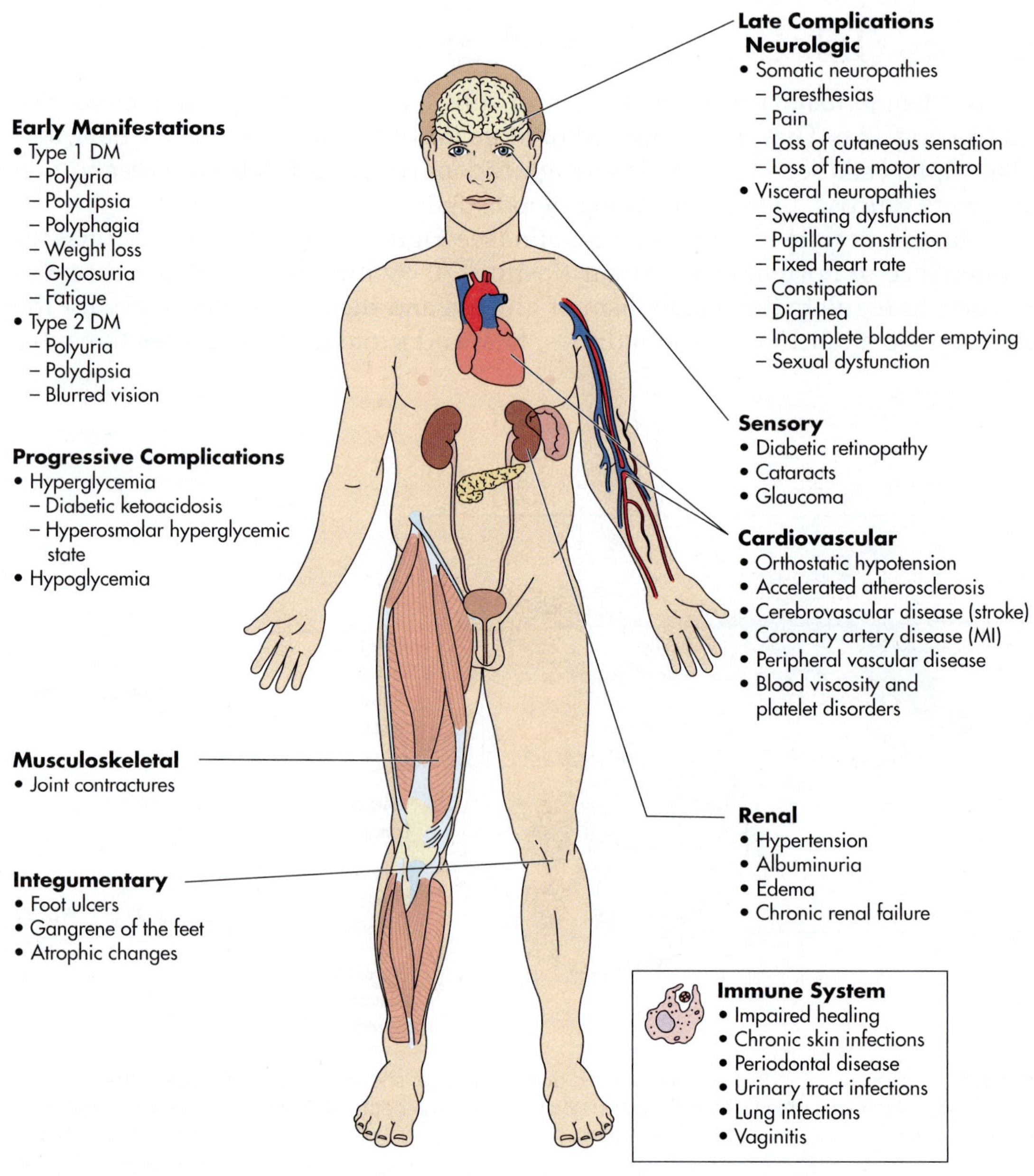

Figure 13.7 Multisystem effects of diabetes mellitus.

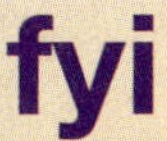

Type 1 diabetes mellitus is usually diagnosed in children and young adults and was previously known as juvenile diabetes. In type 1 DM, the body does not produce insulin. Insulin is a hormone that is needed to convert sugar (glucose), starches, and other food into energy needed for daily life. The classic symptoms of diabetes mellitus (DM)—**polyuria** (frequent urination), **polydipsia** (excessive thirst), and **polyphagia** (extreme hunger)—appear more rapidly in children.

DM is the most common endocrine system disorder of childhood. The rate of occurrence is higher among 5- to 7-year-olds and 11- to 15-year-olds. It is noted that childhood obesity predisposes to insulin resistance and **type 2 diabetes mellitus**, a chronic metabolic disorder characterized by high blood sugar, insulin resistance, and lack of insulin. Obesity in children is a complex disorder. Its prevalence has increased so significantly in recent years that many consider it a major health concern of the developed world.

The American Medical Association has reclassified obesity from a condition to a disease. More than one-third of the adult population of the United States is obese. The Centers for Disease Control and Prevention (CDC) now defines normal weight, overweight, and obesity according to body mass index (BMI) rather than the traditional height/weight charts. BMI is a person's weight in kilograms (kg) divided by his or her height in meters squared. *Obesity* is defined as excessive amount of body fat with a BMI of 30 or above. *Overweight* is defined as a BMI between 25 and 29.9 in adults.

insights In ICD-10-CM, *morbid (severe) obesity*, coded E66.01, is due to excess calories. The term *overweight* is not recognized as a clinical term for high-adiposity obesity.

Adrenal Glands (Suprarenals)

The **adrenal glands** are two small, triangular-shaped glands located on top of each kidney. Each gland weighs about 5 g and consists of an outer portion or *cortex* and an inner portion called the *medulla*. See Figures 13.1 and 13.8.

Adrenal Cortex

The **adrenal cortex** is essential to life due to its secretion of a group of hormones, the glucocorticoids, the mineralocorticoids, and the androgens. The hormones secreted by the adrenal cortex and their functions are described in Table 13.2 and a discussion of these substances and their effects on the body follows.

GLUCOCORTICOIDS

The two glucocorticoid hormones are *cortisol* and *corticosterone*. Cortisol (hydrocortisone) is the principal steroid hormone secreted by the cortex. Hyposecretion of cortisol can result in **Addison disease**; hypersecretion can result in **Cushing disease**.

Corticosterone is a steroid hormone secreted by the adrenal cortex. It is essential for the normal use of carbohydrates, the absorption of glucose, and the formation of glycogen in the liver and tissues. It also influences potassium and sodium metabolism.

MINERALOCORTICOIDS

Aldosterone is the principal **mineralocorticoid** secreted by the adrenal cortex. It is essential in regulating electrolyte and water balance by promoting sodium and chloride reabsorption and potassium excretion. Hyposecretion of this hormone can result in a **reduced plasma volume**, and hypersecretion can result in a condition known as **primary aldosteronism**. In

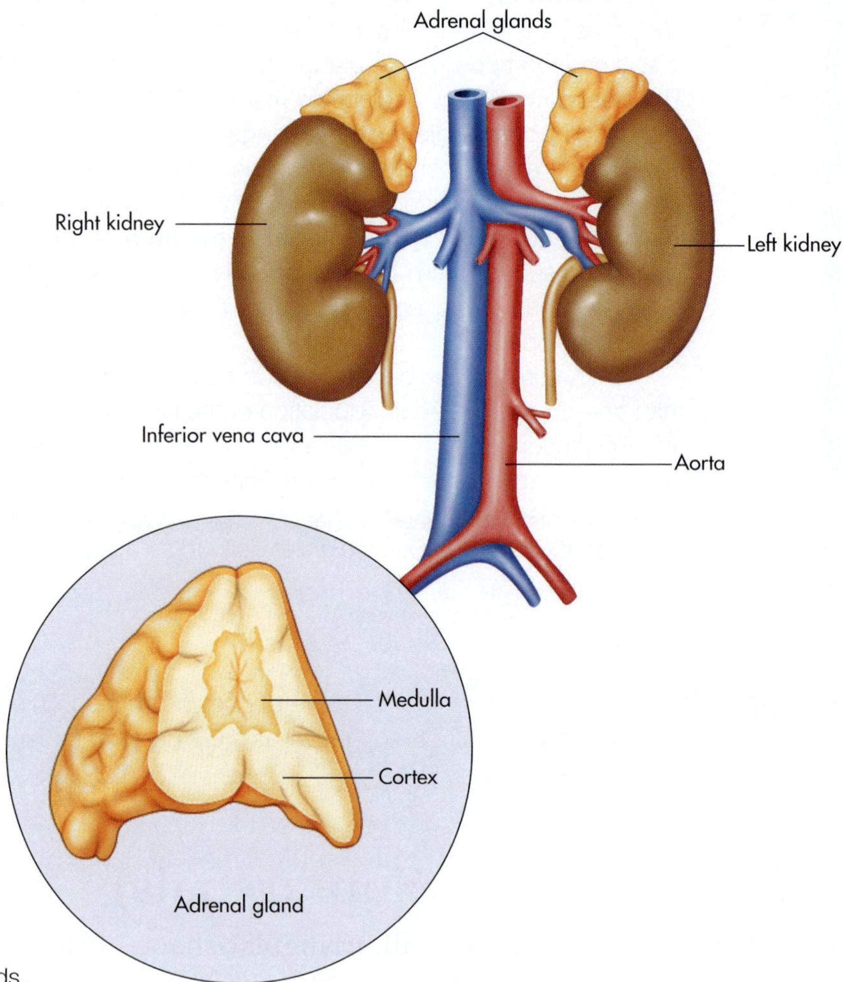

Figure 13.8 Adrenal glands.

primary aldosteronism, the adrenal glands produce too much aldosterone, causing one to lose potassium and retain sodium. The excess sodium in turn holds onto water, increasing the blood volume and blood pressure. Treatment options for people with primary aldosteronism include medications, lifestyle modifications, and surgery.

ANDROGENS

Androgen refers to a substance or hormone that promotes the development of male characteristics. The two main androgen hormones are *testosterone* and *androsterone*. They are essential for the development of the male secondary sex characteristics.

Adrenal Medulla

The **adrenal medulla** synthesizes, secretes, and stores catecholamines, specifically dopamine, epinephrine, and norepinephrine. The hormones secreted by the adrenal medulla and their functions are described in Table 13.2 and a discussion of these substances and their effects on the body follows.

DOPAMINE

Dopamine is a naturally occurring sympathetic nervous system neurotransmitter that is a precursor of norepinephrine. Dopamine can be supplied as a medication that acts on the sympathetic nervous system. It can be given to increase the amount of dopamine in the brains of patients with Parkinson disease. Dopamine has varying vasoactive effects depending on the dose at which it is administered. It can act to dilate systemic arteries, increase cardiac output, and increase urinary output.

EPINEPHRINE

Epinephrine (*adrenaline*) acts as a vasoconstrictor, vasopressor, cardiac stimulant, antispasmodic, and sympathomimetic. Its main function is to assist in regulating the sympathetic branch of the autonomic nervous system. It can be synthetically produced and administered *parenterally* (by an injection), *topically* (on a local area of the skin), or by *inhalation* (by nose or mouth). The following are some of the known influences and functions of epinephrine:

- Elevates the systolic blood pressure
- Increases the heart rate and cardiac output
- Increases glycogenolysis (conversion of glycogen into glucose), thereby hastening the release of glucose from the liver; this action elevates the blood sugar level and provides the body a spurt of energy; referred to as the *fight-or-flight response*
- Dilates the bronchial tubes and relaxes air passageways
- Dilates the pupils to see more clearly

NOREPINEPHRINE

Norepinephrine (*noradrenaline*) acts as a vasoconstrictor, vasopressor, and neurotransmitter. It elevates systolic and diastolic blood pressure, increases the heart rate and cardiac output, and increases glycogenolysis.

Ovaries

The **ovaries** (see Figure 13.1) produce *estrogens* (*estradiol*, *estrone*, and *estriol*) and *progesterone*. Estrogen is the female sex hormone secreted by the graafian follicles of the ovaries. Progesterone is a steroid hormone secreted by the corpus luteum.

Testes

The **testes** (see Figure 13.1) produce the male sex hormone *testosterone*, which is important for sexual development and sexual behavior and libido, supporting spermatogenesis and erectile function.

Placenta

During pregnancy, the **placenta**, containing separate vascular systems of the mother and fetus, serves as an endocrine gland. It produces *chorionic gonadotropin hormone*, *estrogen*, and *progesterone*.

Gastrointestinal Mucosa

The **mucosa** of the pyloric area of the stomach secretes the hormone *gastrin*, which stimulates gastric acid secretion. Gastrin also affects the gallbladder, pancreas, and small intestine secretory activities.

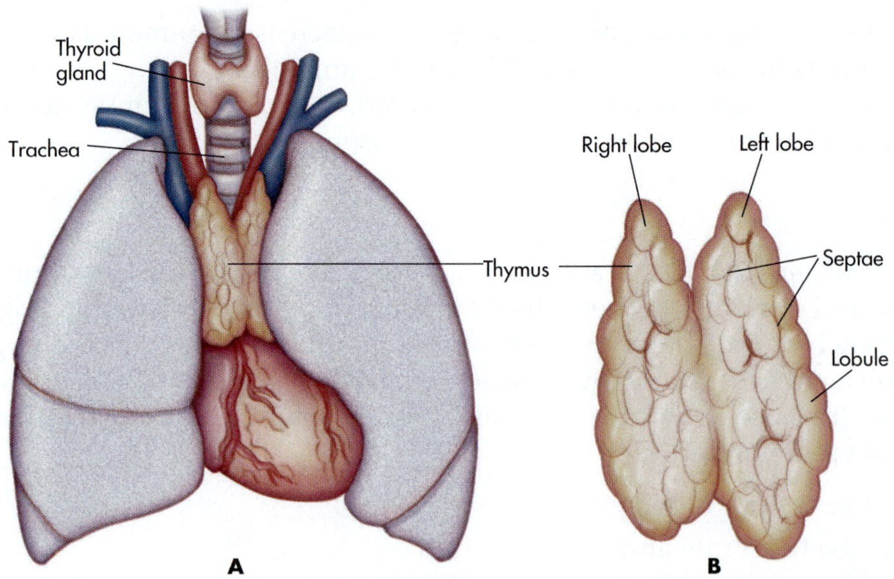

Figure 13.9 Thymus gland. (A) Appearance and position; (B) with anatomic structures.

The mucosa of the duodenum and jejunum secretes the hormone *secretin*, which stimulates pancreatic juice, bile, and intestinal secretion. The mucosa of the duodenum also secretes *cholecystokinin*, which stimulates the pancreas. *Enterogastrone*, a hormone that regulates gastric secretions, is also secreted by the duodenal mucosa.

Thymus

The **thymus** is a bilobed body located in the mediastinal cavity in front of and above the heart. See Figure 13.9. It is composed of lymphoid tissue and is a part of the lymphatic system. It is a ductless glandlike body and secretes the hormones *thymosin* and *thymopoietin*. Thymosin promotes the maturation process of T lymphocytes (thymus dependent), white blood cells that play an important role in cell-mediated immunity. Thymopoietin is a hormone that influences the production of lymphocyte precursors and aids in their process of becoming T lymphocytes.

Leptin and Ghrelin: Different Types of Hormones

As a growing number of people suffer from obesity, understanding the mechanisms by which various hormones and neurotransmitters have influence on energy balance has been a subject of intensive research. *Leptin* and *grehlin* are two hormones recognized to have a major influence on energy level. These hormones are not produced by endocrine cells or glands, but are secreted by adipose tissue throughout the body. Leptin is a peptide hormone that is produced by fat cells and plays a role in body weight regulation by acting on the hypothalamus to suppress appetite and burn fat stored in adipose tissue. Ghrelin, on the other hand, is a fast-acting hormone that seems to play a role in meal initiation. In obese subjects, the circulating level of leptin is increased. It is now established that obese patients are leptin-resistant. However, the manner in which both leptin and ghrelin contribute to the development or maintenance of obesity is as yet unclear.

Study and Review I

Anatomy and Physiology

Write your answers to the following questions.

1. Name the primary glands of the endocrine system.

   a. ______________________ b. ______________________

   c. ______________________ d. ______________________

   e. ______________________ f. ______________________

   g. ______________________ h. ______________________

2. State the vital function of the endocrine system.______________________

   ____

3. Define hormone.______________________

4. State the vital role of the hypothalamus in regulating endocrine functions.______________________

   ____

   ____

   ____

5. Why is the pituitary gland known as the master gland of the body? ______________________

   ____

6. Name the hormones secreted by the anterior lobe (*adenohypophysis*) of the pituitary gland.

   a. ______________________ b. ______________________

   c. ______________________ d. ______________________

   e. ______________________ f. ______________________

   g. ______________________

7. Name the hormones secreted by the posterior lobe (*neurohypophysis*) of the pituitary gland.

   a. ______________________ b. ______________________

8. The pineal gland secretes the hormones ______________________ and ______________________.

9. State the vital role of the thyroid gland. ______________________

10. Name the hormones stored and secreted by the thyroid gland.

a. ______________________________ **b.** ______________________________

c. ______________________________

11. Parathyroid hormone (*parathormone*) is essential for the maintenance of a normal level of ______________________________ and also plays a role in the metabolism of ______________________________.

12. Insulin is essential for the maintenance of a normal level of ______________________________.

13. The adrenal cortex secretes a group of hormones known as the ____________________, the ____________________________, and the ____________________________.

14. Name four functions of cortisol.

a. ______________________________ **b.** ______________________________

c. ______________________________ **d.** ______________________________

15. Name four functions of corticosterone.

a. ______________________________ **b.** ______________________________

c. ______________________________ **d.** ______________________________

16. ______________________________ is the principal mineralocorticoid secreted by the adrenal cortex.

17. Define androgen. ____

18. Name the three main catecholamines synthesized, secreted, and stored by the adrenal medulla.

a. ______________________________ **b.** ______________________________

c. ______________________________

19. Name three functions of the hormone epinephrine.

a. ____

b. ____

c. ____

20. The ovaries produce the hormones ______________________________ and ______________________________.

21. The testes produce the hormone ________________________.

22. Name the two hormones secreted by the thymus.

a. ______________________________ **b.** ______________________________

23. Name the four hormones secreted by the gastrointestinal mucosa.

a. ______________________ **b.** ______________________

c. ______________________ **d.** ______________________

ANATOMY LABELING

Identify the structures shown below by filling in the blanks.

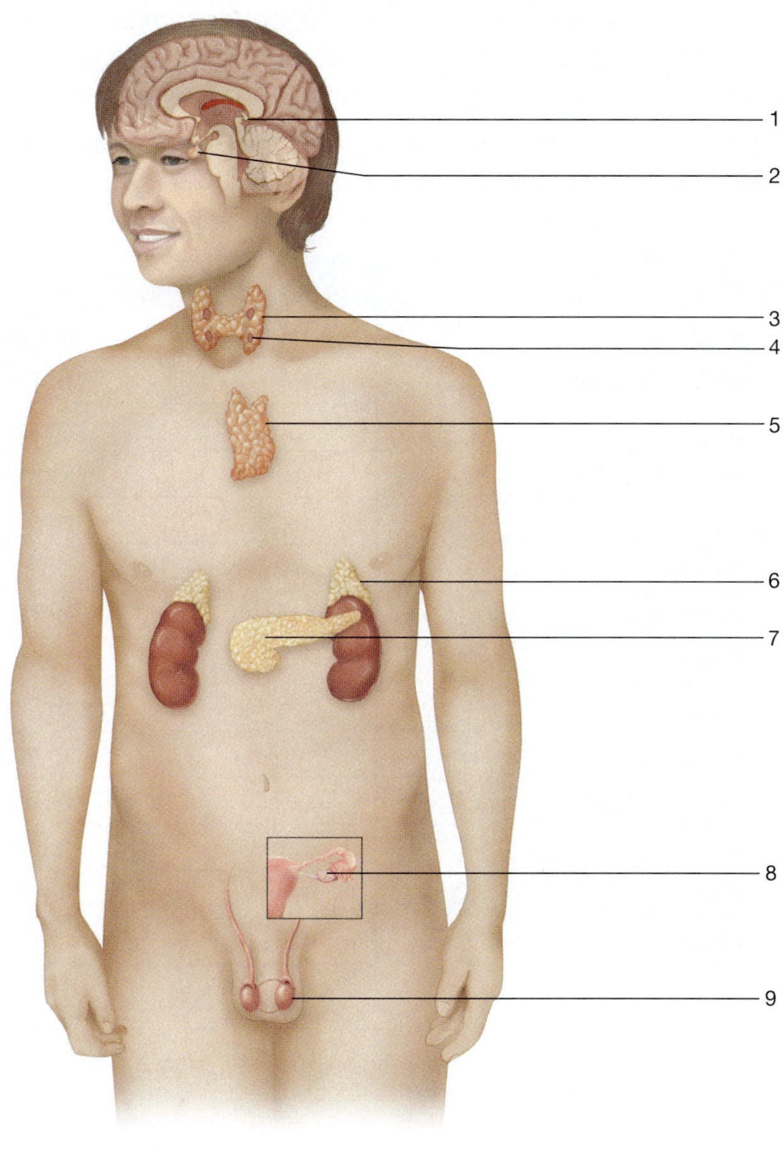

Building Your Medical Vocabulary

This section provides the foundation for learning medical terminology. Review the following alphabetized word list. Note how common prefixes and suffixes are repeatedly applied to word roots and combining forms to create different meanings. The word parts are color-coded: prefixes are yellow, suffixes are blue, roots/combining forms are red. A combining form is a word root plus a vowel. The chart below lists the combining forms for the word roots in this chapter and can help to strengthen your understanding of how medical words are built and spelled.

Remember These Guidelines

1. If the suffix begins with a vowel, drop the combining vowel from the combining form and add the suffix. For example, thym/o (*thymus*) + -itis (*inflammation*) becomes thymitis.
2. If the suffix begins with a consonant, keep the combining vowel and add the suffix to the combining form. For example, andr/o (*man*) + -gen (*formation, production*) becomes androgen.

You will find that some terms have not been divided into word parts. These are common words or specialized terms that are included to enhance your medical vocabulary.

Combining Forms of the Endocrine System

acid/o	acid	**insulin/o**	insulin
acr/o	extremity, point	**kal/i**	potassium (K)
aden/o	gland	**myx/o**	mucus
adren/o	adrenal gland	**nephr/o**	kidney
andr/o	man	**ophthalm/o**	eye
cortic/o	cortex	**pancreat/o**	pancreas
crin/o	to secrete	**somat/o**	body
estr/o	female	**test/o**	testicle
ger/o	old age	**thym/o**	thymus
gigant/o	giant	**thyr/o**	thyroid, shield
gluc/o	sweet, sugar	**toxic/o**	poison
gonad/o	seed	**trop/o**	turning
hirsut/o	hairy	**vas/o**	vessel
hydr/o	water	**viril/o**	masculine

Medical Word	Word Parts		Definition
	Part	**Meaning**	
acidosis (ăs″ ĭ-dō′ sĭs)	acid -osis	acid condition	Condition of excessive acidity of body fluids
acromegaly (ăk″ rō-mĕg′ ă-lē)	acr/o -megaly	extremity enlargement, large	Characterized (in the adult) by marked enlargement and elongation of the bones of the face, jaw, and extremities. It is caused by an overproduction of growth hormone and is treated by surgery, medications, or radiotherapy.
Addison disease (ăd′ ĭ-sŭn)			Results from a deficiency in the secretion of adrenocortical hormones; also called *adrenal insufficiency*. The most common cause of this condition is the result of the body attacking itself (autoimmune disease). For unknown reasons, the immune system views the adrenal cortex as a foreign body, something to attack and destroy. Other causes of Addison disease include infections of the adrenal glands, spread of cancer to the glands, and hemorrhage into the glands.
adenectomy (ăd″ ĕn-ĕk′ tō-mē)	aden -ectomy	gland surgical excision	Surgical excision of a gland
adenoma (ăd″ ĕ-nō′ mă)	aden -oma	gland tumor	Tumor of a gland

! ALERT

The root ***aden*** means *gland* and the root ***adren*** means *adrenal gland*. What a difference a letter makes!

Medical Word	Part	Meaning	Definition
adrenal (ăd-rē′ năl)	adren -al	adrenal gland pertaining to	Pertaining to the adrenal glands, triangular bodies that cover the superior surface of the kidneys; also called *suprarenal glands*
adrenalectomy (ăd-rē″ năl-ĕk′ tō-mē)	adren -al -ectomy	adrenal gland pertaining to surgical excision	Surgical excision of an adrenal gland
androgen (ăn′ drō-jĕn)	andr/o -gen	man formation, produce	Hormones that produce or stimulate the development of male characteristics. The two major androgens are testosterone and androsterone.

RULE REMINDER

This term keeps the combining vowel ***o*** because the suffix begins with a consonant.

Medical Word	Word Parts		Definition
	Part	**Meaning**	
cortisone (kŏr´ tĭ-sōn)	cortis -one	cortex hormone	Glucocorticoid (steroid) hormone secreted by the adrenal cortex; used as an anti-inflammatory agent
cretinism (krē´ tĭn-ĭzm)	cretin -ism	cretin condition	Congenital condition caused by deficiency in secretion of the thyroid hormones and characterized by arrested physical and mental development. Treatment consists of appropriate thyroid replacement therapy.
Cushing disease (koosh´ ĭng)			Results from hypersecretion of cortisol; symptoms include fatigue, muscular weakness, and changes in body appearance. Prolonged administration of large doses of ACTH can cause Cushing syndrome. A *buffalo hump* and a *moon face* are characteristic signs of this condition. See Figure 13.10.

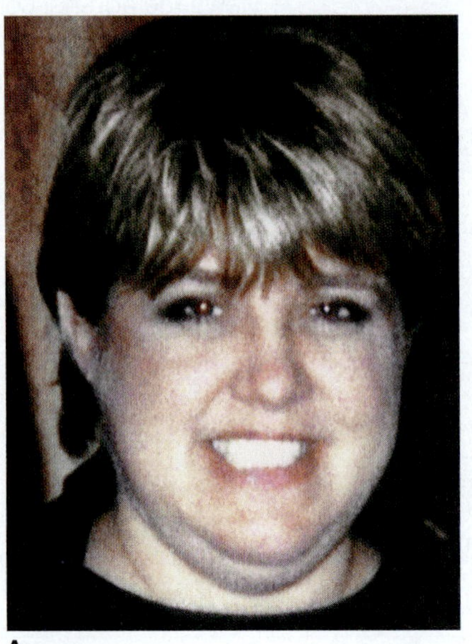

A

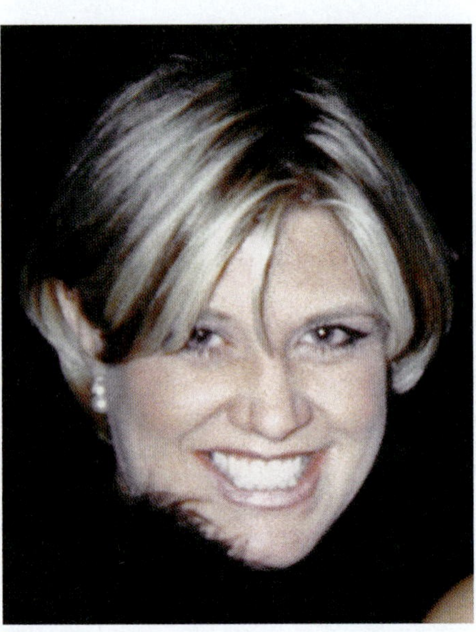

B

Figure 13.10 A woman with Cushing syndrome (A) before and (B) after treatment. (Courtesy Sharmyn McGraw)

Medical Word	Part	Meaning	Definition
diabetes (dī″ ă-bē´ tēz)	dia- -betes	through to go	General term used to describe diseases characterized by polyuria (excessive discharge of urine)
diabetes mellitus (DM) (dī″ ă-bē´ tēz)	dia- -betes	through to go	Group of metabolic diseases characterized by hyperglycemia resulting from defects in insulin production, insulin secretion, or both. There are three major types of diabetes mellitus: type 1, type 2, and gestational diabetes, which occurs as a result of pregnancy. DM is the seventh highest cause of death in the United States.

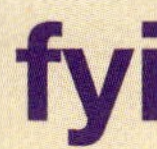

fyi In the second century, Aretaeus the Cappadocian, a Greek physician of Alexandria, Egypt, was confronted with a patient who had polyuria (excessive urination). He chose a Greek word, *diabetes* (that which passes through), to define what he considered to be the most dominant clinical sign in his patient. Later, the word *diabetes* was combined with *mellitus*, a word of Latin origin that means "honey." In 1670, in those suffering from polyuria, a distinction was made between those patients who had sweet-tasting urine (diabetes mellitus [DM]) and those patients whose urine had no taste (diabetes insipidus [DI]).

In DM the body is no longer able to control blood glucose, leading to abnormally high levels of blood sugar (hyperglycemia). Most of the food that we eat is turned into glucose, a simple sugar, for the body to use for energy. Insulin, made by the pancreas, helps glucose get into the cells of the body. When a person has DM, the body either does not make enough insulin or cannot use insulin as well as it should, causing sugar to build up in the blood. Persistently elevated blood glucose levels can cause damage to the body's tissues, including the nerves (neuropathy), blood vessels, and tissues in the eyes. **Sensory neuropathy** occurs if the body's sensory nerves become damaged. It may also be called *polyneuropathy* (poly- [*many*], neuro [*nerve*], -pathy [*disease*]) as it affects a number of different nerve centers. Sensory neuropathy starts from the feet or hands and can develop to affect the legs and arms. The following are symptoms of sensory neuropathy:

- Numbness
- Reduced ability to sense pain or extreme temperatures
- Tingling feeling
- Unexplained burning sensations
- Sharp stabbing pains, which may be more noticeable at night
- Dysesthesia (dys- [*difficult, painful*], esthes [*sensation*], -ia [condition])

In addition, poor circulation may occur in the legs and feet, which can weaken the healing process, contribute to infection, and lead to the formation of ulcers. The possibility of amputation of an extremity is a great concern for diabetics.

See Figure 13.7 for the multisystem effects of diabetes mellitus.

insights In the ICD-10-CM, a significant change has occurred from the previous edition in the classification and coding of diabetes mellitus. Combination codes are now used that include the type of DM, the body system affected, and the complications affecting that body system. All of the codes within the particular category (E08–E13) that are necessary to describe all of the complications and associated conditions that the patient has should be used. The codes should be sequenced based on the reason(s) for the particular visit or encounter.

Medical Word	Word Parts		Definition
	Part	**Meaning**	
dwarfism (dwor´ fĭzm)	dwarf -ism	small condition	Condition of being abnormally small. It is a medical disorder characterized by an adult height less than 4 feet 10 inches (147 cm) and is usually classified as to the underlying condition that is the cause for the short stature. Dwarfism is not necessarily caused by any specific disease or disorder; it can simply be a naturally occurring consequence of a person's genetic makeup.

Medical Word	Word Parts		Definition
	Part	**Meaning**	
endocrinologist (ĕn″ dō-krĭn-ŏl′ ō-gĭst)	endo- crin/o log -ist	within to secrete study of one who specializes	Physician who specializes in the study of the endocrine system
endocrinology (ĕn″ dō-krĭn-ŏl′ ō-jē)	endo- crin/o -logy	within to secrete study of	Study of the endocrine system
epinephrine (ĕp″ ĭ-nĕf′ rĭn)	epi- nephr -ine	upon kidney substance	Hormone produced by the adrenal medulla; used as a vasoconstrictor and cardiac stimulant to relax bronchospasm and to relieve allergic symptoms; also called *adrenaline*
estrogen (ĕs′ trō-jĕn)	estr/o -gen	female formation, production	Hormones produced by the ovaries, including estradiol, estrone, and estriol; female sex hormones important in the development of secondary sex characteristics and regulation of the menstrual cycle

RULE REMINDER

This term keeps the combining vowel **o** because the suffix begins with a consonant.

Medical Word	Part	Meaning	Definition
euthyroid (ū-thī′ royd)	eu- thyr -oid	good, normal thyroid, shield resemble	Normal activity of the thyroid gland
exocrine (ĕks′ ō-krĭn)	exo- -crine	out, away from to secrete	Pertains to a type of gland that secretes into ducts (duct glands); examples include sweat glands, salivary glands, mammary glands, stomach, liver, and pancreas
exophthalmic (ĕks″ ŏf-thăl′ mĭk)	ex- ophthalm -ic	out, away from eye pertaining to	Pertaining to an abnormal condition characterized by a marked protrusion of the eyeballs as often seen in exophthalmic goiter or exophthalmos seen in Graves disease. People with Graves ophthalmopathy develop eye problems, including bulging, red, or swollen eyes, sensitivity to light, and blurring or double vision.
gigantism (jī′ găn-tĭzm)	gigant -ism	giant condition	Pathological condition of being abnormally large
glandular (glăn′ dū-lăr)	glandul -ar	little acorn pertaining to	Pertaining to a gland

Medical Word	Word Parts		Definition
	Part	**Meaning**	
glucocorticoid (glū″ kō-kŏrt′ ĭ-koyd)	gluc/o cortic -oid	sweet, sugar cortex resemble	General classification of the adrenal cortical hormones: cortisol (hydrocortisone) and corticosterone
hirsutism (hŭr′ sūt-ĭzm)	hirsut -ism	hairy condition	Abnormal condition characterized by excessive growth of hair, especially as occurring in women. See Figure 13.11.

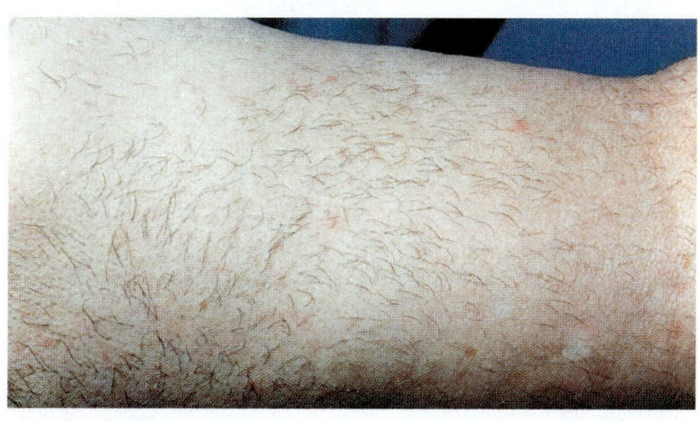

Figure 13.11 Hirsutism.
(Courtesy Jason L. Smith, MD)

Medical Word	Part	Meaning	Definition
hydrocortisone (hī′ drō-kŏr′ tĭ-sōn)	hydr/o cortis -one	water cortex hormone	Glucocorticoid (steroid) hormone produced by the adrenal cortex; used as an anti-inflammatory agent
hypergonadism (hī″ pĕr-gō′ năd-ĭzm)	hyper- gonad -ism	excessive seed condition	Condition of excessive secretion of the sex glands
hyperinsulinism (hī″ pĕr-ĭn′ sū-lĭn-ĭzm)	hyper- insulin -ism	excessive insulin condition	Condition of excessive amounts of insulin in the blood, causing low blood sugar
hyperkalemia (hī″ pĕr-kă-lē′ mĭ-ă)	hyper- kal -emia	excessive potassium (K) blood condition	Condition of excessive amounts of potassium in the blood
hyperthyroidism (hī″ pĕr-thī′ royd-ĭzm)	hyper- thyr -oid -ism	excessive thyroid, shield resemble condition	Excessive secretion of thyroid hormone (TH), a condition that can affect many body systems. The most common etiologies of hyperthyroidism are Graves disease and toxic multinodular goiter. *Graves disease* is an autoimmune disease in which antibodies produced by the immune system stimulate the thyroid to produce too much thyroxine. Other forms of hyperthyroidism can be caused by **thyroiditis**, or inflammation of the thyroid gland. Certain benign or malignant tumors can also produce too much thyroid hormone. See Figure 13.12.

(*continued*)

Medical Word	Word Parts		Definition
	Part	Meaning	

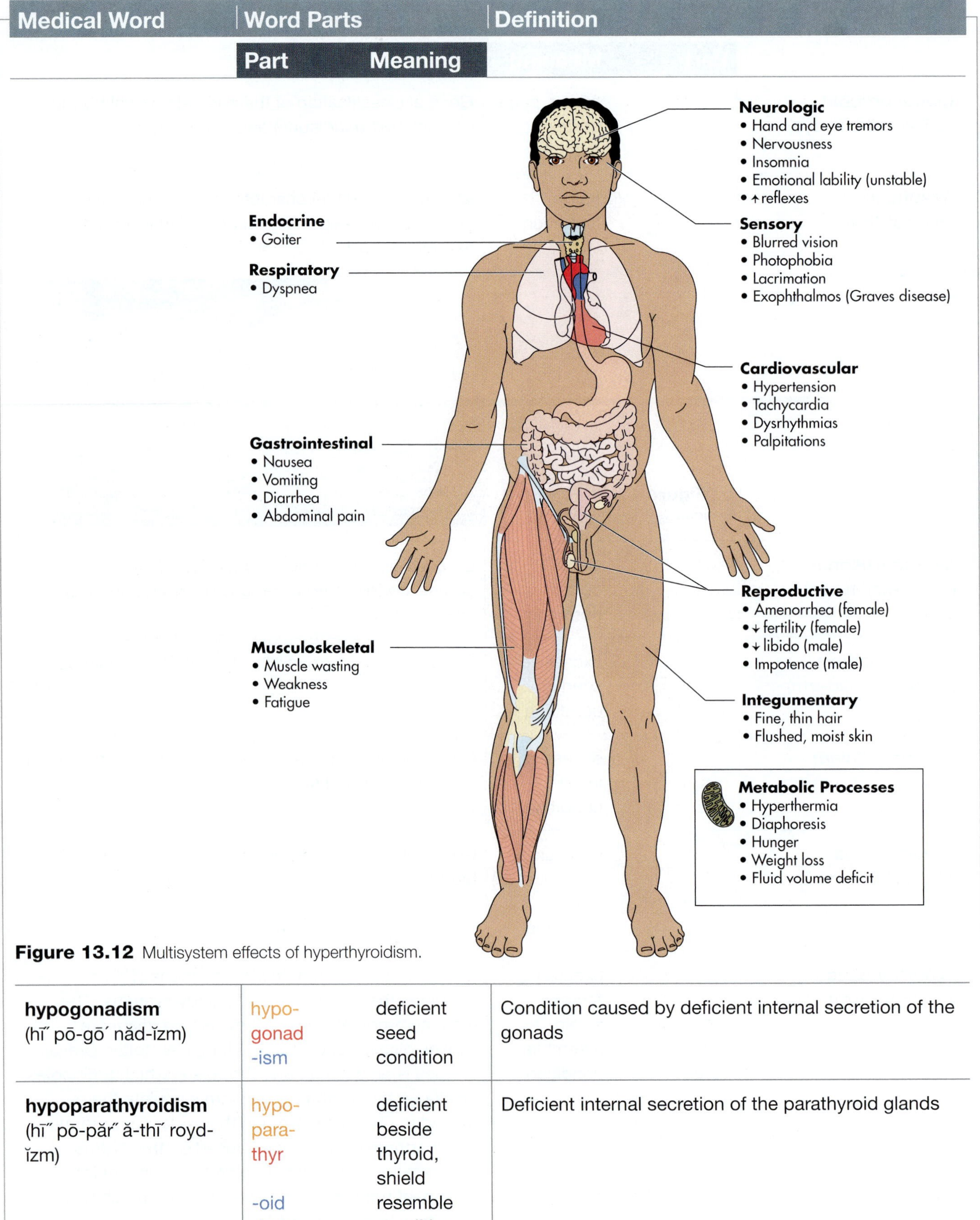

Figure 13.12 Multisystem effects of hyperthyroidism.

hypogonadism (hī″ pō-gō′ năd-ĭzm)	hypo- gonad -ism	deficient seed condition	Condition caused by deficient internal secretion of the gonads
hypoparathyroidism (hī″ pō-păr″ ă-thī′ royd-ĭzm)	hypo- para- thyr -oid -ism	deficient beside thyroid, shield resemble condition	Deficient internal secretion of the parathyroid glands

Medical Word	Word Parts		Definition
	Part	**Meaning**	
hypophysis (hī-pŏf´ ĭ-sĭs)	hypo- -physis	deficient, under growth	Literally means *any undergrowth*; also called the pituitary gland
hypothyroidism (hī˝ pō-thī˝ royd-ĭzm)	hypo- thyr -oid -ism	deficient thyroid, shield resemble condition	Pathological condition in which the thyroid gland produces inadequate amounts of thyroid hormone. It can affect many body systems. See Figure 13.13.

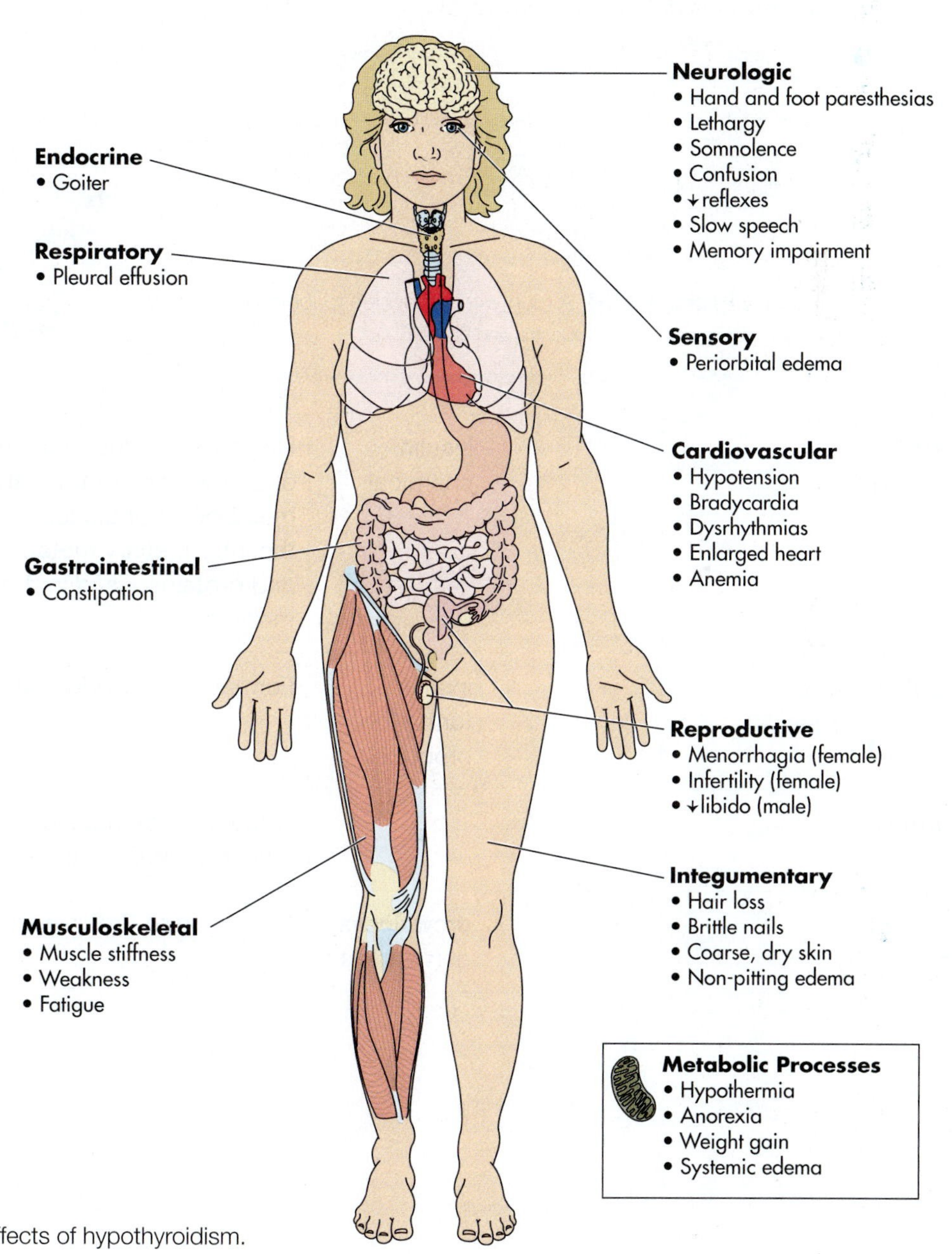

Figure 13.13 Multisystem effects of hypothyroidism.

fyi Untreated hypothyroidism can lead to a number of health problems. Constant stimulation of the thyroid to release more hormones can cause the gland to become larger, a condition known as **goiter**. Hashimoto thyroiditis, an autoimmune disease of the thyroid, is one of the most common causes of goiter. Another type of goiter is an *endemic goiter* that develops in certain geographic regions where the iodine content in food and water is deficient (Figure 13.14).

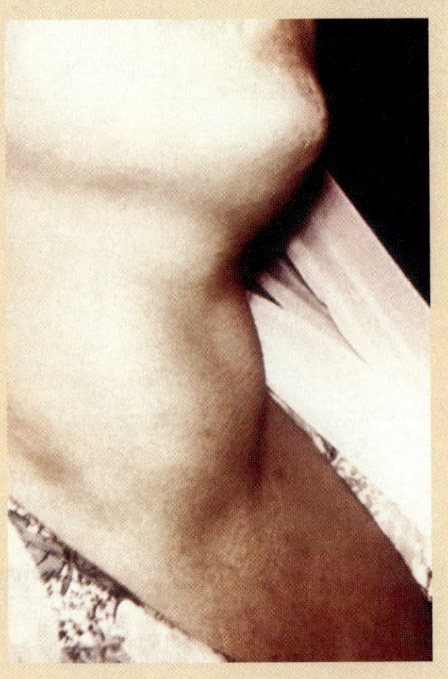

Figure 13.14 A man with goiter due to iodine deficiency.
(Centers for Disease Control and Prevention)

Medical Word	Word Parts: Part	Word Parts: Meaning	Definition
insulin (in´ sū-lĭn)	insul -in	insulin chemical	Hormone produced by the beta cells of the islets of Langerhans of the pancreas; acts to regulate the metabolism of glucose and the process necessary for the intermediary metabolism of carbohydrates, fats, and proteins; used in the management of diabetes mellitus
insulinogenic (ĭn″ sū-lĭn″ ō-jĕn´ ĭk)	insulin/o -genic	insulin formation, produce	Formation or production of insulin
iodine (ī´ ō-dīn)			Trace mineral that aids in the development and functioning of the thyroid gland
lethargic (lĕ-thar´ jĭk)	letharg -ic	drowsiness pertaining to	Pertaining to drowsiness; sluggish

Medical Word	Word Parts		Definition
	Part	**Meaning**	
myxedema (mĭks″ ĕ-dē′ mă)	myx -edema	mucus swelling	Literally means *condition of mucus swelling*; it is the most severe form of hypothyroidism, characterized by marked edema of the face, a somnolent look, and hair that is stiff and without luster. Without treatment, coma and death can occur. See Figure 13.15.

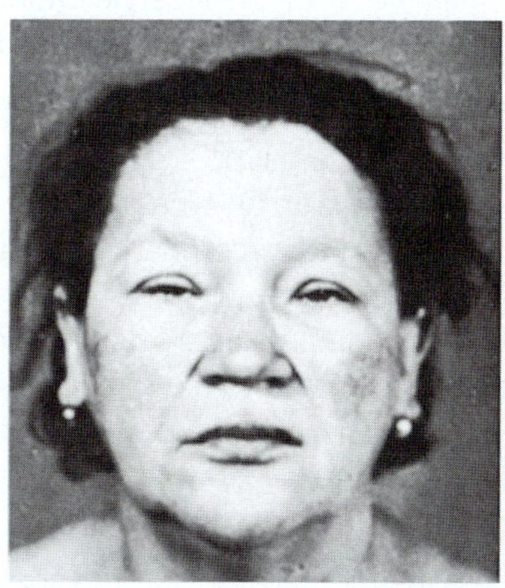

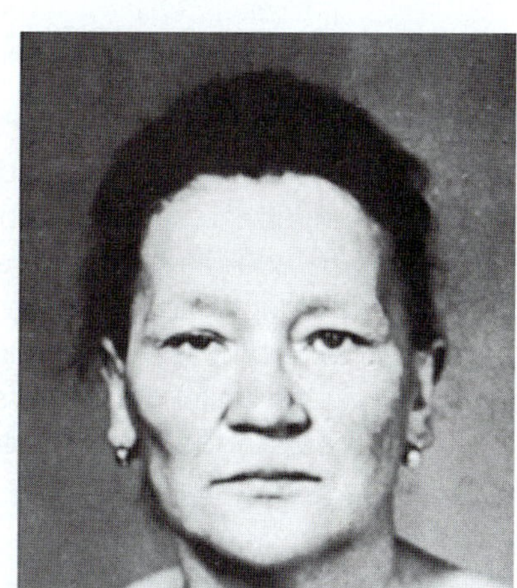

Figure 13.15 (A) A 62-year-old patient with myxedema exhibiting marked edema of the face and a somnolent look. The hair is stiff and without luster. (B) The same patient after 3 months of treatment with thyroxine.

Source: Pearson Education, Inc.

Medical Word	Part	Meaning	Definition
norepinephrine (nor-ĕp″ ĭ-nĕf′ rĭn)	nor- epi- nephr -ine	not upon kidney substance	Hormone produced by the adrenal medulla; used as a vasoconstrictor of peripheral blood vessels in acute hypotensive states
pancreatic (păn″ krē-ăt′ ĭk)	pancreat -ic	pancreas pertaining to	Pertaining to the pancreas
parathyroid glands (păr″ ă-thī′ royd)	para- thyr -oid	beside thyroid, shield resemble	Endocrine glands located beside the thyroid gland
pineal (pĭn′ ē-ăl)	pine -al	pine cone pertaining to	Endocrine gland shaped like a small pine cone
pituitarism (pĭt-ū′ ĭ-tă-rĭzm)	pituitar -ism	pituitary gland condition	Any condition of the pituitary gland
pituitary (pĭ-tū′ ĭ-tăr″ ē)	pituitar -y	pituitary gland pertaining to	Pertaining to the pituitary gland, the hypophysis

Medical Word	Word Parts: Part	Word Parts: Meaning	Definition
prediabetes (prē´dī´ ă-bē´ tēz)	pre- dia- -betes	before through to go	Condition that occurs when a person's blood glucose levels are higher than normal but not high enough for a diagnosis of type 2 diabetes. It is estimated that at least 86 million Americans have prediabetes, in addition to the 29 million with diabetes. Without lifestyle changes, most people who have prediabetes will progress to type 2 diabetes within 10 years.

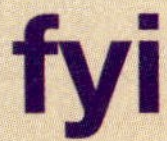

Another precursor condition to developing type 2 diabetes is called **metabolic syndrome**. The underlying causes are overweight, obesity, physical inactivity, and genetic factors. People with metabolic syndrome are at increased risk of coronary heart disease, other diseases related to plaque buildup in artery walls (e.g., stroke and peripheral vascular disease), and type 2 diabetes. Metabolic syndrome is characterized by a group of metabolic risk factors and has become increasingly common in the United States. It is closely associated with a generalized metabolic disorder called **insulin resistance syndrome**, in which the body can't use insulin efficiently.

insights In the ICD-10-CM, the code for prediabetes/prediabetic is R73.09. For metabolic syndrome, the code is E88.81. Additional codes for associated manifestations such as obesity (E66.9) also should be used. *Note:* There are subcategories listed under obesity with their own codes.

Medical Word	Part	Meaning	Definition
progeria (prō-jē´ rĭ-ă)	pro- ger -ia	before old age condition	Pathological condition of premature old age occurring in childhood
progesterone (prō-jĕs´ tĕr-ōn)	pro- gester -one	before to bear hormone	Hormone produced by the corpus luteum of the ovary, the adrenal cortex, or the placenta; released during the second half of the menstrual cycle
Simmonds disease (sĭm´ mŏnds)			Pathological condition in which complete atrophy of the pituitary gland causes loss of function of the thyroid, adrenals, and gonads; symptoms include premature aging, hair loss, and cachexia; also called *panhypopituitarism*
somatotropin (sō-măt´ ō-trō˝ pĭn)	somat/o trop -in	body turning chemical	Growth-stimulating hormone produced by the anterior lobe of the pituitary gland
steroids (stĕr´ oydz)	ster -oid	solid resemble	Group of chemical substances that includes hormones, vitamins, sterols, cardiac glycosides, and certain drugs
testosterone (tĕs-tŏs´ tĕr-ōn)	test/o ster -one	testicle solid hormone	Hormone produced by the testes; male sex hormone important in the development of secondary sex characteristics and masculinization

Medical Word	Word Parts		Definition
	Part	**Meaning**	
thymectomy (thī-mĕk´ tō-mē)	thym -ectomy	thymus surgical excision	Surgical excision of the thymus gland
thymitis (thī-mī´ tĭs)	thym -itis	thymus inflammation	Inflammation of the thymus gland
thyroid (thī´ royd)	thyr -oid	thyroid, shield resemble	Endocrine gland located in the neck; its shape resembles a shield. See Figure 13.16.

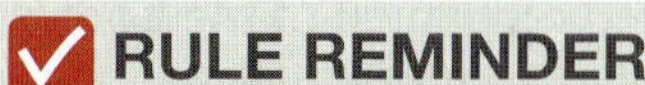

RULE REMINDER

The ***o*** has been removed from the combining form because the suffix begins with a vowel.

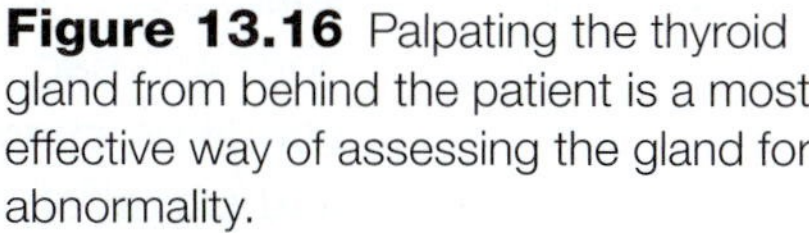

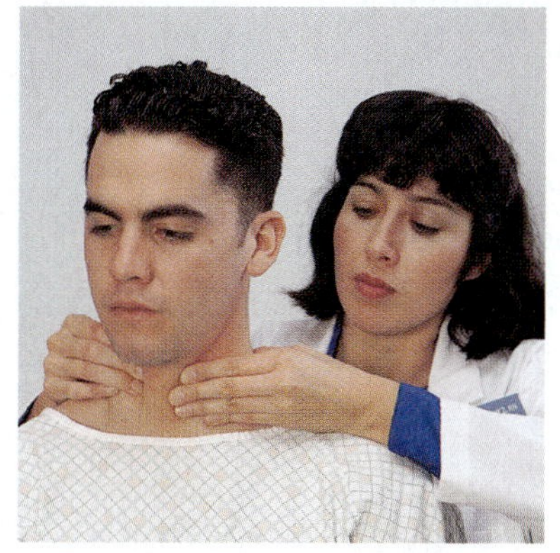

Figure 13.16 Palpating the thyroid gland from behind the patient is a most effective way of assessing the gland for abnormality.

Source: Pearson Education, Inc.

Medical Word	Word Parts		Definition
thyroidectomy (thī″ royd-ĕk´ tō-mē)	thyr -oid -ectomy	thyroid, shield resemble surgical excision	Surgical excision of the thyroid gland. See Figure 13.17.

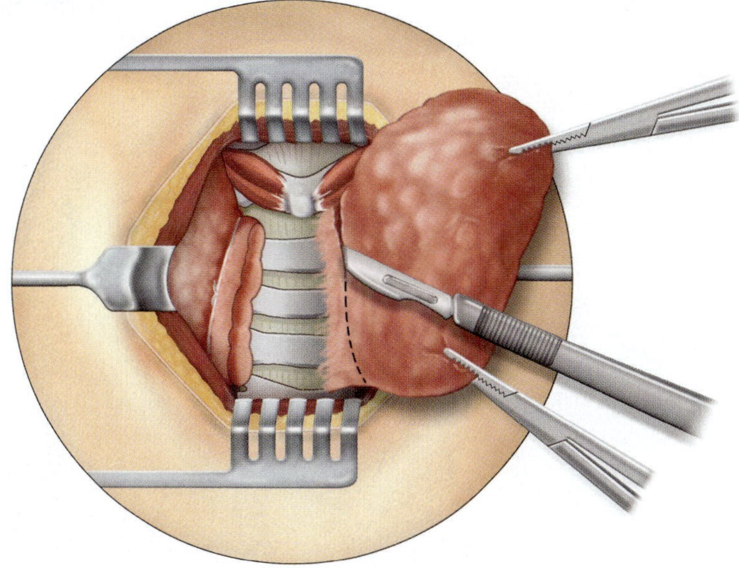

Figure 13.17 Thyroidectomy.

Medical Word	Word Parts		Definition
	Part	Meaning	
thyroiditis (thī″ royd-ī′ tĭs)	thyr -oid -itis	thyroid, shield resemble inflammation	Inflammation of the thyroid gland
thyrotoxicosis (thī″ rō-tŏks″ ĭ-kō′ sĭs)	thyr/o toxic -osis	thyroid, shield poison condition	Literally means *a poisonous condition of the thyroid gland*; pathological condition caused by an acute oversecretion of thyroid hormones
thyroxine (T_4) (thī-rŏks′ ēn)	thyro(x) -ine	thyroid, shield substance	Hormone produced by the thyroid gland; important in growth and development and regulation of the body's metabolic rate and metabolism of carbohydrates, fats, and proteins
vasopressin (VP) (văs″ ō-prĕs′ ĭn)	vas/o press -in	vessel to press chemical	Hormone produced by the hypothalamus and stored in the posterior lobe of the pituitary gland; also called *antidiuretic hormone (ADH)*. Hyposecretion of this hormone can result in **diabetes insipidus (DI)**, a condition characterized by excessive thirst (*polydipsia*) and excretion of large amounts of diluted urine (*polyuria*). *Insipidus* means *tasteless*, reflecting very dilute and watery urine.
virilism (vĭr′ ĭl-ĭzm)	viril -ism	masculine condition	Pathological condition in which secondary male characteristics, such as growth of hair on face and/or body and deepening of the voice, are produced in a female, usually as the result of adrenal dysfunction or hormonal imbalance or taking medications (androgens)

Study and Review II

Word Parts

Prefixes

Give the definitions of the following prefixes.

1. dia- ______________________
2. endo- ______________________
3. eu- ______________________
4. ex- ______________________
5. exo- ______________________
6. hyper- ______________________
7. hypo- ______________________
8. para- ______________________
9. pro- ______________________
10. epi- ______________________

Combining Forms

Give the definitions of the following combining forms.

1. acid/o ______________________
2. acr/o ______________________
3. aden/o ______________________
4. adren/o ______________________
5. andr/o ______________________
6. cortic/o ______________________
7. crin/o ______________________
8. estr/o ______________________
9. ger/o ______________________
10. gigant/o ______________________
11. gluc/o ______________________
12. gonad/o ______________________
13. hirsut/o ______________________
14. insulin/o ______________________
15. kal/i ______________________
16. myx/o ______________________
17. pancreat/o ______________________
18. test/o ______________________
19. thym/o ______________________
20. thyr/o ______________________
21. toxic/o ______________________
22. viril/o ______________________

Suffixes

Give the definitions of the following suffixes.

1. -al ______________________ 2. -gen ______________________
3. -ar ______________________ 4. -betes ______________________
5. -ectomy ______________________ 6. -edema ______________________
7. -emia ______________________ 8. -genic ______________________
9. -ia ______________________ 10. -ic ______________________
11. -ism ______________________ 12. -ist ______________________
13. -itis ______________________ 14. -logy ______________________
15. -one ______________________ 16. -megaly ______________________
17. -oid ______________________ 18. -oma ______________________
19. -osis ______________________ 20. -pathy ______________________
21. -ine ______________________ 22. -physis ______________________
23. -in ______________________ 24. -y ______________________

Identifying Medical Terms

In the spaces provided, write the medical terms for the following meanings.

1. ______________________ Tumor of a gland
2. ______________________ Congenital deficiency in secretion of the thyroid hormones characterized by arrested physical and mental development
3. ______________________ General term used to describe diseases characterized by excessive discharge of urine
4. ______________________ Study of the endocrine system
5. ______________________ Normal activity of the thyroid gland
6. ______________________ Pertains to a type of gland that secretes into ducts (duct glands)
7. ______________________ Pathological condition of being abnormally large
8. ______________________ General classification of the adrenal cortex hormones
9. ______________________ Condition of excessive amounts of potassium in the blood

10. ______________________________ Condition caused by deficient internal secretion of the gonads

11. ______________________________ Pertaining to drowsiness; sluggishness

12. ______________________________ Inflammation of the thymus

Matching

Select the appropriate lettered meaning for each of the following words.

____________ **1.** aldosterone

____________ **2.** androgen

____________ **3.** progesterone

____________ **4.** cortisone

____________ **5.** dopamine

____________ **6.** epinephrine

____________ **7.** insulin

____________ **8.** iodine

____________ **9.** thyroxine

____________ **10.** vasopressin

a. Also called *antidiuretic hormone*, *ADH*

b. Hormone released during the second half of the menstrual cycle

c. Acts to regulate the metabolism of glucose

d. Hormone produced by the thyroid gland

e. Essential in regulating electrolyte and water balance by promoting sodium and chloride reabsorption and potassium excretion

f. Hormones that produce or stimulate the development of male characteristics

g. Glucocorticoid (steroid) hormone used as an anti-inflammatory agent

h. Intermediate substance in the synthesis of norepinephrine

i. Also called *adrenaline*

j. Trace mineral that aids in the development and functioning of the thyroid gland

k. Hormone produced by the testes

MEDICAL CASE SNAPSHOTS

This learning activity provides an opportunity to relate the medical terminology you are learning to a precise patient case presentation. In the spaces provided, write in your answers.

Case 1

A 54-year-old female presents with fatigue, muscular weakness, and a round, red face. These are symptoms associated with ________________ (disease that results from the hypersecretion of cortisol). Prolonged administration of large doses of ACTH can also cause this condition. Two characteristic signs of this condition are: a ________________ ________________ and a moon face.

Case 2

A 15-year-old male complains of being "thirsty, hungry, and frequent urination." The medical terms for his complaints are: _______________ or excessive thirst, _______________ or extreme hunger, and _______________ or frequent urination.

Case 3

The patient is a 48-year-old female presenting with marked protrusion of the eyeballs indicative of _______________ goiter, sometimes called _______________ disease. People with this condition develop eye problems including bulging, red, or _______________ eyes, sensitivity to _______________, and _______________ or double vision.

Drug Highlights

Type of Drug	Description and Examples
thyroid hormones	Increase metabolic rate, cardiac output, oxygen consumption, body temperature, respiratory rate, blood volume, and carbohydrate, fat, and protein metabolism; influence growth and development at cellular level. Thyroid hormones are used as supplements or replacement therapy in hypothyroidism, myxedema, and cretinism. EXAMPLES: Levothroid and Synthroid (levothyroxine sodium), Cytomel (liothyronine sodium), and Thyrolar (liotrix)
antithyroid hormones	Inhibit the synthesis of thyroid hormones by decreasing iodine use in manufacture of thyroglobin and iodothyronine; do not inactivate or inhibit thyroxine or triiodothyronine. They are used in the treatment of hyperthyroidism. EXAMPLES: Tapazole (methimazole), potassium iodide solution, and propylthiouracil
insulin preparations for injection	Insulin is given by subcutaneous injection and is available in various forms such as rapid-acting, intermediate-acting, and long-acting preparations. See Table 13.3.

Table 13.3 Injectible Insulin Preparations and Their Onsets

Type of Insulin and Brand Name	Onset
RAPID-ACTING	
Apidra	15 min
Humalog	15–30 min
Novolog	10–20 min
*PREMIXED**	
Novolin 70/30	30 min
Novolog 70/30	10–20 min
Humalog mix 75/25	15 min
LONG-ACTING	
Lantus	1–$1\frac{1}{2}$ hr

*Premixed insulins are a combination of specific proportions of intermediate-acting and short-acting insulin in one bottle or insulin pen.

Type of Drug	Description and Examples
oral hypoglycemic agents	Stimulate insulin secretion from pancreatic cells in noninsulin-dependent diabetics with some pancreatic function. They are agents of the sulfonylurea class. EXAMPLES: Diabinese (chlorpropamide), Glucotrol (glipizide), DiaBeta (glyburide), and Glucophage (metformin)
hyperglycemic agents	Cause an increase in blood glucose of diabetic patients with severe hypoglycemia (insulin shock). In patients with mild hypoglycemia, the administration of an oral carbohydrate such as orange juice, candy, or a lump of sugar generally corrects the condition. If comatose, the patient is given dextrose solution IV. For management of severe hypoglycemia, the following agents may be used. EXAMPLES: Glucagon (an insulin antagonist), Proglycem (diazoxide), and glucose

Diagnostic and Laboratory Tests

Test	Description
catecholamines (kăt″ ĕ-kōl′ ă-mēns)	Test performed on urine to determine the amount of epinephrine and norepinephrine present. These adrenal hormones increase in times of stress.
corticotropin, corticotropin-releasing factor (kor″ tĭ-kō-trō′ pin)	Test performed on blood plasma to determine the amount of corticotropin present. Increased levels can indicate stress, adrenal cortical hypofunction, and/or pituitary tumors. Decreased **corticotropin-releasing factor (CRF)** levels can indicate adrenal neoplasms and/or Cushing syndrome.
fasting blood sugar (FBS)	Test performed on blood to determine the level of sugar in the bloodstream. It is done after fasting 8–12 hrs (NPO after midnight) and should be performed the next morning. A FBS of 100–125 mg/dL indicates prediabetes. A FBS of 126 mg/dL may indicate diabetes mellitus. Also referred to as *fasting blood glucose (FBG).*
glucose tolerance test (GTT) (gloo′ kōs)	Blood sugar test performed at specified intervals after the patient has been given a significant amount of glucose. Blood samples are drawn, and the glucose level of each sample is measured. It is more accurate than other blood sugar tests and is used to diagnose diabetes mellitus. A GTT of 140–199 mg/dL indicates prediabetes. A GTT at 200 mg/dL or higher indicates diabetes mellitus.
Hb A1C test	The Hb A1C test is a blood test used to diagnose diabetes, to identify people at risk of developing diabetes, and to monitor how well blood sugar levels are being controlled by the diabetic patient. For someone who doesn't have diabetes, a normal A1C level can range from 4.5% to 6%. An A1C level of 6.5% or higher on two separate tests indicates diabetes. A result between 5.7% and 6.4% is considered prediabetes, which indicates a high risk of developing diabetes. For most people who have previously diagnosed diabetes, an A1C level of 7% or less is a common treatment target.
17-hydroxycorticosteroids (17-OHCS) (hī-drŏk″ sē-kor tĭ-kō-stĕr′ oyds)	Test performed on urine to identify adrenocorticosteroid hormones and to determine adrenal cortical function.
17-ketosteroids (17-KS) (kē″ tō-stĕr′ oyds)	Test performed on urine to determine the amount of 17-KS present, the end product of androgens that are secreted from the adrenal glands and testes. It is used to diagnose adrenal tumors.
protein-bound iodine (PBI)	Test performed on serum to indicate the amount of iodine that is attached to serum protein. It can be used to indicate thyroid function.
radioactive iodine uptake (RAIU) (rā″ dē-ō-ăk′ tĭv ī′ ō-dīn)	Test to measure the ability of the thyroid gland to concentrate ingested iodine. Increased level can indicate hyperthyroidism, cirrhosis, and/or thyroiditis. Decreased level can indicate hypothyroidism.
radioimmunoassay (RIA) (rā″ dē-ō-ĭm′ ū-nō-ăs′ ā)	Standard assay method used to measure minute quantities of specific antibodies and/or antigens. It can be used for clinical laboratory measurements of hormones, therapeutic drug monitoring, and substance abuse screening.

Test	Description
thyroid scan (thī′ royd)	Test to detect tumors of the thyroid gland. The patient is given radioactive iodine 131, which localizes in the thyroid gland, which is then visualized with a scanner device.
thyroxine (T_4) (thī-rŏks′ ĭn)	Test performed on blood serum to determine the amount of thyroxine present. Increased levels can indicate hyperthyroidism; decreased levels can indicate hypothyroidism.
total calcium	Test performed on blood serum to determine the amount of calcium present. Increased levels can indicate hyperparathyroidism; decreased levels can indicate hypoparathyroidism.
triiodothyronine uptake (T_3U) (trī′ ī-ō″ dō-thī′ rō-nĭn)	Test performed on blood serum to determine the amount of triiodothyronine present. Increased levels can indicate thyrotoxicosis, toxic adenoma, and/or Hashimoto thyroiditis. Decreased levels can indicate starvation, severe infection, and severe trauma.
ultrasonography (ŭl-tră-sŏn-ŏg′ ră-fē)	Use of high-frequency sound waves as a screening test or as a diagnostic tool to visualize the structure being studied; can be used to visualize the pancreas, thyroid, and any other gland

Abbreviations

Abbreviation	Meaning
17-KS	17-ketosteroids
17-OHCS	17-hydroxycorticosteroids
ACTH	adrenocorticotropin hormone
ADH	antidiuretic hormone
BG	blood glucose
BMI	body mass index
BMR	basal metabolic rate
cm	centimeter
CRF	corticotropin-releasing factor
DI	diabetes insipidus
DM	diabetes mellitus
FBG	fasting blood glucose
FBS	fasting blood sugar
FSH	follicle-stimulating hormone
g	gram
GH	growth hormone
GHRF	growth hormone-releasing factor
GnRF	gonadotropin-releasing factor
GTT	glucose tolerance test
IDDM	insulin-dependent diabetes mellitus
K	potassium
LH	luteinizing hormone
LTH	lactogenic hormone
MIF	melanocyte-stimulating hormone release-inhibiting factor
MRF	melanocyte-stimulating hormone-releasing factor
MSH	melanocyte-stimulating hormone
Na	sodium
NIDDM	non-insulin-dependent diabetes mellitus
PBI	protein-bound iodine
PIF	prolactin release-inhibiting factor
PRF	prolactin-releasing factor
PRL	prolactin hormone
PTH	parathyroid hormone
RAIU	radioactive iodine uptake
RIA	radioimmunoassay
STH	somatotropin hormone
T_3	triiodothyronine
T_3U	triiodothyronine uptake
T_4	thyroxine
TH	thyroid hormone
TRH	thyrotropin-releasing hormone
TSH	thyroid-stimulating hormone
VP	vasopressin

Study and Review III

Building Medical Terms

Using the following word parts, fill in the blanks to build the correct medical terms.

hypo-	letharg	-in
adren	-one	-edema
dwarf	-ism	-al

Definition	Medical Term
1. Pertaining to the adrenal glands; also called suprarenal glands	___________al
2. Glucocorticoid hormone secreted by the adrenal cortex	cortis________
3. Condition of being abnormally small	__________ism
4. Pathological condition of being abnormally large	gigant________
5. Abnormal condition characterized by excessive growth of hair	hirsut________
6. Literally means *any undergrowth*; also called the pituitary gland	________physis
7. Hormone produced by the beta cells of the islets of Langerhans	insul_________
8. Pertaining to drowsiness, sluggish	___________ic
9. Literally means *condition of mucus swelling*	myx_________
10. Endocrine gland shaped like a small pine cone	pine_________

Combining Form Challenge

Using the combining forms provided, write the medical term correctly.

aden/o	estr/o	thym/o
andr/o	insulin/o	thyr/o

1. Any disease condition of a gland: _______osis
2. Hormone that produces the development of male characteristics: _______gen
3. Female sex hormone produced in the ovaries: ______gen
4. Formation or production of insulin: _______genic
5. Surgical excision of the thymus gland: _______ectomy
6. Endocrine gland located in the neck: _______oid

Select the Right Term

Select the correct answer, and write it on the line provided.

1. Characterized (in the adult) by marked enlargement and elongation of the bones of the face, jaw, and extremities is __________.

   Addison disease **acidosis** **acromegaly** **adenoma**

2. General term used to describe diseases characterized by excessive discharge of urine is ___________.

   diabetes **cretinism** **Cushing** **exophthalmic**

3. Hormone produced by the adrenal medulla, also called adrenaline, is __________.

   dopamine **epinephrine** **estrogen** **norepinephrine**

4. Pathological condition in which the thyroid gland produces inadequate amounts of thyroid hormone is __________.

   hyperthyroidism **hypophysis** **hypothyroidism** **hypogonadism**

5. Pathological condition of premature old age occurring in childhood is __________.

   myxedema **lethargic** **pituitarism** **progeria**

6. Pathological condition in which secondary male characteristics are produced in a female is ___________.

   thyrotoxicosis **progeria** **hypoparathyroidism** **virilism**

Diagnostic and Laboratory Tests

Select the best answer to each multiple-choice question. Circle the letter of your choice.

1. A test performed on urine to determine the amount of epinephrine and norepinephrine present.
   a. catecholamines
   b. corticotropin
   c. protein-bound iodine
   d. total calcium

2. Increased levels can indicate prediabetes or diabetes mellitus.
   a. protein-bound iodine
   b. total calcium
   c. fasting blood sugar
   d. thyroid scan

3. Test used to detect tumors of the thyroid gland.
   a. thyroxine
   b. total calcium
   c. thyroid scan
   d. protein-bound iodine

4. Blood sugar test performed at specific intervals after the patient has been given a certain amount of glucose.
   a. fasting blood sugar
   b. glucose tolerance test
   c. protein-bound iodine
   d. corticotropin

5. A test used in the diagnosing of adrenal tumors.
   a. 17-HCS
   b. 17-OHCS
   c. 17-KS
   d. 17-HDL

Abbreviations

Place the correct word, phrase, or abbreviation in the space provided.

1. basal metabolic rate ______________________
2. diabetes mellitus ______________________
3. FBS ______________________
4. GTT ______________________
5. protein-bound iodine ______________________
6. PTH ______________________
7. RIA ______________________
8. somatotropin hormone ______________________
9. TSH ______________________
10. VP ______________________

Practical Application

Case Study Analysis

This exercise contains information, abbreviations, and medical terminology from an actual medical record or case study that has been adapted for this text. The names and any personal information have been created by the author. Read and study each form or case study and then answer the questions that follow. You may refer to Appendix III, *Abbreviations and Symbols*.

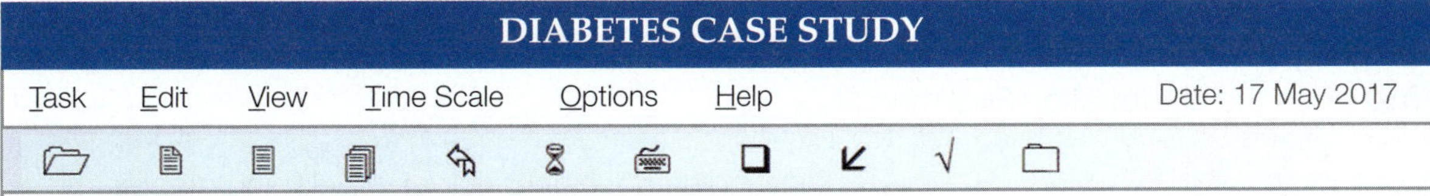

Meet Matthew J. Marshall

Matthew is a 15 y/o white male c/o being "thirsty, hungry, and urinating a lot." He states, "I am tired and just don't have any energy. I eat like a horse, but I stay hungry. I am afraid that I have 'sugar.' My dad and my grandfather both take insulin."

Signs and Symptoms: Polydipsia, polyphagia, polyuria, and fatigue.
Family history is notable for type 1 diabetes in father and paternal grandfather; his maternal grandmother has heart disease. **Allergies:** NKDA. Typically, for a patient with this complaint and history, type 2 diabetes would be considered.

The pertinent findings on physical exam:

Vital Signs: T: 98.4 F; P: 78; R: 18; BP: 132/70

Ht: 5′ 5″

Wt: 160 lb

General Appearance: Overweight for age. BMI: 26.6

Heart: Regular rate and rhythm. No murmurs. Lungs: CTA. Abd: Noted excessive adipose tissue. Soft, nontender, no masses, no liver enlargement. Skin: Warm and dry, no lesions, no discoloration of lower extremities.

The Plan for Diagnosis and Treatment:

1. Send to lab for Hb A1C and schedule FBS, ASAP.
2. Recommend that Matthew attend the next health education seminar. One or both parents are to attend the seminar with him. Explain that individuals who are overweight, have a BMI greater than or equal to 25, and who have immediate family members with diabetes are at a higher risk of developing diabetes. Note: For more information on diabetes, call (800) DIABETES.
3. Patient is to return in 1 week for test results. If indicated, proper medication regimen will be initiated for Matthew.

Case Study Questions

Place the correct answer in the space provided

1. Why is Matthew concerned that he may have “sugar”?____________________

2. To rule out diabetes mellitus, the physician ordered a ____________________ test and a ____________________ ASAP.

3. What are the three classic symptoms of diabetes mellitus that Matthew stated?
____________________ ____________________ ____________________

4. What does the abbreviation *FBS* mean? ____________________

5. A BMI over ____________________ may indicate a higher risk of developing diabetes.

Chapter 14

Nervous System

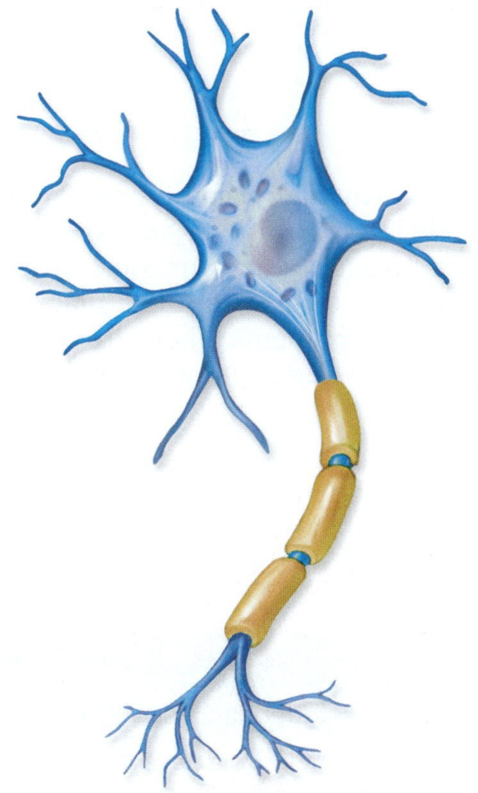

Learning Outcomes

On completion of this chapter, you will be able to:

1. Describe the nervous system.
2. State the description and primary functions of the organs/structures of the nervous system.
3. List the major divisions of the brain and their functions.
4. Recognize terminology included in the ICD-10-CM.
5. Analyze, build, spell, and pronounce medical words.
6. Comprehend the drugs highlighted in this chapter.
7. Describe diagnostic and laboratory tests related to the nervous system.
8. Identify and define selected abbreviations.
9. Apply your acquired knowledge of medical terms by successfully completing the *Practical Application* exercise.

Anatomy and Physiology

The nervous system is usually described as having two interconnected divisions: the central nervous system (CNS) and the peripheral nervous system (PNS). The CNS includes the brain and spinal cord. It is enclosed by the bones of the skull and spinal column. The PNS consists of the network of nerves and neural tissues branching throughout the body from 12 pairs of cranial nerves and 31 pairs of spinal nerves. Table 14.1 provides an at-a-glance look at the nervous system. See Figure 14.1.

Tissues of the Nervous System

The nervous system has two principal tissue types. These tissues are made up of **neurons** or nerve cells and their supporting tissues, collectively called **neuroglia**. See Figure 14.2. Neurons are the structural and functional units of the nervous system. These cells are specialized conductors of impulses that enable the body to interact with its internal and external environments. There are several types of neurons, three of which are described in the following sections.

Motor Neurons

Motor neurons cause contractions in muscles and secretions from glands and organs. They also act to inhibit the actions of glands and organs, thereby controlling most of the body's functions. Motor neurons can be described as being *efferent processes* because

Table 14.1 Nervous System at-a-Glance

Organ/Structure	Primary Functions/Description
Neurons (nerve cells)	Structural and functional units of the nervous system act as specialized conductors of impulses that enable the body to interact with its internal and external environments
Neuroglia	Act as supporting tissue
Nerve fibers and tracts	Conduct impulses from one location to another
Central nervous system	Receives impulses from throughout the body, processes the information, and responds with an appropriate action
Brain	Governs sensory perception, emotions, consciousness, memory, and voluntary movements
Spinal cord	Conducts sensory impulses to the brain and motor impulses from the brain to body parts; also serves as a reflex center for impulses entering and leaving the spinal cord without involvement of the brain
Peripheral nervous system	Links the central nervous system with other parts of the body
Cranial nerves (12 pairs)	Provide sensory input and motor control or a combination of these
Spinal nerves (31 pairs)	Carry impulses to the spinal cord and to muscles, organs, and glands
Autonomic nervous system (sympathetic division and parasympathetic division)	Controls involuntary bodily functions such as sweating, secretion of glands, arterial blood pressure, smooth muscle tissue, and the heart. Also stimulates the adrenal gland to release epinephrine (adrenaline), the hormone that causes the familiar adrenaline rush or the "fight-or-flight" response.

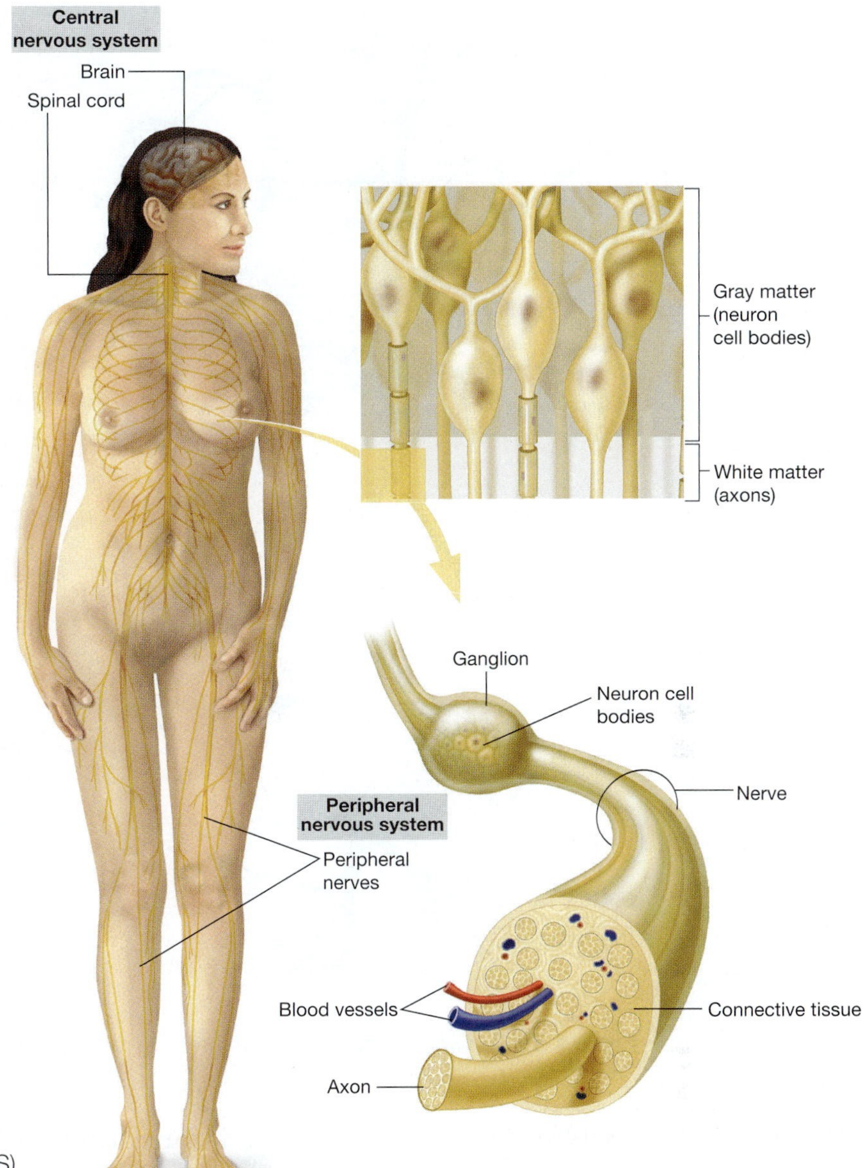

Figure 14.1 The nervous system is described as having two interconnected divisions: the central nervous system (CNS) consisting of the brain and spinal cord and the peripheral nervous system (PNS) consisting of peripheral nerves.

they transmit impulses away from the neural cell body to the muscles or organs to be innervated. Motor neurons consist of a nucleated cell body with protoplasmic processes extending away from it in several directions. These processes are known as the **axons** and **dendrites**. Most axons are long and are covered with a fatty substance, the myelin sheath, which acts as an insulator and increases the transmission velocity of the nerve fiber it surrounds. Axons may be as long as several feet and reach from the cell body to the area to be activated. Dendrites resemble the branches of a tree, are short, unsheathed, and transmit impulses to the cell body. Neurons usually have several dendrites and only one axon.

Sensory Neurons

Sensory neurons differ in structure from motor neurons because they do not have true dendrites. The processes transmitting sensory information to the cell bodies of these neurons are called *peripheral processes*, are sheathed, and resemble axons. They are attached to sensory receptors and transmit impulses to the central nervous system

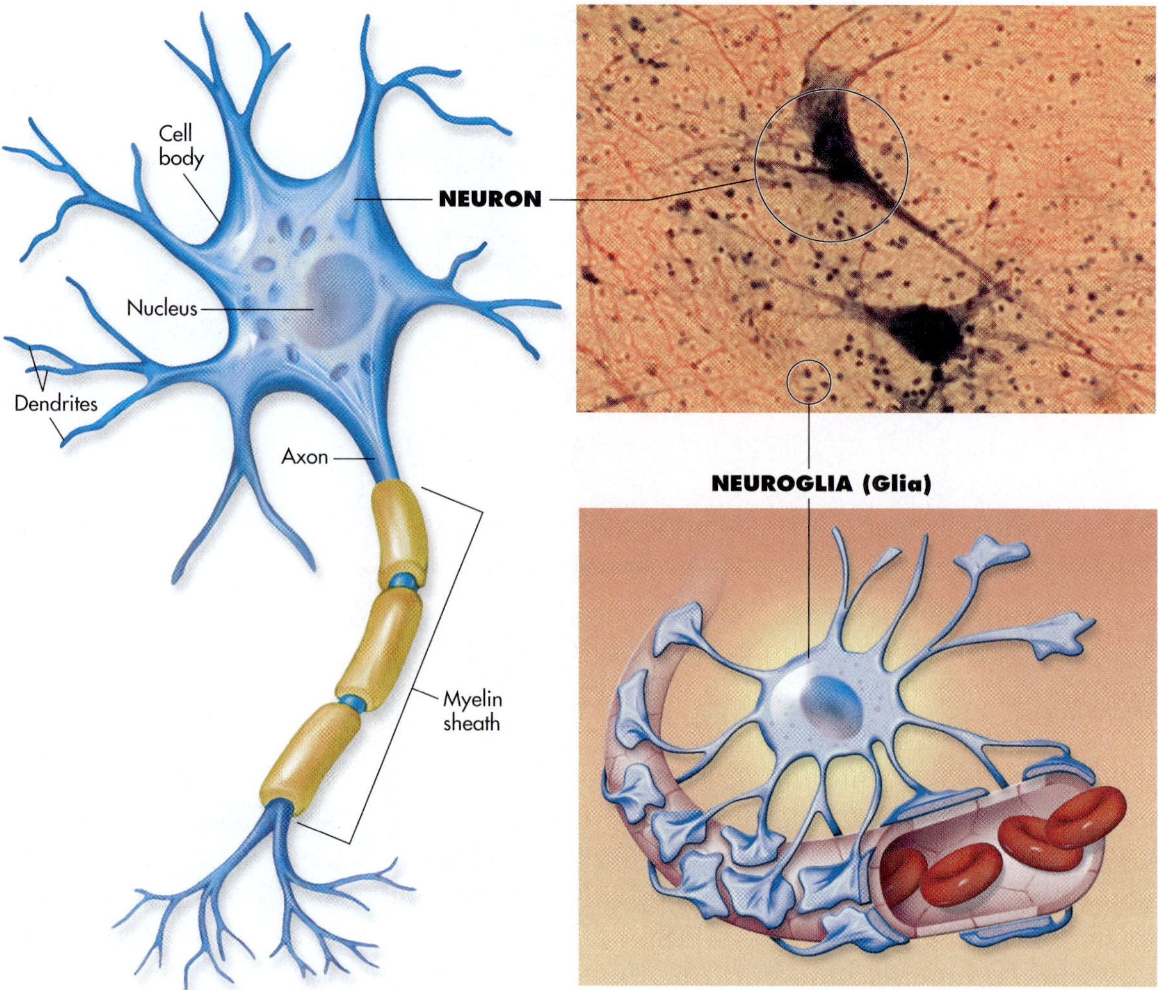

Figure 14.2 Two main types of nerve cells.

(CNS). After processing the information, the CNS can stimulate motor neurons in response to this sensory information. Sensory neurons are referred to as *afferent nerves* because they carry impulses from the sensory receptors to the synaptic endings in the central nervous system.

Interneurons

Interneurons are called *central* or *associative neurons* and are located entirely within the central nervous system. They function to mediate impulses between sensory and motor neurons.

Nerve Fibers, Nerves, and Tracts

The terms *nerve fiber*, *nerve*, and *tract* are used to describe neuronal processes conducting impulses from one location to another.

Nerve Fibers

A **nerve fiber** is a single elongated process, the axon of a neuron. Nerve fibers of the peripheral nervous system are wrapped by protective membranes called **sheaths**. The PNS has two types of sheaths: *myelinated* and *unmyelinated*, which are formed by accessory cells. Myelinated fibers have an inner sheath of myelin, a thick, fatty substance, and an outer sheath, or **neurilemma**, composed of *Schwann cells*. Unmyelinated fibers lack myelin and are sheathed only by the neurilemma. Nerve fibers of the central nervous system do not contain Schwann cells. Therefore, damage to fibers of the CNS is permanent, whereas damage to a peripheral nerve can be reversible.

Nerves

A **nerve** is a collection of nerve fibers, outside the central nervous system. Nerves are usually described as being sensory or **afferent** (conducting to the CNS) or motor or **efferent** (conducting away from the CNS to muscles, organs, and glands).

Tracts

Groups of nerve fibers within the central nervous system are sometimes referred to as **tracts** when they have the same origin, function, and termination. The spinal cord contains afferent sensory tracts ascending to the brain and efferent motor tracts descending from the brain. The brain itself contains numerous tracts, the largest of which is the *corpus callosum* joining the left and right hemispheres.

Transmission of Nerve Impulses

Stimulation of nerves occurs at *sensory receptors*, which are nerve endings that receive and relay responses to stimuli. There are distinct sensory receptors, ranging from the simplest, which are free nerve endings for pain, to the most complex, as in the retina of the eye for vision. Sensory receptors are specialized to specific types of stimulation such as heat, cold, light, pressure, or pain and react by initiating a chemical change or impulse. The transmission of an impulse by a nerve fiber is based on the **all-or-none principle**. This means that no transmission occurs until the stimulus reaches a set minimum strength, which can vary for different receptors. Once the minimum stimulus or threshold is reached, a maximum impulse is produced. The impulse is then transmitted via a **synapse**, a specialized knoblike branch ending, with the help of certain chemical agents, across a space separating the axon's end knobs from the dendrites of the next neuron or from a motor end plate attached to a muscle. This space is called a **synaptic cleft**, and the chemical agents released are called **neurotransmitters**.

Central Nervous System

Consisting of the brain and spinal cord, the **central nervous system (CNS)** receives impulses from throughout the body, processes the information, and responds with an appropriate action. This activity can be at the conscious or unconscious level, depending on the source of the sensory stimulus. Both the brain and spinal cord can be divided into **gray matter** and **white matter**. The gray matter consists of unsheathed cell bodies and true dendrites. The white matter is composed of myelinated nerve fibers. In the spinal cord, the arrangement of white and gray matter results in an H-shaped core of gray cell bodies surrounded by tracts of nerve fibers interconnected to the brain. The reverse is generally true of the brain where the surface layer or cortex is gray matter and most of the internal structures are white matter.

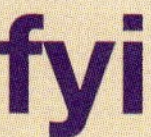

Neural tube development occurs about the third to fourth week of embryonic life. This development becomes the central nervous system. At 6 weeks, a developing fetus's brain waves are measurable. At 28 weeks, the fetal nervous system begins some regulatory functions. By 32 weeks, the developing fetal nervous system is capable of sustaining rhythmic respirations and regulating body temperature. The growth rate of brain and nerve cells is at its most rapid pace up to about 4 years of age.

While the brain of an infant resembles that of an adult, one area is relatively unrefined. In an infant, the right and left hemispheres of the brain have yet to develop their own specific tasks. However, by the time a child is 3 years old, the two sides of the brain are well on their way to becoming specialized for different tasks.

Brain

The nervous tissue of the **brain** consists of millions of nerve cells and fibers. It is the largest mass of nervous tissue in the body, weighing about 1380 g in the male and 1250 g in the female. The brain is enclosed by three membranes known collectively as the **meninges**. See Figure 14.3. From the outside in, these are the *dura mater*, *arachnoid*, and *pia mater*. The major structures of the brain are the *cerebrum*, *cerebellum*, *diencephalon*, and the *brainstem*, which is composed of the *midbrain*, *pons*, and *medulla oblongata*. See Figure 14.4 and Table 14.2.

CEREBRUM

Representing seven-eighths of the brain's total weight, the **cerebrum** contains nerve centers that evaluate and control all sensory and motor activity, including sensory perception, emotions, consciousness, memory, and voluntary movements.

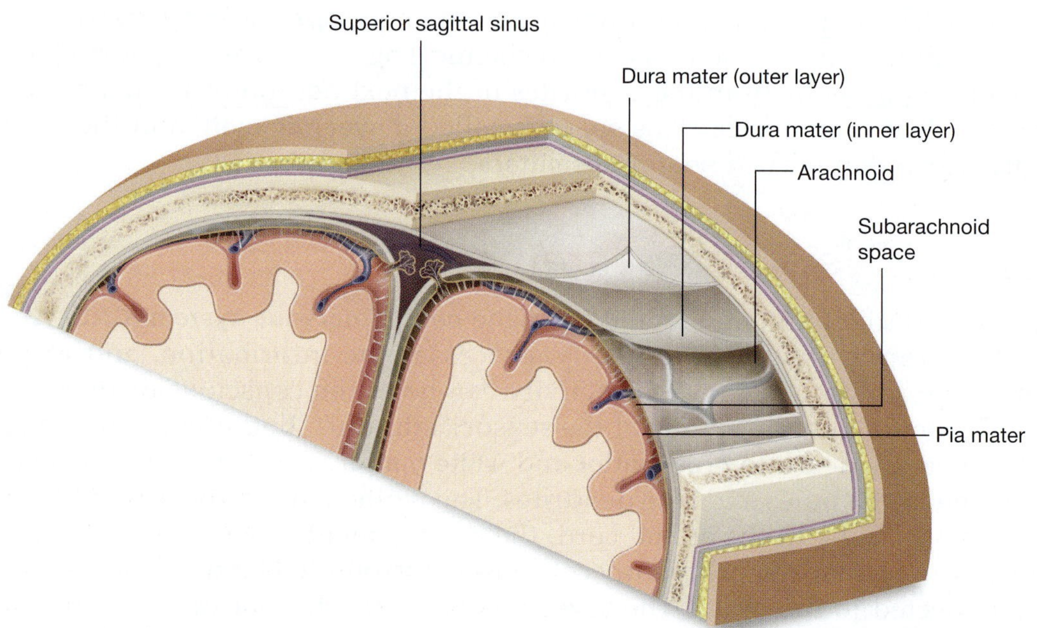

Figure 14.3 The meninges from the outside in: dura mater, arachnoid, and pia mater. Also showing the subarachnoid space and superior sagittal sinus.

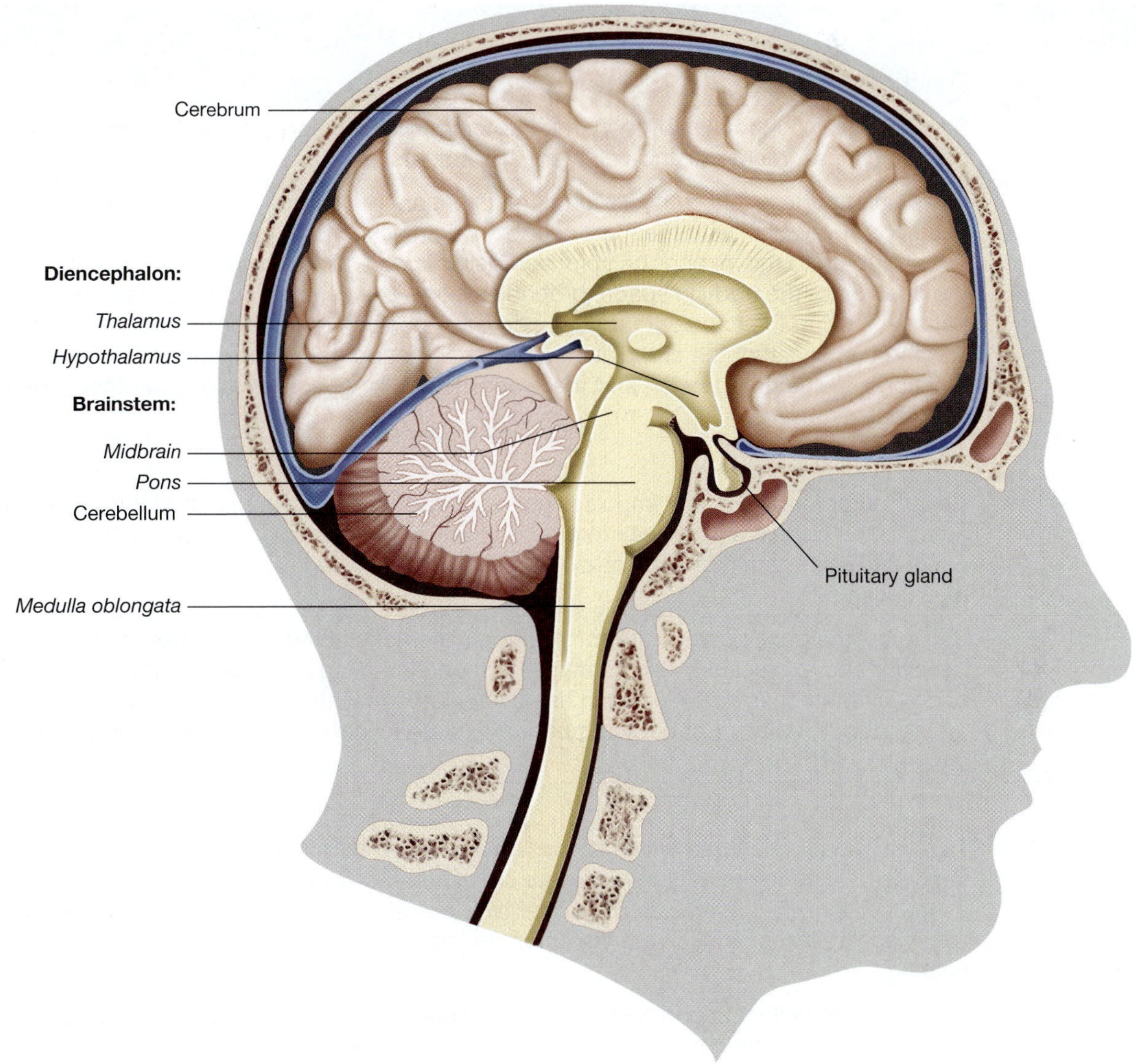

Figure 14.4 Major structures of the brain.

The cerebrum is divided by the longitudinal fissure into two cerebral hemispheres, the right and left, that are joined by large fiber tracts (*corpus callosum*) that allow information to pass from one hemisphere to the other. The surface or *cortex* of each hemisphere is arranged in folds creating bulges and shallow furrows. Each bulge is called a **gyrus** or **convolution**. A furrow is known as a **sulcus**. This surface is composed of gray, unmyelinated cell bodies and is known as the **cerebral cortex**. The cortex has been divided into lobes as a means of identifying certain locations. These lobes correspond to the overlying bones of the skull and are the *frontal*, *parietal*, *temporal*, and *occipital lobes*.

Electrical stimulation of the various areas of the cortex during neurosurgery has identified specialized cell activity within the different lobes. The **frontal lobe** has been identified as the brain's major motor area and the site for personality and speech. The **parietal lobe** contains centers for sensory input from all parts of the body and is known as the *somesthetic area* and the site for the interpretation of language. Temperature, pressure, touch, and an awareness of muscle control are some of the sensory activities localized in this area. The **temporal lobe** contains centers for hearing, smell,

Table 14.2 Major Divisions of the Brain and Their Functions

Brain Area	Functions
Cerebrum	Evaluates and controls all sensory and motor activity; sensory perception, emotions, consciousness, memory, and voluntary movements
Cerebellum	Plays an important role in the integration of sensory perception and motor output. Its neural pathways link with the motor cortex, which sends information to the muscles causing them to move, and the spinocerebellar tract, which provides feedback on the position of the body in space (proprioception). The cerebellum integrates these pathways using the constant feedback on body position to fine-tune motor movements. Research shows that the cerebellum also has a broader role in a number of key cognitive functions, including attention and the processing of language, music, and other sensory temporal stimuli.
Diencephalon	
Thalamus	Relay center for all sensory impulses (except olfactory) being transmitted to the sensory areas of the cortex, and relays motor impulses from the cerebellum and the basal ganglia to motor areas of the cortex, thought to be involved with emotions and arousal mechanisms
Hypothalamus	Serves as the principal regulator of autonomic nervous activity that is associated with behavior and expression; also contains hormones that are important for the control of certain metabolic activities such as maintenance of water balance, sugar and fat metabolism, regulation of body temperature, sleep-cycle control, appetite, and sexual arousal.
Brainstem	
Midbrain	Two-way conduction pathway that acts as a relay center for visual and auditory impulses; found in the midbrain are four small masses of gray cells known collectively as the *corpora quadrigemina*. The upper two, called the *superior colliculi*, are associated with visual reflexes. The lower two, or *inferior colliculi*, are involved with the sense of hearing.
Pons	Links the cerebellum and medulla to higher cortical areas; plays a role in somatic and visceral motor control; contains important centers for regulating breathing.
Medulla oblongata	Acts as the cardiac, respiratory, and vasomotor control center; regulates and controls breathing, swallowing, coughing, sneezing, and vomiting as well as heartbeat and arterial blood pressure, thereby exerting control over the circulation of blood

and language input, and the **occipital lobe** is the primary interpretive processing area for vision. The occipital lobe is directly posterior to the temporal lobe. See Table 14.2 and Figure 14.5.

CEREBELLUM

The **cerebellum** is the second largest part of the brain. It occupies a space in the back of the skull, inferior to the cerebrum and dorsal to the pons and medulla oblongata. The cerebellum is oval in shape and divided into lobes by deep fissures. It has a cortex of gray cell bodies, and its interior contains nerve fibers and white matter connecting it to every part of the central nervous system. The cerebellum plays an important part in the coordination of voluntary and involuntary complex patterns of movement and adjusts muscles to maintain posture. See Table 14.2.

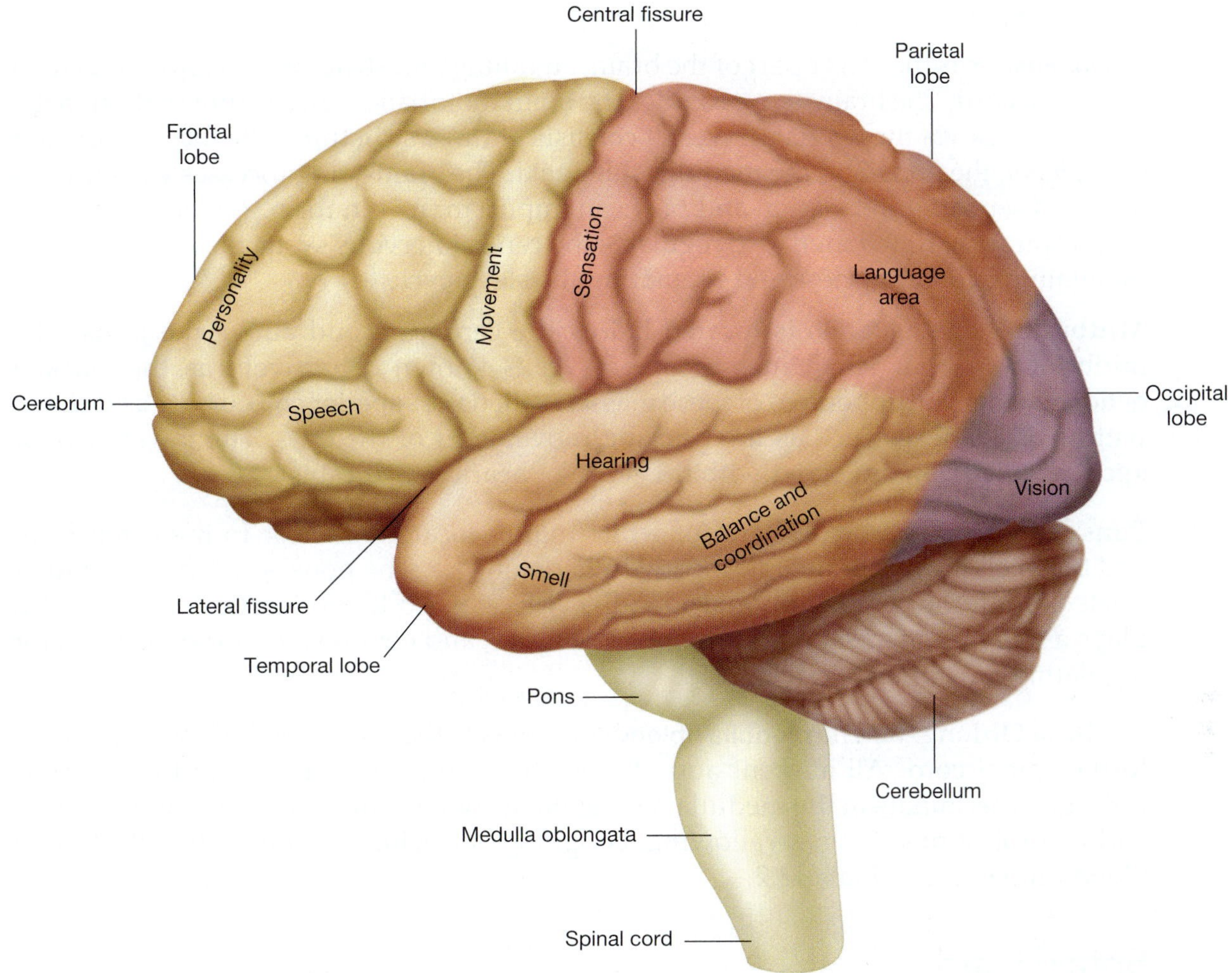

Figure 14.5 The brain, showing the cerebrum and its lobes with their functional centers identified.

DIENCEPHALON

The word ***diencephalon*** means *second portion of the brain* and refers to the thalamus and hypothalamus.

Thalamus. The **thalamus** is the larger of the two divisions of the diencephalon and is actually two large masses of gray cell bodies joined by a third or intermediate mass. The thalamus serves as a relay center for all sensory impulses (except olfactory) being transmitted to the sensory areas of the cortex. Besides its sensory function, the thalamus also relays motor impulses from the cerebellum and the basal ganglia to motor areas of the cortex. Some impulses related to emotional behavior are also passed from the hypothalamus, through the thalamus, to the cerebral cortex. See Table 14.2.

Hypothalamus. The **hypothalamus** lies beneath the thalamus and is a principal regulator of autonomic nervous activity that is associated with behavior and emotional expression. It also produces neurosecretions for the control of water balance, sugar and fat metabolism, regulation of body temperature, and other metabolic activities. See Table 14.2. The pituitary gland is attached to the hypothalamus by a narrow stalk, the *infundibulum*.

Brainstem

The **brainstem** is the lower part of the brain, adjoining and structurally continuous with the spinal cord. The brainstem provides the main motor and sensory innervation to the face and neck via the cranial nerves. It consists of three structures: the mesencephalon or *midbrain*, the pons, and the medulla oblongata. The brainstem processes visual, auditory, and sensory information and plays an important role in the regulation of cardiac and respiratory function. It also regulates the central nervous system and is pivotal in maintaining consciousness and regulating the sleep cycle.

Midbrain. The **midbrain** is located below the cerebrum and above the pons. The midbrain has four small masses of gray cells known collectively as the **corpora quadrigemina**. The upper two of these masses, called the **superior colliculi**, are associated with visual reflexes such as the tracking movements of the eyes. The lower two, or **inferior colliculi**, are involved with the sense of hearing. See Table 14.2.

Pons. The **pons** is a broad band of white matter located anterior to the cerebellum and between the midbrain and the medulla oblongata. The pons is composed of fiber tracts linking the cerebellum and medulla oblongata to higher cortical areas. It also plays a role in somatic and visceral motor control, and contains important centers for regulating breathing. See Table 14.2.

Medulla Oblongata. The **medulla oblongata** connects the pons and the rest of the brain to the spinal cord. All afferent and efferent tracts from the spinal cord either pass through or terminate in the medulla oblongata. It contains nerve centers for regulation and control of breathing, swallowing, coughing, sneezing, vomiting, heartbeat, and blood pressure. See Table 14.2.

Spinal Cord

The **spinal cord** has an H-shaped gray area of cell bodies encircled by an outer region of white matter. The white matter consists of nerve tracts and fibers providing sensory input to the brain and conducting motor impulses from the brain to spinal neurons. The adult spinal cord is about 44 centimeters (cm) long and extends down the vertebral canal from the medulla oblongata to terminate near the junction of the first (L1) and second (L2) lumbar vertebrae. See Figure 14.6. Between the 12th thoracic vertebra (T12) and L1 is a region known as the **conus medullaris**, where the spinal cord becomes conically tapered. The **filum terminale** or terminal thread of fibrous tissue extends from the conus medullaris to the second sacral vertebra. The **cauda equina** (known as the horse's tail) is the terminal portion of the spinal cord that forms the nerve fibers that are the lumbar, sacral, and coccygeal spinal nerves. The functions of the spinal cord are to conduct sensory impulses to the brain, to conduct motor impulses from the brain, and to serve as a reflex center for impulses entering and leaving the spinal cord without direct involvement of the brain.

Cerebrospinal Fluid

The brain and spinal cord are surrounded by **cerebrospinal fluid (CSF)**. This colorless fluid is produced as a filtrate of blood by the *choroid plexuses* within the *ventricles* of the brain. Cerebrospinal fluid circulates through the ventricles, the central canal, and the subarachnoid space. Cerebrospinal fluid is removed from circulation by the **arachnoid villi**, which are small projections of the arachnoid membrane that penetrate the tough outer membrane, the dura mater. The arachnoid villi allow the fluid to drain into the superior sagittal sinus. The normal adult will have between 120 and 150 milliliters (mL)

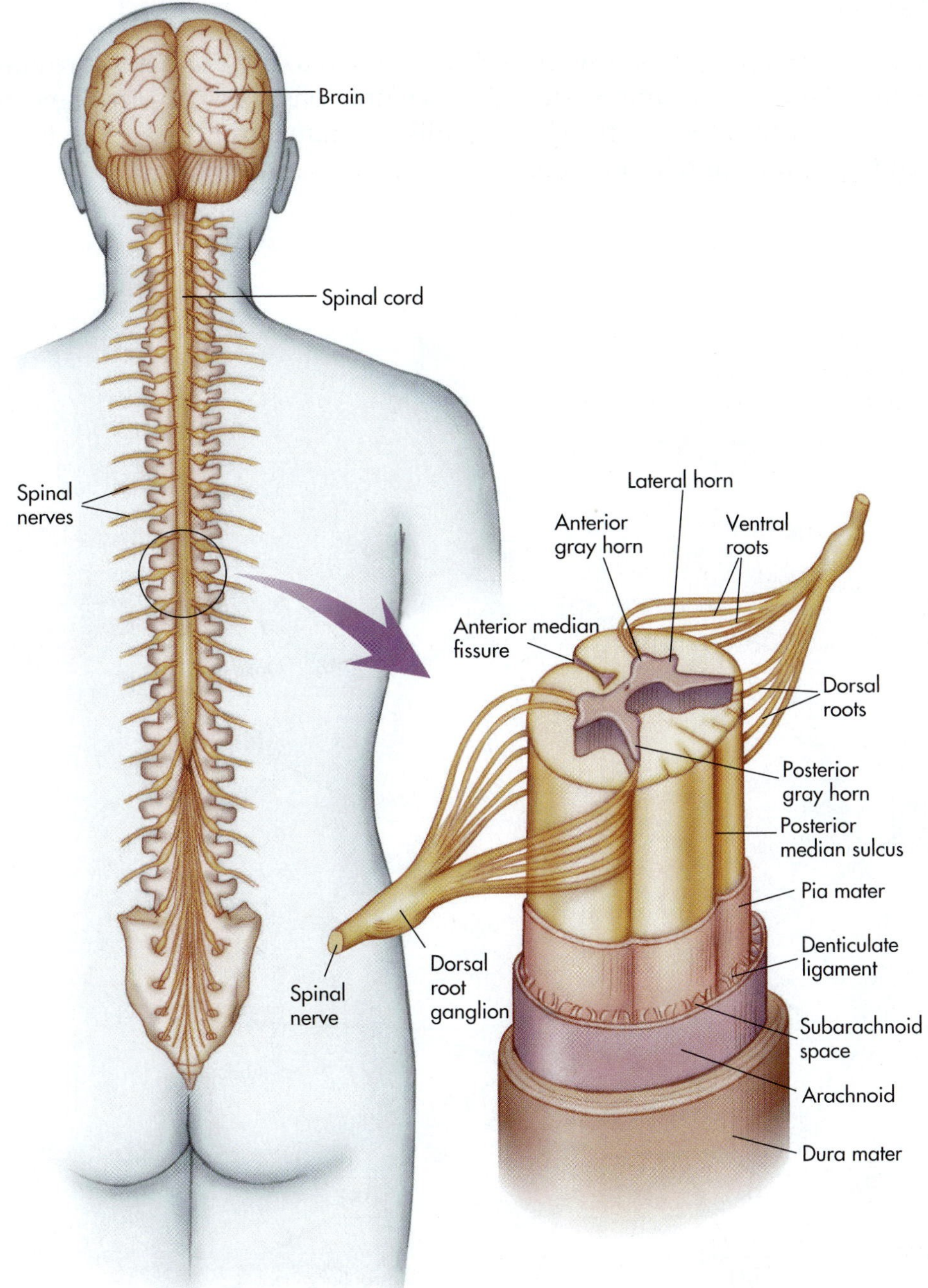

Figure 14.6 Brain, spinal cord, and spinal nerves with an expanded view of a spinal nerve.

of cerebrospinal fluid in circulation. The fluid serves to cushion the brain and spinal cord from shocks that could cause injury. It also helps to support the brain by allowing it to float within the supporting liquid. It also contains neurotransmitters such as monoamines, acetylcholine (ACh), and neuropeptides.

Peripheral Nervous System

The network of nerves branching throughout the body from the brain and spinal cord is known as the **peripheral nervous system (PNS)**. There are 12 pairs of cranial nerves that attach to the brain and 31 pairs of spinal nerves connected to the spinal cord.

Cranial Nerves

The nerves described in the following sections attach to the brain and provide sensory input, motor control, or a combination of these functions. They are arranged symmetrically, 12 to each side of the brain, and generally are named for the area or function they serve. See Figure 14.7 and Table 14.3.

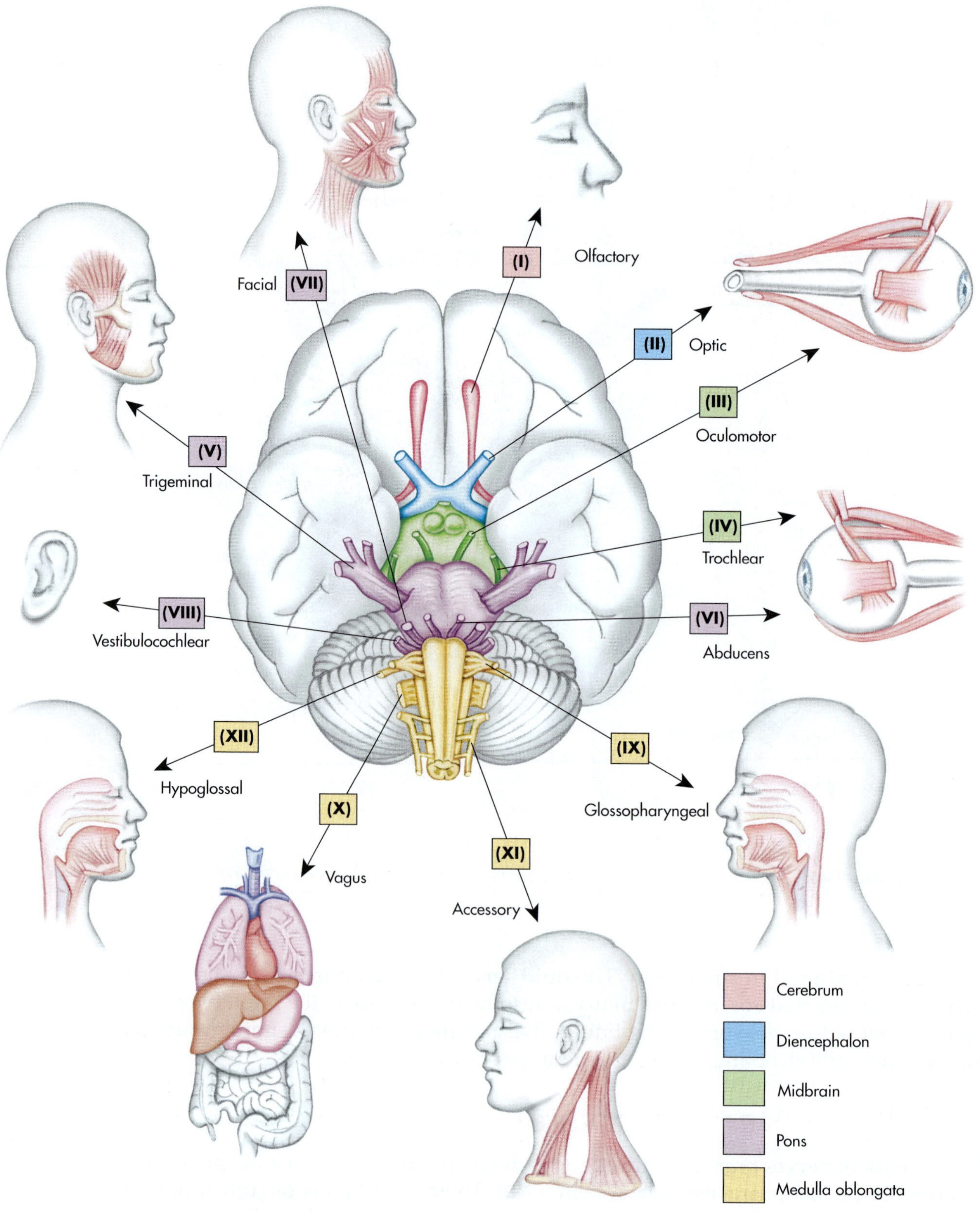

Figure 14.7 Relationship of the 12 cranial nerves to specific regions of the brain.

Table 14.3 Cranial Nerves and Functions

Nerve/Number	Function
Olfactory (I)	Detects and provides the sense of smell
Optic (II)	Provides vision
Oculomotor (III)	Conducts motor impulses to four of the six external muscles of the eye and to the muscle that raises the eyelid
Trochlear (IV)	Conducts motor impulses to control the superior oblique muscle of the eyeball
Trigeminal (V)	Provides sensory input from the face, nose, mouth, forehead, and top of the head; motor fibers to the muscles of the jaw (chewing)
Abducens (VI)	Conducts motor impulses to the lateral rectus muscle of the eyeball
Facial (VII)	Controls the muscles of the face and scalp; the lacrimal glands of the eye and the submandibular and sublingual salivary glands; input from the tongue for the sense of taste
Vestibulocochlear (Acoustic) (VIII)	Provides input for hearing and equilibrium
Glossopharyngeal (IX)	Provides general sense of taste; regulates swallowing; controls secretion of saliva
Vagus (X)	Controls muscles of the pharynx, larynx, thoracic, and abdominal organs; swallowing, voice production, slowing of heartbeat, acceleration of peristalsis
Accessory (XI)	Controls the trapezius and sternocleidomastoid muscles, permitting movement of the head and shoulders
Hypoglossal (XII)	Controls the tongue; tongue movements

Spinal Nerves

There are 31 pairs of **spinal nerves** distributed along the length of the spinal cord and emerging from the vertebral canal on either side through the intervertebral foramina. At the point of attachment, each nerve is divided into two roots (see Figure 14.6). The **dorsal** or **sensory root** is composed of afferent fibers carrying impulses to the cord, and the **ventral root** contains motor fibers carrying efferent impulses to muscles and organs. Named for the region of the vertebral column from which they exit, there are eight pairs of **cervical spinal nerves**, 12 pairs of **thoracic spinal nerves**, five pairs of **lumbar spinal nerves**, five pairs of **sacral spinal nerves**, and one pair of **coccygeal spinal nerves**. See Figure 14.8.

A short distance from the cord, the fibers of the two roots unite to form a spinal nerve. Having formed a single nerve composed of afferent and efferent fibers, each spinal nerve then branches into several smaller nerves. The two primary branches from each spinal nerve are the **dorsal rami** and **ventral rami**. The dorsal rami (*branches*) carry motor and sensory fibers to the muscles and skin of the back and serve an area from the back of the head to the coccyx. The ventral rami, serving a much larger area, carry both motor and sensory fibers to the muscles and organs of the body, including the arms, legs, hands, and feet.

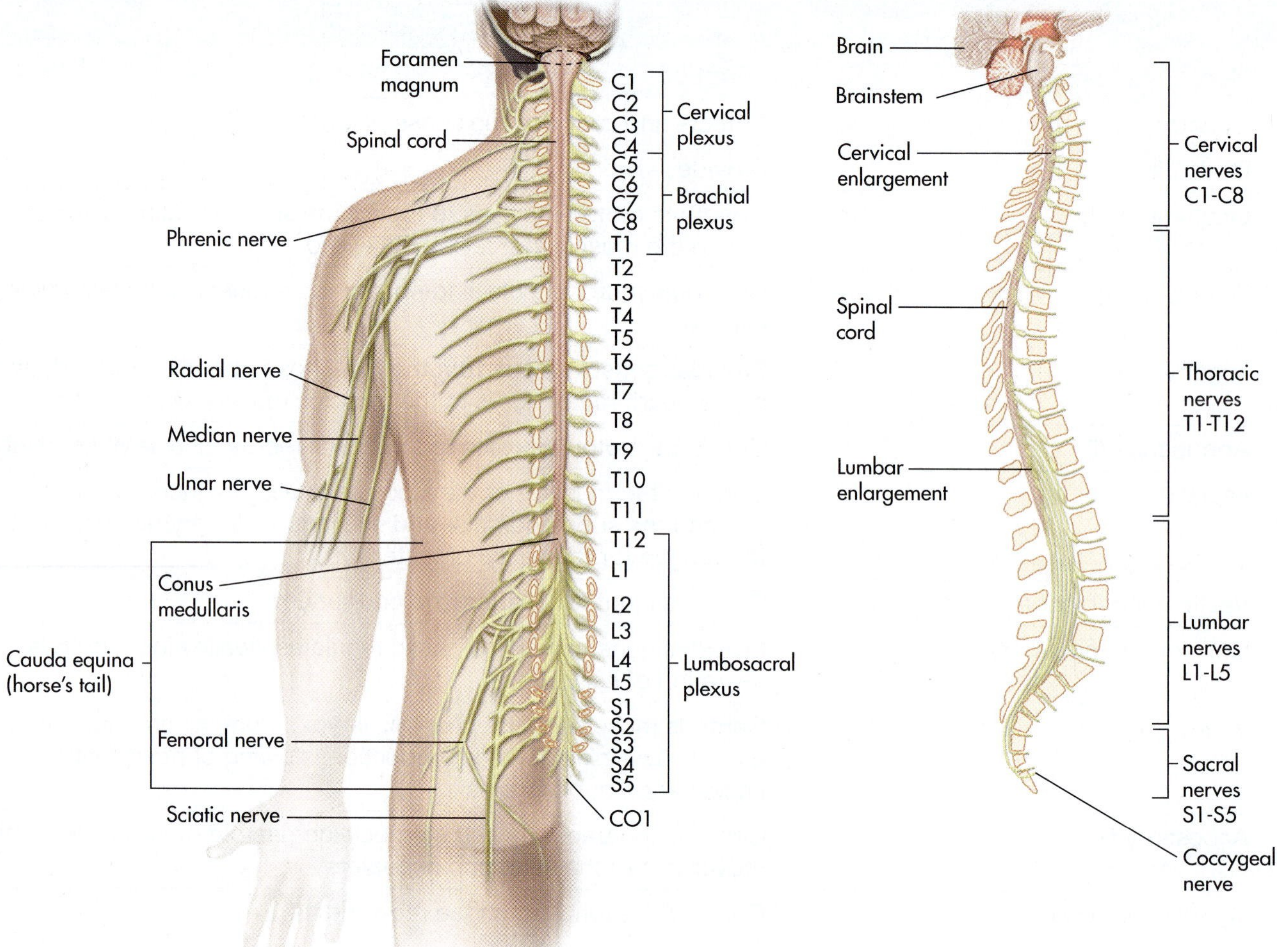

Figure 14.8 The 31 pairs of spinal nerves.

Autonomic Nervous System

Actually a part of the peripheral nervous system, the **autonomic nervous system (ANS)** controls involuntary bodily functions such as sweating, secretions of glands, arterial blood pressure, smooth muscle tissue, and the heart. The autonomic nervous system is primarily composed of efferent fibers from certain cranial and spinal nerves and can be functionally divided into two divisions, the **sympathetic** and **parasympathetic**. These two divisions counteract each other's activity to keep the body in a state of homeostasis. See Figure 14.9.

Sympathetic Division

Branches from the ventral roots of the 12 thoracic and the first three lumbar spinal nerves form the first part of the **sympathetic division**. The cell bodies of these nerve fibers are located in the *gray matter* of the spinal cord. Just outside the spinal cord, axons of these nerve cells leave the spinal nerves and enter almost immediately into masses of nerve cell bodies, the **sympathetic ganglia**, which form a chain that runs next to the vertebral column. This chain of about 23 ganglia runs from the base of the head to the coccyx and is known as the **sympathetic trunk**. Within the ganglia of the sympathetic trunk, fibers from the spinal nerves synapse with ganglionic nerve cell bodies.

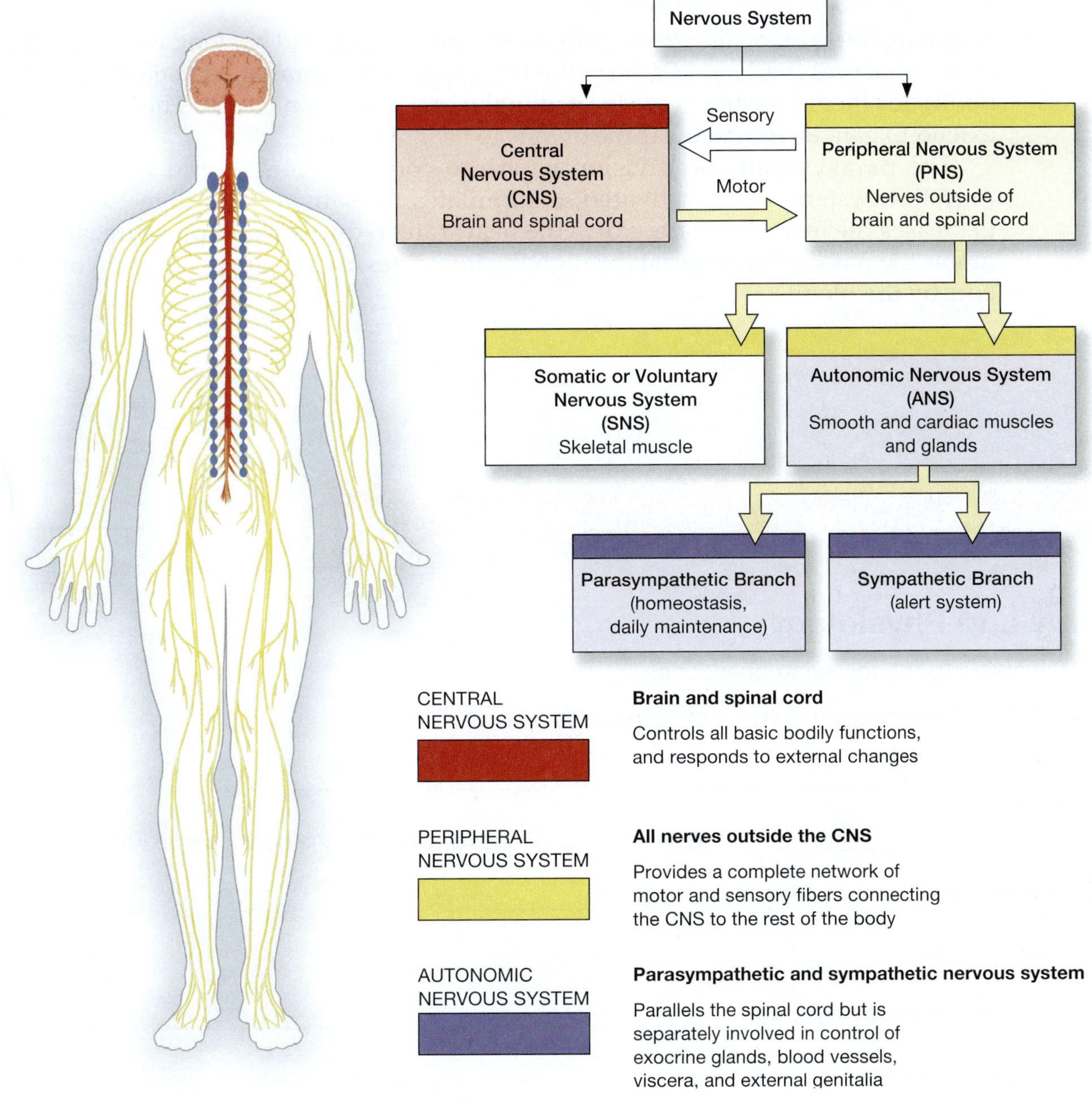

Figure 14.9 General representation of the nervous system.

These ganglionic neurons produce long axons that reach to the parts of the body to be innervated. This arrangement, characteristic of autonomic nerves, creates a two-neuron chain as opposed to single-neuron control of regular motor nerves.

Because of the arrangement in which *sympathetic fibers* from spinal nerves synapse with many cell bodies in the sympathetic ganglia, they tend to produce widespread innervation when activated. This condition has been described as preparing the individual for fight or flight. During the *fight-or-flight response*, a person experiences increased alertness, increased metabolic rate, decreased digestive and urinary function, an increase in respiration, blood pressure, and heart rate, and a corresponding warming of the body that can activate the sweat glands. The sympathetic system stimulates the adrenal glands to release epinephrine (adrenaline), the hormone that causes the familiar adrenaline rush.

Parasympathetic Division

Very long fibers branching from cranial nerves III, VII, IX, and X, along with long fibers of sacral nerves II, III, and IV, form the first stage of the **parasympathetic division**. Cell bodies for these long fibers are located in the brain and spinal cord. These long fibers extend to ganglia located near the organs to be innervated.

The parasympathetic division works to conserve energy and innervate the digestive system. When activated, it stimulates the salivary and digestive glands, decreases the metabolic rate, slows the heart rate, reduces blood pressure, and promotes the passage of material through the intestines along with absorption of nutrients by the blood.

Study and Review I

Anatomy and Physiology

Write your answers to the following questions.

1. Name the two interconnected divisions of the nervous system.

a. ______________________ **b.** ______________________

2. ______________________ are the structural and functional units of the nervous system.

3. Describe an axon. ______________________

4. Describe a dendrite. ______________________

5. State an action of sensory neurons. ______________________

6. Define the following terms:

a. Nerve fiber ______________________

b. Nerve ______________________

c. Tracts ______________________

7. The central nervous system consists of the ______________________ and the ______________________.

8. Name the three meninges enclosing the brain.

a. ______________________ **b.** ______________________

c. ______________________

9. Name four major structures of the brain.

a. ______________________________ **b.** ______________________________

c. ______________________________ **d.** ______________________________

10. The ____________________________ has been identified as the brain's major motor area.

11. The parietal lobe is also known as the ____________________________

12. The temporal lobe contains centers for ____________________________ and ____________________________ input.

13. The occipital lobe is the primary area for ____________________________.

14. State the functions of the thalamus.

a. ______________________________ **b.** ______________________________

15. State three functions of the hypothalamus.

a. ______________________________ **b.** ______________________________

c. ______________________________

16. The cerebellum plays an important role in the integration of ____________________________ and ____________________________.

17. State five functions of the medulla oblongata.

a. ______________________________ **b.** ______________________________

c. ______________________________ **d.** ______________________________

e. ______________________________

18. State the three functions of the spinal cord.

a. ______________________________ **b.** ______________________________

c. ______________________________

19. The normal adult has between ____________________________ and ____________________________ mL of cerebrospinal fluid in circulation.

20. State four functions of the autonomic nervous system.

a. ______________________ **b.** ______________________

c. ______________________ **d.** ______________________

21. Name the two divisions of the autonomic nervous system.

a. ______________________ **b.** ______________________

ANATOMY LABELING

Identify the structures shown below by filling in the blanks.

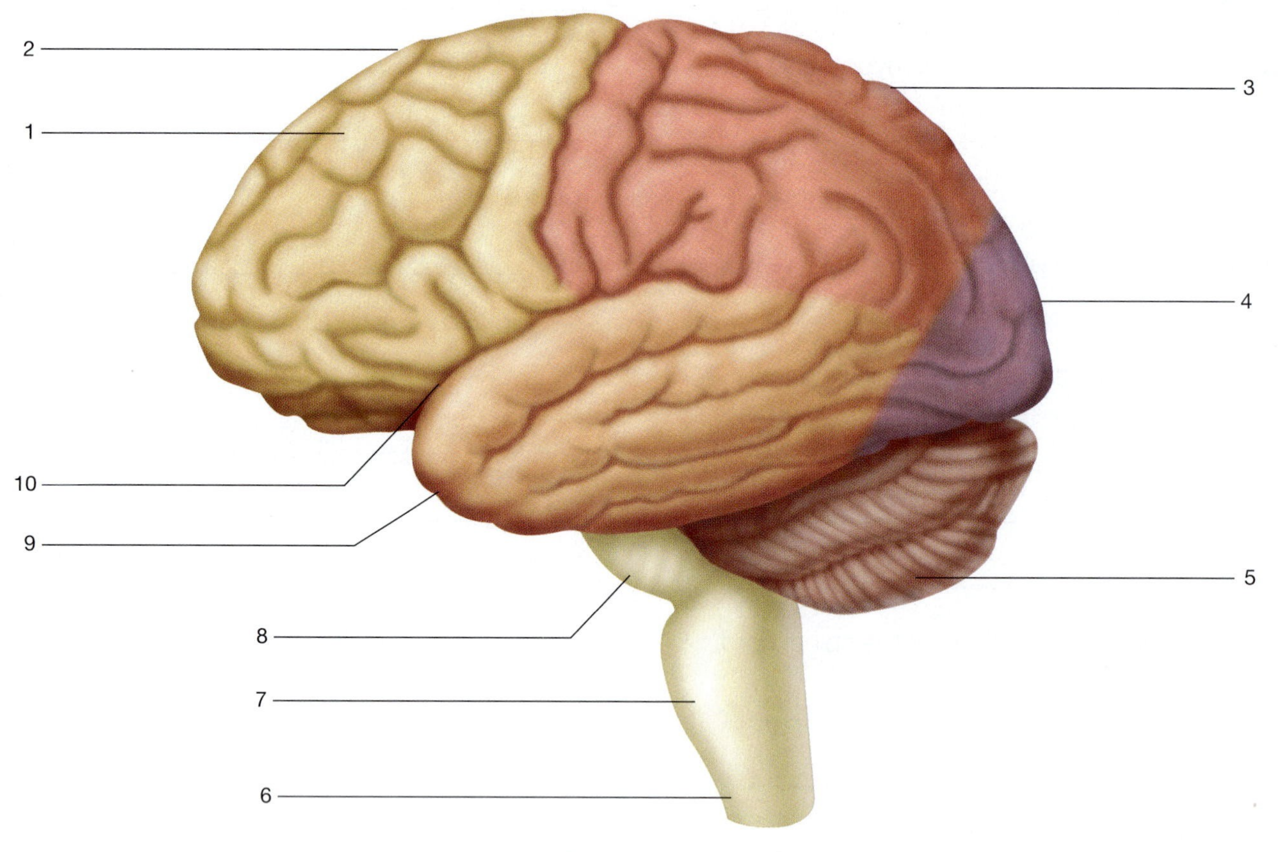

Building Your Medical Vocabulary

This section provides the foundation for learning medical terminology. Review the following alphabetized word list. Note how common prefixes and suffixes are repeatedly applied to word roots and combining forms to create different meanings. The word parts are color-coded: prefixes are yellow, suffixes are blue, roots/combining forms are red. A combining form is a word root plus a vowel. The chart below lists the combining forms for the word roots in this chapter and can help to strengthen your understanding of how medical words are built and spelled.

Remember These Guidelines

1. If the suffix begins with a vowel, drop the combining vowel from the combining form and add the suffix. For example, cephal/o (*head*) + -algia (*pain*) becomes cephalalgia.
2. If the suffix begins with a consonant, keep the combining vowel and add the suffix to the combining form. For example, narc/o (*sleep, stupor*) + -lepsy (*seizure*) becomes narcolepsy.

You will find that some terms have not been divided into word parts. These are common words or specialized terms that are included to enhance your medical vocabulary.

Combining Forms of the Nervous System

cephal/o	head	**lob/o**	lobe
cerebell/o	little brain	**mening/i**	membrane, meninges
cerebr/o	cerebrum	**mening/o**	membrane, meninges
cran/i	skull	**ment/o**	mind
crani/o	skull	**my/o**	muscle
cyt/o	cell	**myel/o**	bone marrow, spinal cord
dendr/o	tree		
disk/o	disk	**narc/o**	numbness, sleep, stupor
dur/o	dura, hard	**neur/o**	nerve
electr/o	electricity	**pallid/o**	globus pallidus
encephal/o	brain	**papill/o**	papilla
esthesi/o	feeling	**poli/o**	gray
fibr/o	fiber	**somn/o**	sleep
gli/o	glue	**spin/o**	thorn, spine
hypn/o	sleep	**spondyl/o**	vertebra
lamin/o	thin plate	**vag/o**	vagus, wandering
later/o	side	**ventricul/o**	ventricle

Medical Word	Word Parts		Definition
	Part	**Meaning**	
acetylcholine (ACh) (ăs″ ĕ-tĭl-kō′ lēn)			Cholinergic neurotransmitter; plays an important role in the transmission of nerve impulses at synapses and myoneural junctions
akathisia (ăk″ ă-thĭ″ zĭ-ă)			Inability to remain still; motor restlessness and anxiety
akinesia (ă″ kĭ-nē′ zĭ-ă)	a- -kinesia	lack of motion, movement	Loss or lack of voluntary motion
Alzheimer disease (AD) (ahlts′ hĭ-mer)			A progressive degeneration of brain tissue that usually begins after age 60. It is the most common cause of dementia among older adults. Symptoms of AD can be described as the 4 A's: anger, aggression, anxiety, and apathy. It is a disease that causes a slow decline in memory, thinking, and reasoning skills.
amnesia (ăm-nē′ zĭ-ă)	a- mnes -ia	lack of memory condition	Condition in which there is a loss or lack of memory
amyotrophic lateral sclerosis (ALS) (ă-mī″ ō-trŏf′ ĭk lăt′ ĕr-ăl sklĕ-rō′ sĭs)	a- my/o -troph(y) -ic later -al scler -osis	lack of muscle nourishment pertaining to side pertaining to hardening condition	Muscular weakness, atrophy, with spasticity caused by degeneration of motor neurons of the spinal cord; also called *Lou Gehrig disease*
analgesia (ăn″ ăl-jē′ zĭ-ă)	an- -algesia	lack of condition of pain	Condition in which there is a lack of the sensation of pain
anesthesia (ăn″ ĕs-thē′ zĭ-ă)	an- -esthesia	lack of feeling	Literally means *loss or lack of the sense of feeling*; a pharmacologically induced reversible state of amnesia, analgesia, loss of responsiveness, loss of skeletal muscle reflexes, and decreased stress response
anesthesiologist (ăn″ ĕs-thē″ zĭ-ŏl′ ō-jĭst)	an- esthesi/o log -ist	lack of feeling study of one who specializes	Physician who specializes in the science of anesthesia

Medical Word	Word Parts		Definition
	Part	**Meaning**	
aphagia (ă-fā´ jĭ-ă)	a- -phagia	lack of to eat, swallow	Loss or lack of the ability to eat or swallow
aphasia (ă-fā´ zĭ-ă)	a- -phasia	lack of to speak, speech	Literally means *a lack of the ability to speak*. It is a language disorder in which there is an impairment of producing or comprehending spoken or written language due to brain damage. It can be caused by a stroke, traumatic brain injury, or other brain injury, or it may develop slowly, as in the case of a brain tumor or progressive neurological disease, such as in Alzheimer or Parkinson diseases.
apraxia (ă-prăks´ ĭ-ă)	a- -praxia	lack of action	Loss or lack of the ability to use objects properly and to recognize common ones; inability to perform motor tasks or activities of daily living (ADL), such as dressing and bathing
asthenia (ăs-thē´ nĭ-ă)	a- -sthenia	lack of strength	Loss or lack of strength
astrocytoma (ăs″ trō-sī-tō´ mă)	astro- cyt -oma	star-shaped cell tumor	A primary tumor of the brain composed of astrocytes (star-shaped neuroglial cells) characterized by slow growth, cyst formation, metastasis, and malignant glioblastoma within the tumor mass. Surgical intervention is possible in the early developmental stage of the tumor; also called *astrocytic glioma*.
ataxia (ă-tăks´ ĭ-ă)	a- -taxia	lack of order, coordination	Literally means *loss or lack of order*; neurological sign and symptom consisting of lack of coordination of muscle movements. It implies dysfunction of parts of the nervous system that coordinate movement, such as the cerebellum.
bradykinesia (brăd″ ĭ-kĭ-nē´ sĭ-ă)	brady- -kinesia	slow motion, movement	Abnormal slowness of motion
cephalalgia (sĕf″ ă-lăl´ jĭ-ă)	cephal -algia	head pain	Head pain; *headache*

Medical Word	Word Parts		Definition
	Part	**Meaning**	
cerebellar (sĕr″ ĕ-bĕl′ ăr)	cerebell -ar	little brain pertaining to	Pertaining to the cerebellum
cerebral palsy (CP) (sĕr′ ă-brĭl pawl′ zē)			Disorder of movement and posture caused by damage to the motor control centers of the developing brain and can occur during pregnancy, during childbirth, or after birth up to about age 3. Most common permanent disorder of childhood involving four motor dysfunctions: spastic, dyskinetic, ataxic, and mixed. See Figure 14.10.

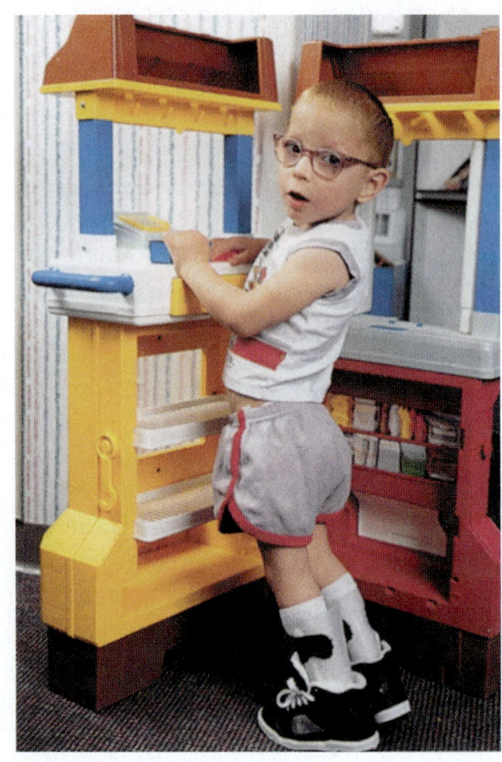

Figure 14.10 Child with cerebral palsy has abnormal muscle tone and lack of physical coordination.

Source: Pearson Education, Inc.

Medical Word	Part	Meaning	Definition
cerebrospinal (sĕr″ ĕ-brō-spī′ năl)	cerebr/o spin -al	cerebrum a thorn, spine pertaining to	Pertaining to the cerebrum and the spinal cord
chorea (kō-rē′ ă)			Abnormal involuntary movement disorder, one of a group of neurological disorders called *dyskinesias*; characterized by episodes of rapid, jerky involuntary muscular twitching of the limbs or facial muscles

Medical Word	Word Parts		Definition
	Part	Meaning	
coma (kō´ mā)			Unconscious state or stupor from which the patient cannot be aroused; may occur as a complication of an underlying illness, or as a result of injuries to the brain. Coma rarely lasts more than 2–4 weeks, although it can last for years. The outcome for coma depends on the cause, severity, and site of the damage.

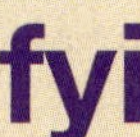

fyi

The **Glasgow Coma Scale (GCS)** is the most common scoring system used to describe the level of consciousness in a person following a traumatic brain injury. It is used to help gauge the severity of an acute brain injury and measures the following functions:

Eye Opening (E)

4 = spontaneous (ICD-10-CM code R40.214)
3 = to voice; sound (R40.213)
2 = to pain (R40.212)
1 = none (R40.211)

Verbal Response (V)

5 = normal; oriented conversation (R40.225)
4 = disoriented; confused conversation (R40.224)
3 = words, but not coherent; inappropriate (R40.223)
2 = incomprehensible; no words, only sounds (R40.222)
1 = none (R40.221)

Motor Response (M)

6 = normal; obeys commands (R40.236)
5 = localized to pain (R40.235)
4 = withdraws to pain (*flexion*) (R40.234)
3 = decorticate posture (an abnormal posture that can include rigidity, clenched fists, legs held straight out, and arms bent inward toward the body with the wrists and fingers bent and held on the chest) (R40.232)
2 = decerebrate (an abnormal posture that can include rigidity, arms and legs held straight out [*extension*], toes pointed downward, head and neck arched backwards) (R40.233)
1 = none (R40.231)

insights

In the ICD-10-CM, coma (R40.20) includes subcategories of motor response (R40.231–R40.236), opening of eyes (R40.211–R40.214), and verbal response (R40.221–R40.225). You will find that the terminology given in the Glasgow Coma Scale correlates to these codes.

Medical Word	Word Parts		Definition
	Part	Meaning	
concussion (brain) (kŏn-kŭsh´ ŭn)	concuss -ion	shaken violently process	Head injury with a transient loss of brain function; may also be called *mild brain injury*, *mild traumatic brain injury (MTBI)*, *mild head injury (MHI)*, and *minor head trauma*

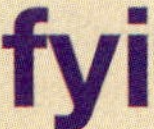

Chronic traumatic encephalopathy (CTE) is a type of traumatic brain injury that can occur in individuals who participate in contact sports and receive repeated blows to the head. CTE injuries are associated with memory disturbances, behavioral and personality changes, Parkinsonism, and speech and gait abnormalities. CTE involves progressive damage to nerve cells, which results in visible changes to the brain.

Over recent years there has been increasing attention focused on the neurological sequelae of sports-related traumatic brain injury, particularly concussion. *Concussion* is a frequent occurrence in contact sports: 1.6 to 3.8 million sports-related concussions occur annually in the United States. Repetitive closed head injury occurs in a wide variety of contact sports, including football, boxing, wrestling, rugby, hockey, lacrosse, soccer, and skiing. Furthermore, in collision sports such as football and boxing, players may experience thousands of subconcussive hits over the course of a single season. *Subconcussive* (below the threshold of concussion) impacts are repetitive, but less forceful impacts to the head. Also at risk are military personnel (and civilians) who experience explosive blasts that may cause subconcussive impacts to the head.

Medical Word	Part	Meaning	Definition
craniectomy (krā″ nĭ-ĕk´ tō-mē)	cran/i -ectomy	skull surgical excision	Surgical excision of a portion of the skull (*cranium*), which encases the brain
craniotomy (krā″ nĭ-ŏt´ ō-mē)	crani/o -tomy	skull incision	Literally means *surgical incision into the skull*. It is a surgical operation in which a bone flap is removed from the skull to access the brain. Used to repair defects associated with traumatic head injuries or to repair a cerebral aneurysm. See Figure 14.11.

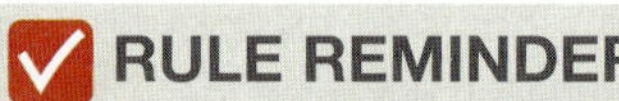

RULE REMINDER

This term keeps the combining vowel ***o*** because the suffix begins with a consonant.

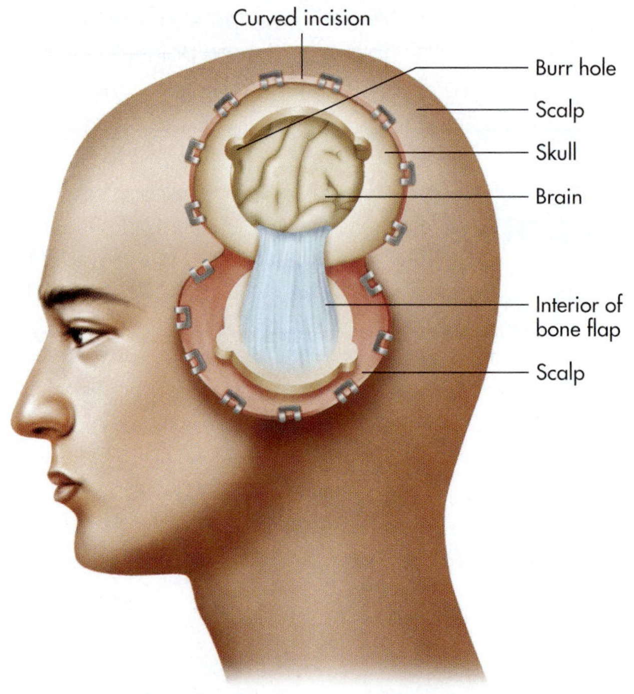

Figure 14.11 In a craniotomy, a portion of the skull and overlying scalp is pulled back to allow access to the brain.

Medical Word	Word Parts		Definition
	Part	**Meaning**	
deep brain stimulation (DBS)			A surgical procedure used to treat a variety of disabling neurological symptoms—most commonly the symptoms of Parkinson disease (PD), such as tremor, rigidity, stiffness, slowed movement, and walking problems; it is also used to treat essential tremor, a common neurological movement disorder. Currently, DBS is used only for patients whose symptoms cannot be adequately controlled with medications.

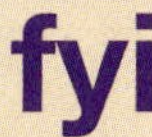

Deep brain stimulation (DBS) employs a surgically implanted, battery-operated medical device called a *neurostimulator*—similar to a heart pacemaker and approximately the size of a stopwatch—to deliver electrical stimulation to targeted areas in the brain that control movement, blocking the abnormal nerve signals that cause neurological problems. Before the DBS procedure, a neurosurgeon uses magnetic resonance imaging (MRI), computed tomography (CT) scanning, or microelectrode recording to locate the exact target(s) within the brain (generally, the thalamus, subthalamic nucleus, and globus pallidus) where electrical nerve signals generate the neurological symptoms. There are three components of a neurotransmitter:

1. The lead (also called an *electrode*)—a thin, insulated wire—is inserted through a small opening in the skull and implanted in the brain. The tip of the electrode is positioned within the targeted brain area.
2. An insulated wire (the *extension*) is passed under the skin of the head, neck, and shoulder, connecting the lead to the neurostimulator.
3. The neurostimulator (the *battery pack*) is usually implanted under the skin near the collarbone, or in some cases, lower in the chest or under the skin over the abdomen.

Once the system is in place, electrical impulses are sent from the neurostimulator up along the extension and the lead and into the brain. These impulses interfere with and block the electrical signals that cause the symptoms and tremors of Parkinson disease, as one example.

Medical Word	Part	Meaning	Definition
dementia (dē-mĕn´ shē-ă)	de- ment -ia	down mind condition	Group of symptoms marked by memory loss and loss of other cognitive functions such as perception, thinking, reasoning, and remembering
diskectomy (dĭs-kĕk´ tō-mē)	disk -ectomy	a disk surgical excision	Surgical excision of an intervertebral disk
dyslexia (dĭs-lĕks´ ĭ-ă)	dys- -lexia	difficult diction, word, phrase	Difficulty reading and writing words even though vision and intelligence are unimpaired
dysphasia (dĭs-fā´ zĭ-ă)	dys- -phasia	difficult speak, speech	Impairment of speech that may be caused by a brain lesion

Medical Word	Word Parts: Part	Word Parts: Meaning	Definition
electromyography (ē-lĕk″ trō-mī-ŏg′ ră-fē)	electr/o my/o -graphy	electricity muscle recording	Process of recording the contraction of a skeletal muscle as a result of electrical stimulation; used in diagnosing disorders of nerves supplying muscles
encephalitis (ĕn-sĕf″ ă-lī′ tĭs)	encephal -itis	brain inflammation	Inflammation of the brain. There are numerous types of encephalitis, many of which are caused by viral infection. Symptoms include sudden fever, headache, vomiting, photophobia (abnormal sensitivity to light), stiff neck and back, confusion, drowsiness, clumsiness, unsteady gait, and irritability.
encephalopathy (ĕn-sĕf″ ă-lŏp′ ă-thē)	encephal/o -pathy	brain disease	Any pathological dysfunction of the brain. HIV encephalopathy is called *AIDS dementia complex*.
endorphins (ĕn-dor′ fĭns)			Chemical substances produced in the brain that act as natural analgesics (opiates) and provide feelings of pleasure
epidural (ĕp″ ĭ-dū′ răl)	epi- dur -al	upon dura, hard pertaining to	Literally means *pertaining to situated on the dura mater*; often used to refer to a form of regional anesthesia involving injection of medication via a catheter into the epidural space. This causes both a loss of sensation (anesthesia) and a loss of pain (analgesia), by blocking the transmission of signals through nerves in or near the spinal cord.

ALERT!

The prefix ***epi-*** means upon. How many words in this chapter begin with ***epi-***?

Medical Word	Part	Meaning	Definition
epiduroscopy (ep″ ĭ-dū-rŏs′ kō-pē)	epi- dur/o -scopy	upon dura, hard visual examination, to view, examine	Minimally invasive form of surgery that introduces medication via an endoscope into the epidural space; used for back pain relief when all other conservative treatments have failed

Medical Word	Word Parts: Part	Word Parts: Meaning	Definition
epilepsy (ĕp´ ĭ-lĕp˝ sē)	epi- -lepsy	upon seizure	A neurological disorder involving repeated seizures of any type. Seizures are episodes of disturbed brain function that cause changes in attention and/or behavior. The types of seizures experienced by those with epilepsy are classified into four main categories: 1. **Partial seizures** (focal seizures)—electrical disturbances are localized to areas of the brain near the source or focal point of the seizure. 2. **Generalized seizures** (bilateral, symmetrical)—widespread electrical discharge that involves both the right and left hemispheres of the brain. 3. **Unilateral seizures**—electrical discharge is predominantly confined to one of the two hemispheres of the brain. 4. **Unclassified seizures**—cannot be placed into one of the other three categories because of incomplete data.

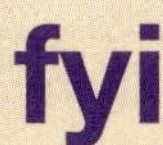

The majority of epilepsy cases are idiopathic (cause not identified) and symptoms begin during childhood or early adolescence. A child who has a seizure while standing should be gently assisted to the floor and placed in a side-lying position. See Figure 14.12. In adults, epilepsy can occur after severe neurological trauma.

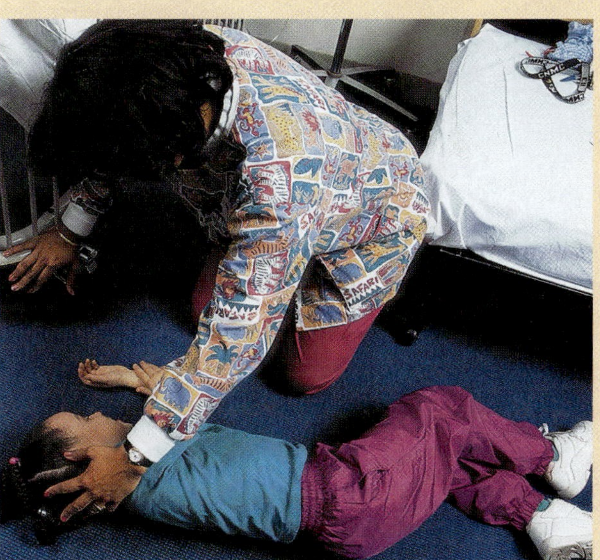

Figure 14.12 A child having a seizure is gently assisted to the floor and placed in a side-lying position.
Source: Pearson Education, Inc.

Medical Word	Word Parts: Part	Word Parts: Meaning	Definition
ganglionectomy (gang˝ lĭ-ō-nĕk´ tō-mē)	ganglion -ectomy	knot surgical excision	Surgical excision of a ganglion (a mass of nerve tissue outside the brain and spinal cord)

Medical Word	Word Parts		Definition
	Part	**Meaning**	
glioma (glī-ō´ mă)	gli -oma	glue tumor	Tumor composed of neuroglial tissue
Guillain-Barré syndrome (gē-yăn´ bă-rā)			Pathological condition in which the myelin sheaths covering peripheral nerves are destroyed, resulting in decreased nerve impulses, loss of reflex response, and sudden muscle weakness. Generally an acute viral infection occurs 1–3 weeks before the onset of the syndrome; also called *infectious polyneuritis*, *acute febrile polyneuritis*, or *acute idiopathic polyneuritis*.
hemiparesis (hĕm″ ĭ-păr´ ĕ-sĭs)	hemi- -paresis	half weakness	Weakness on one side of the body that can be caused by a stroke, cerebral palsy, brain tumor, multiple sclerosis, and other brain and nervous system diseases
hemiplegia (hĕm″ ĭ-plē´ jĭ-ă)	hemi- -plegia	half stroke, paralysis	Paralysis of one-half of the body when it is divided along the median sagittal plane; total paralysis of the arm, leg, and trunk on the same side of the body. Stroke is the most common cause of this condition. See Figure 14.13B.

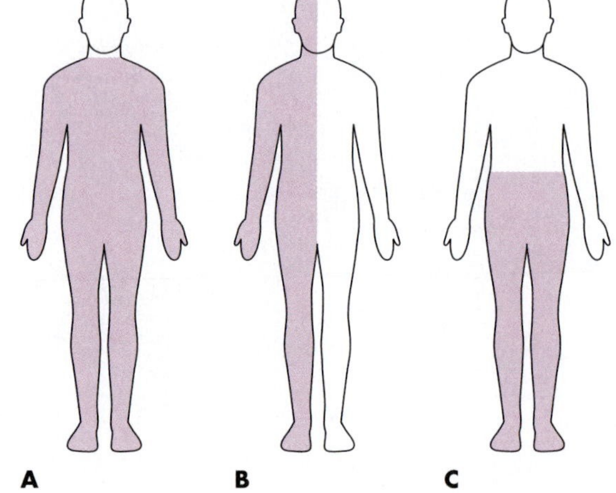

Figure 14.13 Types of paralysis: (A) Quadriplegia is complete or partial paralysis of the upper extremities and complete paralysis of the lower part of the body. (B) Hemiplegia is paralysis of one half of the body when it is divided along the median sagittal plane. (C) Paraplegia is a paralysis of the lower part of the body.

Medical Word	Word Parts		Definition
	Part	Meaning	
herniated disk syndrome (HDS) (hĕr-nē-ā´tĕd)			Condition in which part or all of the soft, gelatinous central portion of an intervertebral disk (the nucleus pulposus) is forced through a weakened part of the disk. Compression on the nerves can cause *sciatica* or severe lumbar back pain that radiates down one or both legs; also called *herniated intervertebral disk*, *ruptured disk*, *herniated nucleus pulposus (HNP)*, or *slipped disk*. See Figure 14.14.

Cross section showing compression of nerve root

Surgical exposure of lower lumbar disc herniation

Dura

Nerve root

Nucleus pulposus

Figure 14.14 Herniated intervertebral disk showing the herniated nucleus pulposus (on the left) applying pressure against the nerve root and surgical intervention (on the right).

Medical Word	Part	Meaning	Definition
herpes zoster (hĕr´ pēz zŏs´ tĕr)			Viral disease characterized by painful vesicular eruptions along a segment of the spinal or cranial nerves; also called *shingles*. See Figure 14.15.

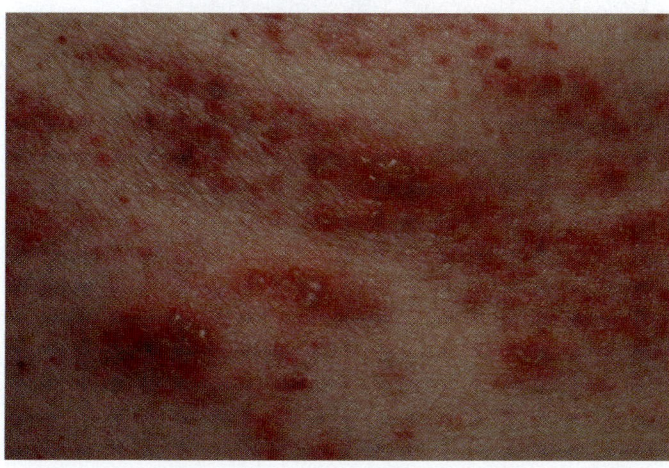

Figure 14.15 Herpes zoster.
(Courtesy of Jason L. Smith, MD)

(continued)

Medical Word	Word Parts		Definition
	Part	**Meaning**	

fyi

Shingles is caused by the varicella-zoster virus, the same virus that causes chickenpox. In people who have had chickenpox, the virus is never fully cleared from the body. Instead, the virus remains dormant in the nerve tissues. When the immune system is weakened, the virus reactivates and spreads along the nerve fibers to the particular area of skin supplied by the involved nerve.

The first sign of shingles is often burning or tingling pain, or sometimes numbness or itch, in one particular location on only one side of the body. After a few days, the painful vesicular eruptions appear.

Zostavax is a vaccine used to help reduce the risk of a person getting shingles in the future. The Centers for Disease Control and Prevention (CDC) recommends that appropriate adults 60 or older get vaccinated to help prevent shingles from reactivating. It works by helping the immune system keep the shingles virus in check. It is given as a single injection once only and cannot be used to treat shingles.

Medical Word	Part	Meaning	Definition
hydrocephalus (hī″ drō-sĕf′ ă-lŭs)	hydro- cephal -us	water head pertaining to	Condition in which there is an increased amount of cerebrospinal fluid within the ventricles of the brain, causing the head to be enlarged. Treatment involves the surgical placement of an artificial shunt, which drains the fluid into the abdominal cavity. See Figure 14.16.

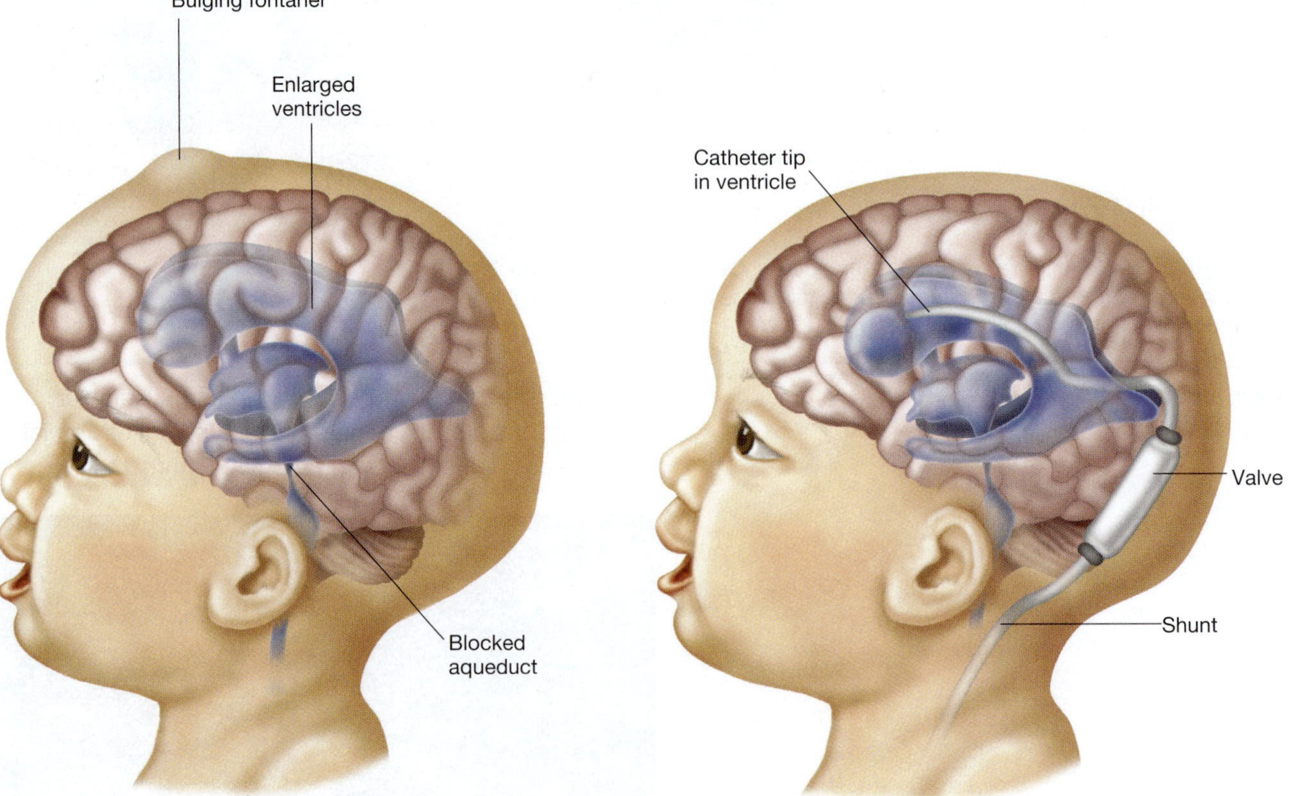

Figure 14.16 Hydrocephalus. The figure on the right shows a shunt inserted to send the excess cerebrospinal fluid to the abdominal cavity.

Medical Word	Word Parts		Definition
	Part	**Meaning**	
hyperesthesia (hī″ pĕr-ĕs-thē′ zĭ-ă)	hyper- -esthesia	excessive feeling	Increased feelings of sensory stimuli, such as pain, touch, or sound
hyperkinesis (hī″ pĕr-kĭn-ē′ sĭs)	hyper- -kinesis	excessive motion	Increased muscular movement and motion; inability to be still; also known as *hyperactivity*
hypnosis (hĭp-nō′ sĭs)	hypn -osis	sleep condition	Artificially induced trancelike state resembling somnambulism (sleepwalking)
intracranial (ĭn″ trăh-krā′ nē-ăl)	intra- crani -al	within skull pertaining to	Pertaining to within the skull
laminectomy (lăm″ ĭ-nĕk′ tō-mē)	lamin -ectomy	thin plate surgical excision	Surgical excision of a vertebral posterior arch
lobotomy (lō-bŏt′ ō-mē)	lob/o -tomy	lobe incision	Surgical incision into the prefrontal or frontal lobe of the brain
meningioma (mĕn-ĭn″ jĭ-ō′ mă)	mening/i -oma	membrane, meninges tumor	Tumor of the meninges that originates in the arachnoidal tissue
meningitis (mĕn″ ĭn-jī′ tĭs)	mening -itis	membrane, meninges inflammation	Inflammation of the meninges of the spinal cord or brain. With early diagnosis and prompt treatment, most patients recover from meningitis. Individuals with bacterial meningitis are usually hospitalized for treatment.

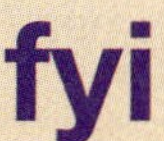

The child with bacterial meningitis assumes an **opisthotonic** (**opisth/o** [*backward*], **ton** [*tone/tension*], **-ic** [*pertaining to*]) **position**, with the neck and head hyperextended to relieve discomfort.

Medical Word	Word Parts: Part	Word Parts: Meaning	Definition
meningocele (mĕn-ĭn´ gō-sēl)	mening/o -cele	membrane, meninges hernia	Congenital hernia (saclike protrusion) in which the meninges protrude through a defect in the skull or spinal column. See Figure 14.17.

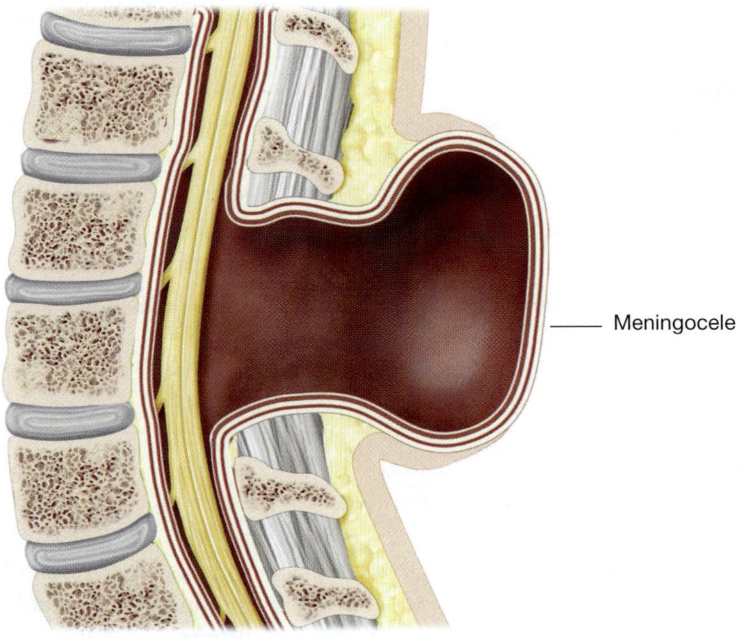

Figure 14.17 Meningocele, a congenital abnormality of the spine.

Medical Word	Part	Meaning	Definition
meningomyelocele (mĕ-nĭng˝ gō-mī˝ ĕ-lō-sēl)	mening/o myel/o -cele	membrane, meninges spinal cord hernia	Congenital herniation of the spinal cord and meninges through a defect in the vertebral column
microcephaly (mī˝ krō-sĕf´ ăl-ē)	micro- cephal -y	small head pertaining to	Abnormally small head; congenital anomaly characterized by an abnormal smallness of the head in relation to the rest of the body

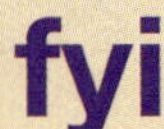

On February 1, 2016, the World Health Organization (WHO) designated the Zika virus (transmitted by *Aedes mosquitoes*) and its suspected complications in newborns as a public health emergency of international concern. The primary reason for the designation was the "strongly suspected" causal relationship between Zika and the rare congenital condition called *microcephaly*. Zika virus, first identified more than 50 years ago, has alarmed public health officials in recent months because of its possible association with thousands of suspected cases of brain damage in babies. The WHO has estimated that the virus will have reached most of the hemisphere and will have infected up to 4 million people by the end of 2016.

Medical Word	Word Parts: Part	Word Parts: Meaning	Definition
multiple sclerosis (MS) (mŭl´ tĭ-pl sklĕ-rō´ sĭs)	scler -osis	hardening condition	Chronic disease of the central nervous system marked by damage to the myelin sheath. Plaques occur in the brain and spinal cord causing tremor, weakness, incoordination, paresthesia, and disturbances in vision and speech. The multiple effects of MS are shown in Figure 14.18.

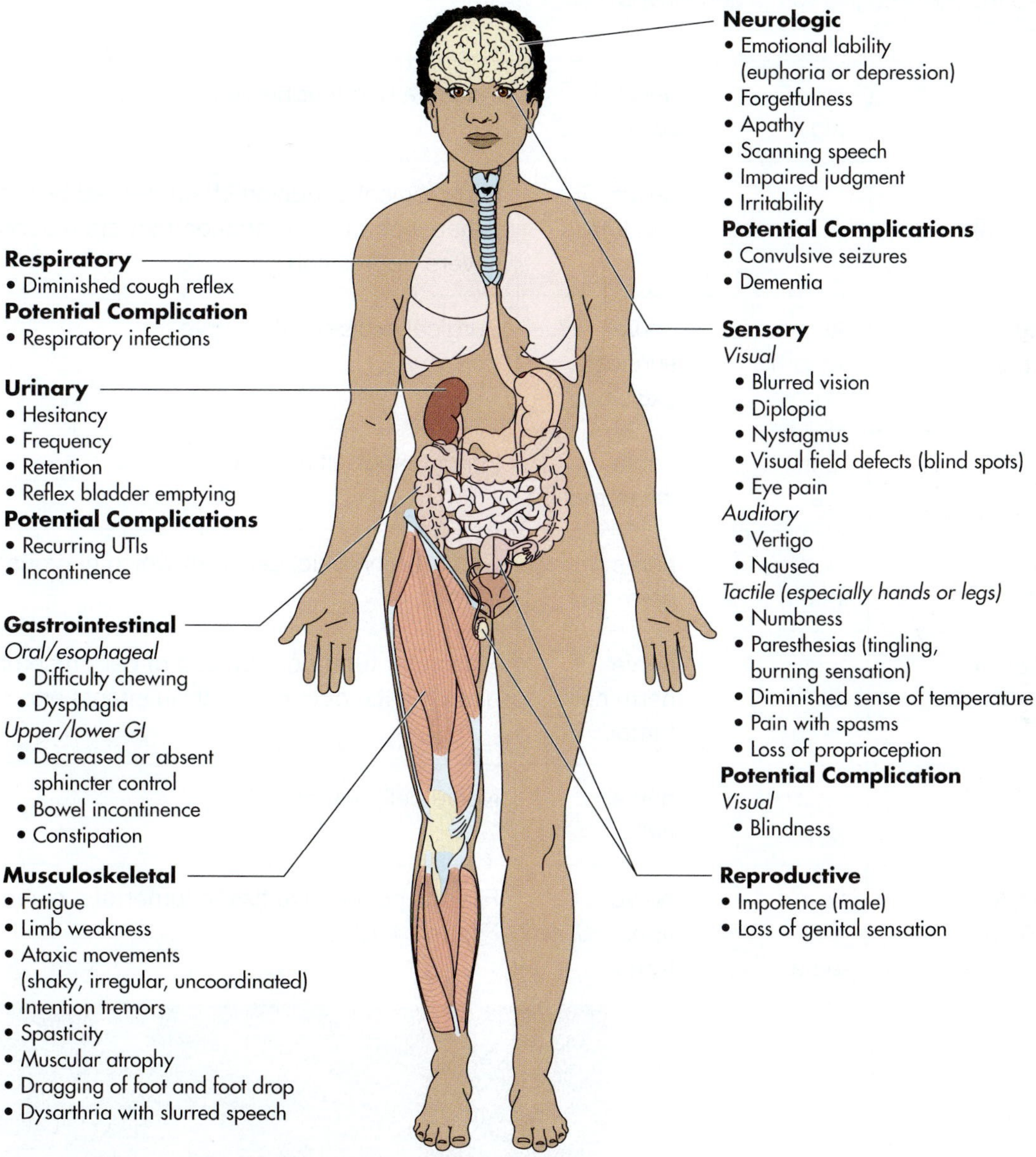

Respiratory
- Diminished cough reflex

Potential Complication
- Respiratory infections

Urinary
- Hesitancy
- Frequency
- Retention
- Reflex bladder emptying

Potential Complications
- Recurring UTIs
- Incontinence

Gastrointestinal
Oral/esophageal
- Difficulty chewing
- Dysphagia

Upper/lower GI
- Decreased or absent sphincter control
- Bowel incontinence
- Constipation

Musculoskeletal
- Fatigue
- Limb weakness
- Ataxic movements (shaky, irregular, uncoordinated)
- Intention tremors
- Spasticity
- Muscular atrophy
- Dragging of foot and foot drop
- Dysarthria with slurred speech

Neurologic
- Emotional lability (euphoria or depression)
- Forgetfulness
- Apathy
- Scanning speech
- Impaired judgment
- Irritability

Potential Complications
- Convulsive seizures
- Dementia

Sensory
Visual
- Blurred vision
- Diplopia
- Nystagmus
- Visual field defects (blind spots)
- Eye pain

Auditory
- Vertigo
- Nausea

Tactile (especially hands or legs)
- Numbness
- Paresthesias (tingling, burning sensation)
- Diminished sense of temperature
- Pain with spasms
- Loss of proprioception

Potential Complication
Visual
- Blindness

Reproductive
- Impotence (male)
- Loss of genital sensation

Figure 14.18 Multisystem effects of multiple sclerosis.

Medical Word	Part	Meaning	Definition
myelitis (mī´ ĕ-lī´ tĭs)	myel -itis	spinal cord inflammation	Inflammation of the spinal cord

Medical Word	Word Parts		Definition
	Part	**Meaning**	
narcolepsy (nār´ kō-lĕp˝ sē)	narc/o -lepsy	numbness, sleep, stupor seizure	Chronic condition with recurrent attacks of uncontrollable drowsiness and sleep
neuralgia (nū-răl´ jĭ-ă)	neur -algia	nerve pain	Pain in a nerve or nerves
neurasthenia (nū˝ răs-thē´ nĭ-ă)	neur -asthenia	nerve weakness	Pathological condition characterized by weakness, exhaustion, and prostration that often accompanies severe depression
neurectomy (nū-rĕk´ tō-mē)	neur -ectomy	nerve surgical excision	Surgical excision of a nerve
neuritis (nū-rī´ tĭs)	neur -itis	nerve inflammation	Inflammation of a nerve
neuroblast (nū´ rō-blăst)	neur/o -blast	nerve germ cell	Germ (embryonic) cell from which nervous tissue is formed
neuroblastoma (nū˝ rō-blăs-tō´ mă)	neur/o -blast -oma	nerve germ cell tumor	Malignant tumor composed of cells resembling neuroblasts; occurs mostly in infants and children
neurocyte (nū´ rō-sīt)	neur/o -cyte	nerve cell	Nerve cell, neuron
neurofibroma (nū˝ rō-fī-brō´ mă)	neur/o fibr -oma	nerve fiber tumor	Fibrous connective tissue tumor of a nerve. See Figure 14.19.

RULE REMINDER

This term keeps the combining vowel for ***o*** because the suffix begins with a consonant.

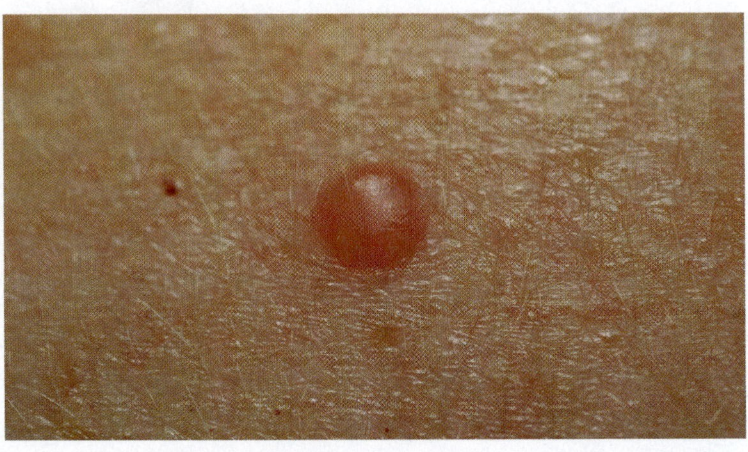

Figure 14.19 Neurofibroma.
(Courtesy of Jason L. Smith, MD)

Medical Word	Word Parts		Definition
	Part	Meaning	
neuroglia (nū-rŏg´ lĭ-ă)	neur/o -glia	nerve glue	Supporting or connective tissue cells of the central nervous system (*astrocytes*, *oligodendroglia*, *microglia*, and *ependymal cells*)
neurologist (nū-rŏl´ ō-jĭst)	neur/o log -ist	nerve study of one who specializes	Physician who specializes in the study of the nervous system
neurology (Neuro) (nū-rŏl´ ō-jē)	neur/o -logy	nerve study of	Study of the nervous system
neuroma (nū-rō´ mă)	neur -oma	nerve tumor	Tumor of nerve cells and nerve fibers
neuropathy (nū-rŏp´ ă-thē)	neur/o -pathy	nerve disease	Any pathological nervous tissue disease
neurotransmitter (nū˝ rō-trăns´ mĭt-ĕr)			Chemical substances, such as dopamine and acetylcholine, that carry electrical impulses across a synapse between two neurons
oligodendroglioma (ŏl˝ ĭ-gō-dĕn˝ drō-glĭ-ō´ mă)	oligo- dendr/o gli -oma	little tree glue tumor	Malignant tumor composed of oligodendroglia (a type of cell that makes up one component of the tissue of the CNS)
pain			A symptom of a physical or emotional condition. The International Association for the Study of Pain defines pain as "the sensory and emotional experience associated with actual or potential tissue damage."

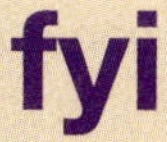

A person's pain may be measured by its threshold and its intensity. *Pain threshold* is the level of stimulus that results in the perception of pain. *Pain tolerance* is the amount of pain a person can manage without disrupting normal functioning and without requiring pain medication. *Intensity* is the degree of pain felt by the individual.

Acute pain comes on suddenly, is severe, and is a warning that something is wrong. Some signs and symptoms of acute pain are increased heart rate and respiratory rate, increased blood pressure, dilated pupils, sweating, nausea, vomiting, anxiety, and fear.

Chronic pain persists beyond the expected time required for the healing of an injury or expected course of recovery; it can last for a long time. Some signs of chronic pain include disturbances in sleep and eating patterns, irritability, constipation, depression, fatigue, and withdrawal from social activities.

insights In the ICD-10-CM, a significant change has occurred in the classification and coding of pain. Codes in category G89, *Pain, not elsewhere classified*, may be used in conjunction with codes from other categories and chapters to provide more detail about *acute* or *chronic pain* and *neoplasm-related pain*. In Chapter 6, Diseases of the Nervous System (G00–G99), there are numerous specific directions and codes for pain.

Medical Word	Word Parts		Definition
	Part	**Meaning**	
pallidotomy (păl″ ĭ-dŏt′ ō-mē)	pallid/o -tomy	globus pallidus incision	Surgical destruction of the globus pallidus of the brain done to treat involuntary movements or muscular rigidity in Parkinson disease
palsy (pawl′ zē)			Pathological loss of sensation or an impairment of motor function; also called *paralysis*. There are many types of palsy; one example is Bell palsy, a unilateral paralysis of the facial (VII) nerve. The facial expression is distorted and the patient may be unable to close an eye or control salivation on the affected side.
papilledema (păp″ ĭl-ĕ-dē′ mă)	papill -edema	papilla swelling	Swelling of the optic disk, usually caused by increased intracranial pressure (ICP); also called *choked disk*
paraplegia (păr″ ă-plē′ jĭ-ă)	para- -plegia	beside stroke, paralysis	Paralysis of the lower part of the body and of both legs. See Figure 14.13C.
paresis (păr′ ĕ-sĭs)			Slight, partial, or incomplete paralysis
paresthesia (păr″ ĕs-thē′ zĭ-ă)	par- -esthesia	beside feeling	Abnormal sensation, feeling of numbness, prickling, or tingling
Parkinson disease (păr′ kĭn-sŭn)			A progressive neurological disorder caused by degeneration of nerve cells in the part of the brain that controls movement. This degeneration creates a shortage of the brain signaling chemical (neurotransmitter) known as *dopamine*, causing the movement impairments that characterize the disease. Often the first symptom of Parkinson disease is tremor (trembling or shaking) of a limb, especially when the body is at rest. The tremor often begins on one side of the body, frequently in one hand. Other common symptoms include slow movement (*bradykinesia*), an inability to move (*akinesia*), rigid limbs, a shuffling gait, and a stooped posture. Also called *paralysis agitans* or *shaking palsy*.

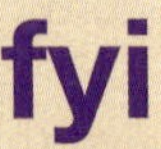

There is no cure for Parkinson disease. Treatment involves drug therapy to replenish dopamine levels and/or inhibit the effects of the neurotransmitter acetylcholine. Surgical interventions that can be used to stop uncontrollable movements include *pallidotomy* and *deep brain stimulation*.

Medical Word	Part	Meaning	Definition
poliomyelitis (pōl″ ĭ-ō-mī″ ĕl-ī′ tĭs)	poli/o myel -itis	gray spinal cord inflammation	Inflammation of the gray matter of the spinal cord
polyneuritis (pŏl″ ē nū-rī′ tĭs)	poly- neur -itis	many nerve inflammation	Literally means *inflammation involving many nerves*

Medical Word	Word Parts		Definition
	Part	Meaning	
quadriplegia (kwŏd″ rĭ plē′ jĭ-ă)	quadri- -plegia	four stroke, paralysis	Paralysis of all four extremities and usually the trunk due to injury to the spinal cord in the cervical spine; also called *tetraplegia*. See Figure 14.13A.
Reye syndrome (rī sĭn′drōm)			Acute disease that causes edema of the brain and increased intracranial pressure, hypoglycemia, and fatty infiltration of the liver and other vital organs; occurs in children and has a relation to aspirin administration; can be viral in origin
sciatica (sī-ăt′ ĭ-kă)			Severe pain along the course of the sciatic nerve
sleep			State of rest for the body and mind; has two distinct types: rapid eye movement (REM), sometimes called *dream sleep*, and no rapid eye movement (NREM)

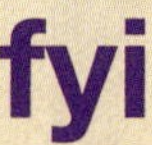

Sleep problems, including snoring, sleep apnea, insomnia, sleep deprivation, and restless legs syndrome, are common. One factor that plays an essential role in sleep is an individual's *circadian* (means around day or *24-hour cycle*) *rhythm* or "body clock." Circadian rhythms are physical, mental and behavioral changes that follow a roughly 24-hour cycle, responding primarily to light and darkness in an organism's environment. They are important in determining human sleep patterns and sleep-wake cycles, hormone release, body temperature, and other important bodily functions. Abnormal circadian rhythms have been associated with sleep disorders, such as insomnia, as well as obesity, diabetes, depression, bipolar disorder, and seasonal affective disorder.

Some Common Circadian Rhythm Disorders and their ICD-10-CM Codes

Jet Lag or Rapid Time Zone Change Syndrome (G47.25): Consists of symptoms that include excessive sleepiness and a lack of daytime alertness in people who travel across time zones.

Shift Work Sleep Disorder (G47.26): Affects people who frequently rotate shifts or work at night.

Delayed Sleep Phase Syndrome (DSPS) (G47.21): Disorder of sleep timing. People with DSPS tend to fall asleep very late at night and have difficulty waking up in the morning.

Advanced Sleep Phase Disorder (ASPD) (G47.22): Disorder in which a person goes to sleep earlier and wakes earlier than desired.

Non 24-Hour Sleep Wake Disorder (G47.29): Frequently affects those who are totally blind since the circadian clock is set by the light and dark cycle over a 24-hour period. The disorder results in drastically reduced sleep time and sleep quality at night and problems with sleepiness during the day.

insights In the ICD-10-CM, sleep disorders are classified according to insomnia, hypersomnia, circadian rhythm sleep disorders, sleep apnea, narcolepsy and cataplexy, parasomnia, and sleep-related movement disorder. The coding G47–G47.9 includes all of the codes used for sleep disorders.

Medical Word	Part	Meaning	Definition
somnambulism (sŏm-năm′ bū-lĭzm)	somn ambul -ism	sleep to walk condition	Condition of sleepwalking
spondylosyndesis (spŏn″ dĭ-lō-sĭn′ dĕ-sĭs)	spondyl/o syn- -desis	vertebra together binding	Surgical procedure to bind vertebrae after removal of a herniated disk; also called *spinal fusion*

Medical Word	Word Parts		Definition
	Part	Meaning	
stroke			Death of focal brain tissue that occurs when the brain does not get sufficient blood and oxygen; also called *cerebrovascular accident (CVA)* or *brain attack*. If the flow of blood in an artery supplying the brain is interrupted for longer than a few seconds, brain cells can die, causing permanent damage. The interruption can be caused either by bleeding (hemorrhagic stroke) or blood clots in the brain. See Figures 14.20 and 14.21. A *transient ischemic attack (TIA)* is a temporary interference in the blood supply to the brain. It sometimes is referred to as a *ministroke*, and symptoms can last for a few minutes or several hours.

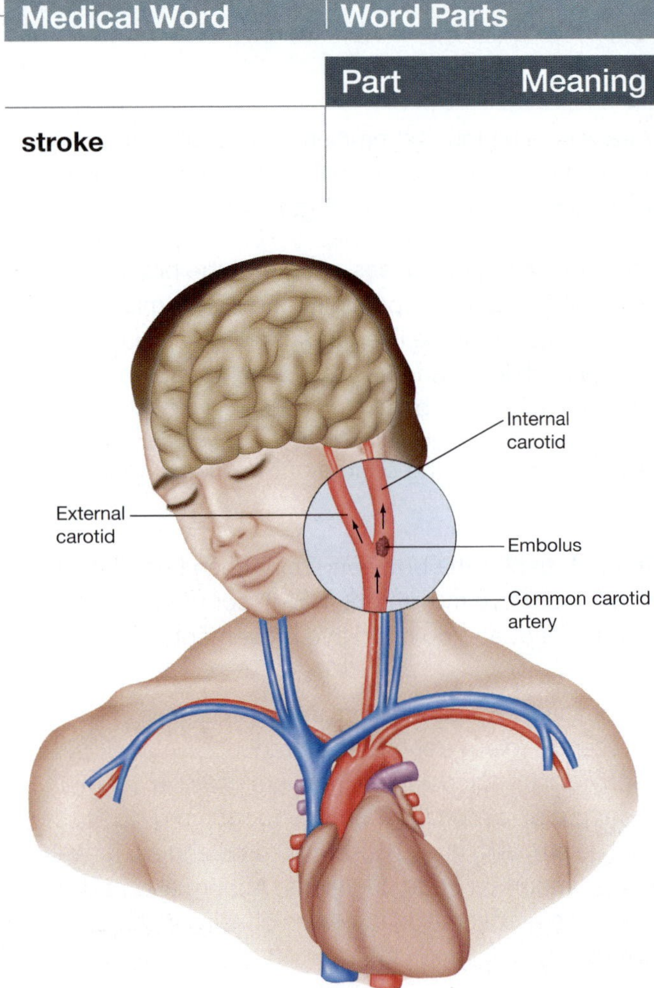

Figure 14.20 Embolus traveling to the brain.

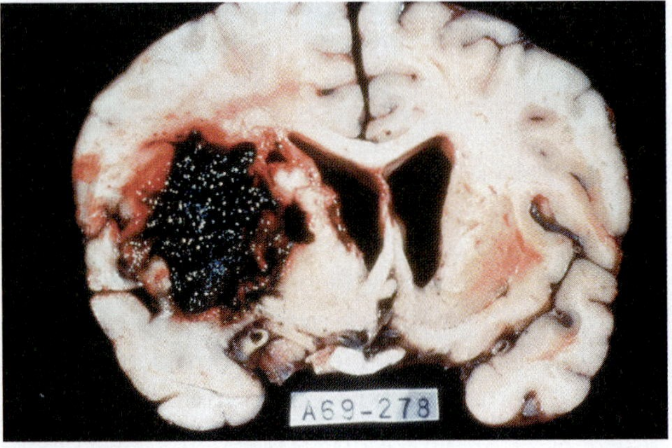

Figure 14.21 Cross section of brain showing cerebrovascular accident.

Source: Pearson Education, Inc.

fyi

The risk of stroke doubles with each decade after age 55. Stroke occurs in men more often than in women. A very common cause of stroke is atherosclerosis. Fatty deposits and blood platelets collect on the wall of the arteries, forming plaques. Over time, the plaques slowly begin to block the flow of blood. The plaque itself can block the artery enough to cause a stroke.

In some cases, the plaque causes the blood to flow abnormally, which leads to a blood clot. A clot can stay at the site of narrowing and prevent blood flow to all of the smaller arteries it supplies. This type of clot, which does not travel, is called a **thrombus**. In other cases, the clot can travel and wedge into a smaller vessel. A clot that travels is called an **embolism** (see Figure 14.20). Strokes caused by embolisms are commonly associated with cardiovascular pathology, especially heart disorders.

The following sudden symptoms are the warning signs of stroke:

- Numbness or weakness of face, arm, or leg, especially on one side of the body.
- Confusion; trouble speaking or understanding.
- Trouble seeing in one or both eyes.
- Trouble walking, dizziness, loss of balance or coordination.
- Severe headache with no known cause.

The FAST test helps spot symptoms of stroke. It stands for:

- **F**ace: Ask for a smile. Does one side droop?
- **A**rms: When raised, does one side drift down?
- **S**peech: Can the person repeat a simple sentence? Does he or she have trouble or slur words?
- **T**ime: Time is critical. Call 911 immediately if any symptoms are present.

Medical Word	Word Parts		Definition
	Part	**Meaning**	
subdural (sŭb-dū′ răl)	sub- dur -al	below dura, hard pertaining to	Pertaining to below the dura mater
sundowning (sŭn′ down-ĭng)			Increased agitation or restlessness that occurs in the late afternoon or early evening in patients with cognitive impairment; most common with Alzheimer-type dementia and Parkinson disease
sympathectomy (sĭm″ pă-thĕk′ tō-mē)	sympath -ectomy	sympathy surgical excision	Surgical excision of a portion of the sympathetic nervous system, such as a nerve or ganglion
syncope (sĭn′ kŭ-pē)			Temporary loss of consciousness caused by a lack of blood supply to the brain; also called *fainting*
tactile (tăk′ tĭl)			Pertaining to the sense of touch
Tay–Sachs disease (tā săks′)			Inherited, progressive disease marked by degeneration of brain tissue; predominantly affects Jewish children of Ashkenazi origin
transcutaneous electrical nerve stimulations (TENS) (trăns-kū-tā′ nē-ŭs)			Use of mild electrical stimulation to interfere with the transmission of painful stimuli; has proved useful in relieving pain in some patients
vagotomy (vā-gŏt′ ō-mē)	vag/o -tomy	vagus, wandering incision	Surgical incision of the vagus nerve
ventriculogram (vĕn-trĭk′ ū-lō-grăm)	ventricul/o -gram	ventricle record	X-ray of the cerebral ventricles

Study and Review II

Word Parts

Prefixes

Give the definitions of the following prefixes.

1. a- _______________
2. an- _______________
3. astro- _______________
4. brady- _______________
5. de- _______________
6. dys- _______________
7. epi- _______________
8. hemi- _______________
9. hydro- _______________
10. hyper- _______________
11. intra- _______________
12. micro- _______________
13. oligo- _______________
14. par- _______________
15. para- _______________
16. poly- _______________
17. quadri- _______________
18. sub- _______________

Combining Forms

Give the definitions of the following combining forms.

1. cephal/o _______________
2. cerebell/o _______________
3. cerebr/o _______________
4. crani/o _______________
5. dendr/o _______________
6. disk/o _______________
7. dur/o _______________
8. electr/o _______________
9. encephal/o _______________
10. esthesi/o _______________
11. hypn/o _______________
12. lamin/o _______________
13. mening/o _______________
14. myel/o _______________
15. narc/o _______________
16. neur/o _______________
17. pallid/o _______________
18. poli/o _______________
19. somn/o _______________
20. spin/o _______________

21. spondyl/o ______________________

22. vag/o ______________________

23. ventricul/o ______________________

Suffixes

Give the definitions of the following suffixes.

1. -al ______________________
2. -algesia ______________________
3. -algia ______________________
4. -ar ______________________
5. -asthenia ______________________
6. -blast ______________________
7. -cele ______________________
8. -cyte ______________________
9. -desis ______________________
10. -ectomy ______________________
11. -edema ______________________
12. -esthesia ______________________
13. -glia ______________________
14. -gram ______________________
15. -graphy ______________________
16. -ia ______________________
17. -ic ______________________
18. -ion ______________________
19. -ism ______________________
20. -ist ______________________
21. -itis ______________________
22. -kinesia ______________________
23. -kinesis ______________________
24. -lepsy ______________________
25. -lexia ______________________
26. -logy ______________________
27. -troph(y) ______________________
28. -scopy ______________________
29. -oma ______________________
30. -osis ______________________
31. -paresis ______________________
32. -pathy ______________________
33. -phagia ______________________
34. -phasia ______________________
35. -praxia ______________________
36. -sthenia ______________________
37. -taxia ______________________
38. -tomy ______________________
39. -us ______________________
40. -y ______________________

Identifying Medical Terms

In the spaces provided, write the medical terms for the following meanings.

1. _______________ Condition in which there is a loss or lack of memory
2. _______________ Condition in which there is a lack of the sensation of pain
3. _______________ Loss or lack of the ability to eat or swallow
4. _______________ Neurological sign and symptom consisting of lack of coordination of muscle movements
5. _______________ Head pain; headache
6. _______________ Pertaining to the cerebellum
7. _______________ Surgical excision of a portion of the skull
8. _______________ Condition in which an individual has difficulty reading and writing words even though vision and intelligence are unimpaired
9. _______________ Inflammation of the brain
10. _______________ Literally means pertaining to situated on the dura mater
11. _______________ Slight paralysis that affects one side of the body
12. _______________ Inflammation of the meninges of the spinal cord or brain
13. _______________ Pain in a nerve or nerves
14. _______________ Inflammation of a nerve
15. _______________ Nerve cell, neuron
16. _______________ The study of the nervous system
17. _______________ Tumor of nerve cells and nerve fibers
18. _______________ Pathological loss of sensation or an impairment of motor function
19. _______________ Literally means *inflammation involving many nerves*
20. _______________ Condition of sleepwalking
21. _______________ Surgical incision of the vagus nerve
22. _______________ X-ray of the cerebral ventricles

Matching

Select the appropriate lettered meaning for each of the following words.

__________ **1.** acetylcholine

__________ **2.** Alzheimer disease

__________ **3.** stroke

__________ **4.** endorphins

__________ **5.** epilepsy

__________ **6.** palsy

__________ **7.** diskectomy

__________ **8.** epiduroscopy

__________ **9.** dementia

__________ **10.** sciatica

a. Group of symptoms marked by memory loss and other cognitive functions

b. Chemical substances produced in the brain that act as natural analgesics (*opiates*) and provide feelings of pleasure

c. Cerebrovascular accident

d. The most common cause of dementia among older adults

e. A neurological disorder involving repeated seizures of any type

f. Used for back pain relief when all other conservative treatments have failed

g. Cholinergic neurotransmitter

h. Pathological loss of sensation or an impairment of motor function

i. Severe pain along the course of the sciatic nerve

j. Surgical excision of an intervertebral disk

k. Anxiety syndrome and panic disorder

Medical Case Snapshots

This learning activity provides an opportunity to relate the medical terminology you are learning to a precise patient case presentation. In the spaces provided, write in your answers.

Case 1

An 8-year-old girl was accompanied by her mother to the doctor's office. The mother states that, about 2 years ago, her daughter was diagnosed with __________ (which is a neurological disorder involving repeated seizures). The majority of diagnosed cases of this disorder are __________ as their causes cannot be identified.

Case 2

The 74-year-old male was seen by his physician. He was in acute pain and complaining of severe itching around his waistline. Examination of his torso revealed evidence of a viral disease characterized by painful vesicular eruptions. This disease, known as __________ __________ is caused by the varicella-zoster virus, the same virus that causes __________. The common name for this condition is __________.

Case 3

A 70-year-old male diagnosed with Parkinson disease was seen by a neurologist. The patient had moderate to severe tremor (worse in the left hand than the right), difficulty in movement with ________ or abnormal slowness of motion, with freezing in place or ____________. The physician discussed with the patient and his wife the possibility of a surgical procedure known as a ________________ wherein there is destruction of the globus pallidus of the brain.

Drug Highlights

Type of Drug	Description and Examples
analgesics	Inhibit ascending pain pathways in the central nervous system. They increase pain threshold and alter pain perception.
narcotic	EXAMPLES: codeine sulfate, Dilaudid (hydromorphone HCl), Demerol (meperidine HCl), morphine sulfate, and Talwin (pentazocine HCl)
non-narcotic	EXAMPLES: butorphanol tartrate and nalbuphine HCl
analgesics–antipyretics	Act to relieve pain (analgesic effect) and reduce fever (antipyretic effect). EXAMPLES: Tylenol (acetaminophen); aspirin; Advil, Motrin, and Naprosyn, Aleve (naproxen)
sedatives and hypnotics	Depress the central nervous system by interfering with the transmission of nerve impulses. Depending on the dosage, barbiturates, benzodiazepines, and certain other drugs can produce either a sedative or a hypnotic effect. When used as a sedative, the dosage is designed to produce a calming effect without causing sleep. Used as a hypnotic, the dosage is sufficient to cause sleep.
barbiturates	EXAMPLE: Seconal sodium (secobarbital)
nonbarbiturates	EXAMPLES: chloral hydrate, lurazepam HCl, Restoril (temazepam), and Halcion (triazolam)
antiparkinsonism drugs	Used for palliative relief from such major symptoms as bradykinesia, rigidity, tremor, and disorder of equilibrium and posture. Therapy involves an attempt to replenish dopamine levels and/or inhibit the effects of the neurotransmitter acetylcholine. EXAMPLES: Sinemet 25–100 (25 mg of carbidopa and 100 mg of levodopa), levodopa, trihexyphenidyl HCl, Cogentin (benztropine mesylate), Requip (ropinirole), Tasmar (tolcapone), and Stalevo (carbidopa, levodopa, and entacapone)

Type of Drug	Description and Examples
anticonvulsants	Inhibit the spread of seizure activity in the motor cortex. EXAMPLES: Dilantin (phenytoin), Depakene (valproic acid), Tegretol (carbamazepine), Klonopin (clonazepam), and Mysoline (primidone) Selected anticonvulsants are used to help control the type of pain caused by damaged nerves and can help quiet the burning, stabbing, or shooting pain often caused by neuropathy.These drugs can be prescribed for diabetic neuropathy, shingles, trigeminal neuralgia, and/or damaged nerves due to chemotherapy, herniated disk, or fibromyalgia. EXAMPLES: Carbatrol, Tegretol (carbamazepine), and Neurontin (gabapentin)
cholinesterase inhibitors	Increase the brain's levels of acetylcholine, which helps to restore communication between brain cells. These medications can be used to improve global functioning (including activities of daily living (ADL), behavior, and cognition) in some patients with Alzheimer disease. EXAMPLES: Aricept (donepezil hydrochloride) and Exelon (rivastigmine tartrate)

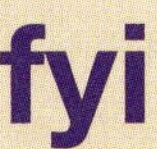

To date, no treatment can stop Alzheimer disease (AD). However, for some people in the early and middle stages of the disease, the drugs donepezil (Aricept), rivastigmine (Exelon), galantamine (Razadyne), or memantine (Namenda) can help prevent some symptoms from becoming worse for a limited time. Also, some medicines can help control behavioral symptoms of AD such as sleeplessness, agitation, wandering, anxiety, and depression.

Type of Drug	Description and Examples
anesthetics	Interfere with the conduction of nerve impulses and are used to produce loss of sensation, loss of pain, muscle relaxation, and/or complete loss of consciousness; block nerve transmission in the area to which they are applied.
local	Block nerve transmission in the area to which they are applied. EXAMPLES: procaine HCl, Xylocaine (lidocaine HCl), and Marcaine (bupivacaine HCl)
general	Affect the central nervous system and produce either partial or complete loss of consciousness. They also produce analgesia, skeletal muscle relaxation, and reduction of reflex activity. EXAMPLES: Suprane (desflurane), isoflurane, Sojourn, Ultane (Sevoflurane)

Diagnostic and Laboratory Tests

Test	Description
cerebral angiography (sĕr´ ĕ-brăl ăn-jē-ŏg´ ră-fē)	Process of making an x-ray record of the cerebral arterial system. A radiopaque substance is injected into an artery of the arm or neck, and x-ray films of the head are taken to visualize cerebral aneurysms, tumors, or ruptured blood vessels.
cerebrospinal fluid (CSF) analysis (sĕr″ ĕ-brŏ-spī´ năl)	Examination of spinal fluid for color, pressure, pH, and the levels of protein, glucose, and leukocytes. Abnormal results can indicate hemorrhage, tumor, and various disease processes.
computed tomography (CT) (kŏm-pū´ tĕd tō-mŏg″ ră-fē)	Diagnostic procedure used to study the structure of the brain. Computerized three-dimensional x-ray images allow the radiologist to differentiate among intracranial tumors, cysts, edema, and hemorrhage.
echoencephalography (ĕk″ ō-ĕn-sĕf-ă-lŏg´ ră-fē)	Process of using ultrasound to determine the presence of a centrally located mass in the brain.
electroencephalography (EEG) (ē-lĕk″ trō-ĕn-sĕf″ ă-lŏg´ ră-fē)	Process of measuring the electrical activity of the brain via an electroencephalograph. Abnormal results can indicate epilepsy, brain tumor, infection, abscess, hemorrhage, and/or coma; brain "death" also can be determined by an EEG.
lumbar puncture (LP) (lŭm´ băr)	Insertion of a needle into the lumbar subarachnoid space for removal of spinal fluid. The fluid is examined for color, pressure, level of protein, chloride, glucose, and leukocytes. See Figure 14.22.

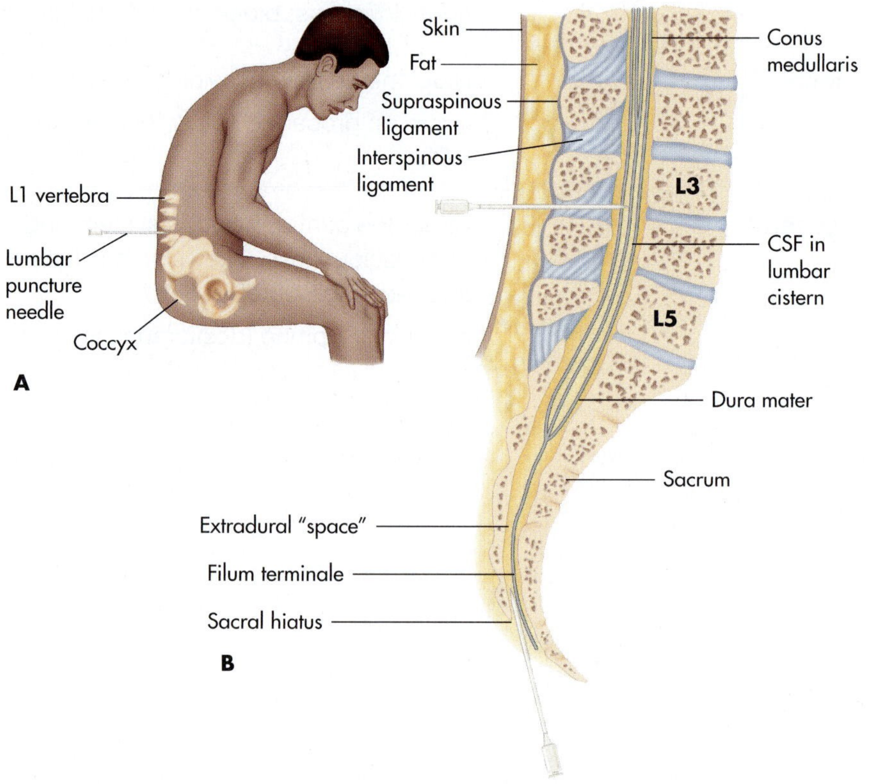

Figure 14.22 (A) Lumbar puncture, also known as *spinal tap*; (B) section of the vertebral column showing the spinal cord and membranes with a lumbar puncture needle at L3–L4 and in the sacral hiatus.

Test	Description
myelogram (mī′ ĕ-lō-grăm)	X-ray of the spinal canal after the injection of a radiopaque dye. Useful in diagnosing spinal lesions, cysts, herniated disks, tumors, and nerve root damage.
neurological examination (nū″ rō-lŏj′ ĭ-kŭl)	Assessment of a patient's vision; hearing; sense of taste, smell, touch, and pain; position; temperature; gait; and muscle strength, coordination, and reflex action to determine neurological status.
positron emission tomography (PET) (pŏz′ ĭ-trŏn ē-mĭsh′ ŭn tō-mŏg′ ră-fē)	Computer-based nuclear imaging procedure that can produce three-dimensional pictures of actual organ functioning. Useful in locating brain lesion, identifying blood flow and oxygen metabolism in stroke patients, showing metabolic changes in Alzheimer disease, and studying biochemical changes associated with mental illness.
ultrasonography, brain (ŭl-tră-sŏn-ŏg′ ră-fē)	Use of high-frequency sound waves to produce an image on a computer screen. Used as a screening test or diagnostic tool.

Abbreviations

Abbreviation	Meaning
ACh	acetylcholine
AD	Alzheimer disease
ADL	activities of daily living
ALS	amyotrophic lateral sclerosis
ANS	autonomic nervous system
ASPD	advanced sleep phase disorder
cm	centimeter
CNS	central nervous system
CP	cerebral palsy
CSF	cerebrospinal fluid
CT	computed tomography
CTE	chronic traumatic encephalopathy
CVA	cerebrovascular accident
DBS	deep brain stimulation
DSPS	delayed sleep phase syndrome
EEG	electroencephalogram
GCS	Glasgow coma scale
HDS	herniated disk syndrome
HNP	herniated nucleus pulposus
ICP	intracranial pressure
LP	lumbar puncture
MHI	mild head injury
MHT	minor head trauma
mL	milliliter
MRI	magnetic resonance imaging
MS	multiple sclerosis
MTBI	mild traumatic brain injury
Neuro	neurology
NREM	no rapid eye movement (sleep)
PD	Parkinson disease
PET	positron emission tomography
PNS	peripheral nervous system
REM	rapid eye movement (sleep)
TENS	transcutaneous electrical nerve stimulation
TIA	transient ischemic attack
WHO	World Health Organization

Study and Review III

Building Medical Terms

Using the following word parts, fill in the blanks to build the correct medical terms.

an-	papill	-esthesia
quadri-	-kinesia	-tomy
concuss	-itis	
neur	-ectomy	

Definition	Medical Term
1. Condition in which there is a lack of the sensation of pain	_______algesia
2. Abnormal slowness of movement	brady ________
3. Head injury with a transient loss of brain function	__________ion
4. Inflammation of the brain	encephal _____
5. Surgical excision of a vertebral posterior arch	lamin ________
6. Pain in a nerve or nerves	_________algia
7. Swelling of the optic disk, usually caused by ICP	_______edema
8. Abnormal sensation, feeling of numbness, or prickling	par _________
9. Paralysis of all four extremities and usually the trunk	________plegia
10. Surgical incision of the vagus nerve	vago ________

Combining Form Challenge

Using the combining forms provided, write the medical term correctly.

cephal/o	encephal/o	mening/o
cran/i	hypn/o	neur/o

1. Head pain; headache: ________algia
2. Surgical excision of a portion of the skull: ________ectomy
3. Any pathological dysfunction of the brain: ________pathy
4. Artificially induced trancelike state resembling sleepwalking: ________osis
5. Inflammation of the meninges of the spinal cord or brain: ________itis
6. Supporting or connective tissue cells of the central nervous system: ________glia

Select the Right Term

Select the correct answer, and write it on the line provided.

1. Inability to remain still; motor restlessness and anxiety is ___________.

akathisia **akinesia** **aphagia** **apraxia**

2. Literally means *loss or lack of the sense of feeling* is ___________.

analgesia **anesthesia** **aphasia** **asthenia**

3. Unconscious state or stupor from which the patient cannot be aroused is ___________.

chorea **concussion** **coma** **epilepsy**

4. Group of symptoms marked by memory loss and other cognitive functions is ___________.

dyslexia **dysphasia** **hypnosis** **dementia**

5. Increased muscular movement and motion is ___________.

hyperesthesia **narcolepsy** **hyperkinesis** **paresis**

6. Death of focal brain tissue that occurs when the brain does not get sufficient blood and oxygen is ___________.

sundowning **stroke** **syncope** **palsy**

Diagnostic and Laboratory Tests

Select the best answer to each multiple-choice question. Circle the letter of your choice.

1. Diagnostic procedure used to study the structure of the brain.

a. computed tomography
b. echoencephalography
c. electroencephalography
d. myelogram

2. Process of using ultrasound to determine the presence of a centrally located mass in the brain.

a. computed tomography
b. echoencephalography
c. electroencephalography
d. myelogram

3. X-ray of the spinal canal after the injection of a radiopaque dye.

a. cerebral angiography
b. computed tomography
c. myelogram
d. ultrasonography

4. Computer-based nuclear imaging procedure that can produce three-dimensional pictures of actual organ functioning.

a. electroencephalography
b. myelogram
c. ultrasonography
d. positron emission tomography

5. Use of high-frequency sound waves to produce an image on a computer screen.

a. electroencephalography
b. myelogram
c. ultrasonography
d. positron emission tomography

Abbreviations

Place the correct word, phrase, or abbreviation in the space provided.

1. Alzheimer disease ______________________________
2. amyotrophic lateral sclerosis ______________________________
3. CNS ______________________________
4. CP ______________________________
5. computed tomography ______________________________
6. herniated disk syndrome ______________________________
7. ICP ______________________________
8. LP ______________________________
9. MS ______________________________
10. positron emission tomography ______________________________

Practical Application

Medical Record Analysis

This exercise contains information, abbreviations, and medical terminology from an actual medical record or case study that has been adapted for this text. The names and any personal information have been created by the author. Read and study each form or case study and then answer the questions that follow. You may refer to Appendix III, *Abbreviations and Symbols*.

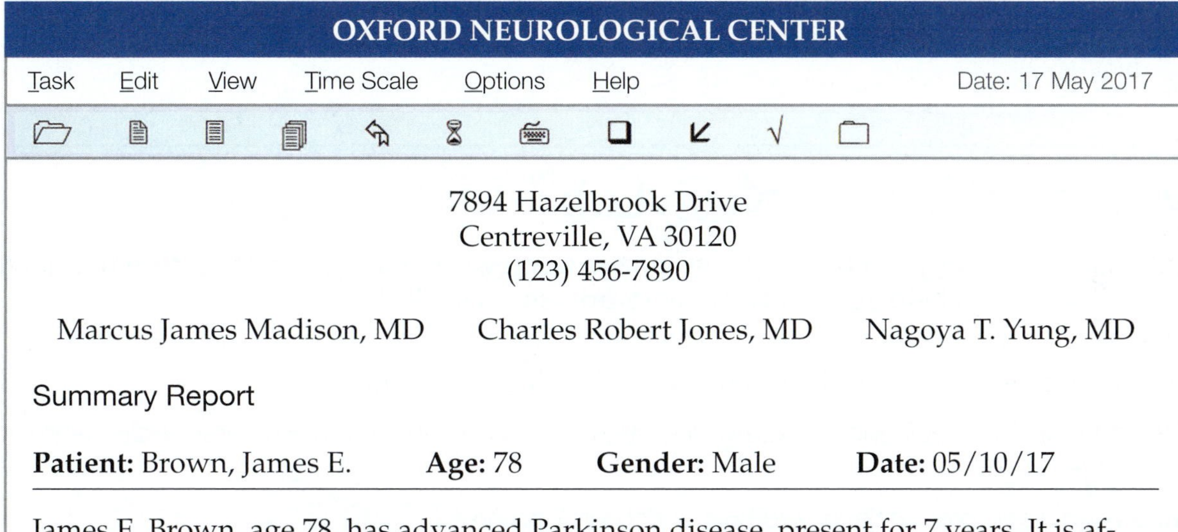

OXFORD NEUROLOGICAL CENTER

Task Edit View Time Scale Options Help Date: 17 May 2017

7894 Hazelbrook Drive
Centreville, VA 30120
(123) 456-7890

Marcus James Madison, MD Charles Robert Jones, MD Nagoya T. Yung, MD

Summary Report

Patient: Brown, James E. **Age:** 78 **Gender:** Male **Date:** 05/10/17

James E. Brown, age 78, has advanced Parkinson disease, present for 7 years. It is affecting his activities of daily living (ADL). He has difficulty bathing, dressing, and has frequent falls. He has marked hesitancy on changing directions and unsteadiness with fatigue. He can brush his teeth and wash his face.

On neurological examination he did have mild to moderate impairment in cognition and short-term memory, although he is oriented to time, place, and person. He has a mild tremor, worse in the left arm than the right. He has rigidity in the upper extremities. He has marked difficulty in movement, with long delays in initiating movement and frequent freezing in place. He has postural instability. He has mild difficulty with articulation of speech, dysarthria. His gait is characterized by shuffling strides. He can arise from a chair with difficulty only after multiple attempts. Deep tendon reflexes are symmetrical, and toes are downgoing. Cranial nerves are unremarkable.

He has been on Sinemet 25–100 mg tid for the last 6 years. I have asked him to increase his Sinemet dose to qid. Mr. Brown is to return to our office in 3 months.

Marcus James Madison, MD

Medical Record Questions

Place the correct answer in the space provided.

1. On neurological examination Mr. Brown did have mild to moderate impairment in ________________ ________________ and short-term memory.
2. Mr. Brown has a mild ________________________________, worse in the left arm than the right.
3. What does *dysarthria* mean? ________________________________
4. Sinemet 25–100 mg is classified as a/an ________________________________ drug.
5. Why is this drug prescribed for Mr. Brown? ________________________________

Chapter 15

Special Senses: The Ear

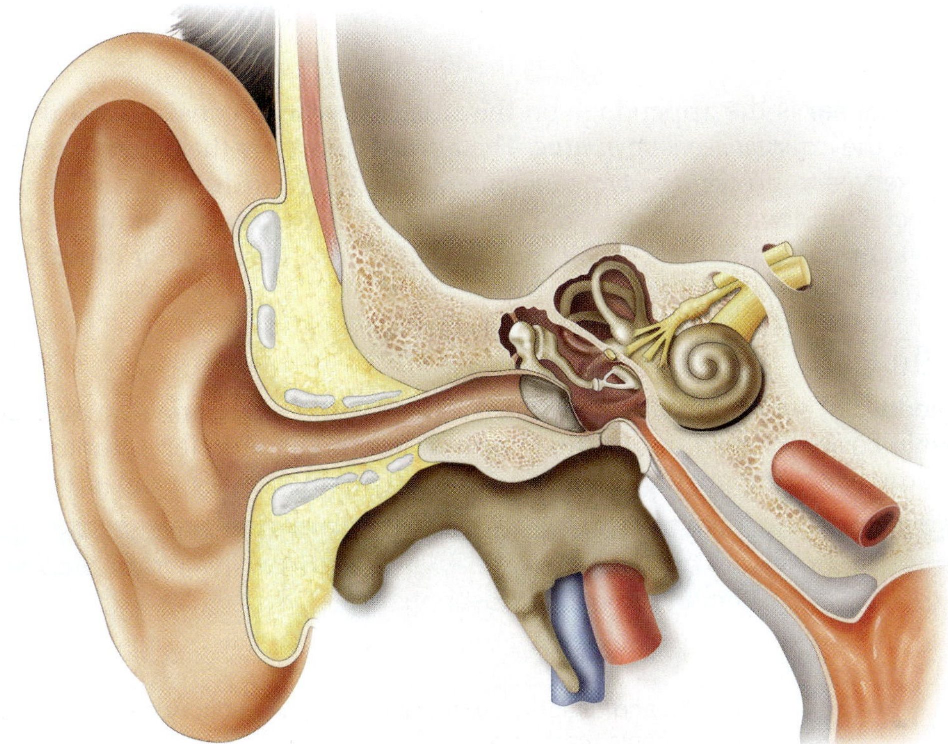

Learning Outcomes

On completion of this chapter, you will be able to:

1. State the description and primary functions of the ear.
2. Recognize terminology included in the ICD-10-CM.
3. Analyze, build, spell, and pronounce medical words.
4. Comprehend the drugs highlighted in this chapter.
5. Describe diagnostic and laboratory tests related to the ear.
6. Identify and define selected abbreviations.
7. Apply your acquired knowledge of medical terms by successfully completing the *Practical Application* exercise.

Anatomy and Physiology

The **ear** is generally described as having three distinct divisions: the external ear, the middle ear, and the inner ear, each with distinct functions. The ear contains structures for both the sense of hearing and the sense of balance. The eighth cranial nerve, also called the acoustic or auditory nerve, carries nerve impulses for both hearing and balance from the ear to the brain. Table 15.1 provides an at-a-glance look at the ear. The ear and its anatomic structures are shown in Figure 15.1.

External Ear

The **external ear** is the appendage on the side of the head consisting of the **auricle** or **pinna** and the *external acoustic meatus*. The auricle (pinna) is the external portion of the ear that serves to protect the **tympanic membrane (TM)** (eardrum), as well as to collect and direct sound waves through the **ear canal** to the eardrum. About 1¼ inches long, the canal contains modified sweat glands that secrete **cerumen**, or *earwax*. Too much cerumen can block sound transmission.

Middle Ear

The **middle ear**, separated from the external ear by the eardrum, is an air-filled cavity (**tympanic cavity**) carved out of the temporal bone. The **attic** (epitympanic recess) of the middle ear is the portion lying above the tympanic cavity proper. It contains the

Table 15.1 Special Senses: The Ear at-a-Glance

Organ/Structure	Primary Functions/Description
External ear	
Auricle (pinna)	Collects and directs sound waves into the auditory canal and then into the tympanic membrane
External acoustic meatus (auditory canal)	Numerous glands line the canal and secrete cerumen (earwax) to lubricate and protect the ear
Tympanic membrane (eardrum)	Separates the external ear from the middle ear and is not actually part of the external ear
Middle ear	
Contains the ossicles: malleus, incus, and stapes; has several openings; is lined with mucous membrane	Transmits sound vibrations from the tympanic membrane to the cochlea
	Equalizes external/internal air pressure on the tympanic membrane
Inner ear	
Cochlea	Located on the basilar membrane is the *organ of Corti* containing hair cell sensory receptors for the sense of hearing
Vestibule	Contains the utricle and saccule, membranous pouches containing perilymph. The utricle communicates with the semicircular canals and contains hair cell sensory receptors connected to fibers from the eighth cranial nerve. These hair cells react to the force of gravity and movement of *otoliths*, and are a part of the sense of equilibrium (state of balance).
Semicircular canals	Contain nerve endings in the form of hair cells that note changes in the position of the head and report such movement to the brain through fibers leading to the eighth cranial nerve

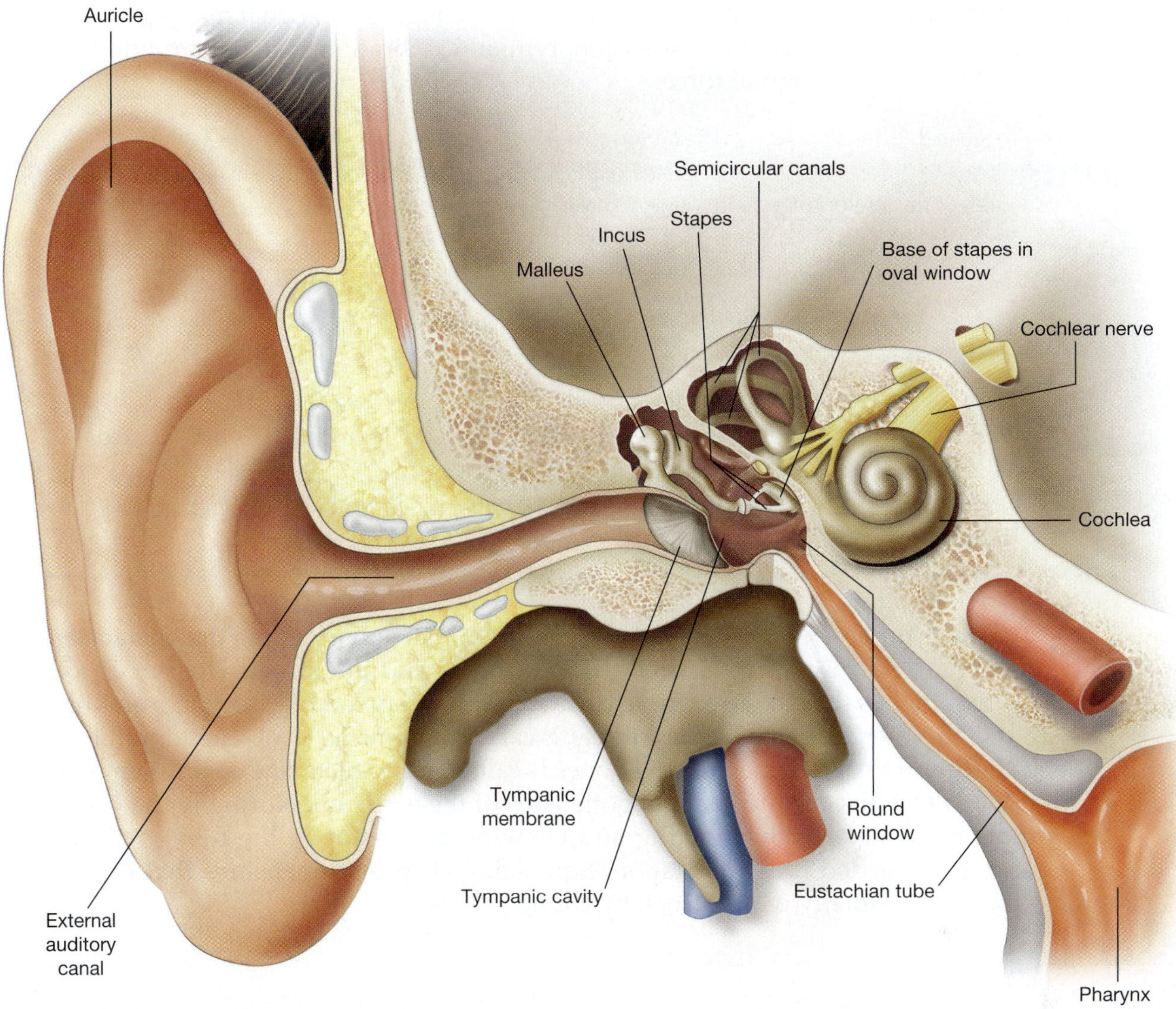

Figure 15.1 The ear and its anatomic structures.

head of the malleus and the short limb of the incus. The tympanic cavity contains three specialized small bones or **ossicles** instrumental to the hearing process. These ossicles are the **malleus (hammer)**, **incus (anvil)**, and **stapes (stirrup)**. See Figure 15.2. These bones mechanically transmit sound vibrations from the tympanic membrane, to which the malleus is attached, through the incus to the stapes, which attaches to a thin membrane

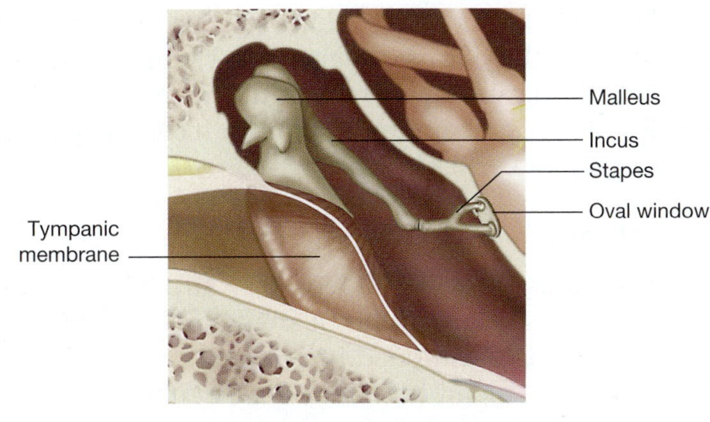

Figure 15.2 The ossicles of the middle ear along with the oval window and tympanic membrane.

covering a small opening, the oval window (see Figure 15.1), that marks the beginning of the inner ear. During transmission, tympanic vibrations can be amplified as much as 22 times their original force.

insights In ICD-10-CM, Chapter 8, *Diseases of the Ear and Mastoid Process* (code numbers H60–H95), categories are arranged into blocks, making it easier to identify the types of conditions that occur in the following:

- External ear (H60–H62) (block 1)
- Middle ear and mastoid process (H65–H75) (block 2)
- Inner ear (H80–H83) (block 3)
- Other disorders of the ear (H90–H94) (block 4)
- Intraoperative and postprocedural complications and disorders of ear and mastoid process, not located elsewhere (H95) (block 5)

Complications are grouped at the end of the chapter rather than scattered throughout different categories.

The tympanic cavity connects to the throat/nasopharynx via the **eustachian tube**, which is a narrow tube between the middle ear and the throat. This ear–throat connection makes the ear susceptible to infection. The spread of infection from the throat along this membrane to the middle ear is called **otitis media (OM)**. The continued spread of infection to one of the mastoid bones is called **mastoiditis**. The eustachian tube functions to equalize air pressure on both sides of the eardrum. Normally the walls of the tube are collapsed. Swallowing and chewing actions open the tube to allow air in or out, as needed for equalization. Equalizing air pressure ensures that the eardrum vibrates maximally when struck by sound waves.

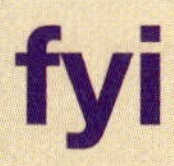

At 36 weeks, the **earlobes** of the fetus are soft and around 40 weeks they become firm. In newborns, the wall of the ear canal is pliable because of underdeveloped cartilage and bone. The eustachian tube in infants is shorter and straighter than in older children and adults. Because of this, an infant or young child is more predisposed to developing an ear infection. When this occurs, the child's ears should be examined very carefully.

Inner Ear

The **inner ear** consists of a membranous labyrinth or mazelike network of canals located within a bony labyrinth. These structures are called **labyrinths** because of their complicated shapes. The bony labyrinth, located in the temporal bone, consists of the *cochlea*, *vestibule*, and three *semicircular canals*. Within the bony labyrinth, but separated from it by a pale fluid called **perilymph**, is the membranous labyrinth, filled with a fluid called **endolymph**. This membranous labyrinth contains the actual hearing cells, the hair cells of the organ of Corti.

Cochlea

The **cochlea** is a spiral-shaped bony structure containing the cochlear duct; it is so named because it resembles a snail shell (see Figure 15.1). The spiral cavity of the bony cochlea is partitioned into three tubelike channels that run the entire length of the spiral. Two membranes form these tubelike areas. The *basilar membrane* forms the lower channel or *scala tympani*, and the *vestibular membrane* (*Reissner membrane*) forms the upper channel, which is called the *scala vestibuli*. Between the two scala is a space, the *cochlear duct*, formed by the vestibular membrane on top and the basilar membrane as a floor. Located on the basilar membrane is the **organ of Corti** containing hair cell sensory receptors for the sense of hearing. The fluid perilymph fills the scala vestibuli and scala tympani. A different fluid, endolymph, fills the cochlear duct.

fyi A cochlear implant is a small, complex electronic device that can help to provide a sense of sound to a person who is profoundly deaf or severely hard of hearing. The implant consists of an external portion that sits behind the ear and a second portion that is surgically placed under the skin. See Figure 15.3. An implant does not restore normal hearing. Instead, it can give a deaf person a useful representation of sounds in the environment and help him or her to understand speech. An implant has the following parts:

- A microphone, which picks up sound from the environment.
- A speech processor, which selects and arranges sounds picked up by the microphone.
- A transmitter and receiver/stimulator, which receive signals from the speech processor and convert them into electric impulses.
- An electrode array, which is a group of electrodes that collects the impulses from the stimulator and sends them to different regions of the auditory nerve.

Children and adults can be fitted for cochlear implants. Adults who have lost all or most of their hearing later in life often can benefit from cochlear implants. Cochlear implants, coupled with intensive postimplantation therapy, can help young children, often between 2 and 6 years old, to acquire speech, language, and social skills. See Figure 15.4.

Ear with Cochlear Implant

Transmitter
Speech processor
Receiver/Stimulator
Microphone
Electrode array

Figure 15.3 Ear with cochlear implant.
(NIH Medical Arts)

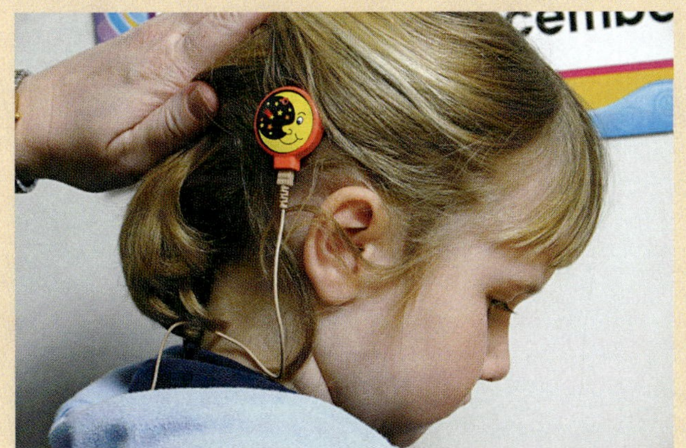

Figure 15.4 A young child with a cochlear implant.
Source: Pearson Education, Inc.

THE PROCESS OF HEARING

In the process of hearing, sound waves are collected by the auricle (pinna) and directed through the external auditory canal to the tympanic membrane (eardrum), causing it to vibrate. These vibrations move the three small bones of the middle ear (malleus, incus, and stapes). The movement of the stapes at the oval window sets up pressure waves in the auditory fluids (perilymph and endolymph). The waves distort the basilar membrane and cause the vibration of the hair cells of the organ of Corti. These vibrations are picked up by auditory nerve fibers that transmit an electric nerve signal to the cerebral cortex of the brain, where it is interpreted as sound. The path of sound vibrations is shown in Figure 15.5.

Vestibule

The **vestibule** is a bony structure located between the cochlea and the three semicircular canals. The bony vestibule contains the **utricle** and **saccule**, membranous pouches containing perilymph. The utricle communicates with the semicircular canals and contains hair cell sensory receptors connected to fibers from the eighth cranial nerve. These hair cells bend to the forces of gravity and movement of **otoliths** and are a part of the sense of *equilibrium*. Receptors in the utricle and saccule respond to gravity and linear acceleration. Because of their orientation in the head, the utricle is sensitive to a change in horizontal movement, and the saccule gives information about vertical acceleration (such as when in an elevator).

The utricle and saccule together make the *otolith organs*. Both of these organs contain a sensory epithelium, the **macula**, which consists of hair cells and associated supporting cells. Overlying the hair cells and their hair bundles is a gelatinous layer, and

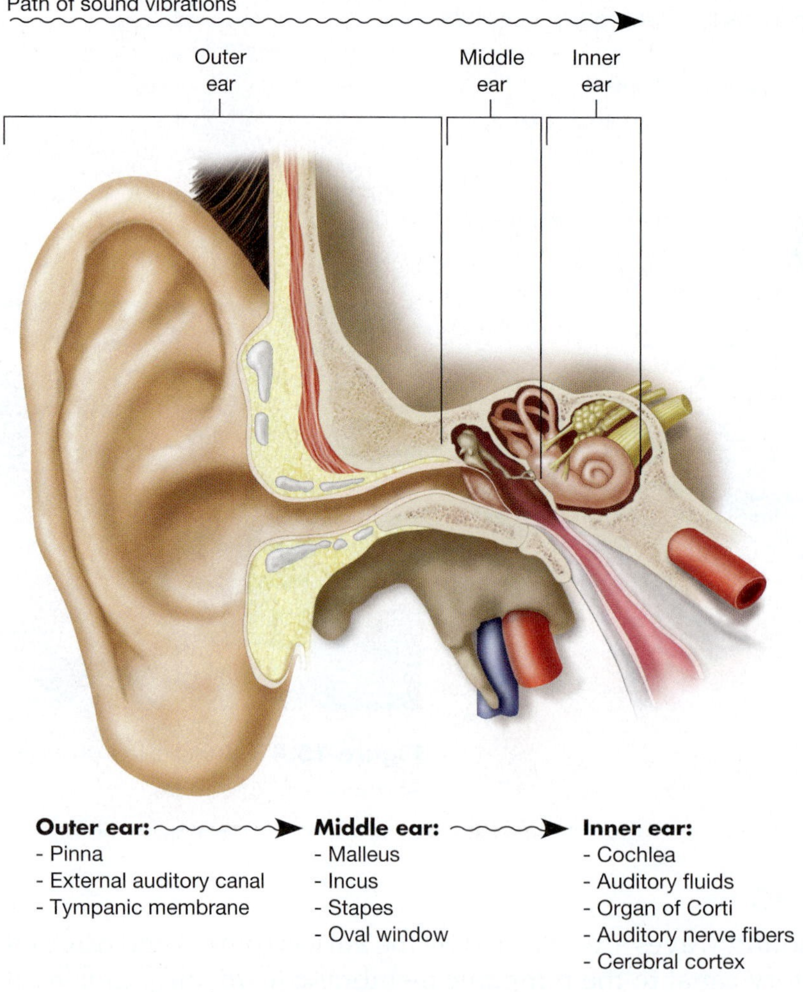

Figure 15.5 Path of sound vibrations.

above this is a fibrous structure, the **otolithic membrane**, in which are embedded crystals of calcium carbonate called **otoconia**. The crystals give the otolith organs their name: *otolith* is Greek for "ear stones."

Semicircular Canals

Located at right angles to each other are the superior, posterior, and inferior **semicircular canals**. Within the bony canals are the membranous semicircular ducts containing endolymph. At the base of each canal is an enlargement called an **ampulla** containing nerve endings in the form of hair cells. Changes in the position of the head cause the fluid in the canals to flow against these sensory receptors, which, in turn, report such movement to the brain through fibers leading to the eighth cranial nerve. Dizziness and motion sickness are associated with the continued movement of the fluid in the semicircular canals due to gravitational influences and the resulting sensory sensation in these areas.

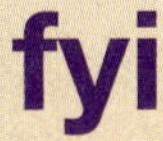

With aging, changes occur in the external, middle, and inner ear. The skin of the auricle can become dry and wrinkled. Production of cerumen declines and it is drier. There is also dryness of the external canal, which causes itching. Hairs in the external canal become coarser and longer, especially in males. The eardrum thickens, and the bony joints in the middle ear degenerate.

Changes in the inner ear affect sensitivity to sound, understanding of speech, and balance. Degenerative changes include atrophy of the cochlea, the cochlear nerve cells, and the organ of Corti. These changes lead to the hearing loss, **presbycusis**, which is common in the older adult. Noisy surroundings make it difficult for older adults to discriminate between sounds, thereby impairing communication and socialization. The hearing distance (HD) of older adults can also be impaired.

Study and Review I

Anatomy and Physiology

Write your answers to the following questions.

1. The ears contain structures for both the sense of ______________ and the sense of ______________.

2. Name the three divisions of the ear.

a. ______________ **b.** ______________

c. ______________

3. The external ear consists of the ______________ and the ______________.

4. Which structure of the external ear collects sound waves? ______________

5. State the two functions of cerumen.

a. ______________ **b.** ______________

6. Name the three ossicles of the middle ear.

a. ______________________________ **b.** ______________________________

c. ______________________________

7. State the function of the ossicles. ____

____

8. State two functions of the middle ear.

a. ______________________________ **b.** ______________________________

9. The bony labyrinth of the inner ear consists of the ________________________,

________________________, and the ________________________.

10. Name the three divisions of the membranous labyrinth.

a. ______________________________ **b.** ______________________________

c. ______________________________

11. Located on the basilar membrane is the ________________________, containing hair cell sensory receptors for the sense of hearing.

12. The ________________________ is a bony structure located between the cochlea and the three semicircular canals.

13. The auditory nerve is also known as the ________________________.

14. Dizziness and ________________________ are associated with the continued movement of the fluid in the semicircular canals due to gravitational influences.

15. Name the two types of fluid found in the ear.

a. ______________________________ **b.** ______________________________

ANATOMY LABELING

Identify the structures shown below by filling in the blanks.

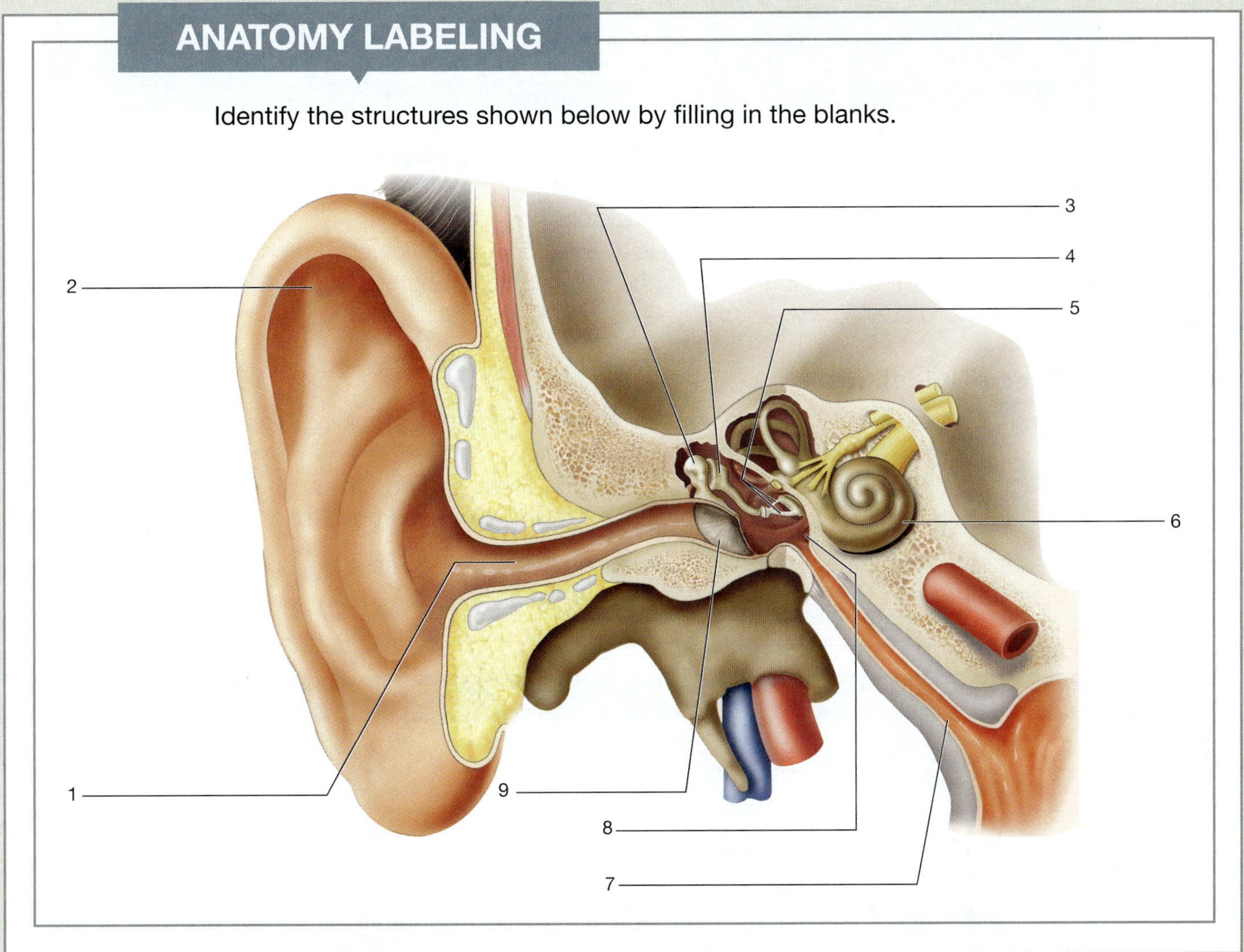

Building Your Medical Vocabulary

This section provides the foundation for learning medical terminology. Review the following alphabetized word list. Note how common prefixes and suffixes are repeatedly applied to word roots and combining forms to create different meanings. The word parts are color-coded: prefixes are yellow, suffixes are blue, roots/combining forms are red. A combining form is a word root plus a vowel. The chart below lists the combining forms for the word roots in this chapter and can help to strengthen your understanding of how medical words are built and spelled.

Remember These Guidelines

1. If the suffix begins with a vowel, drop the combining vowel from the combining form and add the suffix. For example, ot/o (*ear*) + -itis (*inflammation*) becomes otitis.
2. If the suffix begins with a consonant, keep the combining vowel and add the suffix to the combining form. For example, ot/o (*ear*) + -scope (*instrument for examining*) becomes otoscope.

You will find that some terms have not been divided into word parts. These are common words or specialized terms that are included to enhance your medical vocabulary.

Combining Forms of the Ear

audi/o	to hear	**neur/o**	nerve
aur/i	ear	**ot/o**	ear
chol/e	gall or bile	**pharyng/o**	pharynx
cochle/o	land snail	**presby/o**	old
electr/o	electricity	**py/o**	pus
labyrinth/o	maze, inner ear	**scler/o**	hardening
laryng/o	larynx, voice box	**staped/o**	stapes, stirrup
mast/o	mastoid process, breast-shaped	**steat/o**	fat
myring/o	eardrum, tympanic membrane	**tympan/o**	eardrum, tympanic membrane

Medical Word	Word Parts		Definition
	Part	Meaning	
acoustic (ă-koos´ tĭk)	acoust -ic	hearing pertaining to	Pertaining to the sense of hearing
audiogram (ŏ´ dĭ-ō-grăm˝)	audi/o -gram	to hear a mark, record	Record of hearing by audiometry

ALERT!

How many words can you build using the combining form **audi/o**?

Medical Word	Part	Meaning	Definition
audiologist (ŏ˝ dĭ-ŏl´ ō-jĭst)	audi/o log -ist	to hear study of one who specializes	One who specializes in diagnosing disorders of hearing
audiology (ŏ˝ dĭ-ŏl´ ō-jĭ)	audi/o -logy	to hear study of	Study of hearing disorders
audiometer (ŏ˝ dĭ-ŏm´ ĕ-tĕr)	audi/o -meter	to hear instrument to measure	Medical instrument used to measure hearing
audiometry (ŏ˝ dĭ-ŏm´ ĕ-trē)	audi/o -metry	to hear measurement	Measurement of the hearing sense

RULE REMINDER

This term keeps the combining vowel ***o*** because the suffix begins with a consonant.

Medical Word	Part	Meaning	Definition
auditory (ŏ´ dĭ-tō˝ rē)	auditor -y	hearing pertaining to	Pertaining to the sense of hearing
aural (ŏ´ răl)	aur -al	ear pertaining to	Pertaining to the ear
auricle (ŏ´ rĭ-kl)	aur/i -cle	ear small	External portion of the ear; also known as the *pinna*
binaural (bīn-aw´ răl)	bin- aur -al	twice ear pertaining to	Pertaining to both ears
cholesteatoma (kō˝ lē-stē˝ ă-tō´ mă)	chol/e steat -oma	gall or bile fat tumor	Tumorlike mass filled with epithelial cells and cholesterol

Medical Word	Word Parts		Definition
	Part	Meaning	
deafness			Complete or partial loss of the ability to hear. *Hearing impairment* is often used to describe a minimal loss of hearing as compared to the use of the word *deafness* when there is complete or extensive loss of hearing. See Figure 15.6.

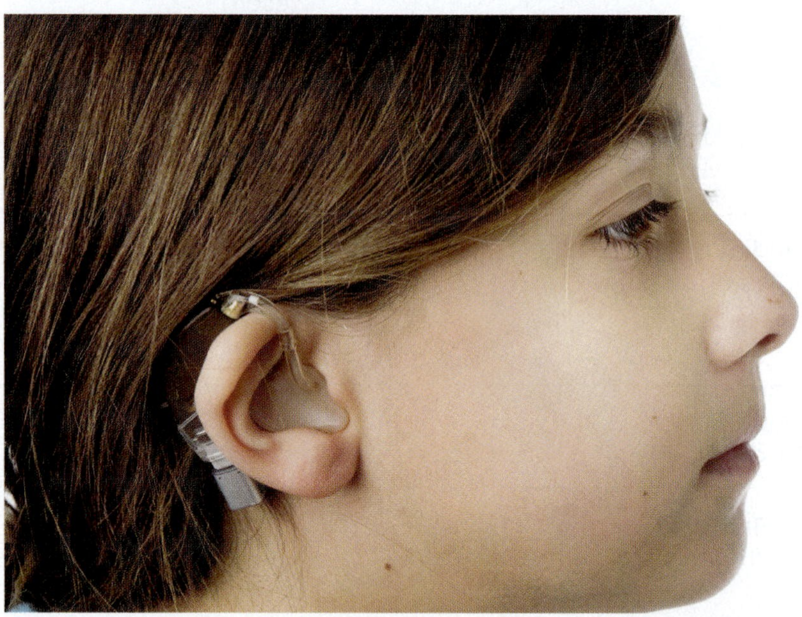

Figure 15.6 A child with a hearing impairment wears a hearing aid in her right ear. (Paul Hill/Fotolia)

fyi Sustained noise over 85 decibels (db, dB) can cause permanent **hearing loss**. Risk doubles with each 5-decibel increase. About two in every 10 teens have lost some of their hearing ability from exposure to noise and are not aware of it, according to a study conducted at the University of Florida. See Figure 15.7. High-pitched sounds are the first to be affected by noise exposure. As hearing loss progresses, a person can start to have difficulty hearing, particularly when there is noise in the background. Excessive noise can permanently damage the hair cell sensory receptors of the organ of Corti. These receptors are instrumental in transmitting sound to the brain.

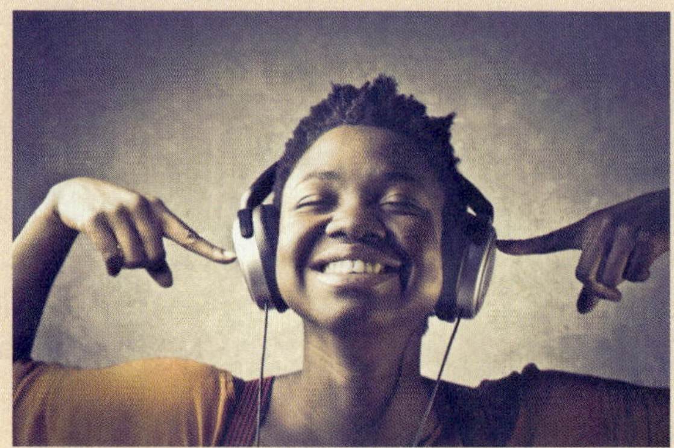

Figure 15.7 Listening to loud music with headphones or at rock concerts is a frequent cause of hearing loss among teenagers and young adults. (ollyy/Shutterstock)

Medical Word	Part	Meaning	Definition
electrocochleography (ē-lĕk″ trō-kŏk″ lē-ŏg′ ră-fē)	electr/o cochle/o -graphy	electricity land snail recording	Recording of the electrical activity produced when the cochlea is stimulated

Medical Word	Word Parts		Definition
	Part	**Meaning**	
endaural (ĕn´ dŏ˝ răl)	end- aur -al	within ear pertaining to	Pertaining to within the ear
endolymph (ĕn´ dō-lĭmf)	endo- -lymph	within serum, clear fluid	Clear fluid contained within the labyrinth of the ear
equilibrium (ē˝ kwĭ-lĭb´ rē-ŭm)			State of balance
fenestration (fĕn˝ ĕs-trā´ shŭn)	fenestrat -ion	window process	Surgical operation in which a new opening is made in the labyrinth of the inner ear to restore hearing
labyrinth (lăb´ ĭ-rĭnth)	labyrinth	maze, inner ear	The inner ear; made up of the *vestibule*, *cochlea*, and *semicircular canals*
labyrinthectomy (lăb˝ ĭ-rĭn-thĕk´ tō-mē)	labyrinth -ectomy	maze, inner ear surgical excision	Surgical excision of the labyrinth
labyrinthitis (lăb˝ ĭ-rĭn-thī˝ tĭs)	labyrinth -itis	maze, inner ear inflammation	Inflammation of the labyrinth
labyrinthotomy (lăb˝ ĭ-rĭn-thŏt´ ō-mē)	labyrinth/o -tomy	maze, inner ear incision	Incision of the labyrinth
malleus (măl´ ē-ŭs)			Largest of the three ossicles; also called the *hammer*
mastoiditis (măs˝ toyd-ī´ tĭs)	mast -oid -itis	mastoid process, breast-shaped resemble inflammation	Inflammation of one of the mastoid bones; characterized by fever, headache, and malaise
Ménière disease (mān˝ ē-ār´)			An abnormality of the inner ear causing a host of symptoms, including vertigo (sensation of spinning), tinnitus (a ringing or roaring sound in the ears), fluctuating hearing loss, and the sensation of pressure or pain in the affected ear. Symptoms are associated with a change in fluid volume within the labyrinth and can occur suddenly and arise daily or as infrequently as once a year.

Medical Word	Word Parts: Part	Word Parts: Meaning	Definition
monaural (mŏn-aw′ răl)	mon(o)- aur -al	one ear pertaining to	Pertaining to one ear
myringectomy (mĭr-ĭn-jĕk′ tō-mē)	myring -ectomy	eardrum, tympanic membrane surgical excision	Surgical excision of the tympanic membrane
myringoplasty (mĭr-ĭn′ gō-plăst″ ē)	myring/o -plasty	eardrum, tympanic membrane surgical repair	Surgical repair of the tympanic membrane
myringoscope (mĭr-ĭn′ gō-skōp)	myring/o -scope	eardrum, tympanic membrane instrument for examining	Medical instrument used to examine the eardrum
myringotome (mĭ-rĭn′ gō-tōm)	myring/o -tome	eardrum, tympanic membrane instrument to cut	Surgical instrument used for cutting the eardrum
myringotomy (mĭr-ĭn-gŏt′ ō-mē)	myring/o -tomy	eardrum, tympanic membrane incision	Surgical incision of the tympanic membrane to remove unwanted fluids from the ear

RULE REMINDER

This term keeps the combining vowel ***o*** because the suffix begins with a consonant.

Medical Word	Part	Meaning	Definition
otalgia (ō″ tăl′ jē-ă)	ot -algia	ear pain	Pain in the ear, earache
otic (ō′ tĭk)	ot -ic	ear pertaining to	Pertaining to the ear
otitis (ō-tī′ tĭs)	ot -itis	ear inflammation	Inflammation of the ear

Medical Word	Word Parts		Definition
	Part	Meaning	
otitis media (ō-tī´ tĭs mē´ dē-ă)	ot -itis med -ia	ear inflammation middle condition	Inflammation of the middle ear. Most middle ear infections are a result of an upper respiratory infection (URI) that has spread through the eustachian tube. See Figure 15.8.

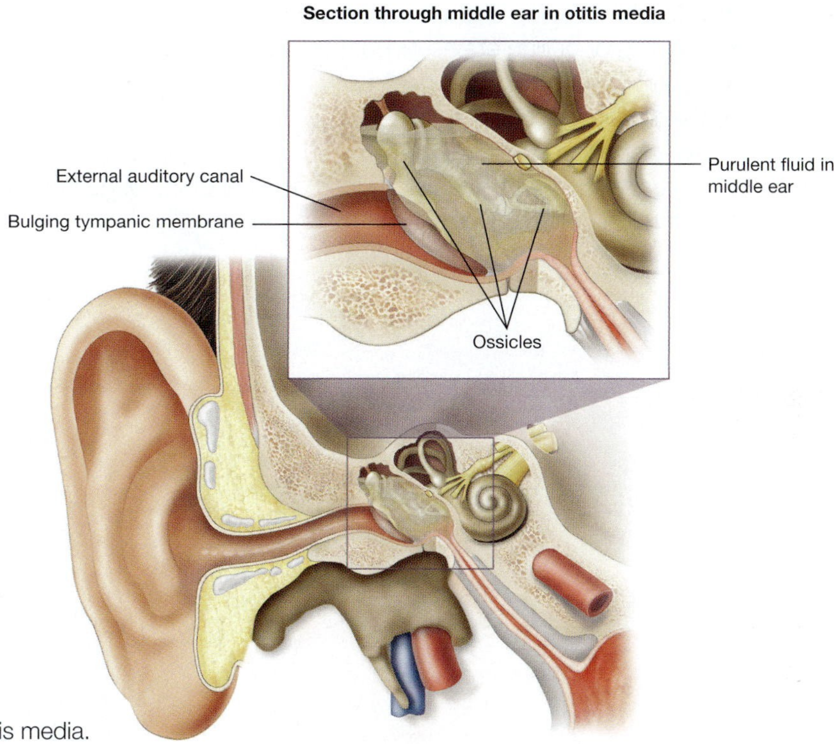

Section through middle ear in otitis media

Figure 15.8 Otitis media.

(continued)

Medical Word	Word Parts		Definition
	Part	**Meaning**	

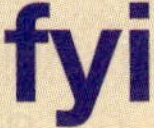

Otitis media is often difficult to detect in children because most children affected by this disorder do not yet have sufficient speech and language skills to tell others what is bothering them. Common signs of otitis media include:

- Unusual irritability; fussiness; crying
- Difficulty sleeping; night awakening
- Tugging or pulling at one or both ears (Figure 15.9)
- Fever
- Fluid draining from the ear
- Loss of balance
- Unresponsiveness to quiet sounds or other signs of hearing difficulty such as sitting too close to the television or being inattentive

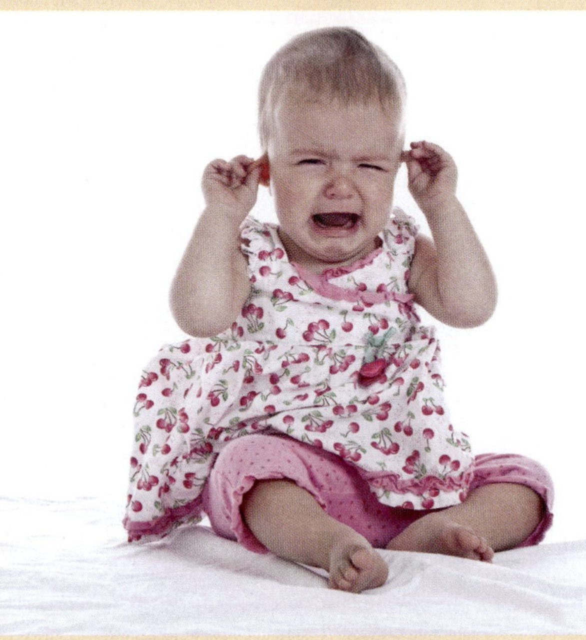

Figure 15.9 This young child is crying and pulling on her ears, two important signs of otitis media.
(Wollwerth Imagery/Fotolia)

insights Terminology included in the ICD-10-CM, otitis media H65–H67 classification:

antrum	a cavity or chamber in a bone
attic	portion of the middle ear lying above the tympanic cavity proper
atticoantral	pertaining to the attic and mastoid antrum of the ear
mastoid antrum	a cavity in the mastoid portion of the temporal bone; tympanic antrum
suppurative	the process of pus formation
tubotympanic	pertaining to the tympanum (middle ear) and the eustachian tube

Medical Word	Part	Meaning	Definition
otolaryngologist (ō″ tō-lar″ ĭn-gŏl′ ō-jĭst)	ot/o laryng/o log -ist	ear larynx, voice box study of one who specializes	Physician who specializes in the study of the ear and larynx (*voice box*)

Medical Word	Word Parts		Definition
	Part	**Meaning**	
otolaryngology (ō″ tō-lar″ ĭn-gŏl′ ō-jē)	ot/o laryng/o -logy	ear larynx, voice box study of	Study of the ear and larynx (*voice box*)
otolith (ō′ tō-lĭth)	ot/o -lith	ear stone	Ear stones
otomycosis (ō″ tō-mī-kō′ sĭs)	ot/o myc -osis	ear fungus condition	Fungal infection of the ear
otoneurology (ō″ tō-nū-rŏl′ ō-jē)	ot/o neur/o -logy	ear nerve study of	Specialized diagnosis and treatment of the ear and its neurological association
otopharyngeal (ō″ tō-far-ĭn′ jē-āl)	ot/o pharynge -al	ear pharynx pertaining to	Pertaining to the ear and pharynx
otoplasty (ō′ tō-plăs″ tē)	ot/o -plasty	ear surgical repair	Surgical repair of the ear
otopyorrhea (ō″ tō-pī″ ō-rē′ă)	ot/o py/o -rrhea	ear pus flow	Pus in the ear
otorhinolaryngology (ENT) (ō″ tō-rī″ nō-lăr″ ĭn-gŏl′ ō-jē)	ot/o rhin/o laryng/o -logy	ear nose larynx study of	Study of the ear, nose, and larynx (*voice box*). The medical specialty is often referred to as *ENT* (*ear, nose, throat*); in this case, *throat* is used in a broad sense instead of *larynx*.
otosclerosis (ō″ tō-sklē-rō′ sĭs)	ot/o scler -osis	ear hardening condition	Hardening (stiffening) condition of the ear structures characterized by progressive deafness
otoscope (ō′ tō-skōp)	ot/o -scope	ear instrument for examining	Medical instrument used to examine the ear. See Figure 15.10. An inspection of the walls of the auditory canal should find no sign of irritation, discharge, or a foreign object. The walls are normally pink and some cerumen is present. The tympanic membrane is usually pearly gray and translucent. It reflects light and the ossicles are visible.

Figure 15.10 The otoscope is positioned in the ear prior to examination of the auditory canal.
(Paul Marcus/Shutterstock)

Medical Word	Word Parts: Part	Word Parts: Meaning	Definition
perilymph (pĕr′ ĭ-lĭmf)	peri- -lymph	around serum, pale fluid	Serum fluid of the inner ear
presbycusis (prĕz″ bĭ-kū′ sĭs)	presby -cusis	old hearing	Impairment of hearing that occurs with aging
stapedectomy (stā″ pē-dĕk′ tō-mē)	staped -ectomy	stapes, stirrup surgical excision	Surgical excision of the stapes in the middle ear to improve hearing, especially in cases of otosclerosis. The stapes is replaced by a prosthesis.
tinnitus (tĭn-ī′ tŭs)			The sensation of ringing or roaring sounds in one or both ears is a symptom associated with damage to the auditory cells in the inner ear. It can also be a symptom of other health problems.

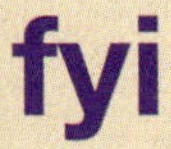

fyi According to estimates by the American Tinnitus Association, over 50 million Americans have tinnitus. Of these, at least 2 million experience it so severely that it interferes with their daily activities, such as hearing, working, and sleeping. There are several possible causes of tinnitus:

- ***Hearing loss.*** Doctors and scientists have discovered that people with different kinds of hearing loss, primarily from presbycusis or trauma-related damage to the inner ear, also have tinnitus.
- ***Loud noise.*** Too much exposure to loud noise can cause noise-induced hearing loss and tinnitus.
- ***Medicine.*** More than 200 medicines can cause tinnitus.
- ***Other health problems.*** Allergies, tumors, and problems in the heart and blood vessels, jaws, and neck can cause tinnitus.

A patient can be referred to an *otolaryngologist* for diagnosis and/or an *audiologist*, who performs hearing tests. Although there is no cure for tinnitus, scientists and doctors have discovered several treatments that can provide some relief such as hearing aids, medications, and maskers, which are small electronic devices that use sound to make tinnitus less noticeable.

Medical Word	Word Parts: Part	Word Parts: Meaning	Definition
tuning fork			Instrument used medically in a hearing test, which, when struck at the forked end, vibrates, producing a musical tone, and thus can be heard and felt. A metal instrument with a handle and two prongs or tines, tuning forks can be made of steel, aluminum, or magnesium alloy. See Figure 15.11.

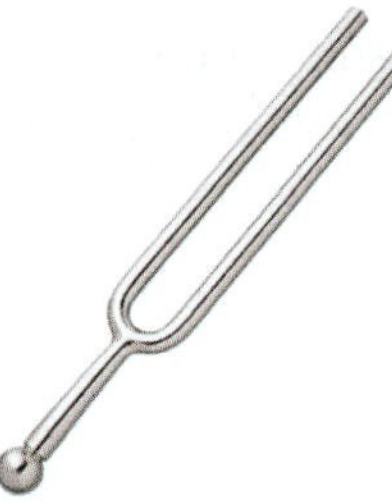

Figure 15.11 Tuning fork. The vibrations and tone produced when the fork is struck can be used to assess a person′s ability to hear various sound frequencies.

Source: Shutswis/Fotolia

Medical Word	Word Parts		Definition
	Part	**Meaning**	
tympanectomy (tĭm″ păn-ĕk′ tō-mē)	tympan -ectomy	eardrum, tympanic membrane surgical excision	Surgical excision of the tympanic membrane (eardrum)

RULE REMINDER

The *o* has been removed from the combining form because the suffix begins with a vowel.

Medical Word	Part	Meaning	Definition
tympanic (tĭm-păn′ ĭk)	tympan -ic	eardrum, tympanic membrane pertaining to	Pertaining to the eardrum (tympanic membrane)
tympanitis (tĭm-păn-ī′ tĭs)	tympan -itis	eardrum, tympanic membrane inflammation	Inflammation of the eardrum (tympanic membrane)
tympanoplasty (tĭm″ păn-ō-plăs′ tē)	tympan/o -plasty	eardrum, tympanic membrane surgical repair	Surgical repair of the tympanic membrane (eardrum)
utricle (ū′ trĭk-l)			Small, saclike structure of the labyrinth of the inner ear
vertigo (ver′ tĭ-gō)			Sensation of instability and loss of equilibrium; patients feel like they are spinning in space or objects around them are spinning. Caused by a disturbance in the semicircular canal of the inner ear or the vestibular nuclei of the brainstem.

Study and Review II

Word Parts

Prefixes

Give the definitions of the following prefixes.

1. end- ______________________
2. endo- ______________________
3. peri- ______________________
4. bin- ______________________
5. mon(o)- ______________________

Combining Forms

Give the definitions of the following combining forms.

1. audi/o ______________________
2. aur/i ______________________
3. chol/e ______________________
4. cochle/o ______________________
5. electr/o ______________________
6. labyrinth/o ______________________
7. laryng/o ______________________
8. mast/o ______________________
9. myring/o ______________________
10. neur/o ______________________
11. ot/o ______________________
12. pharyng/o ______________________
13. presby/o ______________________
14. py/o ______________________
15. scler/o ______________________
16. staped/o ______________________
17. steat/o ______________________
18. tympan/o ______________________

Suffixes

Give the definitions of the following suffixes.

1. -al ______________________
2. -algia ______________________
3. -cusis ______________________
4. -ectomy ______________________
5. -gram ______________________
6. -graphy ______________________
7. -ic ______________________
8. -ist ______________________

9. -itis ______________________

10. -lith ______________________

11. -logy ______________________

12. -lymph ______________________

13. -meter ______________________

14. -metry ______________________

15. -oid ______________________

16. -oma ______________________

17. -osis ______________________

18. -plasty ______________________

19. -rrhea ______________________

20. -scope ______________________

21. -tome ______________________

22. -tomy ______________________

23. -y ______________________

24. -cle ______________________

25. -ion ______________________

26. -ia ______________________

Identifying Medical Terms

In the spaces provided, write the medical terms for the following meanings.

1. ______________________ One who specializes in diagnosing disorders of hearing
2. ______________________ Measurement of the hearing sense
3. ______________________ Pertaining to the sense of hearing
4. ______________________ Pertaining to within the ear
5. ______________________ Inflammation of the labyrinth
6. ______________________ Surgical repair of the tympanic membrane
7. ______________________ Surgical instrument used for cutting the eardrum
8. ______________________ Pain in the ear, earache
9. ______________________ Study of the ear and larynx
10. ______________________ Pertaining to the ear and pharynx
11. ______________________ Medical instrument used to examine the ear
12. ______________________ Serum fluid of the inner ear
13. ______________________ Surgical excision of the stapes of the ear
14. ______________________ Surgical excision of the tympanic membrane
15. ______________________ The sensation of ringing or roaring sounds in one or both ears

Matching

Select the appropriate lettered meaning for each of the following words.

_____________ **1.** auricle
_____________ **2.** binaural
_____________ **3.** acoustic
_____________ **4.** equilibrium
_____________ **5.** fenestration
_____________ **6.** labyrinth
_____________ **7.** myringotomy
_____________ **8.** otoplasty
_____________ **9.** tympanoplasty
_____________ **10.** vertigo

a. State of balance
b. Inner ear
c. Surgical repair of the ear
d. Surgical repair of the tympanic membrane
e. Pertaining to both ears
f. Sensation of instability, loss of equilibrium
g. Surgical operation in which a new opening is made in the labyrinth
h. External portion of the ear
i. Pertaining to the sense of hearing
j. Surgical incision of the tympanic membrane
k. Organ of hearing

Medical Case Snapshots

This learning activity provides an opportunity to relate the medical terminology you are learning to a precise patient case presentation. In the spaces provided, write in your answers.

Case 1

The mother of a 2-year-old baby states that Takeshia has been unusually fussy for 2 days and that last night "she woke me up screaming and she felt so hot." Upon examination of the left ear the physician noted a bulging of the tympanic membrane and the presence of purulent fluid in the middle ear. In the space provided, write the medical term for this condition _____________ ___________. See Figures 15.8 and 15.9.

Case 2

A 15-year-old male is seen by an otolaryngologist. He complains of ringing in the ears and is diagnosed with _____________. When questioned, he admits to listening to loud music with headphones and that he likes going to rock concerts. Excessive noise can do permanent damage to the sensory receptors of the ___________ ___________.

Case 3

The 15-year-old male was referred to an _____________ who specializes in diagnosing disorders of hearing. Using an ____________ (which is a medical instrument used to measure hearing), both ears were tested, one at a time. The patient was diagnosed with a partial loss of the ability to hear in the left ear. Loss of hearing is known as __________.

Drug Highlights

Type of Drug	Description and Examples
analgesic	Used to relieve pain without causing loss of consciousness. EXAMPLES: Tylenol (acetaminophen); Advil, Motrin (ibuprofen); aspirin
antipyretic	Agent that reduces fever. EXAMPLES: Tylenol (acetaminophen), aspirin NOTE: In children, aspirin should not be used as an analgesic or antipyretic because of the risk of Reye syndrome.
antibiotics	Used to treat infectious diseases; can be natural or synthetic substances that inhibit the growth of or destroy microorganisms, especially bacteria
penicillins	Act by interfering with bacterial cell wall synthesis among newly formed bacterial cells. Penicillins are contraindicated in patients who are known to be allergic or hypersensitive to any of its varieties or to any of the cephalosporins. EXAMPLES: penicillin G, ampicillin, penicillin V, piperacillin, and amoxicillin
cephalosporins	Chemically and pharmacologically related to the penicillins, they act by inhibiting bacterial cell wall synthesis, thereby promoting the death of the developing microorganisms. Hypersensitivity to cephalosporins and/or penicillins can result in an allergic reaction. EXAMPLES: cefazolin sodium, cefaclor, Keflex (cephalexin), and Suprax (cefixime)
tetracyclines	Primarily bacteriostatic and active against a wide range of gram-negative and gram-positive microorganisms, they inhibit protein synthesis in the bacterial cell NOTE: Contraindicated in children 8 years of age and younger; they cause permanent discoloration of tooth enamel. EXAMPLES: tetracycline hydrochloride; demeclocycline HCl; and Doryx, Vibramycin (doxycycline)
erythromycin	Works by inhibiting protein synthesis in susceptible bacteria. These drugs can be used for patients who are allergic to penicillin. EXAMPLES: Ery-TabB, E.E.S., EryPed, and Erythrocin
drugs used to treat vertigo	Vertigo is a sensation of movement, when the person is not moving, that can be caused by a lesion or other process affecting the brain, the eighth cranial nerve, or the labyrinthine system of the ear. Drugs used for vertigo include anticholinergics, antihistamines, and antidopamines. EXAMPLES: dimenhydrinate, Benadryl (diphenhydramine HCl), meclizine HCl, Transderm Scop (scopolamine)

Diagnostic and Laboratory Tests

Test	Description
auditory-evoked response (aw´dĭ-tō-rē-ĕ-vōkd´)	Response to auditory stimuli (sound) that can be measured independently of the patient's subjective response. Use of an electroencephalograph can determine the intensity of sound and presence of response. This test is useful to test the hearing of children who are too young for standard tests, autistic, hyperkinetic, and/or developmentally disabled.
electronystagmography (ENG) (ē-lĕk″ trō-nĭs-tăg-mŏg´ ră-fē)	Recording eye movement in response to specific stimuli, such as sound; used to determine the presence and location of a lesion in the vestibule of the ear, to help diagnose unilateral hearing loss of unknown origin, and to help identify the cause of vertigo, tinnitus, and dizziness
pure tone audiometry	Method of testing pure tones by providing calibrated tones to a person via earphones, allowing that person to increase the sound level until it can just be heard. Various strategies are used, but pure tone audiometry with tones starting at about 125 Hz (cycles/second) and increasing by octaves, half-octaves, or third-octaves to about 8000 Hz is typical. Hearing tests of right and left ears are generally done independently. The results of such tests are summarized in audiograms. Audiograms compare hearing to the normal threshold of hearing, which varies with frequency, as illustrated by the hearing curves. The audiogram is normalized to the hearing curve so that a straight horizontal line at 0 represents normal hearing.

Test	Description
otoscopy (ō-tŏs′ kō-pē)	Visual examination of the external auditory canal and the tympanic membrane via an otoscope. Pneumatic otoscopy uses a special attachment on the otoscope. This allows the examiner to direct a light stream of air toward the eardrum. The directed air current should then cause the tympanic membrane to vibrate. With dysfunction there is little or no vibration noted.

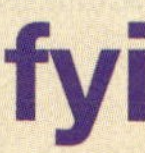

When examining the tympanic membrane with an otoscope, the position, mobility, color, and degree of translucency are evaluated and described. The normal tympanic membrane is in the neutral position (neither retracted nor bulging), pearly gray, translucent, and responds briskly to positive and negative pressure, indicating an air-filled space. An abnormal tympanic membrane can be retracted or bulging and immobile or poorly mobile in pneumatic **otoscopy**. The position of the tympanic membrane is a key for differentiating acute otitis media and otitis media with effusion. In acute otitis media, the tympanic membrane is usually bulging and purulent fluid is present in the middle ear. See Figure 15.12.

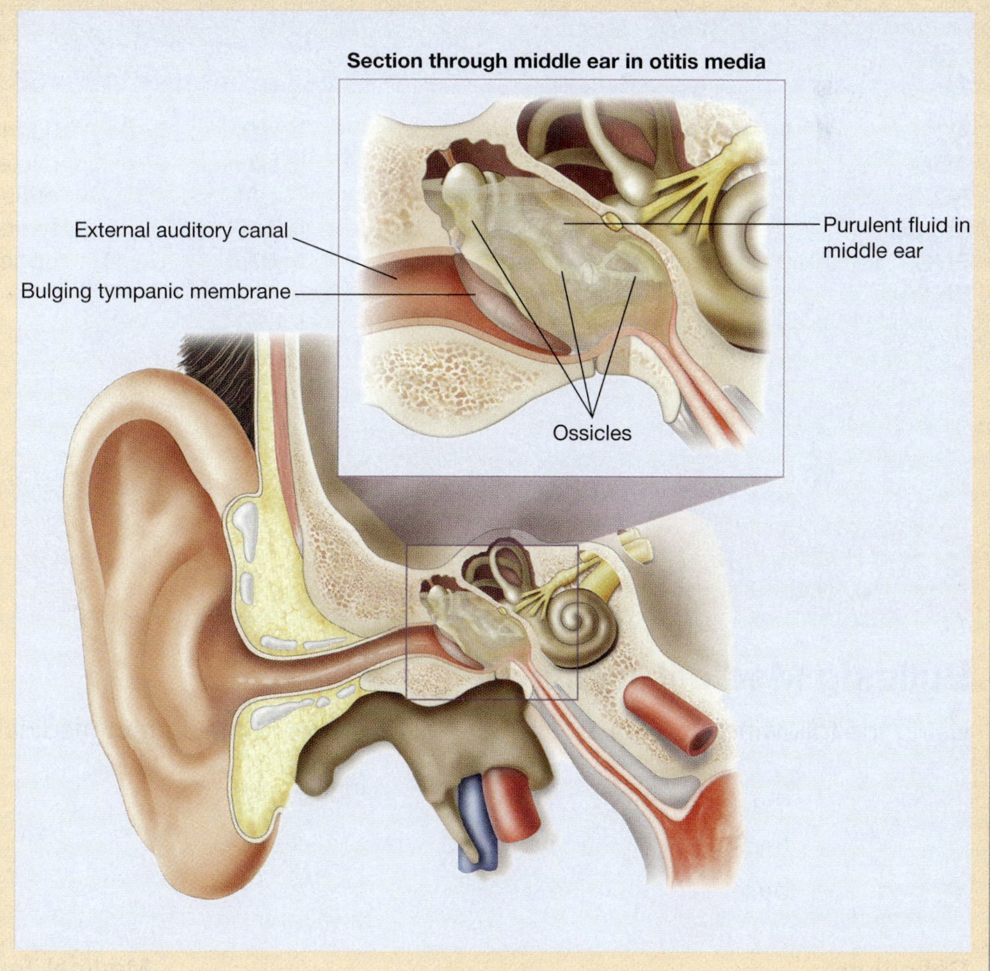

Figure 15.12 In acute otitis media, the tympanic membrane is usually bulging and purulent fluid is present in the middle ear.

Test	Description
tuning fork test	Method of testing hearing by the use of a tuning fork (see Figure 15.11). Two types of hearing loss (conductive and perceptive) can be distinguished through the use of this test. Tuning forks are used in several types of tests: the Rinne, Weber, Bing, and Schwabach tests.
Rinne test (rĭn´ nē)	The Rinne test utilizes a tuning fork to compare bone conduction (BC) hearing with air conduction (AC). After being struck, the vibrating tuning fork is held on the mastoid process until sound is no longer heard. The fork is then immediately placed just outside the ear. Normally, the sound is audible at the ear.
tympanometry (tĭm″ pă-nŏm´ ĕ-trē)	Measurement of the movement of the tympanic membrane and pressure in the middle ear. It is used for detecting middle ear disorders.

Abbreviations

Abbreviation	Meaning	Abbreviation	Meaning
AC	air conduction	**HD**	hearing distance
AOM	acute otitis media	**Hz**	cycles/second
BC	bone conduction	**OM**	otitis media
db, dB	decibel	**TM**	tympanic membrane
ENG	electronystagmography	**URI**	upper respiratory infection
ENT	ear, nose, throat (otorhinolaryngology)		

Study and Review III

Building Medical Terms

Using the following word parts, fill in the blanks to build the correct medical terms.

aur	staped	-lymph
myring/o	tympan/o	-itis
ot/o	-ic	

Definition	**Medical Term**
1. Pertaining to the sense of hearing	acoust________
2. Pertaining to the ear	___________al
3. Clear fluid contained within the labyrinth of the ear	endo________

Definition	Medical Term
4. Surgical instrument used for cutting the eardrum	________tome
5. Inflammation of the ear	ot__________
6. Surgical repair of the ear	________plasty
7. Serum fluid of the inner ear	peri_________
8. Surgical excision of the stapes in the middle ear	_______ectomy
9. Pertaining to the eardrum (tympanic membrane)	tympan______
10. Surgical repair of the tympanic membrane (eardrum)	________plasty

Combining Form Challenge

Using the combining forms provided, write the medical term correctly.

audi/o	labyrinth/o	ot/o
aur/i	myring/o	presby/o

1. Medical instrument used to measure hearing: _______meter
2. External portion of the ear; known as the pinna: _______ cle
3. Surgical excision of the labyrinth: ______ ectomy
4. Surgical repair of the tympanic membrane: ________ plasty
5. Pain in the ear; earache: ______ algia
6. Impairment of hearing that occurs with aging: ________ cusis

Select the Right Term

Select the correct answer, and write it on the line provided.

1. Record of hearing by audiometry is __________.

   acoustic **audiology** **audiogram** **aural**

2. A state of balance is ____________.

   cochlea **equilibrium** **tinnitus** **eustachian**

3. Surgical operation in which a new opening is made in the labyrinth of the inner ear to restore hearing is __________.

   labyrinthotomy **myringectomy** **fenestration** **stapedectomy**

4. Largest of the three ossicles; also called the hammer is _________.

   incus **stapes** **labyrinth** **malleus**

5. The sensation of ringing or roaring sounds in one or both ears is ____________.

tinnitus **tinitus** **presbycusis** **vertigo**

6. Small, saclike structure of the labyrinth of the inner ear is ____________.

oval window **stapes** **utricle** **incus**

Diagnostic and Laboratory Tests

Select the best answer to each multiple-choice question. Circle the letter of your choice.

1. The response to auditory stimuli that can be measured independent of the patient's subjective response.
   a. auditory-evoked response
   b. electronystagmography
   c. tuning fork test
   d. otoscopy
2. Recording of eye movement in response to specific stimuli.
   a. auditory-evoked response
   b. electronystagmography
   c. tympanometry
   d. otoscopy
3. Visual examination of the external auditory canal and the tympanic membrane.
   a. tuning fork test
   b. tympanometry
   c. electronystagmography
   d. otoscopy
4. Measurement of the movement of the tympanic membrane.
   a. tuning fork tests
   b. tympanometry
   c. otoscopy
   d. electronystagmography
5. This test utilizes a tuning fork to compare bone conduction (BC) hearing with air conduction (AC).
   a. Rinne test
   b. tympanometry
   c. otoscopy
   d. electronystagmography

Abbreviations

Place the correct word, phrase, or abbreviation in the space provided.

1. air conduction ____________________
2. bone conduction ____________________
3. db, dB ____________________
4. electronystagmography ____________________
5. ENT ____________________
6. hearing distance ____________________
7. otitis media ____________________

Practical Application

Medical Record Analysis

This exercise contains information, abbreviations, and medical terminology from an actual medical record or case study that has been adapted for this text. The names and any personal information have been created by the author. Read and study each form or case study and then answer the questions that follow. You may refer to Appendix III, *Abbreviations and Symbols*.

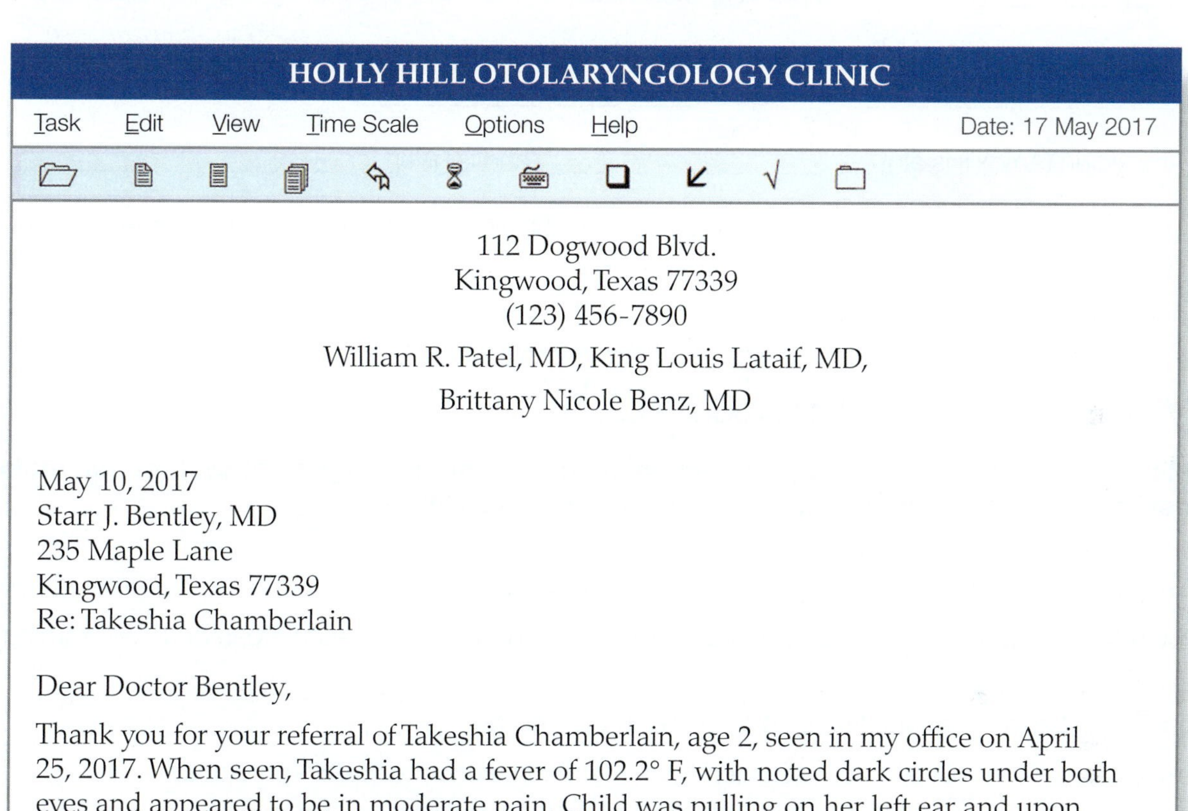

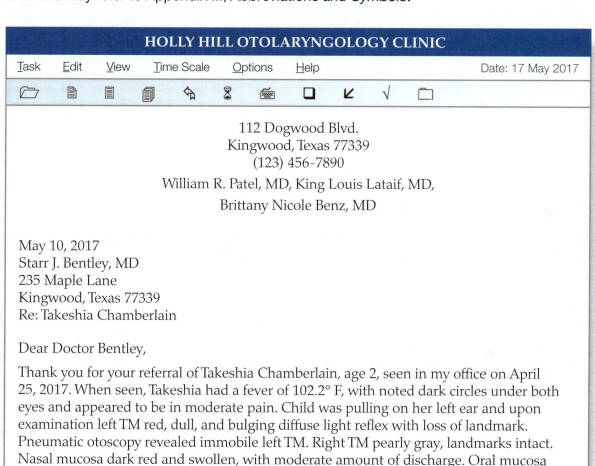

HOLLY HILL OTOLARYNGOLOGY CLINIC

Task Edit View Time Scale Options Help Date: 17 May 2017

112 Dogwood Blvd.
Kingwood, Texas 77339
(123) 456-7890

William R. Patel, MD, King Louis Lataif, MD,
Brittany Nicole Benz, MD

May 10, 2017
Starr J. Bentley, MD
235 Maple Lane
Kingwood, Texas 77339
Re: Takeshia Chamberlain

Dear Doctor Bentley,

Thank you for your referral of Takeshia Chamberlain, age 2, seen in my office on April 25, 2017. When seen, Takeshia had a fever of 102.2° F, with noted dark circles under both eyes and appeared to be in moderate pain. Child was pulling on her left ear and upon examination left TM red, dull, and bulging diffuse light reflex with loss of landmark. Pneumatic otoscopy revealed immobile left TM. Right TM pearly gray, landmarks intact. Nasal mucosa dark red and swollen, with moderate amount of discharge. Oral mucosa erythematous with yellow-white exudates, no lesions. Uvula rises in midline with phonation. Gag reflex present. No lymphadenopathy. Neck supple. Lungs CTA and heart normal rate and rhythm. No murmurs. Skin: no rashes or lesions, warm to the touch.

A diagnosis of acute otitis media (AOM) left ear was confirmed.

I ordered acetaminophen (Tylenol) liquid, 1.6 mL (1 teaspoon) PO every 4 hours prn for pain and fever. Amoxicillin (Amoxil) suspension 40 mg per kg per day, in three divided doses, every 8 hours for 10 days for infection. Instructed the mother on the adverse reactions to penicillin and explained that she should not give the antibiotic with soft drinks or fruit juices because the acid in these products could destroy the effectiveness of the drug. Stressed the importance of the baby taking the antibiotic as ordered for the entire 10 days and around the clock, every 8 hours. Instructed the mother to bring the baby back to the clinic if symptoms do not improve in 48–72 hours. Scheduled a follow-up visit for 3 weeks.

Best regards,

William R. Patel, MD

Medical Record Questions

Place the correct answer in the space provided.

1. In Takeshia the signs and symptoms of acute otitis media included a fever of ______________________ and the child was ______________________ on her left ear.
2. The diagnosis was determined by a visual examination of the ear called pneumatic ______________________, a physical examination of the child, and the signs and symptoms presented.
3. Acetaminophen (Tylenol) is classified as a(n) ______________________ and is given to relieve ______________________ and reduce ______________________.
4. Amoxicillin (Amoxil) is a(n) ______________________ and is given for ______________________.
5. The ______________________ in soft drinks and fruit juices can destroy the effectiveness of the ______________________ drug.

Chapter

Special Senses: The Eye 16

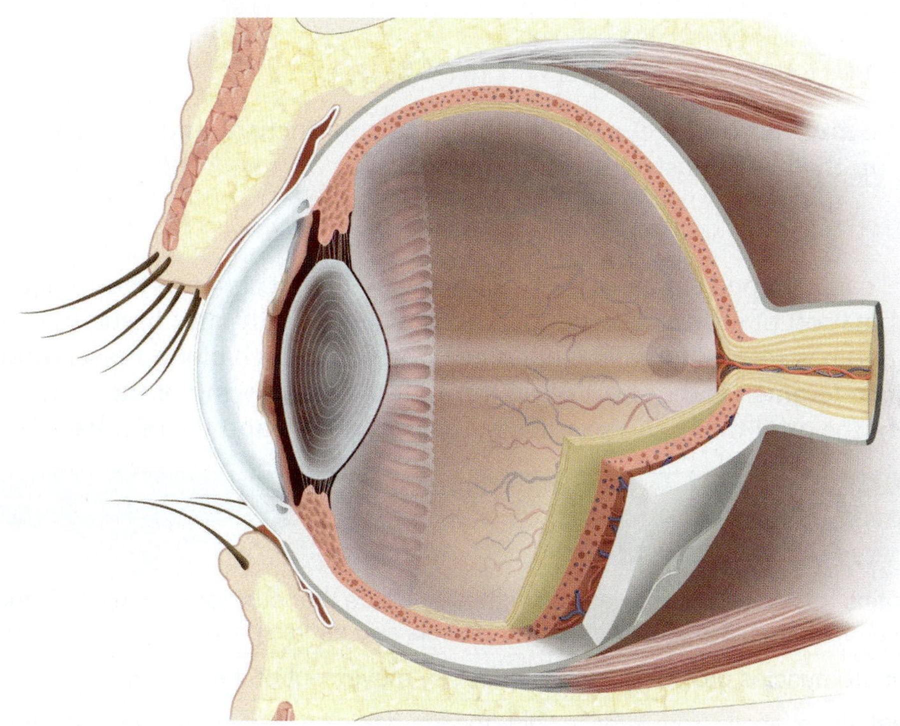

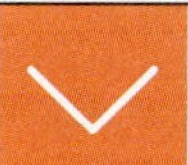

Learning Outcomes

On completion of this chapter, you will be able to:

1. State the description and primary functions of the eye.
2. Recognize terminology included in the ICD-10-CM.
3. Analyze, build, spell, and pronounce medical words.
4. Comprehend the drugs highlighted in this chapter.
5. Describe diagnostic and laboratory tests related to the eye.
6. Identify and define selected abbreviations.
7. Apply your acquired knowledge of medical terms by successfully completing the *Practical Application* exercise.

Anatomy and Physiology

The **eye** is composed of special anatomical structures that work together to facilitate sight. Light passes through the cornea, pupil, lens, and the vitreous body to stimulate sensory receptors (*rods* and *cones*) in the **retina** or innermost layer of the eye. **Vision** is made possible through the coordinated actions of nerves that control the movement of the eyeball, the amount of light admitted by the pupil, the focusing of that light on the retina by the lens, and the transmission of the resulting sensory impulses to the brain by the optic nerve. The brain permits the perception of vision. Table 16.1 provides an at-a-glance look at the eye. Figure 16.1 shows the internal structures of the eye.

External Structures of the Eye

The orbit, the muscles of the eye, the eyelids, the conjunctiva, and the lacrimal apparatus make up the external structures of the eye.

Orbit

The **orbit** is a cone-shaped cavity in the front of the skull that contains the *eyeball*. Formed by the combination of several bones, this cavity is lined with fatty tissue that cushions the eyeball and has several **foramina** (openings) through which blood vessels and nerves pass. The **optic foramen** is the short canal through the lesser wing of the sphenoid bone at the apex of the orbit that gives passage to the optic nerve and the ophthalmic artery.

Table 16.1 Special Senses: The Eye at-a-Glance

Organ/Structure	Primary Functions/Description
Orbit	Contains the eyeball; cavity is lined with fatty tissue that cushions the eyeball and has several openings through which blood vessels and nerves pass
Muscles of the eye	Six short muscles provide support and rotary movement of the eyeball
Eyelids	Protect the eyeballs from intense light, foreign particles, and impact; permits the eye to remain moist
Conjunctiva	Acts as a protective covering for the exposed surface of the eyeball and helps keep the eyelid and eyeball moist
Lacrimal apparatus	Produces, stores, and removes tears that cleanse and lubricate the eye
Eyeball	Organ of vision
Sclera	Outer layer of the eyeball composed of fibrous connective tissue; at the front of the eye, it is visible as the white of the eye and ends at the cornea
Cornea	Transparent anterior portion of the eyeball, which bends light rays and helps to focus them on the surface of the retina
Choroid	Pigmented vascular membrane that prevents internal reflection of light
Ciliary body	Smooth muscle that forms a part of the ciliary body that governs the convexity of the lens; secretes nutrient fluids that nourish the cornea, the lens, and surrounding tissues
Iris	Colored membrane attached to the ciliary body (can appear as blue, brown, green, hazel, or gray) with a circular opening in its center, the pupil, and two muscles that contract; regulates the amount of light admitted by the pupil
Retina	Innermost layer with photoreceptive cells; translates light waves focused on its surface into nerve impulses
Lens	Sharpens the focus of light on the retina (accommodation [Acc])

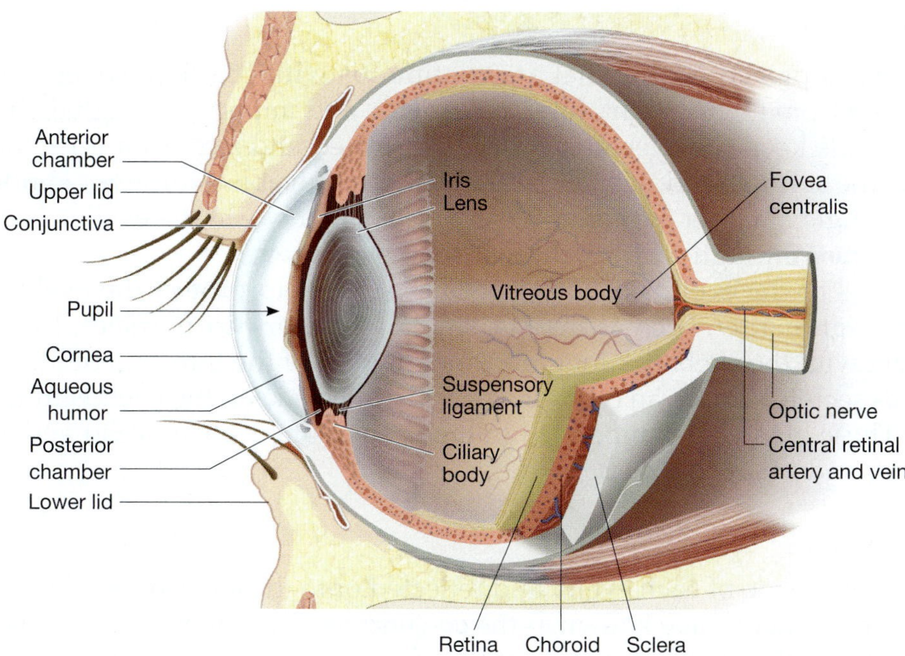

Figure 16.1 Structures of the eye.

Muscles of the Eye

Six eye muscles control movement of the eye, allowing it to follow a moving object and move precisely. Of the six, four are rectus muscles and two are oblique muscles. *Rectus muscles* allow a person to see up, down, right, and left. *Oblique muscles* allow the eyes to turn to see upper left and upper right, lower left and lower right. See Figure 16.2. The eye muscles also help maintain the shape of the eyeball.

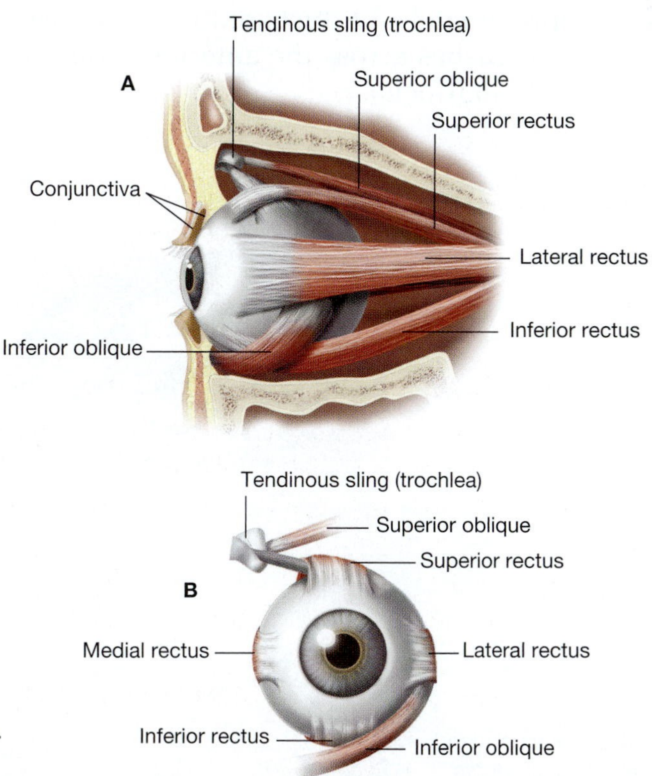

Figure 16.2 Eye muscles. (A) Lateral view, left eye. (B) Anterior view, left eye.

Eyelids

Each eye has a pair of **eyelids** that are continuous with the skin, cover the eyeball, and protect it from intense light, foreign particles, and impact. Through their blinking motion, eyelids keep the eyeball's surface lubricated and free from dust and debris. Known as the *superior* and *inferior palpebrae*, those movable "curtains" join to form a **canthus** or angle at either corner of the eye. The slit between the eyelids is called the **palpebral fissure** through which light reaches the inner eye.

The edges of the eyelids contain eyelashes that help protect the eyeball by preventing foreign matter, such as insects, smoke, dust, or dirt particles, from coming into contact with the eyeball. Along the inner margin of the thin skin of the lid, *meibomian glands* secrete sebum, an oily substance that helps keep the eyelids from sticking together. These glands are embedded in the tarsal plate of each eyelid and are called *tarsal glands* and *palpebral glands*.

Conjunctiva

Lining the underside of each eyelid and reflected onto the anterior portion of the eyeball is a mucous membrane known as the **conjunctiva**. This membrane acts as a protective covering for the exposed surface of the eyeball.

Lacrimal Apparatus

Included in the **lacrimal apparatus** are those structures that produce, store, and remove the tears that cleanse and lubricate the eye. These structures are the lacrimal gland, located in the outer corner of each eyelid, lacrimal canaliculi (ducts), the lacrimal sac, and the nasolacrimal duct, which empties into the nasal cavity. See Figure 16.3.

LACRIMAL GLAND

Located above the outer corner of the eye, the **lacrimal gland** secretes tears through approximately 12 ducts onto the surface of the conjunctiva of the upper lid. This fluid washes across the anterior surface of the eye and is collected by the *lacrimal canaliculi* (ducts).

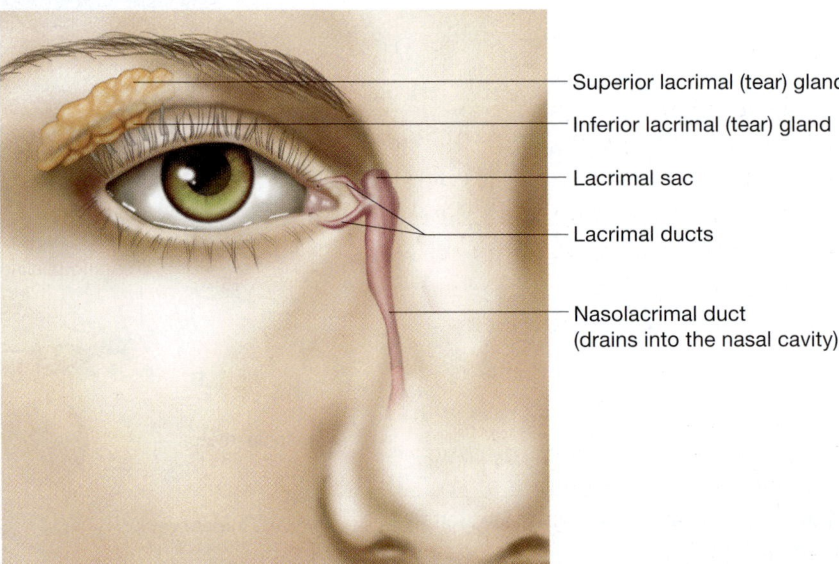

Figure 16.3 Lacrimal glands and lacrimal canaliculi (ducts).

LACRIMAL CANALICULI

The **lacrimal canaliculi** are the two ducts at the inner corner of the eye that collect tears and drain into the lacrimal sac.

LACRIMAL SAC

The enlargement of the upper portion of the lacrimal duct is known as the **lacrimal sac**. Tears secreted by the lacrimal glands are pulled into this sac and subsequently forced into the nasolacrimal duct by the blinking action of the eyelids. The sac is dilated and pulls in fluid as the muscles associated with blinking close the lids. The sac constricts, forcing the fluid down the nasolacrimal duct as the lids are opened.

NASOLACRIMAL DUCT

The passageway draining lacrimal fluid into the nose is known as the **nasolacrimal duct**. The lacrimal sac is the enlarged upper portion of this duct.

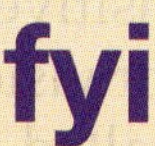

The eyes begin to develop as an outgrowth of the forebrain in the 4-week-old embryo. At 24 weeks, the eyes are structurally complete. At 28 weeks, eyebrows and eyelashes are present, and the eyelids open. The newborn can see, and **visual acuity (VA)** is estimated to be around 20/400. Most newborns appear to have crossed eyes because their eye muscles are not fully developed. At first, the eyes appear to be blue or gray. Permanent coloring becomes fixed between 6 and 12 months of age. Tears do not appear until approximately 1–3 months because the lacrimal gland ducts are immature. Depth perception begins to develop around 9 months of age. Visual acuity testing is recommended for all children starting at 3 years of age. Children are farsighted until about 5 years of age.

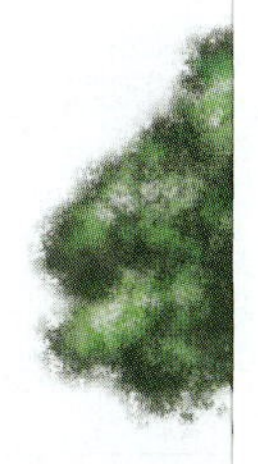

Internal Structures of the Eye

The eyeball, its various structures, and the nerve fibers connecting it to the brain make up the internal eye (see Figure 16.1).

Eyeball

The **eyeball** is the organ of vision. It is globe shaped and is divided into two cavities. The space in front of the lens, called the **ocular cavity**, is further divided by the iris into **anterior** and **posterior chambers**. The anterior chamber is filled with a watery fluid known as the **aqueous humor**. Behind the lens is a much larger cavity filled with a jellylike material, the **vitreous humor**, which maintains the eyeball's spherical shape. The three layers forming the outer, middle, and inner surfaces of the eyeball as well as the lens and its functions are discussed here.

OUTER LAYER

The eyeball's outer layer is composed of the **sclera** or white of the eye and the **cornea** or transparent anterior portion of the eye's fibrous outer surface. The curved surface of the cornea is important because it bends light rays and helps to focus them on the surface of the retina.

Study and Review I

Anatomy and Physiology

Write your answers to the following questions.

1. The external structures of the eye are the ________________,

________________, ________________, ________________,

and the ________________.

2. The orbit is lined with ________________ ________________, which cushions the eyeball.

3. The optic foramen is an opening for the ________________

________________ and ________________

________________.

4. State the functions of the muscles of the eye.

a. ________________________________

b. ________________________________

5. Each eye has a pair of eyelids that function to protect the eyeball from ________________,

________________________, and

________________.

6. Describe the conjunctiva and state its function. ________________

____

7. Define lacrimal apparatus. ________________________________

8. The internal structures of the eye are the ________________,

________________, and the ________________

________________.

9. The eyeball is the organ of ________________.

10. The point at which nerve fibers from the retina converge to form the optic nerve is known as the

________________________.

11. Define accommodation. ________________________________

12. Match the following terms and definitions by placing the correct letter on the line provided.

____________	**1.** aqueous humor	**a.** White of the eye
____________	**2.** vitreous humor	**b.** Colored membrane attached to the ciliary body
____________	**3.** iris	**c.** Watery fluid
____________	**4.** sclera	**d.** Opening in the center of the iris
____________	**5.** uvea	**e.** Jellylike material
____________	**6.** pupil	**f.** Middle layer of the eyeball
____________	**7.** retina	**g.** Transparent anterior portion of the eyeball
____________	**8.** rods and cones	**h.** Innermost layer of the eyeball
____________	**9.** lens	**i.** Photoreceptor cells
____________	**10.** cornea	**j.** Colorless crystalline body

ANATOMY LABELING

Identify the structures shown below by filling in the blanks.

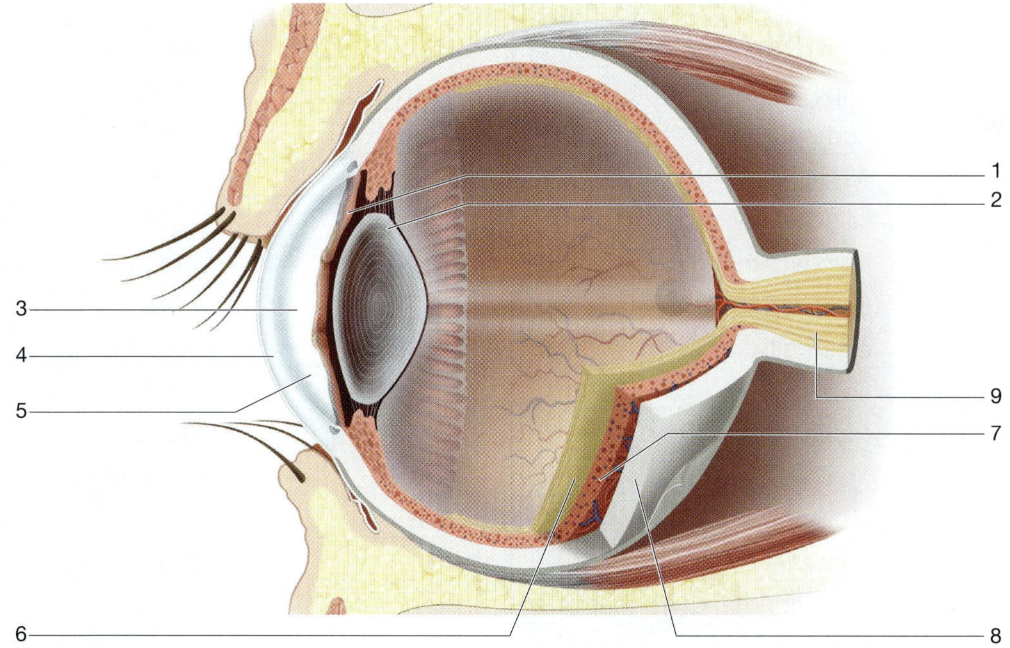

Building Your Medical Vocabulary

This section provides the foundation for learning medical terminology. Review the following alphabetized word list. Note how common prefixes and suffixes are repeatedly applied to word roots and combining forms to create different meanings. The word parts are color-coded: prefixes are yellow, suffixes are blue, roots/combining forms are red. A combining form is a word root plus a vowel. The chart below lists the combining forms for the word roots in this chapter and can help to strengthen your understanding of how medical words are built and spelled.

Remember These Guidelines

1. If the suffix begins with a vowel, drop the combining vowel from the combining form and add the suffix. For example, ambly/o (*dull*) + -opia (*eye*) becomes amblyopia.
2. If the suffix begins with a consonant, keep the combining vowel and add the suffix to the combining form. For example, blephar/o (*eyelid*) + -ptosis (*drooping*) becomes blepharoptosis.

You will find that some terms have not been divided into word parts. These are common words or specialized terms that are included to enhance your medical vocabulary.

Combining Forms of the Eye

ambly/o	dull	**mi/o**	less, small
anis/o	unequal	**my/o**	muscle
blephar/o	eyelid	**ocul/o**	eye
choroid/o	choroid	**ophthalm/o**	eye
conjunctiv/o	to join together, conjunctiva	**opt/o**	eye
cor/o	pupil	**orth/o**	straight
corne/o	cornea	**phac/o**	lens
cry/o	cold	**phak/o**	lens
cycl/o	ciliary body	**phot/o**	light
dacry/o	tear, lacrimal duct, tear duct	**presby/o**	old
dipl/o	double	**pupill/o**	pupil
electr/o	electricity	**retin/o**	retina
fibr/o	fiber	**scler/o**	sclera, hardening
foc/o	focus	**stigmat/o**	point
goni/o	angle	**ton/o**	tone, tension
irid/o	iris	**trich/o**	hair
kerat/o	cornea	**trop/o**	turn
lacrim/o	tear, lacrimal duct, tear duct	**uve/o**	uvea
lent/o	lens	**xen/o**	foreign material
metr/o	measure	**xer/o**	dry

Medical Word	Word Parts		Definition
	Part	**Meaning**	
accommodation (Acc) (ă -kŏm″ ō-dā´ shŭn)			Process by which the eyes make adjustments to see objects at various distances
amblyopia (ăm″ blĭ-ō´ pĭ-ă)	ambly -opia	dull vision	Dullness of vision; reduced or dimness of vision; also called *lazy eye*
anisocoria (ăn-ī″ sō-kō´ rĭ-ă)	anis/o cor -ia	unequal pupil condition	Condition in which the pupils are unequal in size
aphakia (ă-fā´ kĭ-ă)	a- phak -ia	lack of, without lens condition	Condition in which the crystalline lens is absent
astigmatism (ă-stĭg´ mă-tĭzm)	a- stigmat -ism	lack of, without point condition	Defect in the refractive powers of the eye in which a ray of light is not focused on the retina but is spread over an area. It is due to a misshapen curvature of the cornea and lens.
bifocal (bī-fō´ kăl)	bi- foc -al	two focus pertaining to	Pertaining to having two foci, as in bifocal glasses; one focus for near vision and another for far vision
blepharitis (blĕf″ ăr-ī´ tĭs)	blephar -itis	eyelid inflammation	Inflammation of the hair follicles and glands along the edges of the eyelids
blepharoptosis (blĕf″ ă-rŏp-tō´ sĭs)	blephar/o -ptosis	eyelid prolapse, drooping	Drooping of the upper eyelid(s)

insights In ICD-10-CM, visual disturbances, coded H53, include several subcategories of amblyopia, coded H53.0–H53.039.

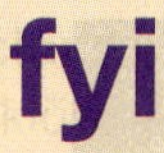

The use of dichoptic therapy (simultaneous training of both eyes), which presents different images to each eye separately, using popular children's movies, has produced improved visual acuity in young children. Dichoptic techniques combined with perceptual-learning tasks or certain video games have been shown to improve visual acuity significantly in people with amblyopia.

RULE REMINDER

The ***o*** has been removed from the combining form because the suffix begins with a vowel.

Medical Word	Word Parts		Definition
	Part	**Meaning**	
esotropia (ET) (ĕs″ ō-trō´ pĭ-ă)	eso- trop -ia	inward turn condition	Condition in which the eye or eyes turn inward; *crossed eyes*
exotropia (XT) (ĕks″ ō-trō´ pē-ă)	ex(o)- trop -ia	out turn condition	Turning outward of one or both eyes
glaucoma (glaw-kō´ mă)			A group of eye diseases that produce increased intraocular pressure (IOP) caused by a backup of fluid in the eye. When the eye pressure is increased, the optic nerve becomes damaged and the retinal ganglion cells undergo a slow process of cell death termed *apoptosis*, resulting in permanent vision loss. See Figure 16.8.

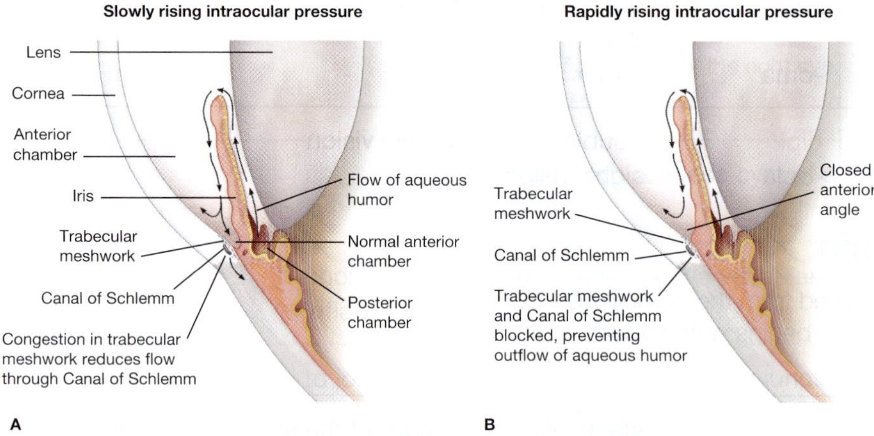

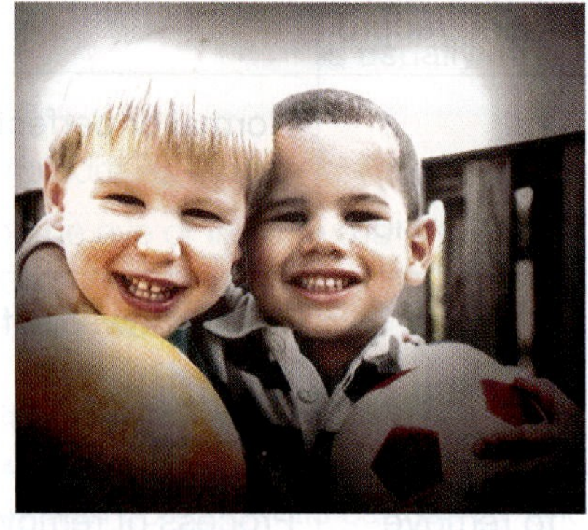

Figure 16.8 In glaucoma, the accumulation of aqueous humor in the anterior chamber of the eye causes pressure to build, resulting in eventual loss of vision. (A) and (B) show two forms of glaucoma; (C) shows the narrowing of the optic field that is a typical symptom of untreated glaucoma. (Pearson Education, Inc.)

(*continued*)

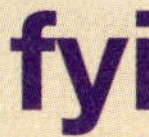

Glaucoma, one of the leading causes of blindness, affects people of all ages and all races. Regular eye exams are very important and should include measurements of the eye's intraocular pressure. If glaucoma is recognized early, vision loss can be slowed or prevented, but once lost, it cannot be recovered. Even with treatment, about 15% of people with glaucoma will become blind in at least one eye within 20 years. The two major categories of glaucoma are open-angle (also known as primary or chronic) and primary angle-closure (acute or chronic). The following are the signs and symptoms of both types of glaucoma:

Open-Angle Glaucoma

- Patchy blind spots in peripheral or central vision, frequently in both eyes
- Tunnel vision in the advanced stages

Acute Angle-Closure Glaucoma

- Severe headaches
- Eye pain
- Nausea and vomiting
- Blurred vision
- Halos around lights
- Eye redness

insights In ICD-10-CM, Chapter 7, *Diseases of the Eye and Adnexa*, it states to "Assign as many codes from category H40, Glaucoma, as needed to identify the type of glaucoma, the affected eye, and the glaucoma stage."

Medical Word	Word Parts: Part	Word Parts: Meaning	Definition
gonioscope (gō′ nĭ-ō-skōp)	goni/o -scope	angle instrument for examining	Instrument used to examine the angle of the anterior chamber of the eye
hemianopia (hĕm″ ē-ă-nō′ pē-ă)	hemi- an- -opia	half lack of sight, vision	Inability (blindness) to see half of the field of vision

Medical Word	Word Parts		Definition
	Part	**Meaning**	
hyperopia (Hy) (hī″ pĕr-ō′ pĭ-ă)	hyper- -opia	beyond sight, vision	Vision defect in which parallel rays come to a focus beyond the retina; *farsightedness*. See Figure 16.9.

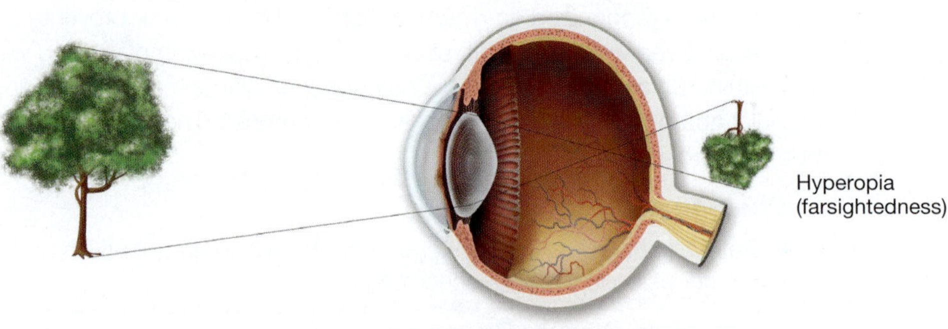

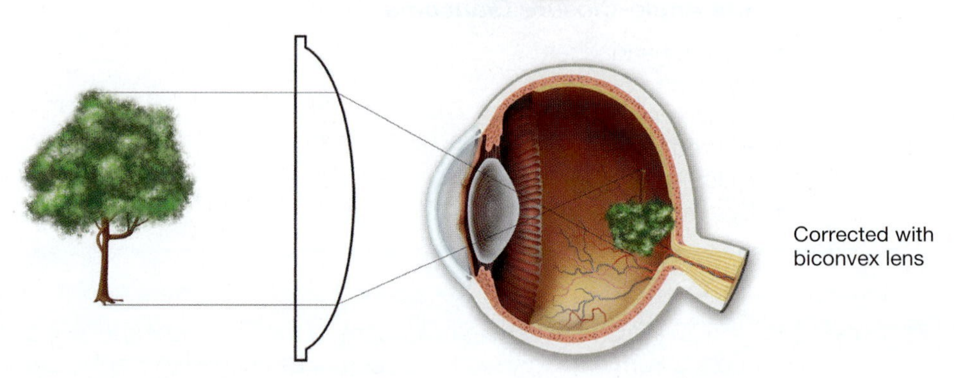

Figure 16.9 Hyperopia is the inability to shorten the focal distance adequately for nearby objects, making the image on the retina blurry. This condition can be corrected by placing a biconvex lens in front of the eyes.

Medical Word	Part	Meaning	Definition
intraocular (ĭn″ trăh-ŏk′ ū-lăr)	intra- ocul -ar	within eye pertaining to	Pertaining to within the eye
iridectomy (ĭr″ ĭ-dĕk′ tō-mē)	irid -ectomy	iris surgical excision	Surgical excision of a portion of the iris
iridocyclitis (ĭr″ ĭd-ō-sī-klī′ tĭs)	irid/o cycl -itis	iris ciliary body inflammation	Inflammation of the iris and ciliary body
keratitis (kĕr″ ă-tī′ tĭs)	kerat -itis	cornea inflammation	Inflammation of the cornea
keratoconjunctivitis (kĕr″ ă-tō-kŏn-jŭnk″ tĭ-vī′ tĭs)	kerat/o conjunctiv -itis	cornea to join together, conjunctiva inflammation	Inflammation of the cornea and the conjunctiva
keratoplasty (kĕr′ ă-tō-plăs″ tē)	kerat/o -plasty	cornea surgical repair	Surgical repair of the cornea

Medical Word	Word Parts		Definition
	Part	**Meaning**	
lacrimal (lăk′ rĭm-ăl)	lacrim -al	tear, lacrimal duct, tear duct pertaining to	Pertaining to the tears
laser (lā′ zĕr)			Acronym for *light amplification by stimulated emission of radiation*

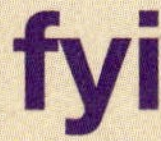

Laser surgery can be used to treat glaucoma, including the following types:

1. Laser peripheral iridotomy (LPI) in which a small hole is made in the iris to allow it to fall back from the fluid channel and help the fluid drain.
2. Argon laser trabeculoplasty (ALT) in which a laser beam opens the fluid channels of the eye, helping the drainage system to work better.
3. Selective laser trabeculoplasty (SLT), a type of laser surgery that uses a combination of frequencies, allowing the laser to work at very low levels. It treats specific cells selectively and leaves untreated portions of the trabecular meshwork (the meshlike drainage canals surrounding the iris) intact.
4. When medication and/or laser surgery does not lower the intraocular pressure of the eye, the doctor could recommend a procedure called *filtering microsurgery*. This procedure makes a tiny drainage hole in the sclera (*sclerostomy*). The new drainage hole allows fluid to flow out of the eye and thereby helps lower eye pressure. This prevents or reduces damage to the optic nerve.

Medical Word	Part	Meaning	Definition
macular degeneration (măk′ ū-lăr dē′ jĕn-ĕr″ ā-shŭn)			Macular degeneration, or age-related macular degeneration (AMD), is a leading cause of vision loss in Americans 55 and older. It causes severe loss of central vision, but peripheral vision is retained. AMD blurs the sharp central vision one needs for straight-ahead activities such as reading, sewing, and driving. AMD causes no pain.

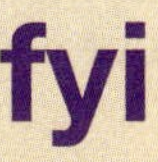

The two basic types of macular degeneration are *dry* and *wet*. The dry form is marked by atrophy (a wasting away) and degeneration of retinal cells with the formation of small yellow deposits (drusen). There is no treatment for the dry form. The wet form results from the growth of new (neovascular) and oozing (exudative) blood vessels under the retina and macula. Wet AMD can be treated with laser surgery, photodynamic therapy, and injections into the eye. Regular comprehensive eye exams can detect macular degeneration before the disease causes vision loss. Treatment can slow vision loss, but it does not restore vision.

Medical Word	Part	Meaning	Definition
miotic (mī-ŏt′ ĭk)	mi/o -tic	less, small pertaining to	Pertaining to an agent that causes the pupil to contract
mydriatic (mĭd″ rĭ-ăt′ ĭk)	mydriat -ic	dilation, widen pertaining to	Pertaining to an agent that causes the pupil to dilate

Medical Word	Word Parts: Part	Word Parts: Meaning	Definition
myopia (MY) (mī-ō´ pē-ă)			Vision defect in which parallel rays come to a focus in front of the retina; *nearsightedness*. See Figure 16.10.

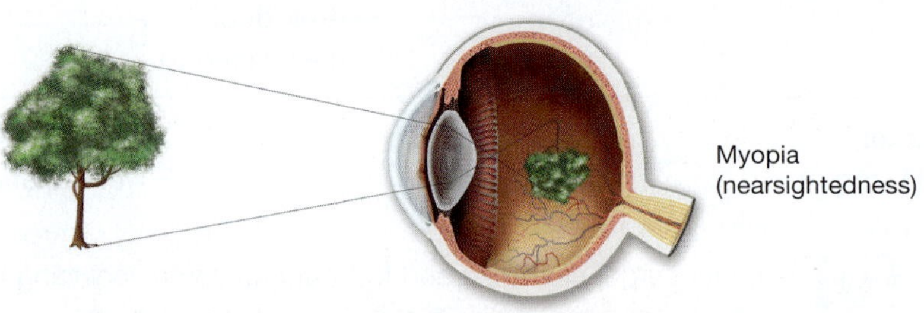

Figure 16.10 Myopia is the inability to lengthen the focal distance adequately for distant objects, making the image on the retina blurry. This condition can be corrected by placing a biconcave lens in front of the eyes.

Medical Word	Word Parts: Part	Word Parts: Meaning	Definition
nyctalopia (nĭk″ tă-lō´ pĭ-ă)	nyctal -opia	night sight, vision	Condition in which the individual has difficulty seeing at night; *night blindness*
nystagmus (nĭs-tăg´ mŭs)			Involuntary, constant, rhythmic movement of the eyeball
ocular (ŏk´ ū-lăr)	ocul -ar	eye pertaining to	Pertaining to the eye
ocular fundus (ŏk´ ū-lăr fŭn-dŭs)			Posterior inner part of the eye as seen with an ophthalmoscope
ophthalmologist (ŏf″ thăl-mŏl´ ō-jĭst)	ophthalm/o log -ist	eye study of one who specializes	Physician who specializes in the study of the eye
ophthalmology (ŏf″ thăl-mŏl´ ō-jē)	ophthalm/o -logy	eye study of	Study of the eye
ophthalmoscope (ŏf″ thăl´ mō-skōp)	ophthalm/o -scope	eye instrument for examining	Medical instrument used to examine the interior of the eye
optic (op´ tĭk)	opt -ic	eye pertaining to	Pertaining to the eye

! ALERT!

How many words can you build using the root **opt** and the combining form **opt/o**?

Medical Word	Word Parts		Definition
	Part	**Meaning**	
optician (ŏp-tĭsh´ ăn)	opt -ician	eye specialist	One who specializes in making optical products and accessories, such as eyeglasses. This person is not a physician.
optometrist (ŏp-tŏm´ ĕ-trĭst)	opt/o metr -ist	eye measure one who specializes	One who specializes in examining the eyes for refractive errors and providing appropriate corrective lenses. This person is not a medical doctor (MD) but is trained and licensed as a doctor of optometry (OD).
orthoptics (or-thŏp´ tĭks)	orth opt -ic(s)	straight eye pertaining to	Study and treatment of defective binocular vision resulting from defects in ocular musculature; also a technique of eye exercises for correcting defective binocular vision
phacoemulsification (fāk″ ō-ē-mŭl´ sĭ-fĭ-kā″ shŭn)	phac/o emulsificat -ion	lens disintegrate process	Process of using ultrasound to disintegrate a cataract by inserting a needle through a small incision and aspirating the disintegrated cataract. See Figure 16.11.

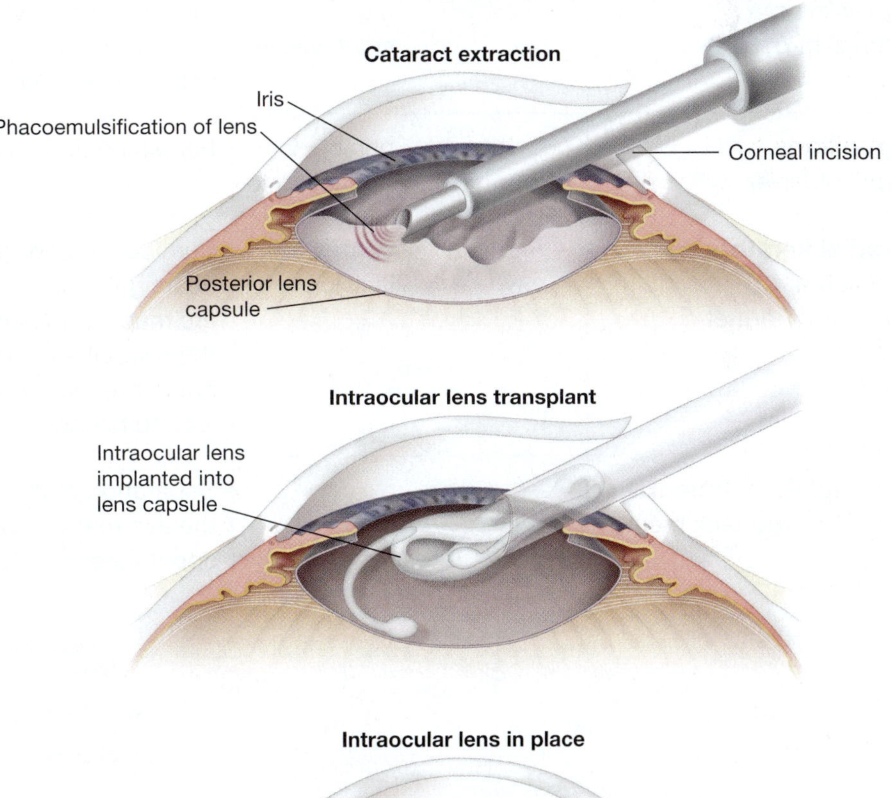

Figure 16.11 Phacoemulsification is used to remove the cataract, then an artificial lens is implanted.

Medical Word	Part	Meaning	Definition
phacolysis (făk-ŏl´ ĭ-sĭs)	phac/o -lysis	lens destruction, to separate	Surgical destruction and removal of the crystalline lens in the treatment of a cataract

Medical Word	Word Parts		Definition
	Part	Meaning	
photocoagulation (fō″ tō-kō-ăg″ ū-lā′ shŭn)	phot/o coagulat -ion	light to clot process	Process of altering proteins in tissue by the use of light energy such as the laser beam; used to treat retinal detachment, retinal bleeding, intraocular tumors, and/or macular degeneration (wet)
photophobia (fō″ tō-fō′ bĭ-ă)	phot/o -phobia	light fear	Unusual intolerance to light

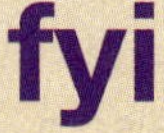

Computer vision syndrome (CVS) is a condition that occurs when eye or vision problems relate to the heavy use of digital devices. Ocular symptoms associated with the syndrome include eye strain, decreased vision, burning, stinging, and photophobia. One may help avoid this syndrome by following the 20-20-20 rule. At least every 20 minutes, take a 20-second break and view something 20 feet away. It is also recommended that one should take a 15-minute break for every two hours spent on computers or other digital devices.

Medical Word	Part	Meaning	Definition
presbyopia (prĕz″ bĭ-ō′ pĭ-ă)	presby -opia	old sight, vision	Vision defect in which parallel rays come to a focus beyond the retina; occurs normally with aging; also called *hyperopia* (farsightedness). See Figure 16.9.
pupillary (pū′ pĭ-lĕr-ē)	pupill -ary	pupil pertaining to	Pertaining to the pupil
radial keratotomy (rā′ dē-ăl kĕr-ă-tŏt′ ō-mē)	kerat/o -tomy	cornea incision	Surgical procedure that can be performed to correct nearsightedness (*myopia*). Delicate spokelike incisions are made in the cornea to flatten it, thereby shortening the eyeball so that light reaches the retina. Vision is not improved for all patients, and complications could lead to blindness.
retinal detachment (rĕt′ ĭ-năl dē-tăch′mĕnt)			Separation of the retina from the choroid layer of the eye that can be caused by trauma or can occur spontaneously. See Figure 16.12.

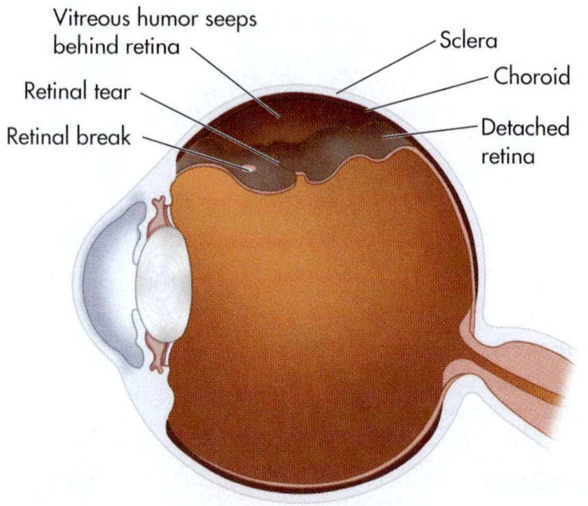

Figure 16.12 Retinal detachment.

Medical Word	Word Parts		Definition
	Part	**Meaning**	
retinitis (rĕt″ ĭ-nī′ tĭs)	retin -itis	retina inflammation	Inflammation of the retina

RULE REMINDER

The ***o*** has been removed from the combining form because the suffix begins with a vowel.

Medical Word	Part	Meaning	Definition
retinitis pigmentosa (rĕt″ ĭ-nī′ tĭs pĭg″ mĕn-tō′ să)			Chronic progressive disease marked by bilateral primary degeneration of the retina beginning in childhood and leading to blindness by middle age. Night blindness and a reduced field of vision are early clinical signs of this disease.
retinoblastoma (rĕt″ ĭ-nō-blăs-tō′ mă)	retin/o -blast -oma	retina germ cell tumor	Malignant tumor arising from the germ cell of the retina
retinopathy (rĕt″ ĭn-ŏp′ ă-thē)	retin/o -pathy	retina disease	Any disease of the retina. In the United States, *diabetic retinopathy* is the leading cause of new blindness in people ages 20–74. See Figure 16.13.

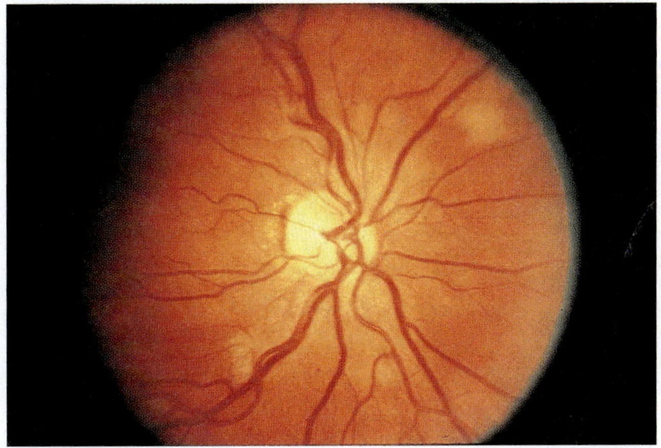

Figure 16.13 Appearance of the ocular fundus in diabetic retinopathy.
(National Eye Institute, National Institutes of Health)

Medical Word	Part	Meaning	Definition
retrolental fibroplasia (RLF) (rĕt″ rō-lĕn′ tăl fī″ brō-plā′ sē-ă)	retro- lent -al fibr/o -plasia	behind lens pertaining to fiber formation	Disease of the retinal vessels present in premature newborns; can be caused by excessive use of oxygen in the incubator; can cause retinal detachment and blindness
scleritis (sklĕ-rī′ tĭs)	scler -itis	hardening, sclera inflammation	Inflammation of the sclera (white of the eye)
strabismus (stră-bĭz′ mŭs)	strabism -us	a squinting structure	Disorder of the eye in which the optic axes cannot be directed to the same object; *squinting*

Medical Word	Word Parts		Definition
	Part	Meaning	
sty(e) (stī)			Inflammation of one or more of the sebaceous glands of the eyelid; also called a *hordeolum*
tonography (tō-nŏg´ ră-fē)	ton/o -graphy	tone recording	Recording of intraocular pressure used in detecting glaucoma

RULE REMINDER

This term keeps the combining vowel ***o*** because the suffix begins with a consonant.

Medical Word	Part	Meaning	Definition
tonometer (tōn-ŏm´ ĕ-tĕr)	ton/o -meter	tone instrument to measure	Medical instrument used to measure intraocular pressure. See Figure 16.14.

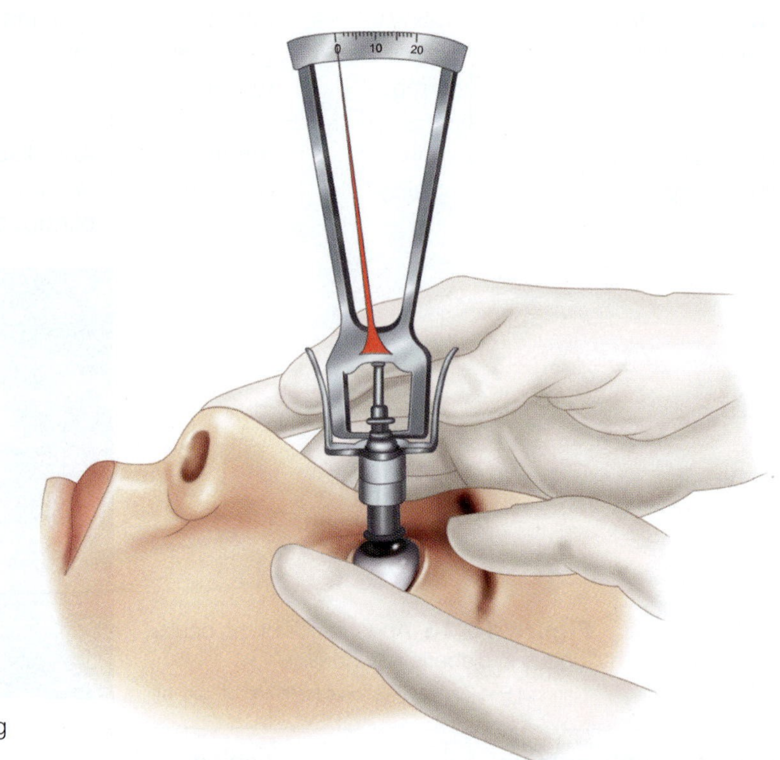

Figure 16.14 Schiötz tonometer for measuring intraocular pressure.

Medical Word	Part	Meaning	Definition
trichiasis (trĭk-ī´ ă-sĭs)	trich -iasis	hair condition	Condition of in-growing eyelashes that rub against the cornea, causing a constant irritation to the eyeball
trifocal (trī-fō´ kăl)	tri- foc -al	three focus pertaining to	Pertaining to having three foci
uveal (ū´ vē-ăl)	uve -al	uvea pertaining to	Pertaining to the second or vascular coat of the eye

Medical Word	Word Parts		Definition
	Part	**Meaning**	
uveitis (ū-vē-ī´ tĭs)	uve -itis	uvea inflammation	Inflammation of the uvea (consists of the iris, ciliary body, and choroid, and forms the pigmented layer)
xenophthalmia (zĕn˝ ŏf-thăl´ mē-ă)	xen ophthalm -ia	foreign material eye condition	Inflamed eye condition caused by foreign material
xerophthalmia (zē-rŏf-thăl´ mē-ă)	xer ophthalm -ia	dry eye condition	Eye condition in which the conjunctiva is dry

Study and Review II

Word Parts

Prefixes

Give the definitions of the following prefixes.

1. a- ______
2. bi- ______
3. en- ______
4. em- ______
5. eso- ______
6. hyper- ______
7. intra- ______
8. tri- ______
9. ex(o)- ______
10. hemi- ______
11. an- ______
12. retro- ______

Combining Forms

Give the definitions of the following combining forms.

1. ambly/o ______
2. anis/o ______
3. blephar/o ______
4. choroid/o ______
5. conjunctiv/o ______
6. cor/o ______
7. corne/o ______
8. cry/o ______
9. cycl/o ______
10. dacry/o ______
11. dipl/o ______
12. irid/o ______
13. kerat/o ______
14. lacrim/o ______
15. lent/o ______
16. mi/o ______
17. ophthalm/o ______
18. opt/o ______
19. orth/o ______
20. phac/o ______
21. phot/o ______
22. retin/o ______
23. xen/o ______
24. xer/o ______

Suffixes

Give the definitions of the following suffixes.

1. -al ______________________
2. -ar ______________________
3. -ary ______________________
4. -blast ______________________
5. -iasis ______________________
6. -ectomy ______________________
7. -gram ______________________
8. -graphy ______________________
9. -ia ______________________
10. -ic ______________________
11. -ician ______________________
12. -ion ______________________
13. -ism ______________________
14. -ist ______________________
15. -itis ______________________
16. -logy ______________________
17. -lysis ______________________
18. -plasia ______________________
19. -meter ______________________
20. -oma ______________________
21. -opia ______________________
22. -osis ______________________
23. -pathy ______________________
24. -phobia ______________________
25. -plasty ______________________
26. -plegia ______________________
27. -ptosis ______________________
28. -scope ______________________
29. -tic ______________________
30. -tomy ______________________
31. -us ______________________

Identifying Medical Terms

In the spaces provided, write the medical terms for the following meanings.

1. ______________________ Dullness of vision
2. ______________________ Pertaining to having two foci
3. ______________________ Drooping of the upper eyelid(s)
4. ______________________ Pertaining to the cornea
5. ______________________ Tumor-like swelling caused by obstruction of the tear duct(s)
6. ______________________ Double vision
7. ______________________ Normal or perfect vision
8. ______________________ Pertaining to within the eye

9. ______________________ Inflammation of the cornea

10. ______________________ Surgical repair of the cornea

11. ______________________ Pertaining to tears

12. ______________________ Pertaining to the eye

13. ______________________ Unusual intolerance to light

Matching

Select the appropriate lettered meaning for each of the following words.

_______ **1.** anisocoria

_______ **2.** entropion

_______ **3.** cataract

_______ **4.** hemianopia

_______ **5.** phacoemulsification

_______ **6.** photocoagulation

_______ **7.** radial keratotomy

_______ **8.** retrolental fibroplasia

_______ **9.** strabismus

_______ **10.** sty(e)

a. Disorder of the eye in which the optic axes cannot be directed to the same object

b. Disease of the retinal vessels present in premature infants

c. Process of using ultrasound to disintegrate a cataract

d. Use of a laser to treat retinal detachment and/or retinal bleeding

e. Condition in which the pupils are unequal

f. Turning inward of the margin of the lower eyelid

g. Surgical procedure performed to correct myopia

h. Inability to see half of the field of vision

i. *Hordeolum*

j. Opacity of the crystalline lens or its capsule

k. Disease characterized by increased intraocular pressure

Medical Case Snapshots

This learning activity provides an opportunity to relate the medical terminology you are learning to a precise patient case presentation. In the spaces provided, write in your answers.

Case 1

A 63-year-old male presents with "trouble driving at night." He states that "bright lights hurt my eyes" and "I see halos around them." When opacity of the crystalline lens occurs in an older adult it is said to be a ________________. With this condition colors seem faded and the only effective treatment is known as ________________, a process of using ultrasound to disintegrate the lens. See Figure 16.11.

Case 2

A 17-year-old male was seen by an ophthalmologist. He complains that his eyes are really bothering him. He has been swimming every day for the past two weeks training for a swim meet. He is diagnosed with _______________ or inflammation of the conjunctiva. With this condition some of the symptoms are _______________ in the white of the eye, an increased amount of tears, a thick _______________ discharge and _______________ vision.

Case 3

A 64-year-old female is seen by her physician. Her medical history includes diagnoses of hypertension and type 2 diabetes mellitus. The results of a comprehensive eye exam revealed an increased intraocular pressure, which is known as _______________. With this condition there are no outward symptoms. Some of the predisposing factors of this condition are being over _______________ years of age, having _______________ ancestry, and diagnoses of _______________ and _______________ diabetes _______________.

Drug Highlights

Type of Drug	Description and Examples
drugs used to treat glaucoma	Work by increasing the outflow of aqueous humor, by decreasing its production, or by producing both of these actions.
prostaglandin analogues	Increase the drainage of intraocular fluid, thereby decreasing intraocular pressure. EXAMPLES: Travatan Z (travoprost ophthalmic solution 0.004%), Lumigan (bimatoprost ophthalmic solution 0.03%), and Xalatan (latanoprost)
adrenergic drugs	Increase the drainage of intraocular fluid. EXAMPLES: Propine ophthalmic solution with 0.1% (epinephrine)
alpha antagonist	Decreases production of intraocular fluid and increases drainage. EXAMPLE: Alphagan P (brimonidine tartrate ophthalmic solution 0.1%)
beta blockers	Decrease production of intraocular fluid. EXAMPLES: Akbeta (levobunolol HCl ophthalmic solution, carteolol HCl ophthalmic solution), Betoptic S (betaxolol HCl 0.25%), Betagan Liquifilm (levobunolol), OptiPranolol (metipranolol), Timoptic-XE, Betimol (timolol hemihydrate), and Ocupress (carteolol HCl)

(continued)

Type of Drug	Description and Examples
carbonic anhydrase inhibitors	Decrease production of intraocular fluid. EXAMPLES: Azopt (brinzolamide ophthalmic suspension 1%), Diamox Sequels, acetazolomide, and Trusopt (dorzolamide)
cholinergic (miotic)	Increases drainage of intraocular fluid. EXAMPLE: pilocarpine HCl (ophthalmic solution)
cholinesterase	Increases drainage of intraocular fluid. EXAMPLE: Phospholine Iodide (echothiophate)
combination of beta blocker and carbonic anhydrase inhibitor	Decreases production of intraocular fluid. EXAMPLE: Cosopt (dorzolomide HCl timolol maleate) (ophthalmic solution)
mydriatics	Agents used to dilate the pupil (mydriasis); can be anticholinergics or sympathomimetics.
anticholinergics	Dilate the pupil and interfere with the ability of the eye to focus properly (cycloplegia). They are used primarily as an aid in refraction, during internal examination of the eye, in intraocular surgery, and in the treatment of anterior uveitis and secondary glaucomas. EXAMPLES: atropine sulfate, Mydriacyl (tropicamide)
sympathomimetics	Produce mydriasis without cycloplegia. Pupil dilation is obtained as the drug causes contraction of the dilator muscle of the iris. They also affect intraocular pressure by decreasing production of aqueous humor while increasing its outflow from the eye. EXAMPLES: epinephrine HCl and phenylephrine HCl
antibiotics	Used to treat infectious diseases, especially those caused by bacteria. Those used for the eye can be in the form of an ointment, cream, or solution. EXAMPLES: chloramphenicol, polymyxin B sulfate, Vigamox (moxifloxacin), and Zymar (gatifloxacin)
antifungal agent	Natacyn (natamycin) is used to treat fungal infections of the eye, such as blepharitis, conjunctivitis, and keratitis.
antiviral agents	Dendrid (idoxuridine) and Herplex (idoxuridine) are potent antiviral agents used to treat keratitis caused by the herpes simplex virus. Viroptic (trifluridine) is also used to treat viral infections of the eye and is effective in the treatment of herpes simplex infections.

Diagnostic and Laboratory Tests

Test	Description
color vision tests	Use of polychromatic (multicolored) charts or an *anomaloscope* (a device for detecting color blindness) to assess an individual's ability to recognize differences in color. A person who is color blind will not see the number 27 in the circle in Figure 16.15.

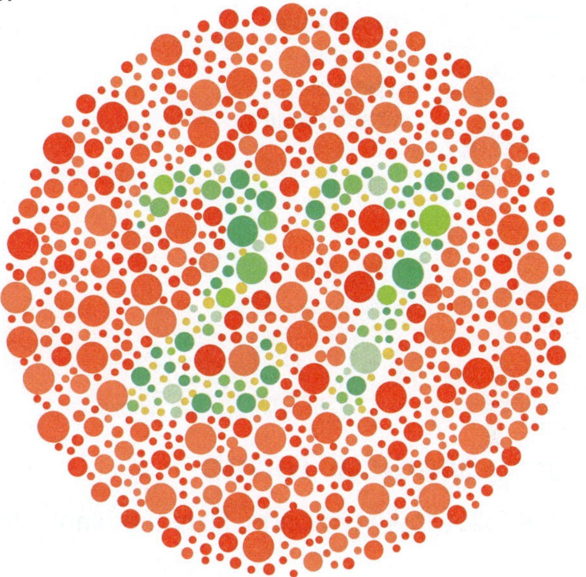

Figure 16.15 Color vision chart. Color blind individuals cannot see the number 27 in the circle.

Test	Description
exophthalmometry (ĕk″ sŏf-thăl-mŏm′ ĕ-trē)	Process of measuring the forward protrusion of the eye via an exophthalmometer; used to evaluate an increase or decrease in *exophthalmos* (abnormal protrusion of the eyeball) usually associated with hyperthyroidism
gonioscopy (gō″ nē-ŏs′ kō-pē)	Examination of the anterior chamber of the eye via a gonioscope; used for determining ocular motility and rotation
keratometry (kĕr″ ă-tŏm′ ĕ-trē)	Process of measuring the cornea via a keratometer
ocular ultrasonography (ŏk′ ū-lăr ŭl-tră-sŏn-ŏg′ ră-fē)	Use of high-frequency sound waves (via a small probe placed on the eye) to measure for intraocular lenses (IOL) and to detect orbital and periorbital lesions; also used to measure the length of the eye and the curvature of the cornea in preparation for surgery
ophthalmoscopy (ŏf-thăl-mŏs′ kō-pē)	Examination of the interior of the eyes via an ophthalmoscope; used to view the retina and identify changes in the blood vessels and to diagnose systemic diseases
tonometry (tōn-ŏm′ ĕ-trē)	Measurement of the intraocular pressure (IOP) of the eye via a tonometer; used to screen for and detect glaucoma. See Figure 16.14.
visual acuity (VA) (vĭzh′ ū-ăl ă-kū′ ĭ-tē)	Acuteness or sharpness of vision. A Snellen eye chart can be used to test it; the patient reads letters of various sizes from a distance of 20 feet. Normal vision is 20/20.

Abbreviations

Abbreviation	Meaning	Abbreviation	Meaning
Acc	accommodation	**IOP**	intraocular pressure
AMD	age-related macular degeneration	**LPI**	laser peripheral iridotomy
ALT	argon laser trabeculoplasty	**MY**	myopia
CVS	computer vision syndrome	**RLF**	retrolental fibroplasia
EM	emmetropia	**SLT**	selective laser trabeculoplasty
ET	esotropia	**STIs**	sexually transmitted infections
Hy	hyperopia	**VA**	visual acuity
IOL	intraocular lens	**XT**	exotropia

Study and Review III

Building Medical Terms

Using the following word parts, fill in the blanks to build the correct medical terms.

dipl-	retin/o	-phobia
lacrim	uve	-iasis
nyctal	-ectomy	
ophthalm/o	-tic	

Definition	Medical Term
1. Double vision	_________opia
2. Surgical excision of a portion of the iris	irid__________
3. Pertains to tears	__________al
4. Pertaining to an agent that causes the pupil to contract	mio__________
5. Condition in which the individual has difficulty seeing at night	_________opia
6. Study of the eye	_________logy
7. Unusual intolerance to light	photo_______
8. Any disease of the retina	________pathy
9. Condition of in-growing eyelashes that rub against the cornea	trich__________
10. Pertaining to the second or vascular coat of the eye	__________al

Combining Form Challenge

Using the combining forms provided, write the medical term correctly.

ambly/o	cycl/o	goni/o
blephar/o	dacry/o	kerat/o

1. Dullness of vision: ___________ opia
2. Drooping of the upper eyelid(s): ___________ ptosis
3. Paralysis of the ciliary muscle: ___________ plegia
4. Tumor-like swelling caused by obstruction of the tear duct(s): ___________ oma
5. Instrument used to examine the angle of the anterior chamber of the eye: ___________ scope
6. Inflammation of the cornea: ___________ itis

Select the Right Term

Select the correct answer, and write it on the line provided.

1. Process by which the eyes make adjustments to see objects at various distances is ___________.

   amblyopia **accommodation** **anisocoria** **astigmatism**

2. Opacity of the crystalline lens or its capsule is ___________.

   cataract **chalazion** **choroiditis** **conjunctivitis**

3. Turning inward of the margin of the lower eyelid is ___________.

   enucleation **esotropia** **entropion** **exotropia**

4. Disease caused by increased intraocular pressure is ___________.

   nystagmus **hemianopia** **gonioscope** **glaucoma**

5. Vision defect in which parallel rays come to a focus beyond the retina is ___________.

   hyperopia **presbyopia** **myopia** **esotropia**

6. Inflammation of one or more of the sebaceous glands of the eyelid is ___________.

   scleritis **strabismus** **sty(e)** **xerophthalmia**

Diagnostic and Laboratory Tests

Select the best answer to each multiple-choice question. Circle the letter of your choice.

1. Process of measuring the forward protrusion of the eye.
   a. gonioscopy
   b. keratometry
   c. exophthalmometry
   d. tonometry

2. Process of measuring the cornea.
   a. gonioscopy
   b. keratometry
   c. exophthalmometry
   d. tonometry

3. Used to identify changes in the blood vessels in the eye and to diagnose systemic diseases.
   a. exophthalmometry
   b. gonioscopy
   c. ophthalmoscopy
   d. tonometry

4. Process of measuring the intraocular pressure of the eye.
   a. exophthalmometry
   b. gonioscopy
   c. ophthalmoscopy
   d. tonometry

5. Process used to measure the acuteness or sharpness of vision.
   a. color vision tests
   b. ultrasonography
   c. tonometry
   d. visual acuity

Abbreviations

Place the correct word, phrase, or abbreviation in the space provided.

1. accommodation ____________________
2. EM ____________________
3. Hy ____________________
4. intraocular lens ____________________
5. esotropia ____________________
6. MY ____________________
7. VA ____________________
8. IOP ____________________
9. retrolental fibroplasia ____________________
10. XT ____________________

Practical Application

Medical Record Analysis

This exercise contains information, abbreviations, and medical terminology from an actual medical record or case study that has been adapted for this text. The names and any personal information have been created by the author. Read and study each form or case study and then answer the questions that follow. You may refer to Appendix III, *Abbreviations and Symbols*.

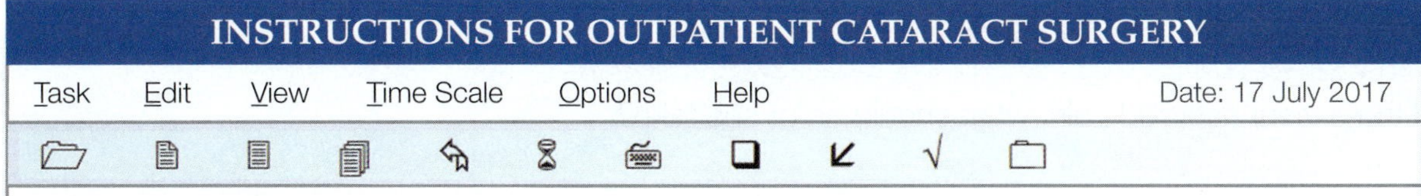

Before Surgery

1. Your surgery has been scheduled for Tuesday, August 2, 2017, as an outpatient at: Dewdrop Surgery Center.
2. Report to the center the day of surgery at 7:10 A.M.
3. The afternoon before surgery and the morning of surgery, use the antibiotics Vigamox and Zymar drops in the right eye to help prevent a bacterial infection. Afternoon and evening before surgery, 1 drop at 3:00, 5:00, 7:00, and 9:00 P.M.
4. Do not eat or drink anything the morning of surgery, except a sip of water to take your medications.
5. Do not wear makeup, fingernail polish, or jewelry to the center.
6. If you are normally taking any medications in the morning, especially heart or blood pressure medications, be sure to take them before you come to the center for surgery. However, if you take insulin or diabetes medication, do not take it until you get home from surgery.
7. Go by the outpatient surgery department at Dewdrop Surgery Center to pre-admit any time before the day of surgery.

After Surgery

1. You may go home shortly after surgery. Be sure to bring someone to drive you home. You may resume normal activities but do not engage in vigorous exercise on the day of surgery. Be careful not to have a fall.
2. The shield may be removed 6 hours after surgery. **DO NOT PUT ANY PRESSURE ON YOUR EYE AND DO NOT RUB YOUR EYE**. Put the Vigamox/Zymar drops in 3 times before you go to bed.
3. Return to Dr. Cedric Emmanuel's office on Wednesday, August 3, 2017, at 10:25 A.M. and further instructions will be given. Bring all your eyedrops to the office with you.
4. Continue any medications that you are taking unless otherwise instructed. Resume your usual diet.
5. If you have mild pain, take Tylenol regular-strength (325 mg) acetaminophen: two tablets every 4–6 hours as needed, not to exceed 12 tablets in 24 hours. If the pain is severe call Dr. Cedric Emmanuel: Office & beeper (123) 456-7890.

Medical Record Questions

Place the correct answer in the space provided.

1. What type of medication is Vigamox and why is it ordered for this patient? ______________________

2. What type of medication is Zymar and why is it ordered for this patient? ______________________

3. Should the patient take his or her heart and blood pressure medicine the morning of surgery? __________ ____________________

4. When should the patient go by the Dewdrop Surgery Center to pre-admit? ______________________

5. If the patient has mild pain, what should he or she take? ______________________

Chapter 17

Female Reproductive System with an Overview of Obstetrics

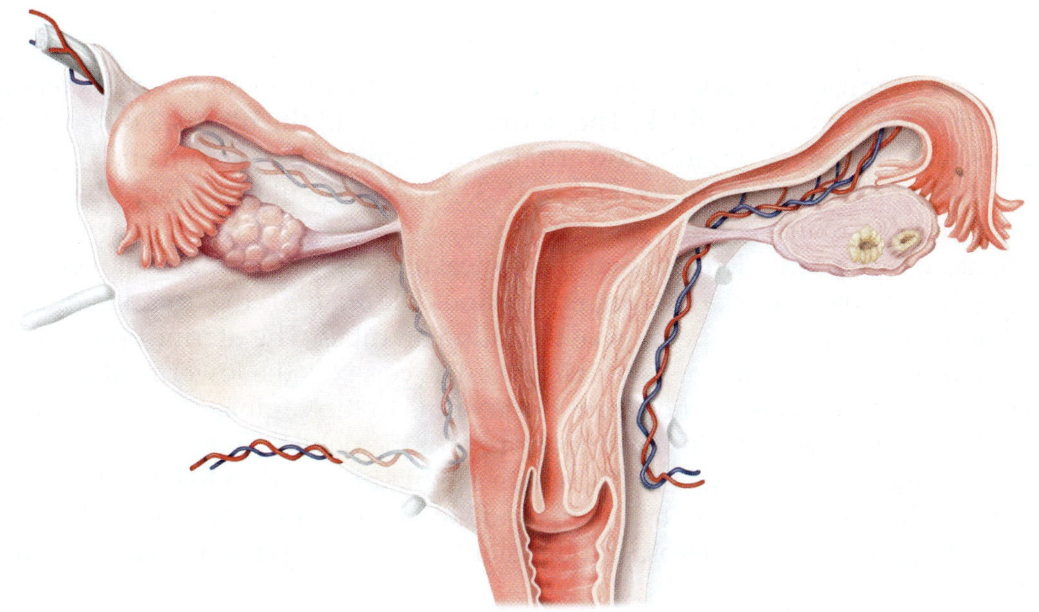

Learning Outcomes

On completion of this chapter, you will be able to:

1. State the description and primary functions of the organs/structures of the female reproductive system.
2. Describe three abnormal positions of the uterus.
3. Describe the menstrual cycle.
4. Define obstetrics and summarize the process of fertilization.
5. State the definition of pregnancy and describe its four stages.
6. Describe the three stages of labor.
7. Recognize terminology included in the ICD-10-CM.
8. Analyze, build, spell, and pronounce medical words.
9. Comprehend the drugs highlighted in this chapter.
10. Describe diagnostic and laboratory tests related to this chapter.
11. Identify and define selected abbreviations.
12. Apply your acquired knowledge of medical terms by successfully completing the *Practical Application* exercise.

Anatomy and Physiology

The female reproductive system consists of a left and a right ovary, which are the female's primary sex organs, and the following accessory sex organs: two fallopian tubes, the uterus, the vagina, the vulva, and two breasts. The vital function of the female reproductive system is to perpetuate the species through sexual or germ cell reproduction. Table 17.1 provides an at-a-glance look at the female reproductive system. See Figures 17.1 and 17.2.

Uterus

The **uterus** is a muscular, hollow, pear-shaped organ that is about 8 centimeters (cm) long, 5 cm wide, and 2.5 cm thick. The normal position of the uterus, known as **anteflexion**, is with the cervix pointing toward the lower end of the sacrum and the fundus toward the suprapubic region. See Figure 17.3. An average uterus weighs between 30 and 40 grams (g), which is 1 and 1.4 ounces (oz).

The uterus can be divided into two anatomical regions: the body and the cervix. The *uterine body* or *corpus* is the larger (upper) portion. The *fundus* is the rounded portion of the uterine body above the openings of the fallopian tubes. The uterine body ends at a constricted central area known as the *isthmus*. The cervix is the lowermost cylindrical portion of the uterus that extends from the isthmus to the vagina.

The uterus is suspended in the anterior part of the pelvic cavity, halfway between the sacrum and the symphysis pubis, above the bladder, and in front of the rectum. A number of ligaments support the uterus and hold it in position: two broad ligaments, two round ligaments, two uterosacral ligaments, and the ligaments that are attached to the bladder.

Table 17.1 Female Reproductive System at-a-Glance

Organ/Structure	Primary Functions/Description
Uterus	Provides a place for the nourishment and development of the fetus during pregnancy; contracts rhythmically and powerfully to help push out the fetus during the process of birthing
Fallopian tubes	Serve as ducts to convey the ovum from the ovary to the uterus and to convey spermatozoa from the uterus toward each ovary
Ovaries	Produce ova and hormones
Vagina	Female organ of copulation (sexual intercourse), serves as a passageway for the discharge of menstruation and a passageway for the birth of a fetus
Vulva	External female genitalia
Mons pubis	Provides pad of fatty tissue
Labia majora	Provides two folds of adipose tissue
Labia minora	Lying within the labia majora, encloses the vestibule
Vestibule	Serves as the entrance to the urethra, the vagina, and two excretory ducts of Bartholin glands located on either side of the vaginal opening at the base of the *labia majora*. These glands secrete mucus for lubrication.
Clitoris	Erectile tissue that is homologous to the penis of the male; produces pleasurable sensations during the sexual act
Breasts	Following childbirth, mammary glands produce milk

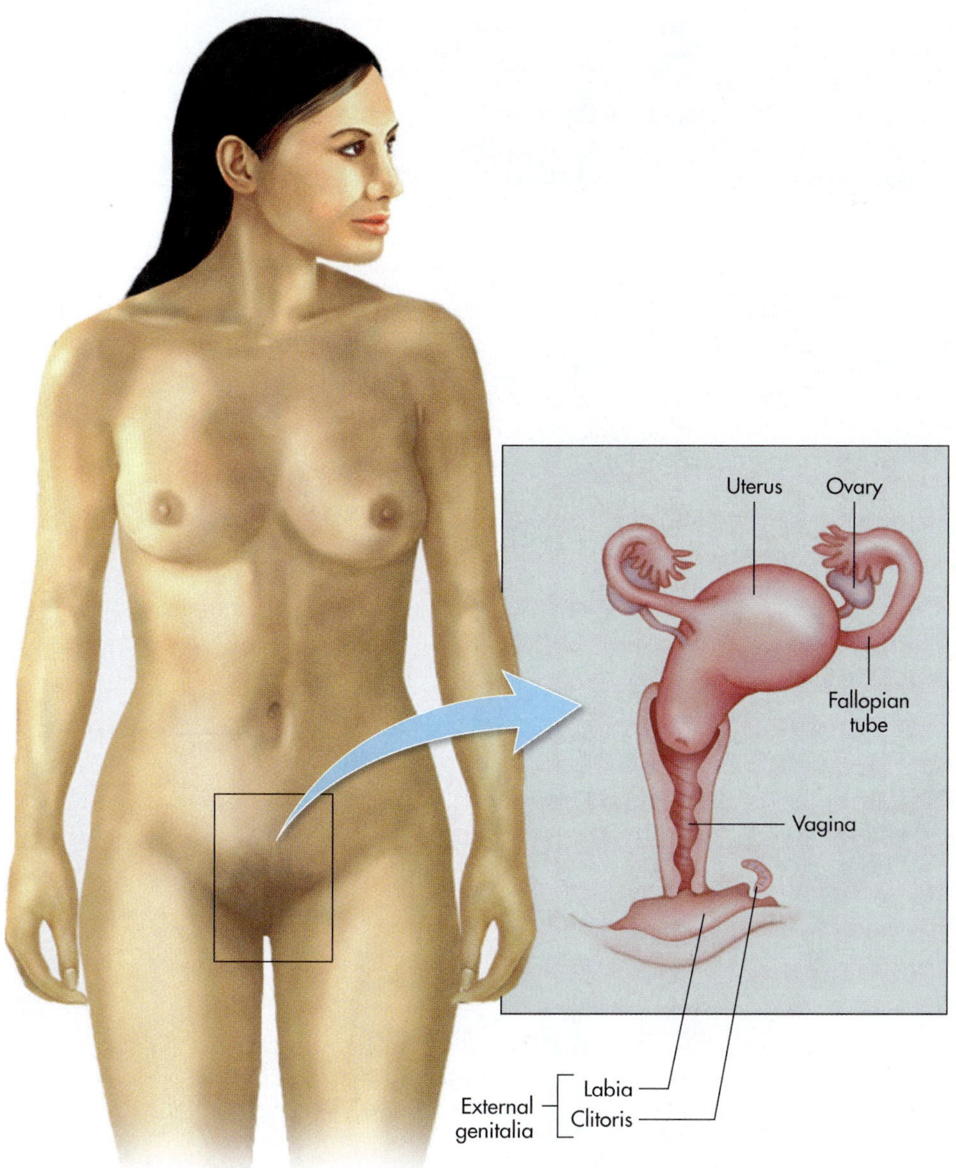

Figure 17.1 Female reproductive system.

Uterine Wall

The wall of the uterus consists of three layers: the **perimetrium** or outer layer, the **myometrium** or muscular middle layer, and the **endometrium**, which is the mucous membrane lining the inner surface of the uterus. See Figure 17.2B. The endometrium is composed of columnar epithelium and connective tissue and is supplied with blood by both straight and spiral arteries. It undergoes marked changes in response to hormonal stimulation during the menstrual cycle.

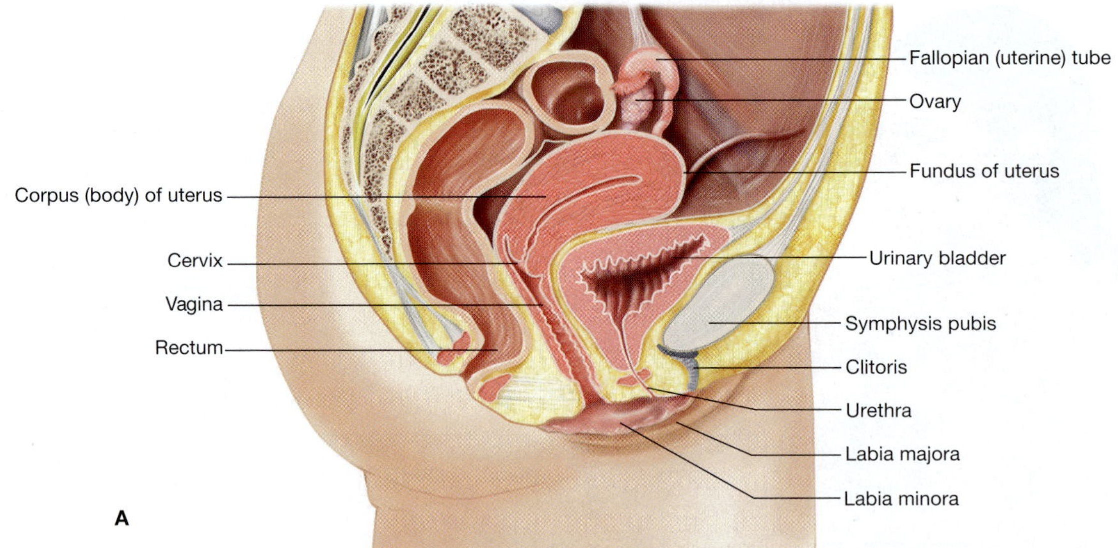

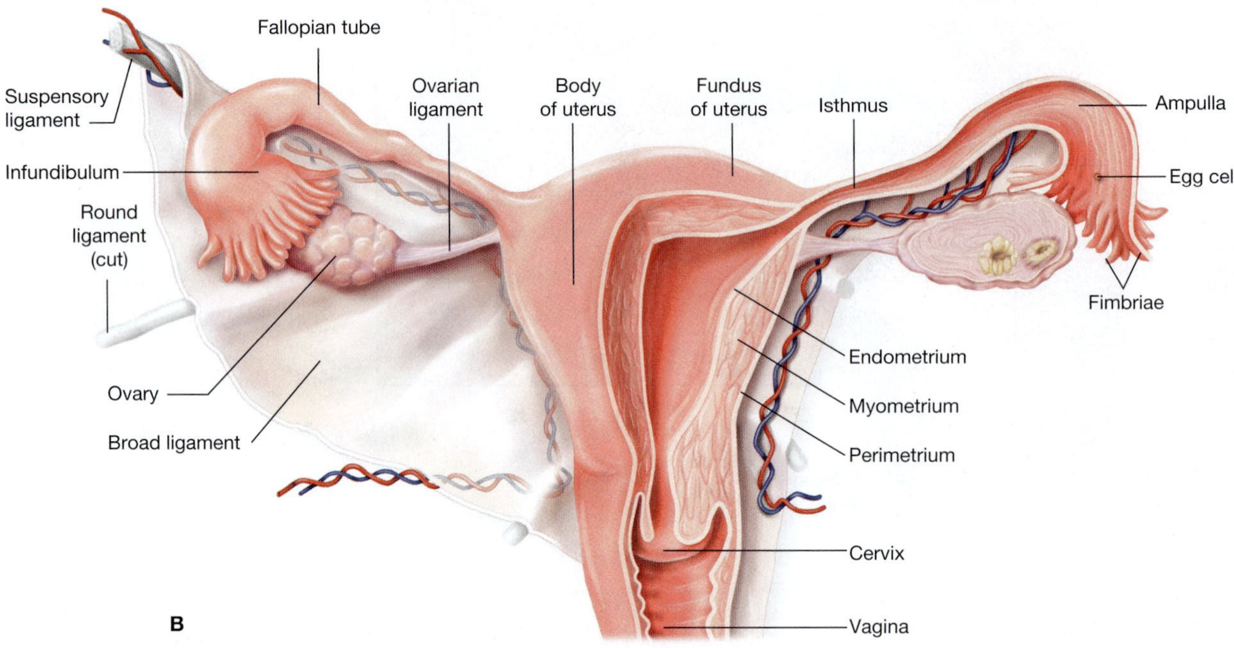

Figure 17.2 Female organs of reproduction and associated structures.

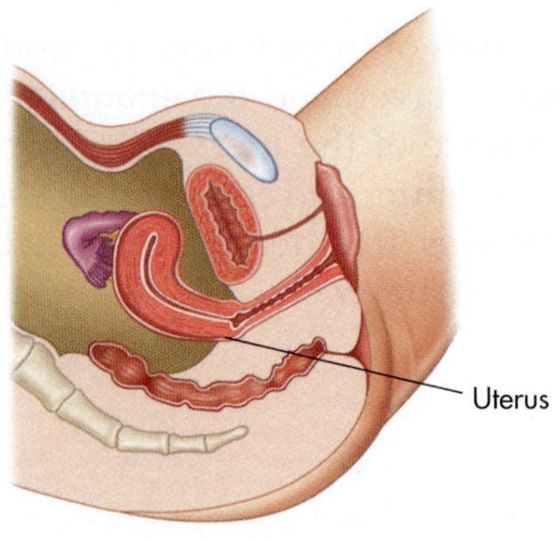

Figure 17.3 Normal position of the uterus, called *anteflexion*.

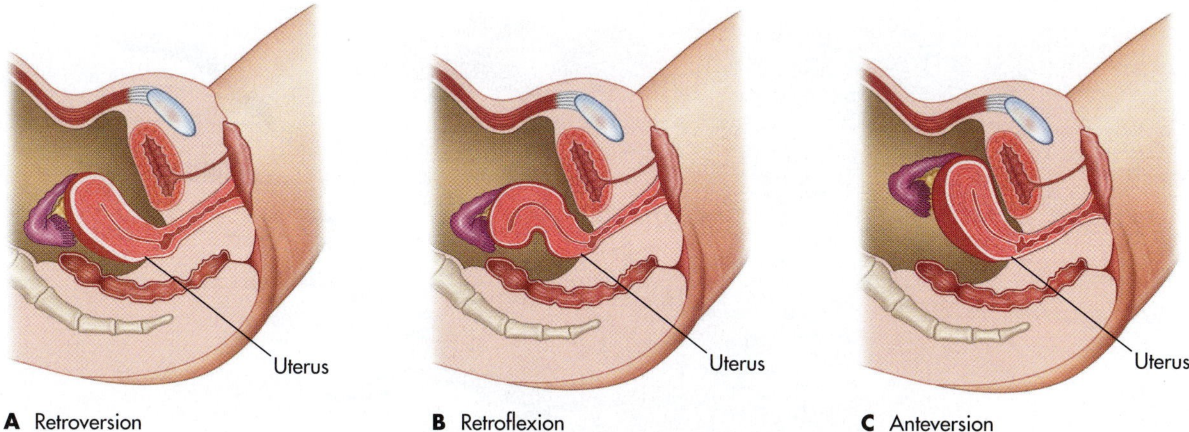

Figure 17.4 Displacement of the uterus within the uterine cavity. (A) Retroversion is a backward tilting. (B) Retroflexion is a backward bending. (C) Anteversion is a forward tilting.

Abnormal Positions of the Uterus

The uterus can become malpositioned because of weakness of any of its supporting ligaments. Trauma, disease processes of the uterus, or multiple pregnancies can contribute to the weakening of the supporting ligaments. The following terms describe some of the abnormal positions (Figure 17.4) of the uterus:

Retroversion. Turned backward with the cervix pointing forward toward the symphysis pubis.

Retroflexion. Bent backward at an angle with the cervix usually unchanged from its normal position.

Anteversion. Fundus turned forward toward the pubis with the cervix tilted up toward the sacrum.

Fallopian Tubes

Also called the **uterine tubes** or **oviducts**, the **fallopian tubes** extend laterally from either side of the uterus and end near each ovary. An average, normal fallopian tube is about 11.5 cm long and 0.6 cm wide. Its wall is composed of three layers: the **serosa** or outermost layer, composed of connective tissue; the **muscular layer**, containing inner circular and outer longitudinal layers of smooth muscle; and the **mucosa** or inner layer, consisting of simple columnar epithelium.

Anatomical Features of the Fallopian Tubes

The **isthmus** is the constricted portion of the fallopian tube nearest the uterus. From the isthmus, the tube continues laterally and widens to form a section called the **ampulla**. Beyond the ampulla, the tube continues to expand and ends as a funnel-shaped opening. This end of the tube is called the **infundibulum**, and its opening is the **ostium**. Surrounding each ostium are **fimbriae** or *fingerlike structures* (see Figure 17.2) that work to propel the discharged ovum into the tube, where ciliary action aids in moving it toward the uterus. Should the ovum become impregnated by a spermatozoon while in the tube, the process of *fertilization* occurs.

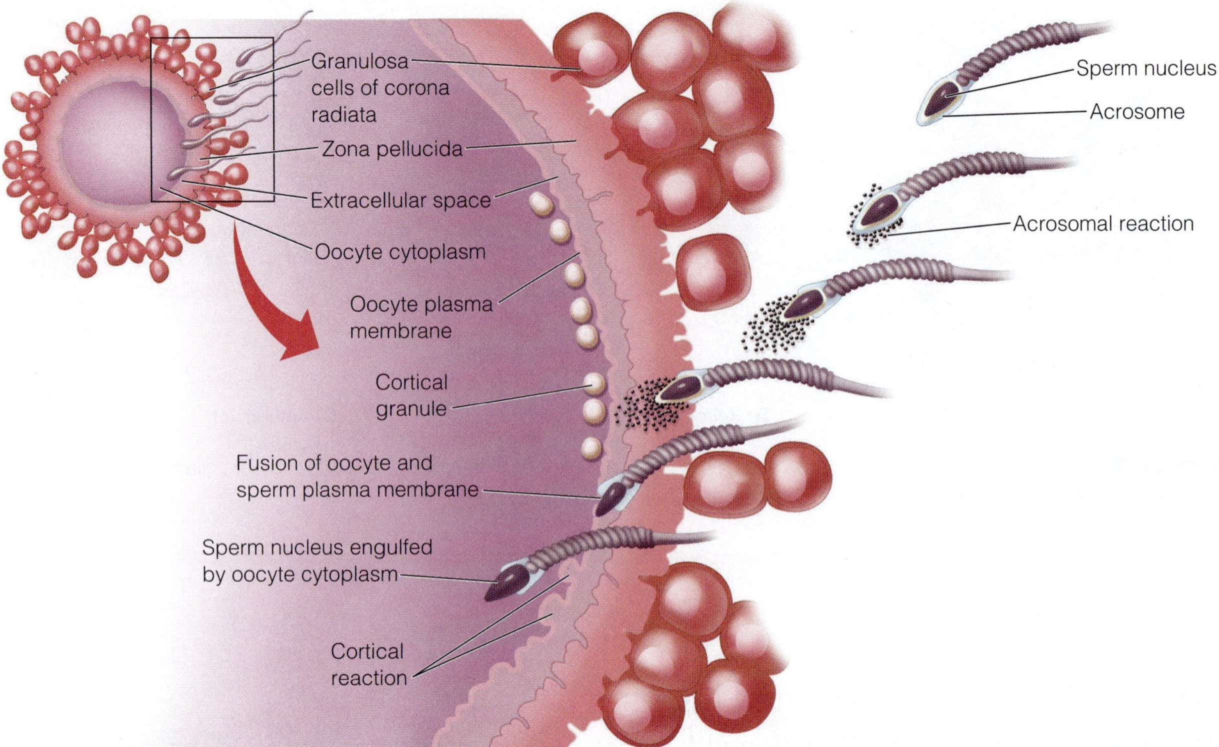

Figure 17.5 Sperm penetration of an ovum. The sequential steps of oocyte penetration by a sperm are depicted moving from top to bottom.

Fertilization

Fertilization is the process in which a sperm penetrates an ovum and unites with it. See Figure 17.5. At this time, the 23 chromosomes from the male combine with the 23 chromosomes from the female to make a new life. Fertilization generally occurs within 24 hours following ovulation and usually takes place in the fallopian tube. A single sperm penetrates the ovum, and the resulting cell is called a **zygote**.

By this event, called **conception**, the gender and other biological traits of the new individual are determined. The fertilized ovum or zygote is genetically complete and immediately begins to divide, forming a solid mass of cells called a **morula**. See Figure 17.6. The cells of the morula continue to divide, and by the time the developing **embryo** (the term for the stage of development between weeks 2 and 8) reaches the uterus, it is a hollow ball of cells known as a **blastocyst**, which consists of an outer layer of cells and an inner cell mass. As the blastocyst develops, it forms a structure with two cavities, the **yolk sac** and **amniotic cavity**. In humans, the yolk sac is the site of formation of the first red blood cells and the cells that will become ovum and sperm.

Ovaries

Located on either side of the uterus, the **ovaries** are almond-shaped organs attached to the uterus by the ovarian ligament. They lie close to the fimbriae of the fallopian tubes. The anterior border of each ovary is connected to the posterior layer of the broad ligament by the **mesovarium** (portion of the peritoneal fold). Each ovary is attached to the side of the pelvis by the **suspensory ligaments**. An average, normal ovary is about 4 cm long, 2 cm wide, and 1.5 cm thick. See Figure 17.8.

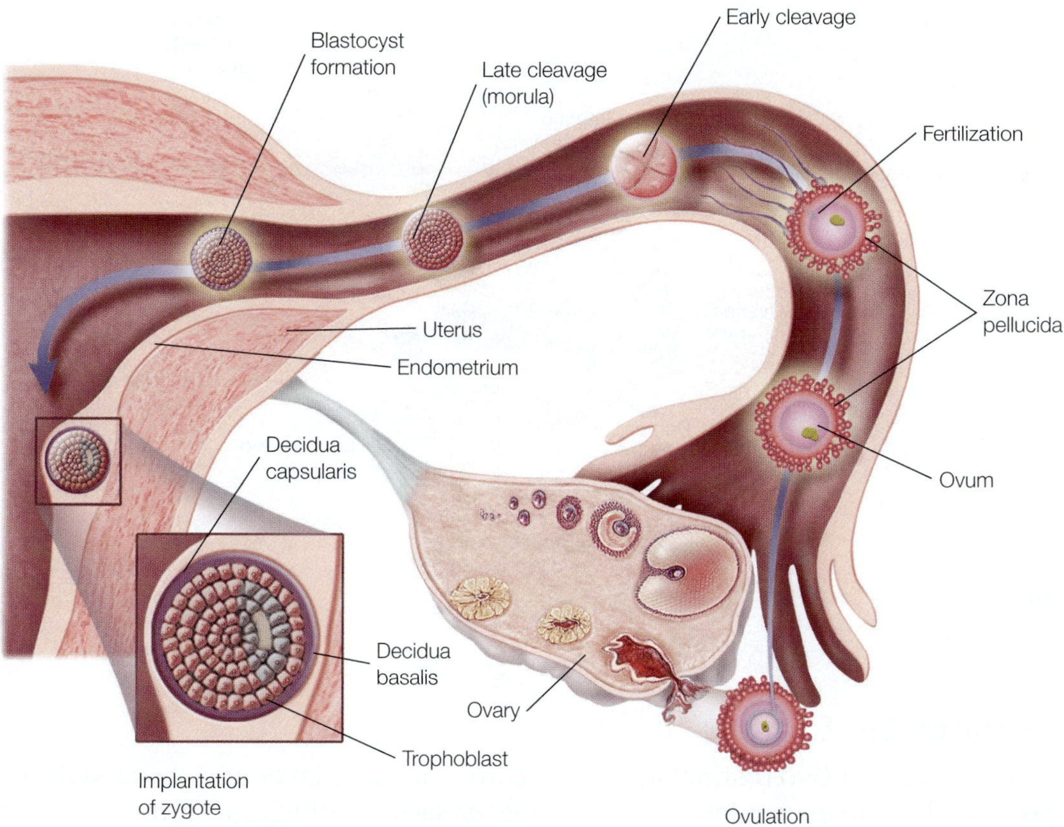

Figure 17.6 During ovulation, the ovum leaves the ovary and enters the fallopian tube. Subsequent changes in the fertilized ovum from conception to implantation are depicted.

fyi

The sex of a child is determined at the time of fertilization. When a spermatozoon carrying the X sex chromosome fertilizes the X-bearing ovum, the result is a female child (X + X = female). When the X-bearing ovum is fertilized by the Y-bearing spermatozoon, a male child is produced (X + Y = male). Sex differentiation occurs early in the embryo. At 16 weeks, the external genitals of the fetus are recognizably male or female. This difference can be seen during ultrasonography. See Figure 17.7.

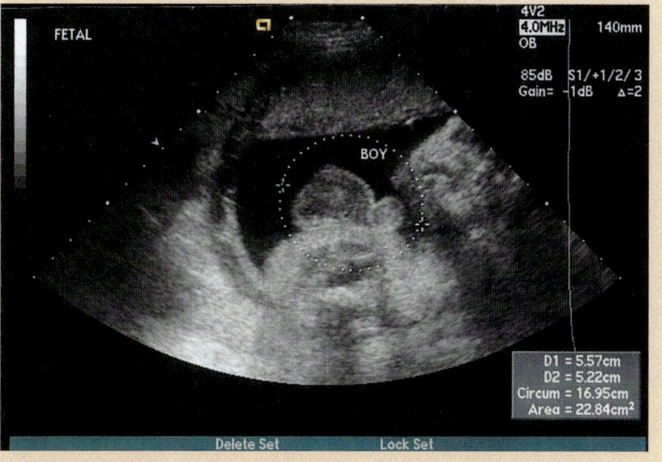

Figure 17.7 Ultrasonogram showing a male fetus.
(Courtesy of Nancy West-Davis)

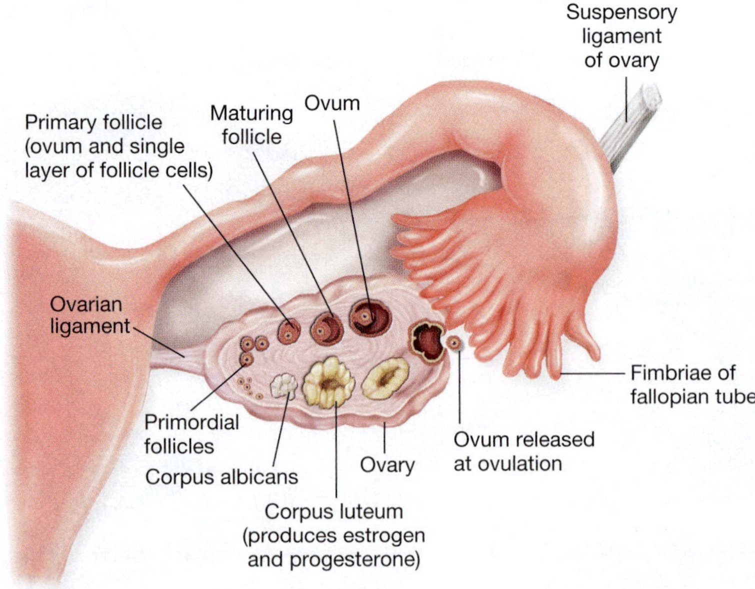

Figure 17.8 Ovary.

Microscopic Anatomy

Each ovary consists of two distinct areas: the **cortex** or outer layer and the **medulla** or inner portion. The cortex contains small secretory sacs or follicles in three stages of development. These stages are known as **primary**, **growing**, and **graafian** or *mature stage*. The ovarian medulla contains connective tissue, nerves, blood and lymphatic vessels, and some smooth muscle tissue in the region of the hilus.

Function of the Ovaries

The anterior lobe of the pituitary gland, which produces the *gonadotropic hormones* FSH and LH, primarily controls the functional activity of the ovaries. These abbreviations are for *follicle-stimulating hormone*, which is instrumental in the development of the ovarian follicles, and *luteinizing hormone*, which stimulates the development of the **corpus luteum**, a small yellow mass of cells that develops within a ruptured ovarian follicle.

Two functions have been identified for the ovary: the production of ova (female reproductive cells) and the production of hormones.

PRODUCTION OF OVA

Each month a *graafian follicle* ruptures on the ovarian cortex, and an **ovum** (singular of ova) discharges into the pelvic cavity, where it enters the fallopian tube. This process is known as **ovulation**. In an average, normal woman more than 400 ova may be produced during her reproductive years (see Figure 17.8).

PRODUCTION OF HORMONES

The ovaries are also endocrine glands, producing **estrogen**, the female sex hormone secreted by the ovarian follicles, and **progesterone**, a steroid hormone secreted by the corpus luteum that is important in the maintenance of pregnancy. These hormones are essential in promoting growth and development and maintaining the female secondary sex organs and characteristics. These hormones also prepare the uterus for pregnancy, promote development of the mammary glands, and play a vital role in a woman's emotional well-being and sexual drive.

Vagina

The **vagina** is a musculomembranous tube extending from the vestibule to the uterus (see Figure 17.2). It is 8–10 cm in length and situated between the bladder and the rectum. It is lined by mucous membrane made up of *squamous epithelium*. A fold of mucous membrane, the **hymen**, partially covers the external opening of the vagina.

Vulva

The **vulva** consists of the following five organs that comprise the external female genitalia (see Figure 17.2):

Mons pubis. A pad of fatty tissue of triangular shape and, after puberty, covered with pubic hair. It may be referred to as the *mons veneris* or *mound of Venus* and is the rounded area over the *symphysis pubis*.

Labia majora. The two folds of adipose tissue, which are large liplike structures, lying on either side of the vaginal opening.

Labia minora. Two thin folds of skin that lie within the labia majora and enclose the vestibule.

Vestibule. The cleft between the labia minora. It is approximately 4–5 cm long and 2 cm wide. Four major structures open into it: the urethra, the vagina, and two excretory ducts of the Bartholin glands.

Clitoris. A small organ consisting of sensitive erectile tissue that is homologous to the penis of the male. It is located between the anterior labial commissure and partially hidden by the anterior portion of the labia minora.

The **perineum** is the region bounded by the inferior edges of the pelvis. In the female, it is located between the vulva and the anus. It is a muscular sheet that forms the pelvic floor, and during childbirth it can be torn and cause injury to the anal sphincter. To avoid such an injury, an *episiotomy*, a surgical procedure to prevent tearing of the perineum and facilitate delivery of the baby, may be performed.

Breasts

The **breasts** or *mammary glands* are compound alveolar structures consisting of 15–20 glandular tissue lobes separated by septa of connective tissue. Most women have two breasts that lie anterior to the pectoral muscles and curve outward from the lateral margins of the sternum to the anterior border of the axilla. See Figure 17.9. The size of the breast can vary greatly according to age, heredity, and adipose (fatty) tissue present.

The **areola** is the dark, pigmented area found in the skin over each breast, and the *nipple* is the elevated area in the center of the areola. During pregnancy, the areola changes from its pinkish color to a dark brown or reddish color. The areola is supplied with a row of small sebaceous glands that secrete an oily substance to keep it resilient. The *lactiferous glands* consist of 20–24 glands in the areola of the nipple, which conveys milk to a suckling baby during **lactation** (the process of milk secretion).

The hormone **prolactin**, which is produced by the anterior lobe of the pituitary, stimulates the mammary glands to produce milk after childbirth. Other hormones playing a role in milk production are insulin and glucocorticoids. **Colostrum**, a thin yellowish secretion, is the *first milk* and contains mainly serum and white blood cells.

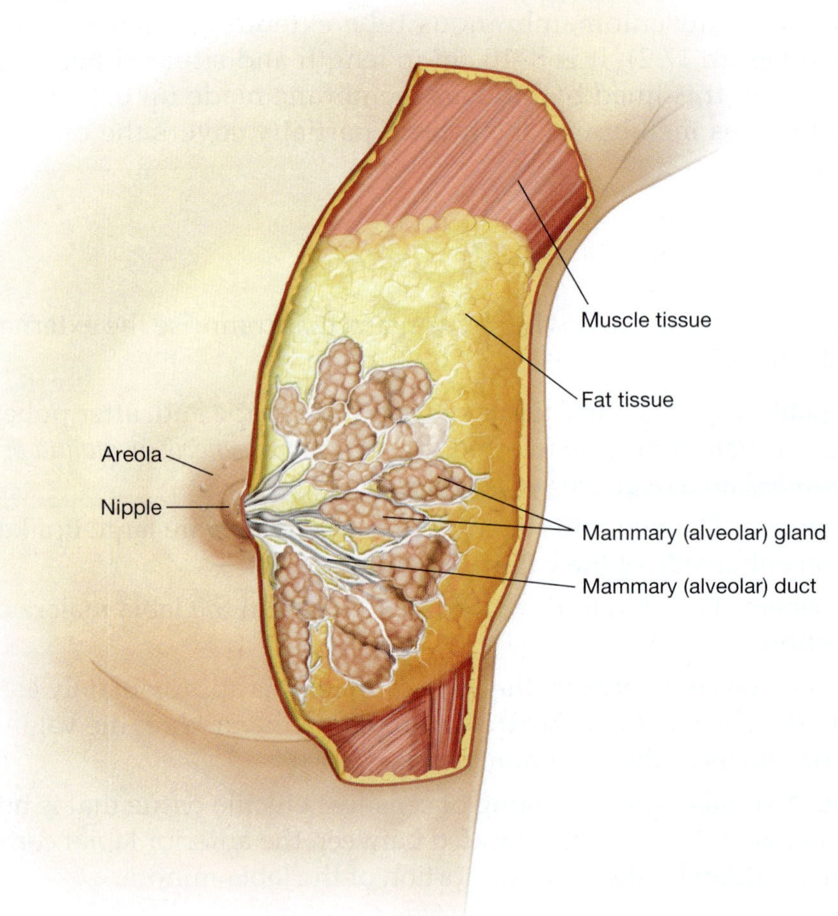

Figure 17.9 Breast.

Breastfeeding

Breastfeeding is the act of providing milk to a baby from the mother's breasts. Mature mother's milk and its precursor, *colostrum*, are considered to be the most balanced foods available for newborns and infants. Breast milk is sterile, easily digested, nonallergenic, and transmits maternal antibodies that protect against various infections and illnesses. In addition, the baby's suckling causes the release of **oxytocin** in the mother, which stimulates uterine contractions and promotes the return of the uterus to its normal nonpregnant size and state.

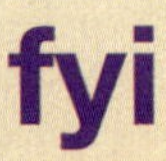

The American Academy of Pediatrics currently recommends that pediatricians and parents be aware that exclusive breastfeeding is sufficient to support optimal growth and development for approximately the first 6 months of life and provides continuing protection against diarrhea and respiratory tract infection. Breastfeeding should be continued for at least the first year of life.

Menstrual Cycle

The menstrual cycle is a periodic recurrent series of changes occurring in the uterus, ovaries, vagina, and breasts. It is regulated by the complex interaction of hormones: luteinizing hormone (LH) and follicle-stimulating hormone (FSH), which are produced by the pituitary gland, and the female sex hormones estrogen and progesterone, which are produced by the ovaries. The onset of the **menstrual cycle**, *menarche*, occurs at the age of **puberty** and ceases at **menopause**. The menstrual cycle occurs during a woman's reproductive years, except during **pregnancy**. The first day of bleeding is counted as the beginning of each menstrual cycle (day 1). The cycle ends just before the next menstrual period. The menstrual cycle occurs approximately every 21–35 days in an adult (the average cycle is 28 days) and has three phases: follicular phase, ovulation, and the luteal phase. See Figure 17.10.

Follicular Phase

Menstruation, which marks the first day of the follicular phase, is characterized by the discharge of a bloody fluid from the uterus accompanied by a shedding of the endometrium. This phase averages 4–5 days and is considered to be the first to the fifth days of the cycle.

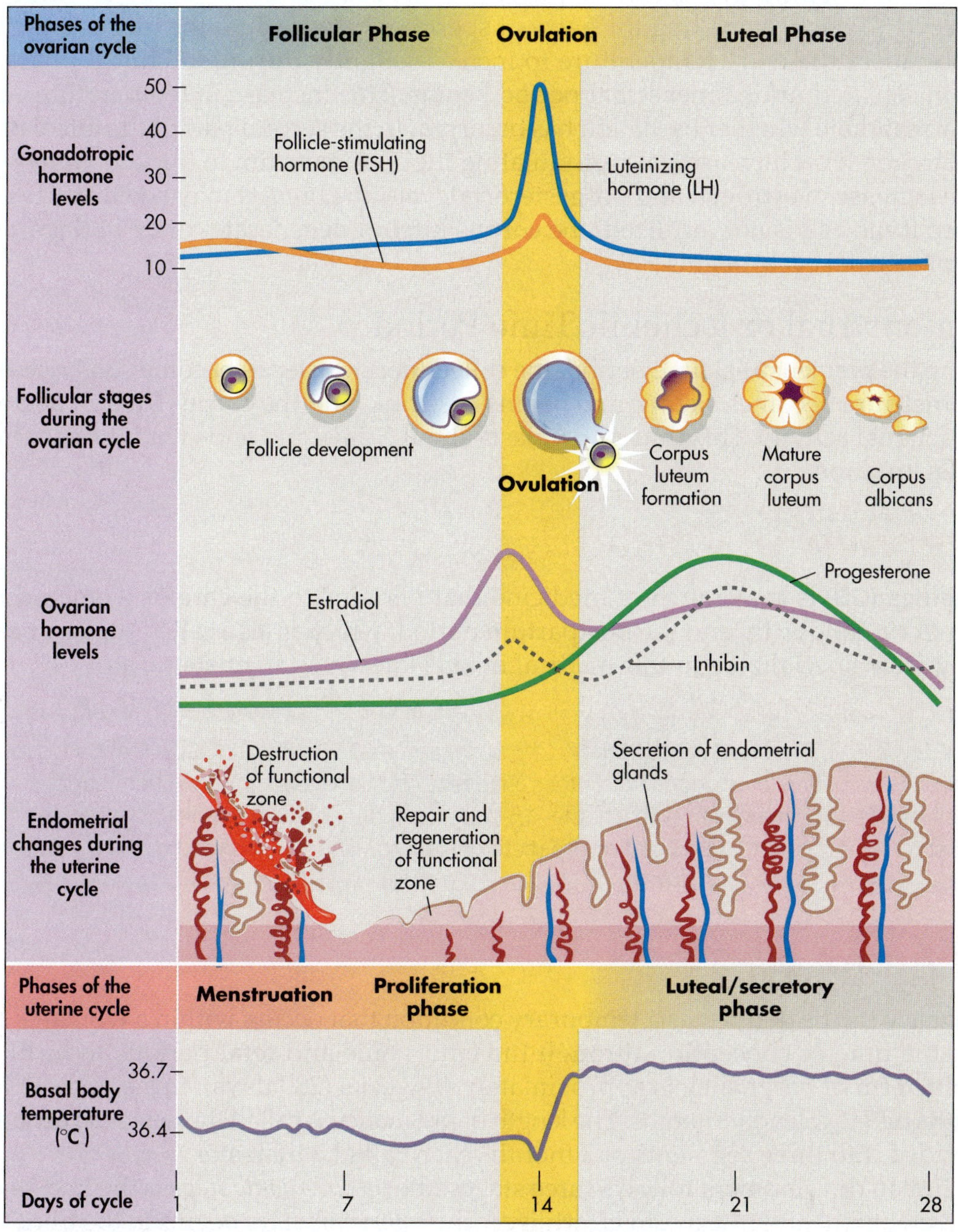

Figure 17.10 Hormonal regulation of the female reproductive cycle.

Ovulatory Phase

The **ovulatory phase** is characterized by the stimulation of estrogen, the thickening and vascularization of the endometrium, along with the maturing of the ovarian follicle. This phase begins about the fifth day and ends at the time of rupture of the graafian follicle (release of the egg), usually 36 hours after the surge in luteinizing hormone begins. About 12–24 hours after the egg is released, this surge can be detected by measuring the luteinizing hormone level in the urine. If the egg is not fertilized within 12–48 hours of being released, it disintegrates. The ovulatory phase occurs about 14 days before the onset of menstruation.

Luteal or Secretory Phase

The **luteal phase** follows ovulation. It lasts about 14 days, unless fertilization occurs, and ends just before a menstrual period. During this phase, the corpus luteum in the ovary is developing and secreting progesterone. Progesterone causes the mucus in the cervix to thicken, making the entry of sperm or bacteria into the uterus less likely. It also causes the body temperature to increase slightly during the luteal phase and remain elevated until a menstrual period begins. This increase in temperature can be used to estimate whether ovulation has occurred. In the second part of the luteal phase, the estrogen level increases, also stimulating the endometrium to thicken. In response to the increase in estrogen and progesterone levels, the breasts may swell and become tender. If the egg is not fertilized, the corpus luteum degenerates after 14 days, and a new menstrual cycle begins.

Premenstrual or Ischemic Time Period

During the **premenstrual** time period, the coiled uterine arteries become constricted, the endometrium becomes anemic and begins to shrink, and the corpus luteum decreases in functional activity. This time period lasts about 2 days and ends with the occurrence of menstruation.

Overview of Obstetrics

Obstetrics (OB) is the branch of medicine that pertains to the care of women during pregnancy, childbirth, and the postpartum period, which is also called the **puerperium**. A physician specializing in this medical field is known as an **obstetrician**.

insights In ICD-10-CM, Chapter 15, *Pregnancy, Childbirth, and the Puerperium* (O00-O9A) codes have sequencing priority over codes from other chapters. Additional codes from other chapters may be used in conjunction with Chapter 15 codes to further specify conditions. Note: Chapter 15 codes are to be used on the maternal record, never on the record of the newborn.

Pregnancy

Pregnancy can be defined as a temporary condition that occurs within a woman's body from the time of conception through the embryonic and fetal periods to birth. The normal term of pregnancy is approximately 40 weeks (280 days); this equals 10 lunar months or $9\frac{1}{3}$ calendar months. The length of pregnancy is called the **gestation period** and is divided into three segments of 3 months each called a **trimester**.

Human development follows three stages: the *preembryonic stage* is the first 14 days of development after the ovum is fertilized; the *embryonic stage* begins in the third week after fertilization; and the *fetal stage* begins in the ninth week. See Figure 17.11.

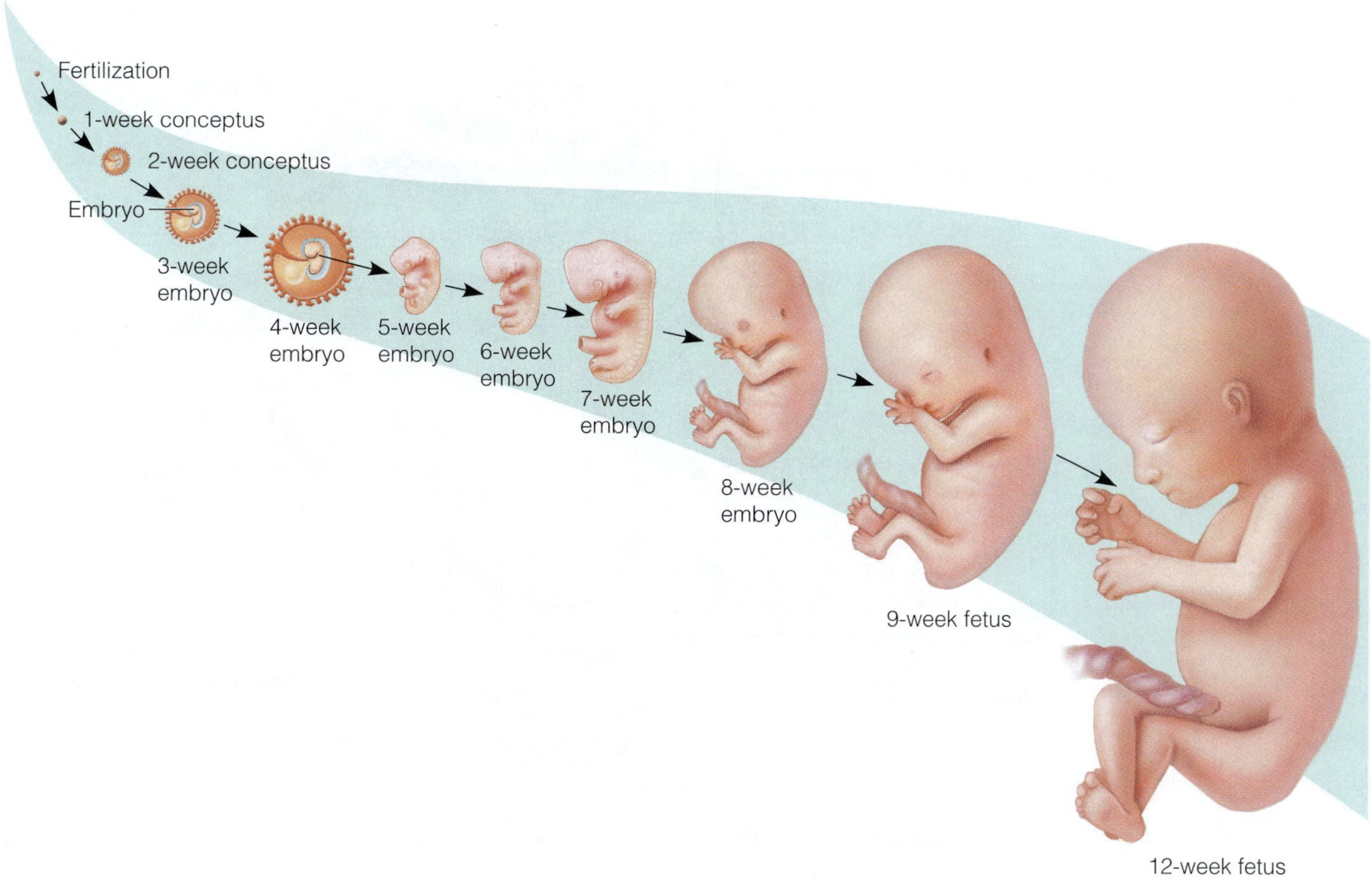

Figure 17.11 Actual size of a human conceptus from fertilization to the early fetal stage. The embryonic stage begins in the third week after fertilization; the fetal stage begins in the ninth week.

During the fifth week of development, the embryo has a marked C-shaped body and a rudimentary tail. At 7 weeks, the head of the embryo is rounded and nearly erect. The eyes have shifted forward and are closer together, and the eyelids begin to form. At 9 weeks, every organ system and external structure is present, and the developing embryo is now called a **fetus**.

At 14 weeks, the skin of the fetus is so transparent that blood vessels are visible beneath it. More muscle tissue and body skeleton have developed and hold the fetus more erect. At 20 weeks, the fetus weighs approximately 312 g and measures crown to rump about 16 cm. The skin is less transparent due to subcutaneous deposits of brown fat. Fingernails and toenails have developed and "woolly" hair may cover the head. See Figure 17.12.

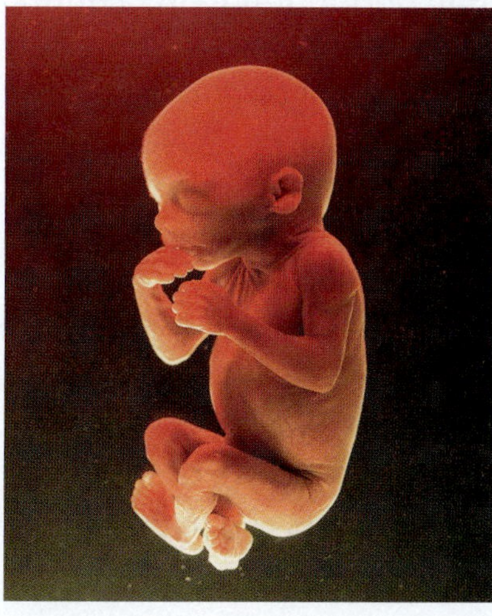

Figure 17.12 Fetus at 20 weeks. The fetus weighs approximately 312 g and measures about 16 cm. Subcutaneous deposits of brown fat make the skin less transparent.

(James Stevenson/Science Source)

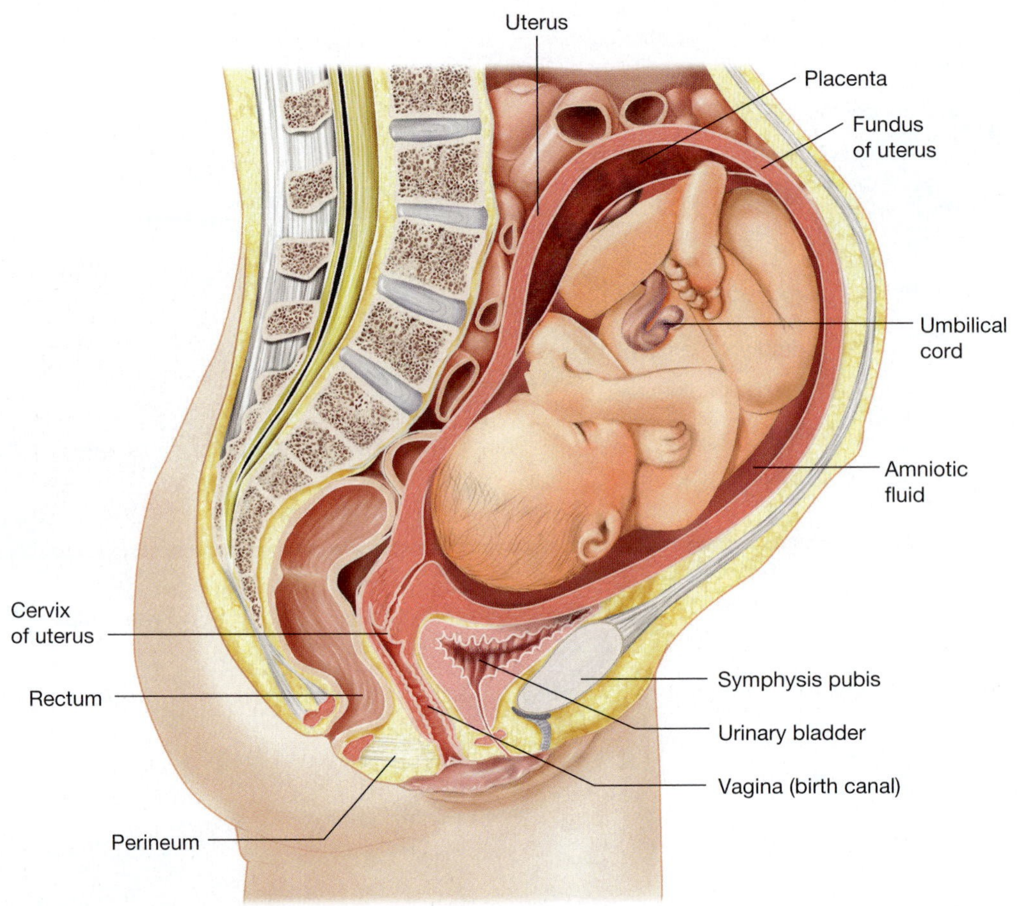

Figure 17.13 Position of fetus in full-term pregnancy.

Pregnancy is divided into four stages:

1. **Prenatal**. Time period between conception and onset of labor; refers to both the care of the woman during pregnancy and the growth and development of the fetus. Figure 17.13 shows the position of the fetus in a full-term pregnancy.
2. **Labor**. Time period during which forceful contractions move the fetus down the birth canal and expel it from the uterus during childbirth.
3. **Parturition**. Time period of actively giving birth; also known as **childbirth** or **delivery**.
4. **Postpartum period** or **puerperium**. Six-week time period following childbirth and expulsion of the placenta. The female reproductive organs usually return to an essentially prepregnant condition in which *involution of the uterus* (return of the uterus to normal size after childbirth) occurs.

Labor and Delivery

Labor is the process by which forceful contractions move the fetus down the birth canal and expel it from the uterus during childbirth. The signs and symptoms that labor is about to start can occur from hours to weeks before the actual onset of labor. Signs of impending labor include:

- ***Braxton Hicks contractions***. Irregular contractions that begin in the second trimester and intensify as full term approaches.

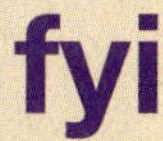

In 2016 the World Health Organization (WHO) designated the Zika virus (transmitted by *Aedes* mosquitoes) and its suspected complications in newborns as a public health emergency of international concern. The primary reason for the designation was the "strongly suspected" causal relationship between the Zika virus and the rare congenital condition called *microcephaly*.

The *Aedes* are the same mosquitoes that spread dengue and chikungunya viruses and typically lay their eggs in and near standing water. The infected mosquitoes spread the virus to people through bites. Spread of the virus through blood transfusions and sexual contact also have been reported.

The Centers for Disease Control and Prevention (CDC) recommends that pregnant women in any trimester, or women trying to or thinking about becoming pregnant, should consider postponing travel to areas where Zika virus transmission is ongoing. These women who must travel to one of these areas should talk to their doctors or other healthcare providers first and strictly follow steps to avoid mosquito bites during the trip.

- ***Increased vaginal discharge***. Normally clear and nonirritating discharge caused by fetal pressure.
- ***Lightening***. The descent of the baby into the pelvis. The expectant mother will notice that she can breathe easier and often states, "The baby has dropped." This may occur 2–3 weeks before the first stage of labor begins.
- ***Bloody show***. Thick mucus mixed with pink or dark-brown blood. As the cervix softens, effaces, and dilates, the mucous plug that has sealed the uterus during pregnancy is dislodged from the cervix and small capillaries are torn, producing the bloody show.
- ***Rupture of the membranes***. Occurs when the amniotic sac (bag of waters) ruptures.

  Note: When the membranes do not rupture on their own, they will be ruptured by the attending physician or midwife. This is known as **AROM**: **a**rtificial **r**upture **o**f **m**embranes.
- ***Energy spurt or nesting***. Occurs in many women shortly before the onset of labor. They may suddenly have the energy to clean their houses and do things that they have not had the energy to do previously.
- ***Weight loss***. Loss of 1–3 pounds shortly before labor can occur as hormone changes cause excretion of extra body water.

Stages of Labor

True labor is characterized by rhythmic contractions that develop a regular pattern and are more frequent, more intense, and last longer. A general feeling of discomfort is felt in the lower back and lower abdomen. A bloody show is often present, and progressive effacement and dilation of the cervix occur. Labor is divided into three stages: dilation, expulsion, and placental. See Figure 17.14.

- ***First stage:* Dilation**. Begins with the onset of true labor and lasts until the cervix is fully dilated to 10 cm.
- ***Second stage:* Expulsion**. Continues after the cervix is dilated to 10 cm until the delivery of the baby. During this stage an **episiotomy**, a surgical procedure performed to prevent tearing of the perineum and to facilitate delivery of the fetus, may be performed.
- ***Third stage:* Placental**. Delivery of the placenta.

The **placenta** is a highly vascular organ that anchors the developing fetus to the uterus and provides the means by which the fetus receives its nourishment and oxygen.

A

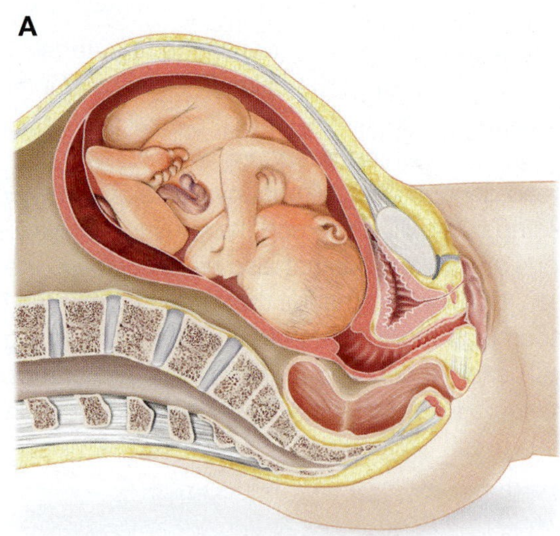

DILATION STAGE:
Uterine contractions dilate cervix

B

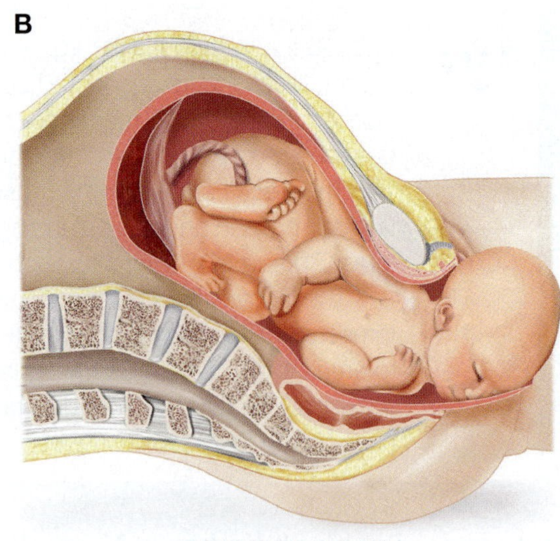

EXPULSION STAGE:
Birth of baby or expulsion

C

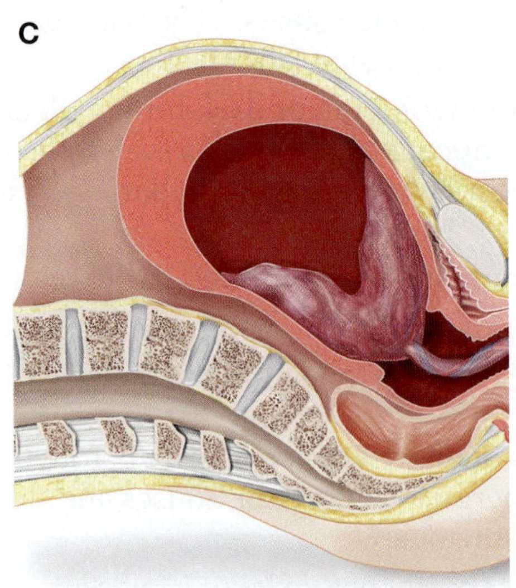

PLACENTAL STAGE:
Delivery of placenta

Figure 17.14 Three stages of labor and delivery.

It also functions as an excretory, respiratory, and endocrine organ, which produces human chorionic gonadotropin (hCG). The placenta consists of a fetal portion and a maternal portion. The fetal portion has a shiny, slightly grayish appearance and is formed by a coming together of chorionic villi in which the umbilical vein and arteries intertwine to form the **umbilical cord**. The maternal portion develops from the decidua basalis of the uterus. It has a red, beefy-looking appearance. The mature placenta is 15–18 centimeters (cm) (6–7 inches) in diameter and weighs approximately 450 grams (about 1 pound). When expelled following parturition, it is known as the **afterbirth**.

fyi The newborn baby usually has a cone-shaped or molded head due to its journey down the birth canal. It is covered with **vernix caseosa**, a protective cheesy substance that covers the fetus during intrauterine life. The baby will present with **lanugo**, fine downy hair that covers the body, especially the shoulders, back, forehead, and temple. The external **genitalia**, the male or female reproductive organs, are usually enlarged.

The time it takes to deliver the placenta is anywhere from 5 to 30 minutes. The placenta is expelled in one of two ways: the **Schultze mechanism**, with the fetal surface presenting, or the **Duncan mechanism** presenting the maternal surface. The placenta is examined to be certain that all of it has been expelled. Any small portion of the placenta that remains in the uterus could interfere with uterine contractions after the birth of the baby and contribute to infection. To control bleeding from the vessels that supplied the placenta during pregnancy, the uterus must contract and remain contracted after placental expulsion.

NEWBORN ASSESSMENT

The first assessment of the newborn involves using the Apgar score. It is performed immediately following the birth of the baby. This method was developed by Virginia Apgar (U.S. anesthesiologist, 1909–1974) as the first objective evaluation of newborns in 1952 and since then, the Apgar score has become the standard tool for assessing newborns. The five assessments of the Apgar score are a mnemonic based on Virginia's last name. Ratings are based on **A**ppearance (color), **P**ulse (heartbeat), **G**rimace (reflex), **A**ctivity (muscle tone), and **R**espiration (breathing). The score is taken at 1 and 5 minutes after birth, the high score being 10 and the low score being 1. See Table 17.2.

Table 17.2 The Apgar Score

Sign	0	1	2
Heart rate	Absent	Less than 100/min	More than 100/min
Respiratory effort	Absent	Slow, irregular	Regular or crying
Reflex irritability	No response	Grimace, frown	Cry, cough
Muscle tone	Limp	Some motion, some flexion of extremities, some resistance to extension of extremities	Active, spontaneous flexion, good tone
Color	Cyanotic or pale	Body pink, extremities cyanotic	Completely pink or good color; no cyanosis

Study and Review I

Anatomy and Physiology

Write your answers to the following questions.

1. List the primary and accessory sex organs of the female reproductive system.

   a. ______________________ b. ______________________

   c. ______________________ d. ______________________

   e. ______________________ f. ______________________

2. The normal position of the uterus is known as ______________________.

3. Define fundus.______________________.

4. Name the three layers of the uterine wall.

   a. ______________________ b. ______________________

   c. ______________________

5. State two primary functions associated with the uterus.

   a. ______________________

   b. ______________________

6. Define the following terms.

   a. Retroflexion ______________________

   ____

   b. Anteversion ______________________

   ____

   c. Retroversion ______________________

   ____

7. The fallopian tubes are also called the ______________ ______________ or ______________.

8. Should the ovum become impregnated by a spermatozoon while in the fallopian tube, the process of ______________ occurs.

9. State the two functions of the ovary.

a. ______________________________ **b.** ______________________________

10. State the three functions of the vagina.

a. ______________________________ **b.** ______________________________

c. ______________________________

11. The breasts or ________________________ ___________________ are compound alveolar structures.

12. The ___________________ is the dark pigmented area found in the skin over each breast, and the ___________________ is the elevated area in its center.

13. Define colostrum. ____

____

14. Name the three phases of the menstrual cycle.

a. ______________________________ **b.** ______________________________

c. ______________________________

Overview of Obstetrics

Write your answers to the following questions.

1. _________________________ is the branch of medicine that pertains to the care of women during pregnancy, childbirth, and the postpartum period.

2. _________________________ is the process in which a sperm penetrates an ovum.

3. The fertilized ovum is also known as a _________________________.

4. As the blastocyst develops, it forms a structure with two cavities, the _________________________ and _________________________.

5. Pregnancy is divided into four stages. Describe each of these stages.

a. Prenatal stage ____

b. Labor ____

c. Parturition ____

d. Postpartum period ____

6. Labor is divided into three stages. Describe each of these stages.

a. First stage ______________________________

b. Second stage ______________________________

c. Third stage ______________________________

ANATOMY LABELING

Identify the structures shown below by filling in the blanks.

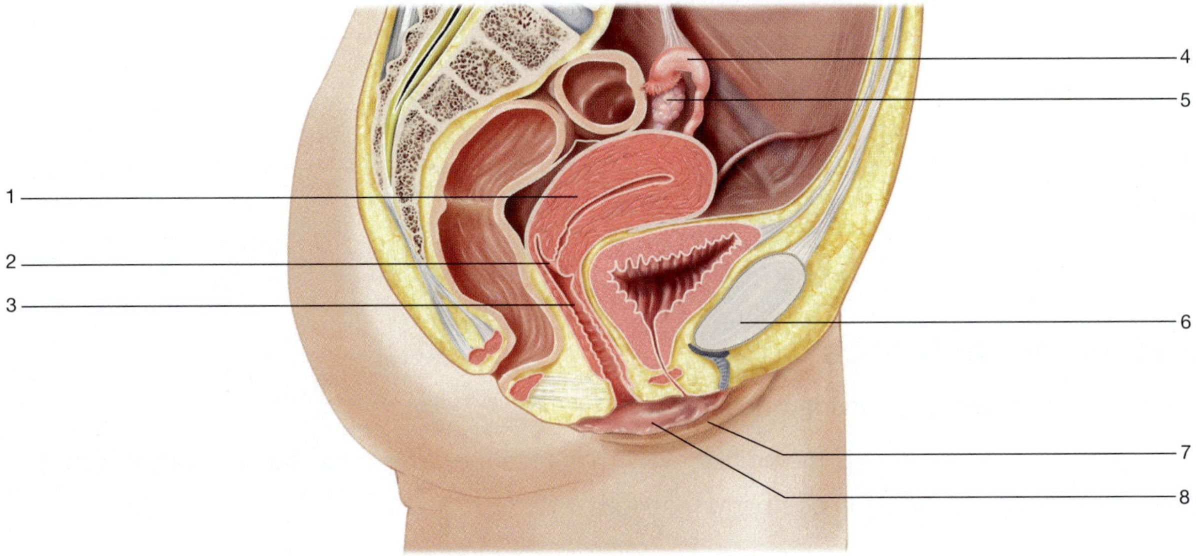

1 ______________________________
2 ______________________________
3 ______________________________
4 ______________________________
5 ______________________________
6 ______________________________
7 ______________________________
8 ______________________________

Building Your Medical Vocabulary

This section provides the foundation for learning medical terminology. Review the following alphabetized word list. Note how common prefixes and suffixes are repeatedly applied to word roots and combining forms to create different meanings. The word parts are color-coded: prefixes are yellow, suffixes are blue, roots/combining forms are red. A combining form is a word root plus a vowel. The chart below lists the combining forms for the word roots in this chapter and can help to strengthen your understanding of how medical words are built and spelled.

Remember These Guidelines

1. If the suffix begins with a vowel, drop the combining vowel from the combining form and add the suffix. For example, abort/o (*to miscarry*) + -ion (*process*) becomes abortion.
2. If the suffix begins with a consonant, keep the combining vowel and add the suffix to the combining form. For example, colp/o (*vagina*) + -scope (*instrument for examining*) becomes colposcope.

You will find that some terms have not been divided into word parts. These are common words or specialized terms that are included to enhance your medical vocabulary.

Combining Forms of the Female Reproductive System

abort/o	to miscarry	**metr/o**	womb, uterus
cervic/o	cervix, neck	**my/o**	muscle
coit/o	a coming together	**o/o**	ovum, egg
colp/o	vagina	**oophor/o**	ovary
culd/o	cul-de-sac	**pareun/o**	lying beside, sexual intercourse
cyst/o	bladder		
fibr/o	fibrous tissue	**rect/o**	rectum
gynec/o	female	**salping/o**	fallopian tube
hyster/o	womb, uterus	**uter/o**	uterus
mamm/o	breast	**vagin/o**	vagina
mast/o	breast	**vers/o**	turning
men/o	month, menses, menstruation		

Medical Word	Word Parts		Definition
	Part	Meaning	
abortion (AB) (ă-bōr´ shŭn)	abort -ion	to miscarry process	Process of miscarrying (either spontaneous or induced); termination of the pregnancy before the fetus is viable (capable of living outside of the uterus). Treatment during or after a miscarriage includes measures to prevent hemorrhage and infection. With any type of miscarriage, the patient should see her healthcare provider as soon as possible. If the abortion is incomplete and not all tissue has been expelled, a dilation and curettage (D&C), which is an expansion of the cervical canal and scraping of the uterine wall, is usually performed.

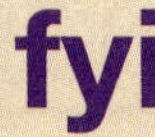

The risk for spontaneous abortion is higher in women over age 35, in women with systemic diseases such as diabetes mellitus or thyroid conditions, and in women with a history of three or more prior spontaneous abortions. The types of spontaneous abortions or miscarriages include the following:

Threatened. Uterine bleeding or spotting is accompanied by cramping or low-back pain. The cervix is not dilated. See Figure 17.15A.

Imminent or inevitable. Uterine bleeding or spotting is accompanied by cramping or low-back pain. The cervix is dilated. Miscarriage is inevitable when there is dilation or effacement of the cervix or rupture of the membranes. See Figure 17.15B.

Incomplete. Some products of conception have been expelled, but some remain in the uterus. Bleeding and cramps may persist when the miscarriage is not complete. See Figure 17.15C.

Complete. All of the products of conception are expelled. A completed miscarriage can be confirmed by an ultrasound.

Missed. A pregnancy demise in which nothing is expelled. It is not known why this occurs. Signs of this would be a loss of pregnancy symptoms and the absence of fetal heart tones.

Recurrent miscarriage (RM). Defined as three or more consecutive first-trimester miscarriages. Also referred to as *habitual abortion.*

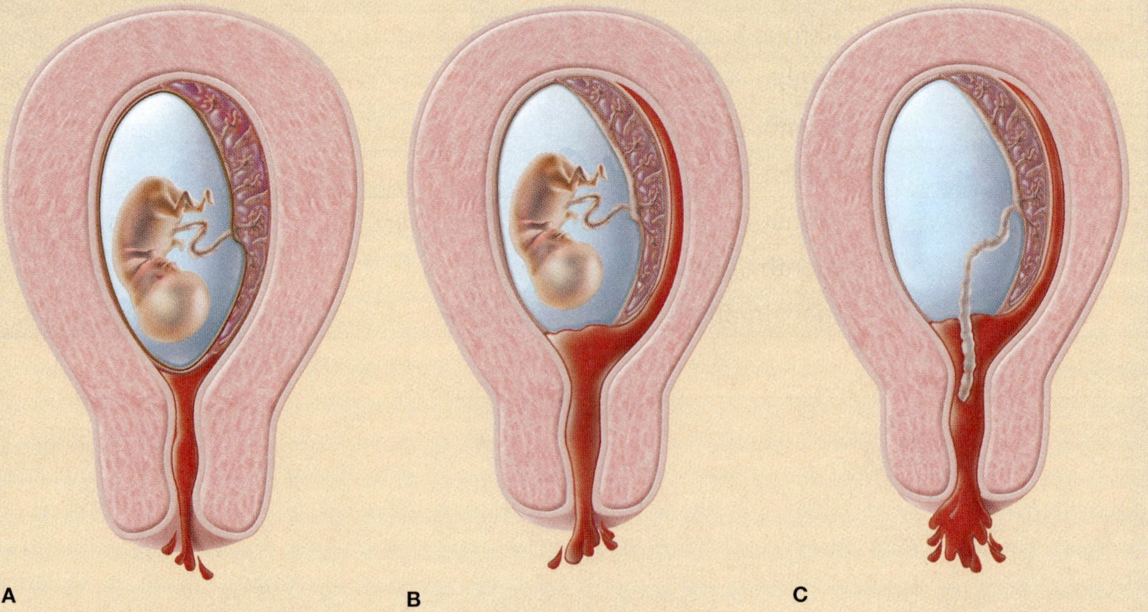

Figure 17.15 Types of spontaneous abortion. (A) Threatened: The cervix is not dilated, and the placenta is still attached to the uterine wall, but some bleeding occurs. (B) Imminent: The placenta has separated from the uterine wall, the cervix has dilated, and the amount of bleeding has increased. (C) Incomplete: The embryo or fetus has passed out of the uterus; however, the placenta remains.

Medical Word	Word Parts		Definition
	Part	**Meaning**	
adnexa (ăd-nĕk´ să)			Accessory parts of a structure; *adnexa uteri* refers to the ovaries and fallopian tubes
amenorrhea (ă-mĕn″ ō-rē´ ă)	a- men/o -rrhea	lack of month, menses, menstruation flow	Lack of the monthly flow (menses or menstruation)
bartholinitis (băr″ tō-lĭn-ī´ tĭs)	bartholin -itis	Bartholin glands inflammation	Inflammation of Bartholin glands. To check for swelling, redness, or tenderness, a Bartholin gland is palpated at the posterior labia majora.
cervicitis (sĕr-vĭ-sī´ tĭs)	cervic -itis	cervix inflammation	Inflammation of the uterine cervix
cesarean section (CS, C-section)			Delivery of the fetus by means of an incision through the abdominal cavity and then into the uterus. Elective C-section is indicated for known cephalopelvic (head to pelvis) disproportion, malpresentations, and active herpes infection. Fetal distress is the most common cause for an emergency C-section.
colposcope (kŏl´ pō-skōp)	colp/o -scope	vagina instrument for examining	Medical instrument used to examine the vagina and cervix by means of a magnifying lens

RULE REMINDER

This term keeps the combining vowel ***o*** because the suffix begins with a consonant.

Medical Word	Part	Meaning	Definition
contraception (kŏn″ tră-sĕp´ shŭn)	contra- cept -ion	against receive process	Process of preventing conception
culdocentesis (kŭl″ dō-sĕn-tē´ sĭs)	culd/o -centesis	cul-de-sac surgical puncture	Surgical puncture of the cul-de-sac for removal of fluid
cystocele (sĭs´ tō-sēl)	cyst/o -cele	bladder hernia	Hernia of the bladder that protrudes into the vagina

Medical Word	Word Parts		Definition
	Part	**Meaning**	
Doppler ultrasound (dŏp′ lĕr ŭl′ trăh-sownd)			Procedure using an audio transformation of high-frequency sounds to monitor the fetal heartbeat (FHB). See Figure 17.16.
dysmenorrhea (dĭs″ mĕn-ō-rē′ ă)	dys- men/o -rrhea	difficult, painful month, menses, menstruation flow	Difficult or painful monthly flow (menses or menstruation)
dyspareunia (dĭs″ pă-rū′ nĭ-ă)	dys- pareun -ia	difficult, painful lying beside, sexual intercourse condition	Difficult or painful sexual intercourse (copulation)
eclampsia (ĕ-klămp′ sē-ă)	ec- lamp(s) -ia	out to shine condition	Complication of severe preeclampsia that involves seizures; also known as *toxemia* or *pregnancy-induced hypertension (PIH)*

Figure 17.16 The fetal heartbeat (FHB) can be monitored with a Doppler device.
(© Artur Steinhagen/Fotolia)

Medical Word	Word Parts: Part	Word Parts: Meaning	Definition
ectopic pregnancy (ĕk-tŏp´ ĭk prĕg´năn-sē)			A pregnancy that occurs when the fertilized egg is implanted in one of various sites, the most common being a fallopian tube; also referred to as a *tubal pregnancy*. See Figure 17.17. This type of pregnancy is life threatening to the mother and almost always fatal to her fetus.

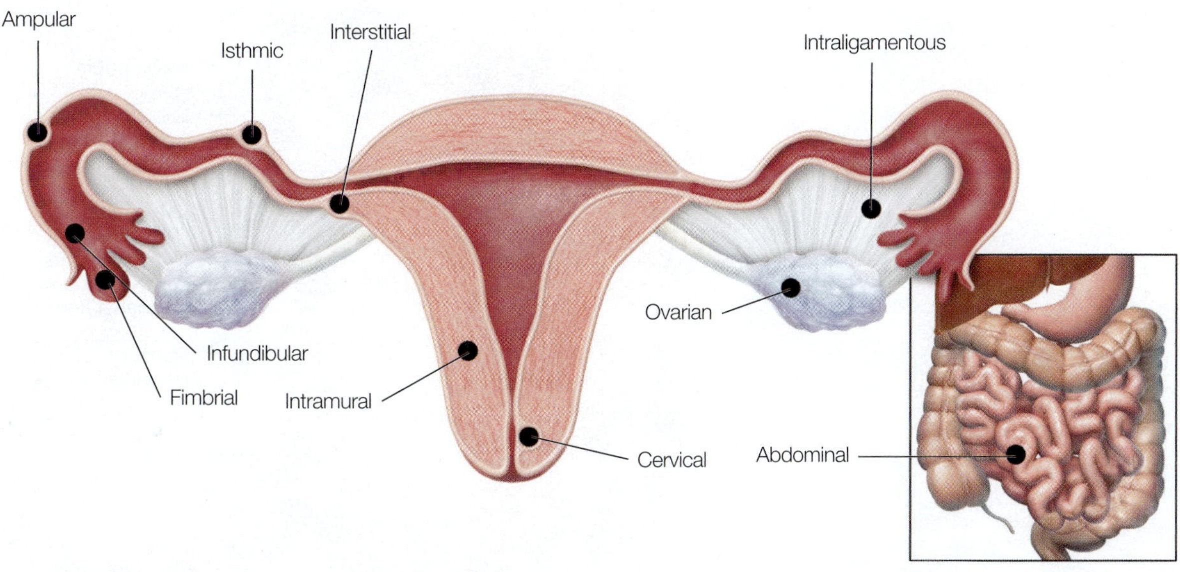

Figure 17.17 Various implantation sites in ectopic pregnancy. The most common site is within the fallopian tube, hence the term *tubal pregnancy*.

Medical Word	Word Parts: Part	Word Parts: Meaning	Definition
endometriosis (ĕn˝ dō-mē˝ trĭ-ō´ sĭs)	endo- metr/i -osis	within uterus condition	Pathological condition in which endometrial tissue has been displaced to various sites in the abdominal or pelvic cavity. This tissue responds to cyclic hormonal signals. Because it is outside the uterus and cannot be cast off each month, the tissue causes bleeding, with the formation of scars and adhesions. This is generally what causes daily or monthly cyclic pain.
fibroma (fī-brō´ mă)	fibr -oma	fibrous tissue tumor	Fibrous tissue tumor; also called *fibroid tumor*, the most common benign tumor found in women. See *uterine fibroid*.

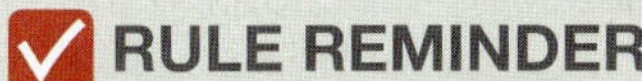

RULE REMINDER

The ***o*** has been removed from the combining form because the suffix begins with a vowel.

Medical Word	Word Parts		Definition
	Part	Meaning	
genitalia (jĕn-ĭ-tăl´ ĭ-ă)	genital -ia	belonging to birth condition	Male or female reproductive organs. See Figure 17.18.

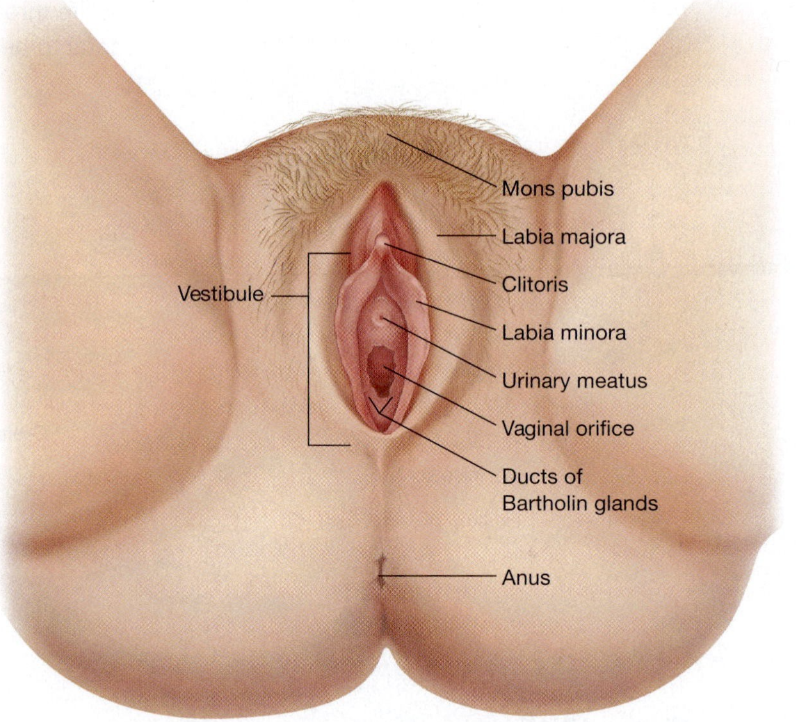

Figure 17.18 External female genitalia (vulva).

Medical Word	Part	Meaning	Definition
gravida (grăv´ ĭ-dă)			Refers to any pregnancy, regardless of duration, including the present one; when used in the recording of an obstetrical history, indicates the number of pregnancies, for example, **nulligravida** refers to a woman who has never been pregnant and is written as gravida 0, **primigravida** refers to a woman who is pregnant for the first time and is written as gravida 1, **multigravida** refers to a woman who has been pregnant more than once and is written as gravida 2 (3, 4, 5, etc.).
group B streptococcus (GBS) (strĕp˝ tō-kŏk´ ŭs)			Type of bacterium commonly found in the vagina and intestinal tract; found in 10%–25% of all pregnant women; it can cause life-threatening infections in the newborn
gynecologist (gī˝ nĕ-kōl´ ō-jĭst)	gynec/o log -ist	female study of one who specializes	Physician who specializes in the study of the female, especially the diseases of the female reproductive organs and the breasts
gynecology (GYN) (gī˝ nĕ-kōl´ ō-jē)	gynec/o -logy	female study of	Study of the female, especially the diseases of the female reproductive organs and the breasts

Medical Word	Word Parts		Definition
	Part	**Meaning**	
hymenectomy (hī″ mĕn-ĕk′ tō-mē)	hymen -ectomy	hymen surgical excision	Surgical excision of the membranous fold of tissue (the hymen) that partially or completely covers the vaginal opening
hysterectomy (hĭs″ tĕr-ĕk′ tō-mē)	hyster -ectomy	womb, uterus surgical excision	Surgical excision of the uterus

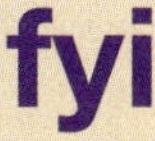

When the entire uterus, including the cervix, fallopian tubes, and ovaries, is removed during a hysterectomy, it is referred to as *total abdominal hysterectomy with bilateral salpingo-oophorectomy (TAH-BSO)*. If a woman has not yet reached menopause, a hysterectomy stops menstruation (monthly periods), and ends her ability to become pregnant. This is referred to as *surgical menopause*.

Medical Word	Part	Meaning	Definition
hysteroscope (hĭs′ tĕr-ō-skōp)	hyster/o -scope	womb, uterus instrument for examining	Instrument used in the biopsy of uterine tissue before 12 weeks of gestation. This tissue is then analyzed for chromosome arrangement, DNA sequence, and genetic defects.
hysterotomy (hĭs″ tĕr-ŏt′ ō-mē)	hyster/o -tomy	womb, uterus incision	Incision into the uterus, commonly combined with a laparotomy (surgical incision into the abdomen) during a cesarean section
intrauterine (ĭn′ tră-ū′ tĕr-ĭn)	intra- uter -ine	within uterus pertaining to	Pertaining to within the uterus
laser ablation (lā′ zĕr ăb-lā′ shŭn)			Procedure that uses a laser to destroy the uterine lining; may also be called *endometrial ablation*. A biopsy is performed before the procedure to make sure no cancer is present. This procedure can be used to reduce excessive menstrual bleeding. It causes sterility.

Medical Word	Word Parts		Definition
	Part	Meaning	
linea nigra (lĭn´ ē-ă nī´ gră)			Dark line on the abdomen that runs from above the umbilicus to the pubis during pregnancy. See Figure 17.19.

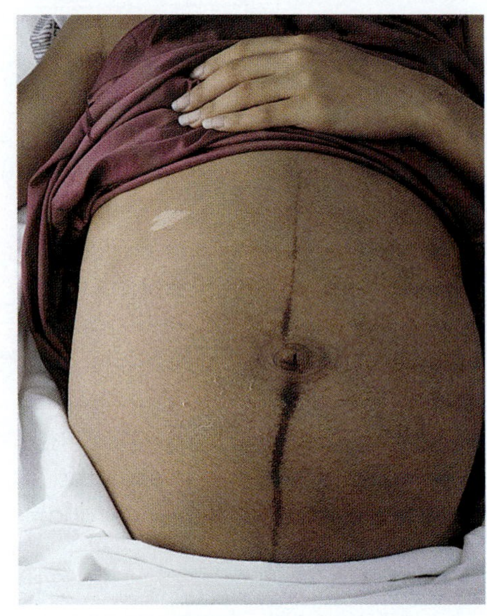

Figure 17.19 Linea nigra.
Source: Pearson Education, Inc.

Medical Word	Part	Meaning	Definition
lochia (lō´ kē-ă)			Vaginal discharge occurring after childbirth. At first it is blood-tinged (*lochia rubra*); then, after three or four days, it becomes pink and brown-tinged (*lochia serosa*); after that, it becomes yellow and then turns to white (*lochia alba*). Lochia typically last 2–4 weeks.
lumpectomy (lŭm-pĕk´ tō-mē)	lump -ectomy	lump surgical excision	Surgical removal of a tumor from the breast. This procedure removes only the tumor and some surrounding tissue but no lymph nodes. See Figure 17.20.

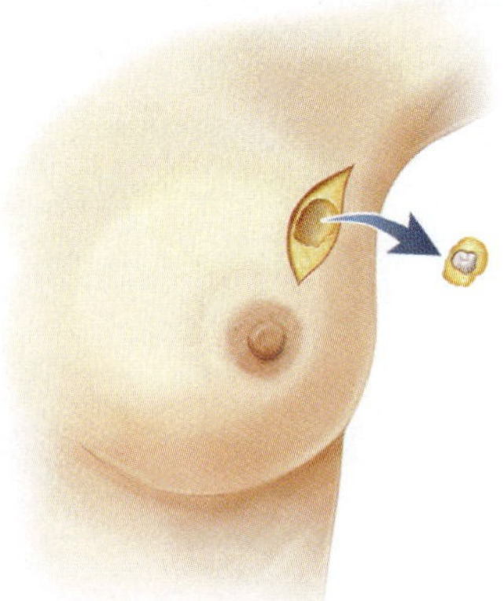

Figure 17.20 A lumpectomy removes only the tumor and a small margin of surrounding tissue.

Medical Word	Word Parts		Definition
	Part	**Meaning**	
mammoplasty (măm´ ō-plăs˝ tē)	mamm/o -plasty	breast surgical repair	Surgical repair of the breast

Rule Reminder

This term keeps the combining vowel ***o*** because the suffix begins with a consonant.

Medical Word	Part	Meaning	Definition
mastectomy (măs-tĕk´ tō-mē)	mast -ectomy	breast surgical excision	Surgical excision of the breast can involve a modified radical or a radical mastectomy. With a modified radical approach, all of the breast tissue and the underarm lymph nodes are removed but the muscles remain intact. See Figure 17.21. In a radical mastectomy (not shown), the chest muscles are removed.

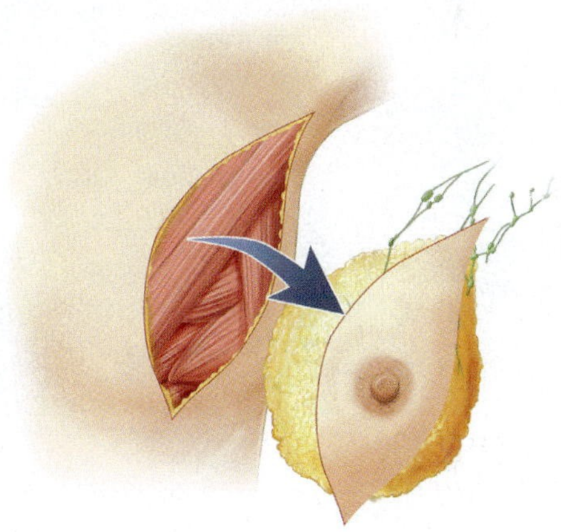

Figure 17.21 A modified radical mastectomy removes all breast tissue and the underarm lymph nodes but leaves the underlying muscles.

Modified radical mastectomy

Medical Word	Word Parts		Definition
	Part	Meaning	
mastitis (măs-tī´ tis)	mast -itis	breast inflammation	Inflammation of the breast that occurs most commonly in women who are breastfeeding. It is caused by bacteria that enter through a crack or abrasion of the nipple. Generalized symptoms include fever, chills, and headache. Localized symptoms include breast pain, redness, tenderness, and swelling. See Figure 17.22.

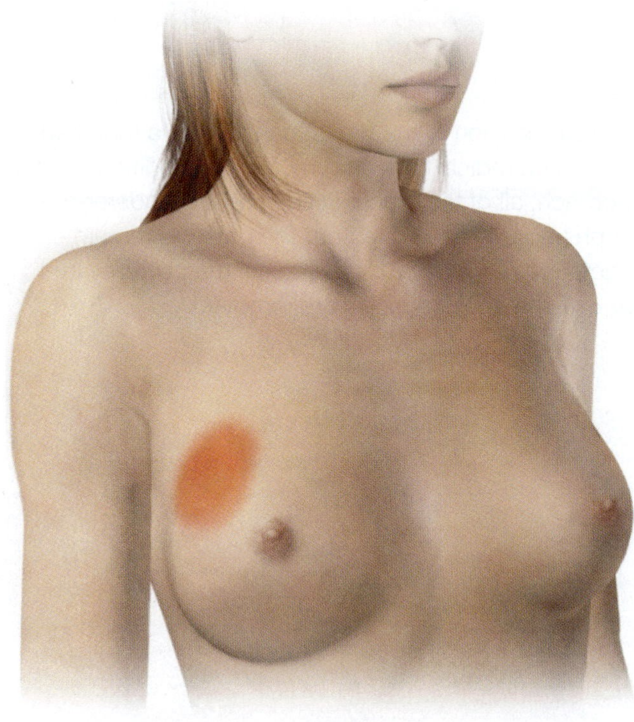

Figure 17.22 Mastitis. Inflammation and swelling are present in the upper outer quadrant of the breast.

insights In ICD-10-CM, the code for mastitis (acute, diffuse, nonpuerperal, subacute, and/or chronic) is N61, which is included in the Inflammatory Disorders of Breast category.

Note: *Diffuse* means to spread, spreading. *Nonpuerperal* means not pertaining to the puerperium (postpartum period). You should have already learned the other terms. If you need to refresh your memory, refer to the Index.

Medical Word	Part	Meaning	Definition
menarche (měn-ar´ kē)	men -arche	month, menses, menstruation beginning	Beginning of the first monthly flow (menses, menstruation)

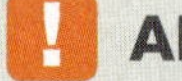 **ALERT!**

How many words can you build using the root **men** and the combining form **men/o**?

Medical Word	Word Parts		Definition
	Part	**Meaning**	
menopause (mĕn´ ō-pawz)	men/o pause	month, menses, menstruation cessation	Cessation of the monthly flow; also called *climacteric*

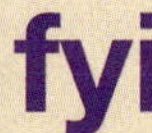

At about 50 years of age, men and women begin experiencing bodily changes that are directly related to **hormonal** production. In women, the ovaries cease to produce estrogen and progesterone. With decreased production of these female hormones, women enter the phase of life known as **menopause**.

The symptoms of menopause vary from being hardly noticeable to being severe and can include irregular periods, hot flashes, vaginal dryness, insomnia, joint pain, headache, mood changes, irritability, and depression. Breast tissue can lose its firmness, and pubic and axillary hair becomes sparse. Without estrogen, the uterus becomes smaller, the vagina shortens, and vaginal tissues become drier. There can be loss of bone mass, leading to **osteoporosis**.

Medical Word	Part	Meaning	Definition
menorrhagia (mĕn″ ō-rā´ jĭ-ă)	men/o -rrhagia	month, menses, menstruation to burst forth	Excessive uterine bleeding at the time of a menstrual period, either in number of days or amount of blood or both. Can be caused by such conditions as uterine fibroid tumors, pelvic inflammatory disease, or an endocrine imbalance.
menorrhea (mĕn″ ō-rē´ă)	men/o -rrhea	month, menses, menstruation flow	Normal monthly flow (menses, menstruation)
mittelschmerz (mĭt´ ĕl-shmārts)			Abdominal pain that occurs midway between the menstrual periods at ovulation
myometritis (mī″ ō-mē-trī´ tĭs)	my/o metr -itis	muscle womb, uterus inflammation	Inflammation of the muscular wall of the uterus
oligomenorrhea (ŏl″ ĭ-gō-mĕn″ ō-rē´ ă)	oligo- men/o -rrhea	scanty month, menses, menstruation flow	Scanty monthly flow (menses, menstruation)
oogenesis (ō″ ō-jĕn´ ĕ-sĭs)	o/o -genesis	ovum, egg formation, produce	Formation of the ovum

Medical Word	Word Parts: Part	Word Parts: Meaning	Definition
oophorectomy (ō″ ŏf-ō-rĕk′ tō-mē)	oophor -ectomy	ovary surgical excision	Surgical excision of an ovary

Rule Reminder

The ***o*** has been removed from the combining form because the suffix begins with a vowel.

Medical Word	Part	Meaning	Definition
ovulation (ŏv″ ū-lā′ shŭn)	ovulat -ion	little egg process	Process in which an ovum is discharged from the cortex of the ovary; periodic ripening and rupture of a mature graafian follicle and the discharge of an ovum from the cortex of the ovary. Occurs approximately 14 days before the onset of the next menstrual period. See Figure 17.23.

Primary follicle | Secondary follicle | Vesicular follicle | Ovulation | Corpus luteum | Degenerating corpus luteum

Follicular phase | Ovulation (Day 14) | Luteal phase

Ovarian cycle

Figure 17.23 Changes in the ovarian follicle during the 28-day ovarian cycle.

Medical Word	Part	Meaning	Definition
para			Means to bear or bring forth; refers to a woman who has given birth after a minimum of 20 weeks' gestation, regardless of whether the infant is born alive or dead

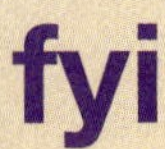

When recording an obstetrical history, *para* is used to indicate the number of births. For example, **multipara** refers to a woman who has given birth to two or more children and is written as Para 2 (3, 4, 5, etc.); **nullipara** refers to a woman who has not given birth after more than 20 weeks of gestation and is written as Para 0; and **primipara** refers to a woman who has had one birth at more than 20 weeks' gestation, regardless of whether the infant was born alive or dead, and is written as Para 1.

Medical Word	Part	Meaning	Definition
pelvic inflammatory disease (PID) (pĕl′ vĭk ĭn-flăm′ ă-tōr″ ē)			Infection of the upper genital area; can affect the uterus, ovaries, and fallopian tubes

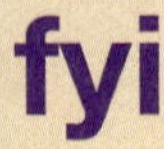

Pelvic inflammatory disease (PID) is the most common and serious complication of sexually transmitted infections (STIs) among women. This infection of the upper genital area occurs when disease-causing organisms migrate upward from the vagina and cervix into the upper genital area. If untreated, it can cause scarring, which can lead to infertility, tubal pregnancy, chronic pelvic pain, and other serious consequences. Infertility occurs in approximately 20% of women who have had PID.

Medical Word	Part	Meaning	Definition
perimenopause (pĕr-ĭ-mĕn′ ō-pawz)	peri- men/o pause	around month, menses, menstruation cessation	Period of gradual changes that lead into menopause, affecting a woman's hormones, body, and feelings. It can be a stop–start process that can take months or years. Hormone levels fluctuate, thereby causing changes in the menstrual cycle, which becomes irregular.

Medical Word	Word Parts		Definition
	Part	**Meaning**	
placenta previa (plă-sĕn´ tă prē´ vē-ă)			In this condition, the placenta is improperly implanted in the lower uterine segment. The fetus receives less oxygen and the expectant mother has an increased risk of hemorrhage and infection. Placenta previa is classified as one of four degrees (Figure 17.24): **i. Low-lying placenta.** The placenta is implanted in the lower segment but does not reach the internal os, although it is in close proximity to it. **ii. Marginal placenta previa.** The edge of the placenta is at the margin of the internal os. **iii. Partial placenta previa.** The placenta partially covers the internal os. **iv. Total placenta previa.** The placenta completely covers the internal os.

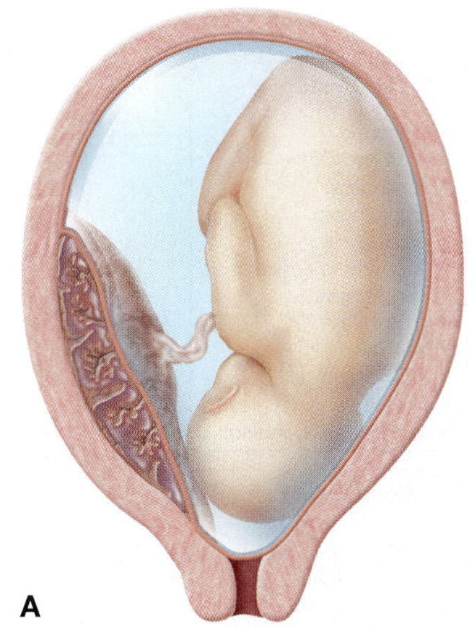

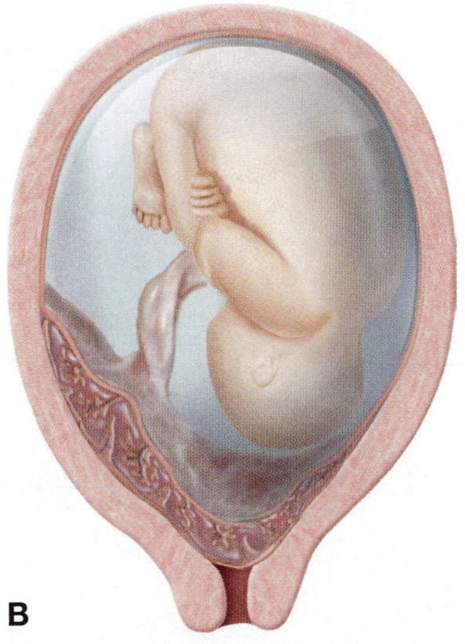

Figure 17.24 Placenta previa. (A) Low placental implantation. (B) Total placenta previa.

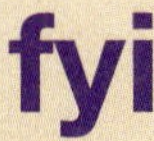

The most common symptom of placenta previa is painless uterine bleeding during the second half of pregnancy. Bleeding can be scanty or profuse (hemorrhage). When this occurs, the expectant mother is advised to go to the hospital.

To determine a diagnosis, a transabdominal ultrasound examination is performed to pinpoint the placenta's location. A vaginal examination is usually avoided because it could trigger heavy bleeding. A woman who has been diagnosed with placenta previa may need to stay in the hospital until delivery. If the bleeding stops, as it often does, her physician continues to monitor the expectant mother and her baby.

Medical Word	Part	Meaning	Definition
postcoital (pōst-kō´ ĭt-ăl)	post- coit -al	after a coming together pertaining to	Pertaining to after sexual intercourse

Medical Word	Word Parts		Definition
	Part	**Meaning**	
preeclampsia (prē″ ĕ-klămp′ sē-ă)	pre- ec- lamp(s) -ia	before out to shine condition	Serious complication of pregnancy characterized by increasing hypertension, proteinuria (abnormal concentrations of urinary protein), and edema, also known as *toxemia* or *pregnancy-induced hypertension (PIH)*
premenstrual syndrome (PMS) (prē-mĕn′ stroo-ăl)			Condition that affects certain women and can cause distressful symptoms that begin 2 weeks before the onset of menstruation. The cause is unknown but may be due to the amount of prostaglandin produced, a deficient or excessive amount of estrogen or progesterone, or an interrelationship between these factors. The multisystem effects of premenstrual syndrome are presented in Figure 17.25.

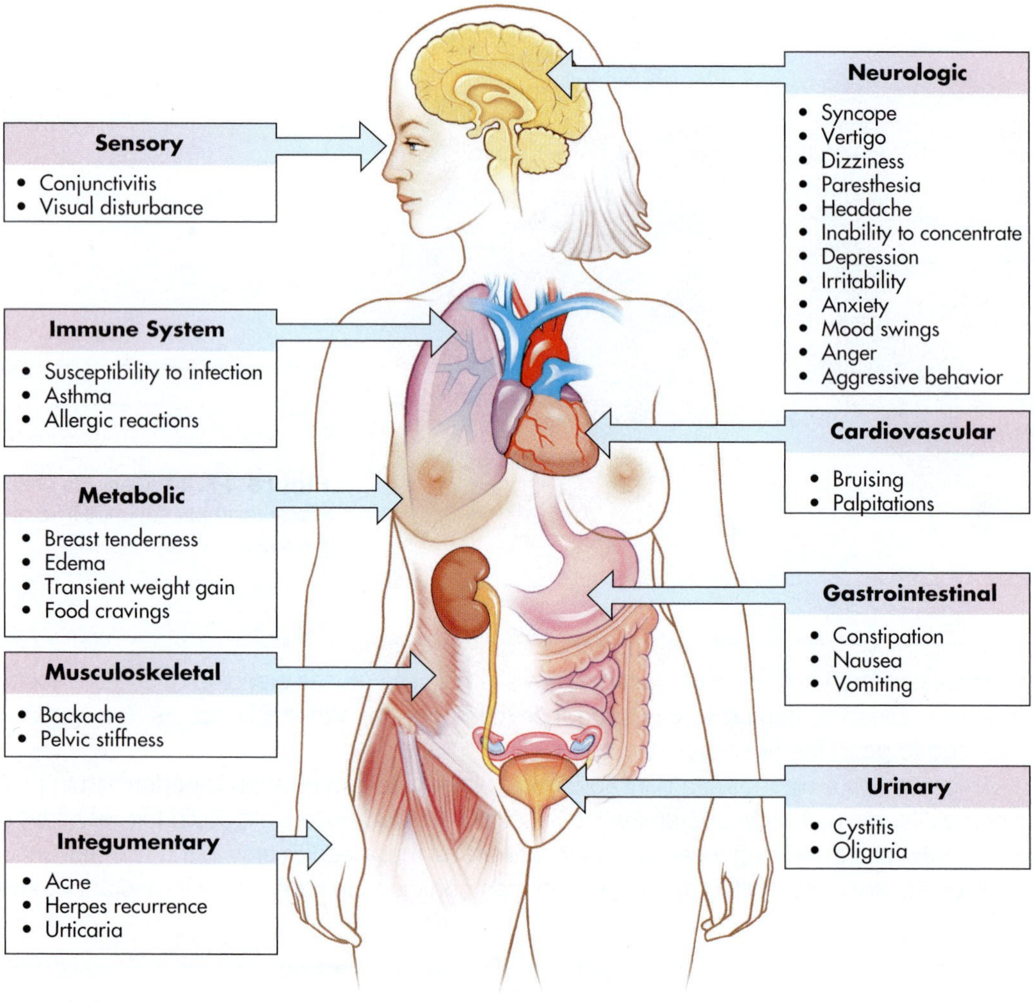

Figure 17.25 Multisystem effects of premenstrual syndrome.

Medical Word	Word Parts		Definition
	Part	**Meaning**	
rectovaginal (rĕk″ tō-văj′ ĭ-năl)	rect/o vagin -al	rectum vagina pertaining to	Pertaining to the rectum and vagina
retroversion (rĕt″ rō-vur′ shĭn)	retro- vers -ion	backward turning process	Process of being turned backward, such as the displacement of the uterus with the cervix pointed forward. See Figure 17.4A.
salpingectomy (săl″ pĭn-jĕk′ tō-mē)	salping -ectomy	fallopian tube surgical excision	Surgical excision of a fallopian tube
salpingitis (săl″ pĭn-jī′ tĭs)	salping -itis	fallopian tube inflammation	Inflammation of a fallopian tube
salpingo-oophorectomy (săl′ pĭng″ gō-ō″ ŏf-ō- rĕk′ tō-mē)	salping/o oophor -ectomy	fallopian tube ovary surgical excision	Surgical excision of an ovary and a fallopian tube
toxic shock syndrome (TSS)			A serious bacterial infection caused by *staphylococcus aureus* bacteria. Symptoms of TSS start suddenly with vomiting, high fever (temperature at least 102°F [38.8°C]), a rapid drop in blood pressure (with lightheadedness or fainting), watery diarrhea, headache, sore throat, and muscle aches.

Medical Word	Word Parts: Part	Word Parts: Meaning	Definition
uterine fibroid (ū´ tĕr-ĭn fī-broyd)	uter -ine fibr -oid	uterus pertaining to fibrous tissue resemble	Benign fibrous tumor of the uterus made up of muscle cells and other tissues that grow within the wall of the uterus; the most common benign tumors in women of childbearing age; also called *uterine leiomyoma*. Fibroids are classified into three groups based on where they grow, such as just underneath the lining of the uterus, between the muscles of the uterus, or on the outside of the uterus. Most fibroids grow within the wall of the uterus, and some grow on stalks (called *peduncles*) that grow out from the surface of the uterus or into the cavity of the uterus. See Figure 17.26.

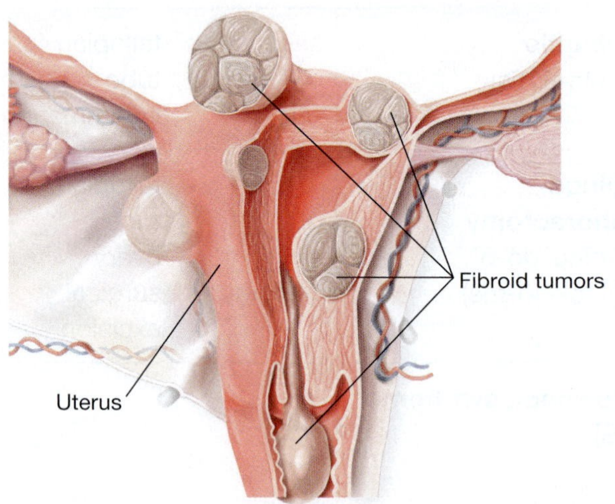

Figure 17.26 Types of uterine fibroid tumors.

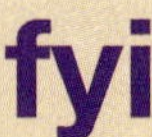

Types of surgery used to treat uterine fibroids include:

- *Dilation and curettage (D&C)* is a procedure that involves enlarging the cervix (dilation) and then scraping (curettage) out portions of the lining of the uterus. It is considered to be minor surgery performed in a hospital, ambulatory surgery center, or clinic.
- *Myomectomy* is a surgery to remove fibroids without taking out the healthy tissue of the uterus. It can be major surgery (with an abdominal incision) or minor surgery. The type, size, and location of the fibroids determine what type of procedure is done.
- *Hysterectomy* is a surgery to remove the uterus and is the only sure way to cure uterine fibroids. This surgery is used when a woman's fibroids are large or if she has heavy bleeding and is either near or past menopause and/or does not want to become pregnant in the future.

Medical Word	Part	Meaning	Definition
vaginitis (văj˝ ĭn-ī´ tĭs)	vagin -itis	vagina inflammation	Inflammation of the vagina

Study and Review II

Word Parts

Prefixes

Give the definitions of the following prefixes.

1. a- ______________________
2. contra- ______________________
3. dys- ______________________
4. ec- ______________________
5. endo- ______________________
6. intra- ______________________
7. oligo- ______________________
8. peri- ______________________
9. post- ______________________
10. retro- ______________________
11. pre- ______________________

Combining Forms

Give the definitions of the following combining forms.

1. abort/o ______________________
2. cervic/o ______________________
3. coit/o ______________________
4. colp/o ______________________
5. culd/o ______________________
6. cyst/o ______________________
7. fibr/o ______________________
8. gynec/o ______________________
9. hyster/o ______________________
10. mamm/o ______________________
11. mast/o ______________________
12. men/o ______________________
13. metr/o ______________________
14. my/o ______________________
15. o/o ______________________
16. oophor/o ______________________
17. pareun/o ______________________
18. rect/o ______________________
19. salping/o ______________________
20. uter/o ______________________
21. vagin/o ______________________
22. vers/o ______________________

Suffixes

Give the definitions of the following suffixes.

1. -al ________________
2. -arche ________________
3. -cele ________________
4. -centesis ________________
5. -ectomy ________________
6. -genesis ________________
7. -ia ________________
8. -ine ________________
9. -ion ________________
10. -ist ________________
11. -itis ________________
12. -oma ________________
13. -osis ________________
14. -plasty ________________
15. -rrhagia ________________
16. -rrhea ________________
17. -scope ________________
18. -oid ________________

Identifying Medical Terms

In the spaces provided, write the medical terms for the following meanings.

1. ________________ Inflammation of the uterine cervix
2. ________________ Difficult or painful monthly flow
3. ________________ Fibrous tissue tumor
4. ________________ Study of the female
5. ________________ Surgical excision of the hymen
6. ________________ Surgical repair of the breast
7. ________________ Normal monthly flow
8. ________________ Formation of the ovum
9. ________________ Difficult or painful sexual intercourse
10. ________________ Male or female reproductive organs

Matching

Select the appropriate lettered meaning for each of the following words.

______	**1.** laser ablation	**a.** Beginning of the first monthly flow (menses, menstruation)
______	**2.** lumpectomy	**b.** Surgical removal of a tumor from the breast
______	**3.** menarche	**c.** Abdominal pain that occurs midway between the menstrual periods at ovulation
______	**4.** mittelschmerz	**d.** Process in which an ovum is discharged from the cortex of the ovary
______	**5.** ovulation	**e.** Procedure that uses a laser to destroy the uterine lining
______	**6.** gynecologist	**f.** Pertaining to the rectum and vagina
______	**7.** contraception	**g.** Period of gradual changes that lead into menopause
______	**8.** perimenopause	**h.** Physician who specializes in the study of the female
______	**9.** hysterotomy	**i.** Incision into the uterus
______	**10.** rectovaginal	**j.** Process of preventing conception
		k. Lack of monthly flow (menses, menstruation)

Medical Case Snapshots

This learning activity provides an opportunity to relate the medical terminology you are learning to a precise patient case presentation. In the spaces provided, write in your answers.

Case 1

A pregnant 36-year-old woman calls her obstetrician's office, stating, "I am passing bright-red blood and I am cramping. Please tell me what to do. I don't want to lose my baby." The woman was advised to immediately come to the doctor's office. A threatened abortion is one with ______ bleeding or spotting accompanied by ______ or low-back pain. The ______ is not dilated.

Case 2

A 21-year-old female is seen in the emergency room. She has missed her last two periods and feels sick. An ultrasound is ordered stat (immediately). The ultrasound confirmed an ______ pregnancy or tubal ______. An ______ or physician specializing in the care of women during pregnancy, childbirth, and the postpartum period is notified of this patient's condition.

Case 3

A 52-year-old female complains of irregular periods (menses), hot flashes, insomnia, difficult or painful sexual intercourse, and moodiness. The medical term for painful sexual intercourse is ______________. Her condition is known as ______________ (or period of gradual changes that lead into menopause).

Drug Highlights

Type of Drug	Description and Examples
female hormones	
estrogens	Natural female sex hormone secreted by the ovarian follicles. Used for a variety of conditions including amenorrhea, dysfunctional uterine bleeding (DUB), and hirsutism as well as in palliative therapy for breast cancer in women and prostatic cancer in men. They are also used as hormone therapy (HT) in the treatment of uncomfortable symptoms that are related to menopause. EXAMPLES: Premarin (conjugated estrogens), estradiol, Estraderm (estradiol) transdermal system, Ogen (estropipate), and Menest (esterified estrogens)
progestogens/progestins	Natural female steroid hormone secreted by the corpus luteum. When produced synthetically, progesterones can be used to prevent uterine bleeding; combined with estrogen they can be used for treatment of amenorrhea. They may be used in cases of infertility and threatened or habitual miscarriage. Progesterone is responsible for changes in the uterine endometrium during the second half of the menstrual cycle, development of maternal placenta after implantation, and development of mammary glands. EXAMPLES: Provera (medroxyprogesterone acetate), norethindrone acetate, and Prometrium (natural progesterone)
contraceptives	
combined oral contraceptives (COCs)	Oral contraceptives (also called *birth control pills*) containing mixtures of estrogen and progestin in various levels of strength that are nearly 100% effective when used as directed. The estrogen in the pill inhibits ovulation, and the progestin inhibits pituitary secretion of luteinizing hormone (LH), causes changes in the cervical mucus that renders it unfavorable to penetration by sperm, and alters the nature of the endometrium. EXAMPLES: Micronor, Brevicon, Lo/Ovral, and Nor-QD
minipill	Another oral contraceptive is the minipill, which contains only progestin. It is taken daily and continuously. It acts by interfering with sperm and ovum transport and by adversely affecting the suitability of the endometrium for ovum implant. EXAMPLES: Nexplanon, Depo-Provera (injectable)

Type of Drug	Description and Examples
birth control patch	Ortho Evra is the first transdermal birth control patch that continuously delivers two synthetic hormones, progestin (norelgestromin) and estrogen (ethinyl estradiol). The patch impedes pregnancy by preventing the ovaries from releasing eggs (ovulation) and thickening the cervical mucus. The patch is applied directly to the skin (buttocks, abdomen, upper torso, or upper outer arm) and has an effectiveness rate of 95%.
injectable	Depo-Provera is an injectable contraceptive that is given four times a year. It contains medroxyprogesterone acetate, a synthetic drug that is similar to progesterone. Depo-Provera prevents pregnancy by stopping the ovaries from releasing eggs (ovulation) and thickens the cervical mucus. When used correctly, it can prevent pregnancy over 99% of the time.
intrauterine device (IUD)	Small device that is placed within the uterus to prevent pregnancy. It is usually made of soft, flexible, ultralight plastic and is 99.2%– 99.9% effective as birth control. Two types are available: ParaGard and Mirena. ParaGard uses copper around the plastic. Anyone allergic to copper should not use it. Mirena releases small amounts of a synthetic progesterone over time and can be left in place for up to 5 years. IUDs do not protect against sexually transmitted infections (STIs) or the human immunodeficiency virus (HIV). See Figure 17.27.

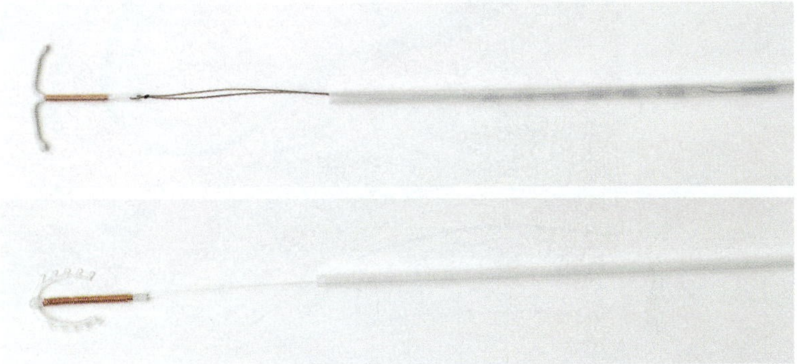

Figure 17.27 Examples of intrauterine devices (IUDs).
(Jules Selmes and Debi Treloar/Dorling Kindersley Limited)

Diagnostic and Laboratory Tests

Test	Description
amniocentesis (ăm″ nĭ-ō -sĕn-tē′ sĭs)	Surgical puncture of the amniotic sac to obtain a sample of amniotic fluid containing fetal cells that are examined. It can be determined whether the fetus has Down syndrome, neural tube defects, Tay–Sachs disease, or other genetic defects. Determines chromosomal abnormalities and biochemical disorders. See Figure 17.28.

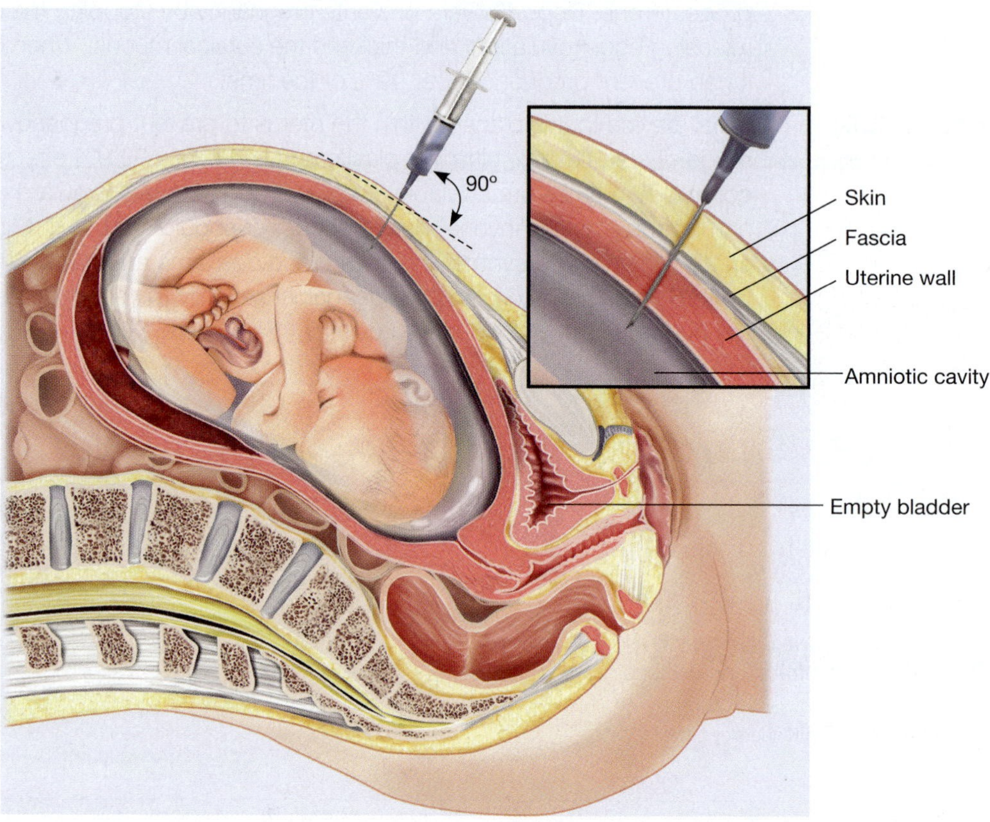

Figure 17.28 Amniocentesis. The woman is usually scanned by ultrasound to determine the placental site and to locate a pocket of fluid. As the needle is inserted, three levels of resistance are felt when the needle penetrates the skin, fascia, and uterine wall. When the needle is placed within the amniotic cavity, amniotic fluid is withdrawn.

Test	Description
blood grouping (A, B, AB, and O)	Determines blood type.
breast examination	Visual inspection and manual examination of the breast for changes in contour, symmetry, dimpling of skin, retraction of the nipple, and the presence of lumps.
chorionic villus sampling (CVS) (kō″ rē-ŏn′ ĭk vĭl′ŭs)	Removal of a small sample of the placenta to determine chromosomal abnormalities and biochemical disorders (Down syndrome, Tay–Sachs disease, and cystic fibrosis). Unlike amniocentesis, CVS does not test for neural tube defects.

Test	Description
colposcopy (kŏl-pŏs′ kō-pē)	Visual examination of the vagina and cervix via a colposcope. Abnormal results can indicate cervical or vaginal erosion, tumors, and dysplasia.
complete blood count	Check for anemia, infection, and cell abnormalities.
cordocentesis (kor-dō-sĕn-tē′sĭs)	Examine blood from the fetus to detect fetal abnormalities (Down syndrome and fetal blood disorders); also known as fetal blood sampling, percutaneous umbilical blood sampling (PUBS), and umbilical vein sampling.
culdoscopy (kŭl-dŏs′ kō-pē)	Direct visual examination of the viscera of the female pelvis through a culdoscope. The instrument is introduced into the pelvic cavity through the posterior vaginal fornix. Can be used to diagnose ectopic pregnancy and to determine the cause of pelvic pain and to check for pelvic masses.
estrogen (es′ trō-jĕn)	Test done on urine or blood serum to determine the level of estrone, estradiol, and estriol.
group B streptococcus (GBS) screening (strĕp″ tō-kŏk′ ŭs)	Screen for vaginal strep B infection. It is to be performed between the 35th and 37th week of pregnancy. Any time other than this will not be significant to show if the expectant mother is carrying GBS during her time of delivery. Note: When the expectant mother tests positive, intravenous antibiotics are recommended during delivery to reduce the chance of the baby becoming infected with GBS.
hematocrit (hē-măt′ ō-krĭt)	Check for anemia during pregnancy.
hemoglobin (hēm″ ō-glō′ bĭn)	Check for anemia during pregnancy.
hepatitis B screen (hĕp″ ă-tī′ tĭs)	Identify carriers of hepatitis.
human chorionic gonadotropin (hCG) (kō″ rē-ŏn-ĭk gŏn″ ă-dō-trō′ pĭn)	Determine the presence of hCG, which is secreted by the placenta. A positive result usually indicates pregnancy.
human immunodeficiency virus (HIV) screen (ĭm″ ū-nō-dĕ-fĭsh′ ĕn-sē)	Identify HIV infection.
hysterosalpingography (HSG) (hĭs″ tĕr-ō -săl″ pĭn-gŏg′ ră-fē)	X-ray of the uterus and fallopian tubes after the injection of a radiopaque substance. Size and structure of the uterus and fallopian tubes can be evaluated. Uterine tumors, fibroids, tubal pregnancy, and tubal occlusion can be observed. Also used for treatment of an occluded fallopian tube.
laparoscopy (lăp-ăr-ŏs′ kō-pē)	Visual examination of the abdominal cavity. A flexible, lighted instrument (laparoscope) is inserted through a periumbilical incision to examine the ovaries and fallopian tubes.

Test	Description
ultrasound (ŭl´ tră-sownd)	Uses during pregnancy include the following: • Confirming viable pregnancy • Confirming fetal heartbeat (FHB) • Measuring the crown–rump length or gestational age of the fetus • Confirming ectopic pregnancy • Confirming molar pregnancy (hydatidiform mole or hydatid mole) • Assessing abnormal gestation • Diagnosing fetal malformation and structural abnormalities • Confirming multiple fetuses • Determining sex of the baby • Identifying placenta location • Confirming intrauterine death • Observing fetal presentation and movements • Identifying uterine and pelvic abnormalities of the mother during pregnancy
urinalysis (ū″ rĭ-năl´ ĭ-sĭs)	Check for infection, renal disease, or diabetes.
wet mount or wet prep	Examination of vaginal discharge for the presence of bacteria and yeast. Vaginal smear is placed on a microscopic slide, wet with normal saline, and then viewed under a microscope by the physician.

Abbreviations

Abbreviation	Meaning
AB	abortion
AFP	alpha-fetoprotein
AROM	artificial rupture of membranes
Ascus	atypical squamous cells of undetermined significance
CDC	Centers for Disease Control and Prevention
CIN	cervical intraepithelial neoplasia
CMV	cytomegalovirus
COCs	combined oral contraceptives
CS, C-section	cesarean section
CVS	chorionic villus sampling
D&C	dilation and curettage
DUB	dysfunctional uterine bleeding
FHB	fetal heartbeat
FSH	follicle-stimulating hormone
GBS	group B streptococcus
GTT	glucose tolerance test
GYN	gynecology
hCG	human chorionic gonadotropin
HIV	human immunodeficiency virus
HSG	hysterosalpingography
HSV	herpes simplex virus
HT	hormone therapy
IUD	intrauterine device
LH	luteinizing hormone
LMP	last menstrual period
NST	nonstress test
OB	obstetrics
OTC	over-the-counter
Pap	Papanicolaou (smear)
PID	pelvic inflammatory disease
PIH	pregnancy-induced hypertension
PMS	premenstrual syndrome
PUBS	percutaneous umbilical blood sampling
STIs	sexually transmitted infections
TAH-BSO	total abdominal hysterectomy with bilateral salpingo-oophorectomy
TORCH	toxoplasmosis, rubella, cytomegalovirus, herpes simplex virus
TSS	toxic shock syndrome
UE	unconjugated estriol
WNL	within normal limits

Study and Review III

Building Medical Terms

Using the following word parts, fill in the blanks to build the correct medical terms.

bartholin	salping	-genesis
hyster	-al	-pause
mast	-centesis	
men/o	-ectomy	

Definition	Medical Term
1. Inflammation of the Bartholin glands	_________itis
2. Surgical puncture of the cul-de-sac for removal of fluid	culdo________
3. Surgical excision of the uterus	______ectomy
4. Surgical removal of a tumor from the breast	lump ________
5. Surgical excision of the breast	_______ectomy
6. Cessation of the monthly flow	meno_________
7. Normal monthly flow (menses, menstruation)	________rrhea
8. Formation of the ovum	oo___________
9. Inflammation of a fallopian tube	_________itis
10. Pertaining to after sexual intercourse	postcoit _______

Combining Form Challenge

Using the combining forms provided, write the medical term correctly.

cervic/o	cyst/o	genital/o
colp/o	fibr/o	gynec/o

1. Inflammation of the uterine cervix: _________ itis
2. Medical instrument used to examine the vagina and cervix: _________scope
3. Hernia of the bladder that protrudes into the vagina: ________cele
4. Fibrous tissue tumor: ________ oma
5. Male or female reproductive organs: ________ ia
6. Study of the female, especially the diseases of the female reproductive organs and the breast: _______ logy

Chapter

18 Male Reproductive System

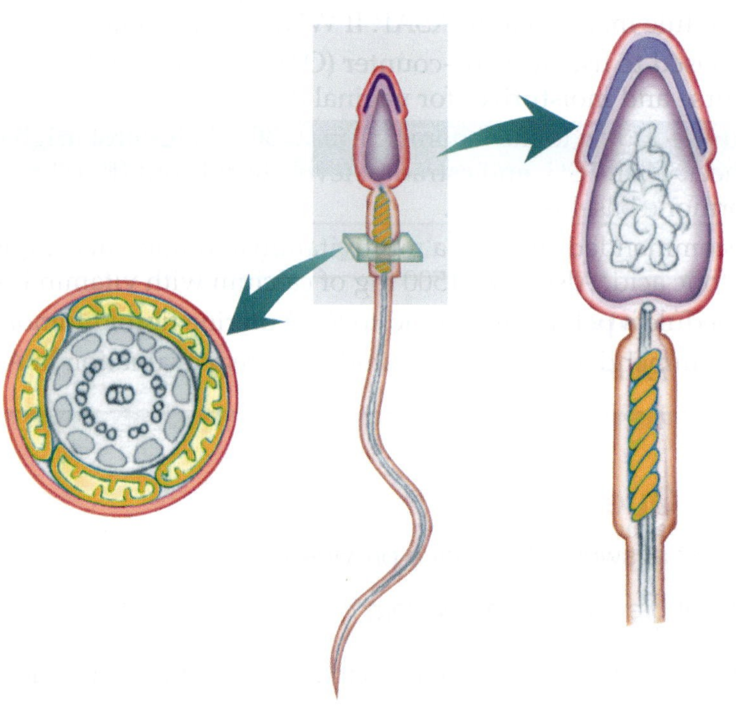

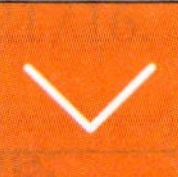

Learning Outcomes

On completion of this chapter, you will be able to:

1. State the description and primary functions of the organs/structures of the male reproductive system.
2. Recognize terminology included in the ICD-10-CM.
3. Analyze, build, spell, and pronounce medical words.
4. Explain the causes, symptoms, and treatments of selected sexually transmitted infections.
5. Comprehend the drugs highlighted in this chapter.
6. Provide the description of diagnostic and laboratory tests related to the male reproductive system.
7. Identify and define selected abbreviations.
8. Apply your acquired knowledge of medical terms by successfully completing the *Practical Application* exercise.

Anatomy and Physiology

The male reproductive system consists of the testes, epididymis, vas deferens, urethra, and the following accessory glands: bulbourethral, prostate, and the seminal vesicles. The supporting structures and accessory sex organs are the scrotum and the penis. The vital function of the male reproductive system is to provide the sperm cells necessary to fertilize the ovum, thereby perpetuating the species. Table 18.1 provides an at-a-glance look at the male reproductive system. See Figure 18.1.

External Organs

In the male, the scrotum, the testes, and the penis are the external organs of reproduction. See Figures 18.1 and 18.2.

Scrotum

The **scrotum** is a pouchlike structure located behind and below the penis. It is suspended from the perineal region and is divided by a septum into two sacs, each containing one of the testes along with its connecting tube called the **epididymis**. Within the tissues of the scrotum are fibers of smooth muscle that contract in the absence of sufficient heat, giving the scrotum a wrinkled appearance. This contractile action brings the testes closer to the perineum where they can absorb sufficient body heat to maintain the viability of the **spermatozoa**. These changes in the scrotum illustrate its primary function, which is to act as a natural climate control center for the testicles.

The temperature in the scrotum is a degree or two lower than the usual body temperature of 98.6°F. The testicles need this lower temperature in order to carry out their job of producing viable sperm. If the testicles are kept at body temperature or higher for

Table 18.1 Male Reproductive System at-a-Glance

Organ/Structure	Primary Functions/Description
Scrotum	Acts as a natural climate control center for the testicles in order to maintain viability of sperm. The temperature in the scrotum is a degree or two lower than the usual body temperature of 98.6°F, which would kill sperm.
Penis	Acts as male organ of copulation and urination; site of the orifice for the elimination of urine and semen from the body. **Semen** is the fluid-transporting medium for spermatozoa discharged during ejaculation.
Testes (also called *testicles*)	Provide the male sex hormone, testosterone, produced by cells within them; contain seminiferous tubules that are the site of sperm formation and development
Epididymis	Acts as site for the maturation of sperm
Vas deferens	Acts as excretory duct of the testis
Seminal vesicles	Produce a slightly alkaline fluid that becomes a part of the seminal fluid or semen
Prostate gland	Secretes an alkaline fluid that aids in maintaining the viability of spermatozoa
Bulbourethral or Cowper glands	Produce a mucous secretion before ejaculation that becomes a part of the semen
Urethra	Transmits urine and semen out of the body

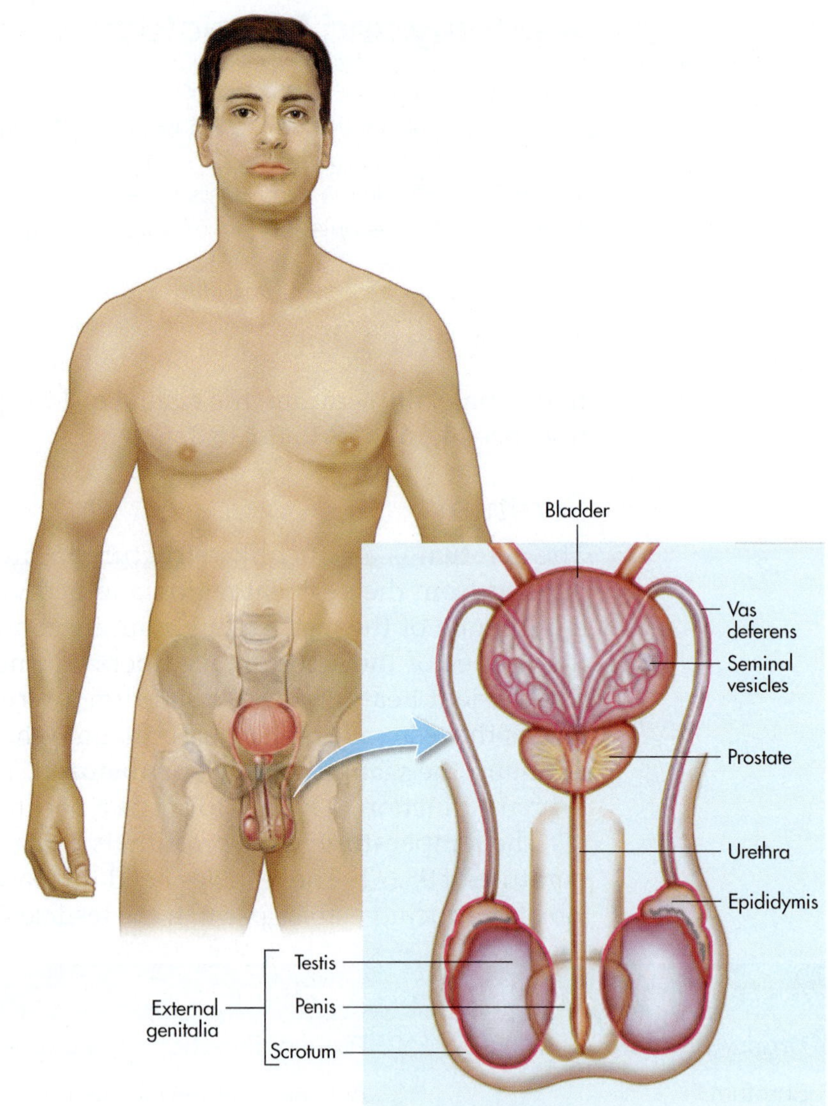

Figure 18.1 Male reproductive system: seminal vesicles, prostate, urethra, vas deferens, epididymis, and external genitalia.

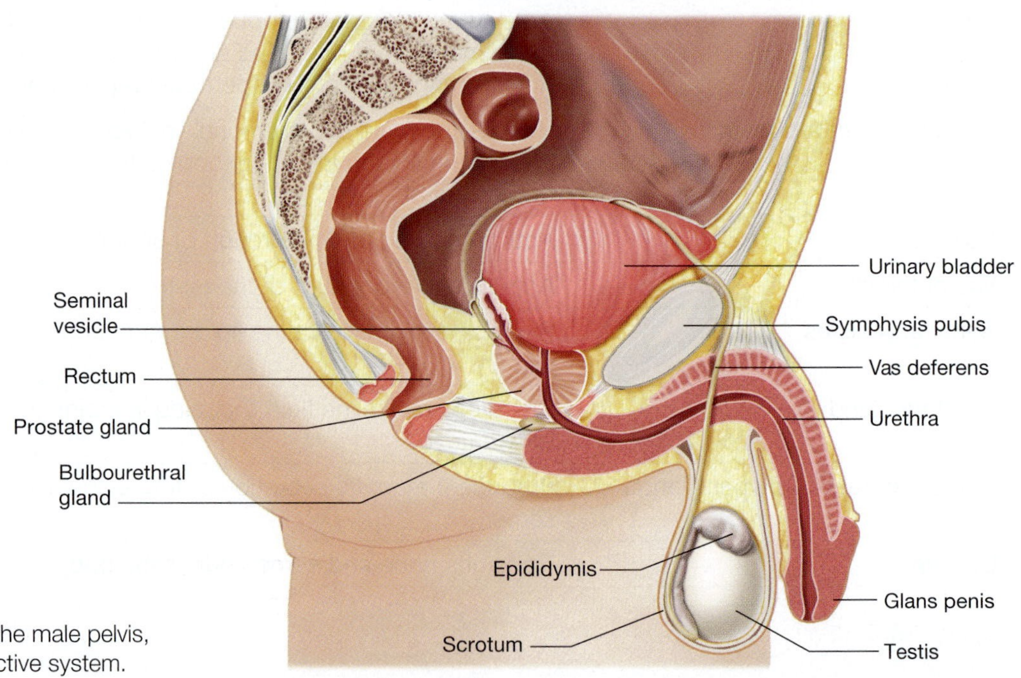

Figure 18.2 Sagittal section of the male pelvis, showing the organs of the reproductive system.

a prolonged period, infertility or sterility can result. The scrotum continually monitors the environment for temperature changes and responds automatically in the way that is best for the production of healthy sperm.

Under normal conditions, the walls of the scrotum are generally free of wrinkles, and it hangs loosely between the thighs (Figure 18.1).

Testes

The male has two ovoid-shaped organs, the **testes**, located within the scrotum. See Figure 18.3. Each testis is about 4 cm long and 2.5 cm wide. The interior of each testis is divided into about 250 wedge-shaped lobes by fibrous tissues. Coiled within each lobe are one to three small tubes called the **seminiferous tubules**, which are the site of the development of male reproductive cells, the **spermatozoa**. Cells within the testes also produce the male sex hormone, **testosterone**, which is responsible for the development of secondary male sexual characteristics during puberty and maintaining them through adulthood.

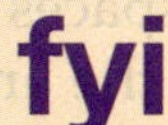

Puberty is defined as a period of rapid change in the lives of boys and girls during which time the reproductive organs mature and become functionally capable of reproduction. In the male, puberty generally begins around 12 years of age when the genitals start to increase in size and the shoulders broaden and become muscular. As testosterone is released, secondary sexual characteristics develop, such as pubic and axillary hair, increase in size of the penis and testes, voice changes (deepening), facial hair, erections, and nocturnal emissions.

Testosterone is essential for normal growth and development of the male accessory sex organs. It plays a vital role in the erection process of the penis and thus is necessary for the reproductive act, or copulation. Additionally, testosterone affects the growth of hair on the face, muscular development, and vocal timbre. The *seminiferous tubules* form a plexus or network called the *rete testis* from which 15–20 small ducts, the efferent ductules, leave the testis and open into the epididymis (see Figure 18.3).

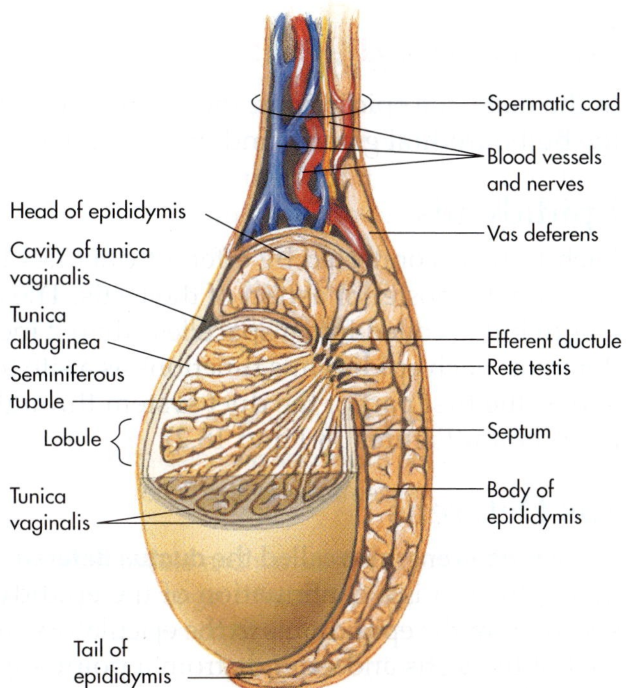

Figure 18.3 Sagittal view of a testis showing interior anatomy.

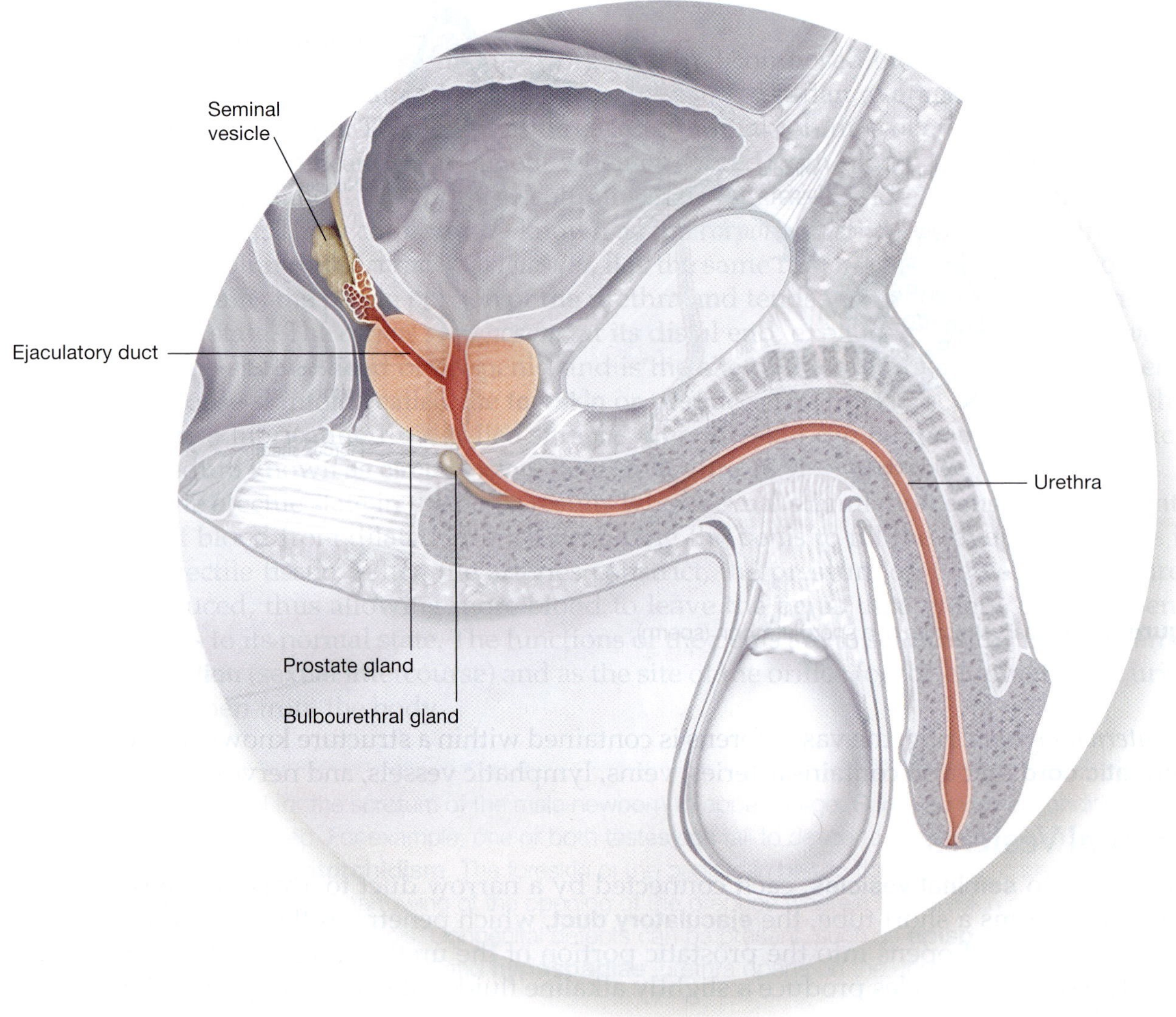

Figure 18.5 Sagittal view of the male pelvis showing the seminal vesicle, ejaculatory duct, prostate gland, bulbourethral glands, and urethra.

Bulbourethral Glands

The **bulbourethral glands**, or *Cowper glands*, are two small pea-sized glands located below the prostate and on either side of the urethra. A duct about 2.5 cm long connects them with the wall of the urethra. The bulbourethral glands produce a mucous secretion before ejaculation, which becomes a component of semen.

Urethra

The male **urethra** is approximately 20 cm long and is divided into three sections: prostatic, membranous, and penile. It extends from the urinary bladder to the external urethral orifice at the head of the penis. It serves the dual function of transmitting urine and semen out of the body.

Sexually Transmitted Infections

Sexually transmitted infections (STIs) can occur in men, women, and children. They are passed from person to person through sexual contact or from mother to child. Table 18.2 is a summary of the most common sexually transmitted infections.

Table 18.2 Sexually Transmitted Infections

Infection	Cause	Symptoms	Treatment
Chlamydia (klă-mĭd´ ē-ă)	*Chlamydia trachomatis* (bacterium)	Can be asymptomatic or exhibit the following: **MALE**: Mucopurulent discharge from penis; burning, itching in genital area; dysuria; swollen testes; can cause nongonococcal urethritis (NGU) and sterility **FEMALE:** Mucopurulent discharge from vagina, cystitis, pelvic pain, cervicitis; can lead to pelvic inflammatory disease (PID) and sterility **NEWBORN:** Eye infection, pneumonia; can cause death	Antibiotics—Zithromax (azithromycin) and doxycycline, tetracycline, or erythromycin
Genital warts (jĕn´ ĭ-tăl)	Human papillomavirus (HPV)	**MALE:** Cauliflowerlike growths on the penis and perianal area **FEMALE:** Cauliflowerlike growths around vagina and perianal area	Laser surgery, chemotherapy, cryosurgery, cauterization **Note:** Gardasil is the only HPV vaccine that helps protect against four types of HPV. In girls and young women ages 9–26, it helps protect against two types of HPV that cause about 75% of cervical cancer cases, and two more types that cause 90% of genital warts cases. In boys and young men ages 9–26, Gardasil helps protect against 90% of genital warts cases. Gardasil also helps protect girls and young women ages 9–26 against 70% of vaginal cancer cases and up to 50% of vulvar cancer cases.
Gonorrhea (gŏn˝ ŏ-rē´ā)	*Neisseria gonorrhoeae* (bacterium)	**MALE:** Purulent urethral discharge, dysuria, urinary frequency **FEMALE**: Purulent vaginal discharge, dysuria, urinary frequency, abnormal menstrual bleeding, abdominal tenderness; can lead to PID and sterility **NEWBORN:** Gonorrheal ophthalmia neonatorum, purulent eye discharge; can cause blindness	Antibiotics—ceftriaxone, cefixime, ciprofloxacin, ofloxacin

(*continued*)

Table 18.2 Sexually Transmitted Infections (*continued*)

Infection	Cause	Symptoms	Treatment
Herpes genitalis (hĕr´ pēz jĕn-ĭ-tāl´ ĭs)	Herpes simplex virus–2 (HSV-2)	**ACTIVE PHASE** **MALE:** Fluid-filled vesicles (blisters) on penis; acute pain and itching **FEMALE:** Blisters in and around vagina **NEWBORN:** Can be infected during vaginal delivery; severe infection, physical and mental damage **GENERALIZED:** Flulike symptoms, fever, headache, malaise, anorexia, muscle pain	No cure; antiviral drugs Zovirax (acyclovir), Famvir (famciclovir), or Valtrex (valacyclovir hydrochloride) can be used to relieve symptoms during acute phase
Syphilis (sĭf´ ĭ-lĭs)	*Treponema pallidum* (bacterium)	**PRIMARY STAGE:** Chancre at point of infection. See Figure 18.6. **MALE:** penis, anus, rectum **FEMALE:** vagina, cervix **BOTH:** lips, tongue, fingers, nipples	Antibotics—penicillin, tetracycline, erythromycin

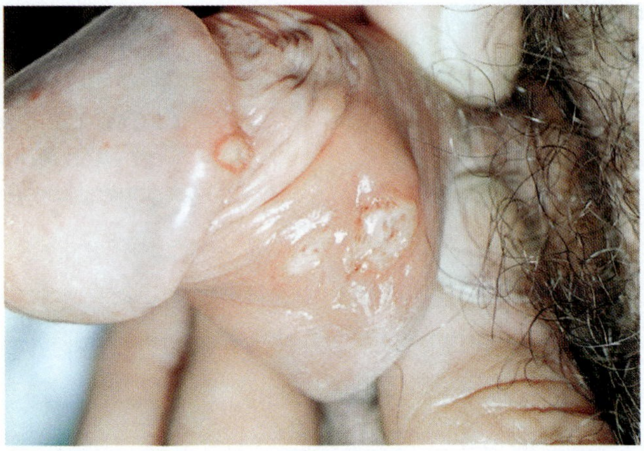

Figure 18.6 Chancre.
(Courtesy of Jason L. Smith, MD)

(*continued*)

Table 18.2 Sexually Transmitted Infections (*continued*)

Infection	Cause	Symptoms	Treatment
		SECONDARY STAGE: Flulike symptoms with a skin rash over moist, fatty areas of the body. See Figure 18.7. **Figure 18.7** Secondary syphilis. (Courtesy of Jason L. Smith, MD) **LATE STAGE:** Difficulty coordinating muscle movements, paralysis, numbness, gradual blindness, and dementia; this damage can be serious enough to cause death **NEWBORN:** Congenital syphilis—heart defect, bone or other deformities	
Trichomoniasis (trĭk″ ō-mō-nī′ ă-sĭs)	*Trichomonas* (parasitic protozoa)	**MALE:** Usually asymptomatic; can lead to cystitis, urethritis, prostatitis, and nongonococcal urethritis (NGU) **FEMALE:** White frothy vaginal discharge, burning and itching of vulva; can lead to cystitis, urethritis, vaginitis	Flagyl (metronidazole)

Study and Review I

Anatomy and Physiology

Write your answers to the following questions.

1. List the primary and accessory glands of the male reproductive system.

a. ______________________ **b.** ______________________

c. ______________________ **d.** ______________________

e. ______________________ **f.** ______________________

2. Name the supporting structure and accessory sex organs of the male reproductive system.

a. ______________________ **b.** ______________________

3. State the vital function of the male reproductive system. ______________________

4. The ______________________ ______________________ is the cone-shaped head of the penis.

5. Define prepuce. ______________________

6. Define smegma. ______________________

7. State two functions of the penis.

a. ______________________ **b.** ______________________

8. ______________________ ______________________ is the site of the development of spermatozoa.

9. List five effects of testosterone regarding male development.

a. ______________________ **b.** ______________________

c. ______________________ **d.** ______________________

e. ______________________

10. State two functions of the epididymis.

a. ______________________ **b.** ______________________

11. The excretory duct of the testes is known by two names, ______________________ ______________________ or ______________________ ______________________.

12. State the function of the seminal vesicles. ______________________________

13. Describe the prostate gland. ______________________________
____

14. Define the condition known as benign prostatic hyperplasia. ______________________________
____

15. The two small pea-sized glands located below the prostate and on either side of the urethra are known as the ______________________ glands or as ______________________ glands.

16. Name the three sections of the male urethra.

  a. ______________________________ b. ______________________________

  c. ______________________________

17. State a function of the male urethra. ______________________________

18. The male urethra is approximately ______________________________ cm long.

ANATOMY LABELING

Identify the structures shown below by filling in the blanks.

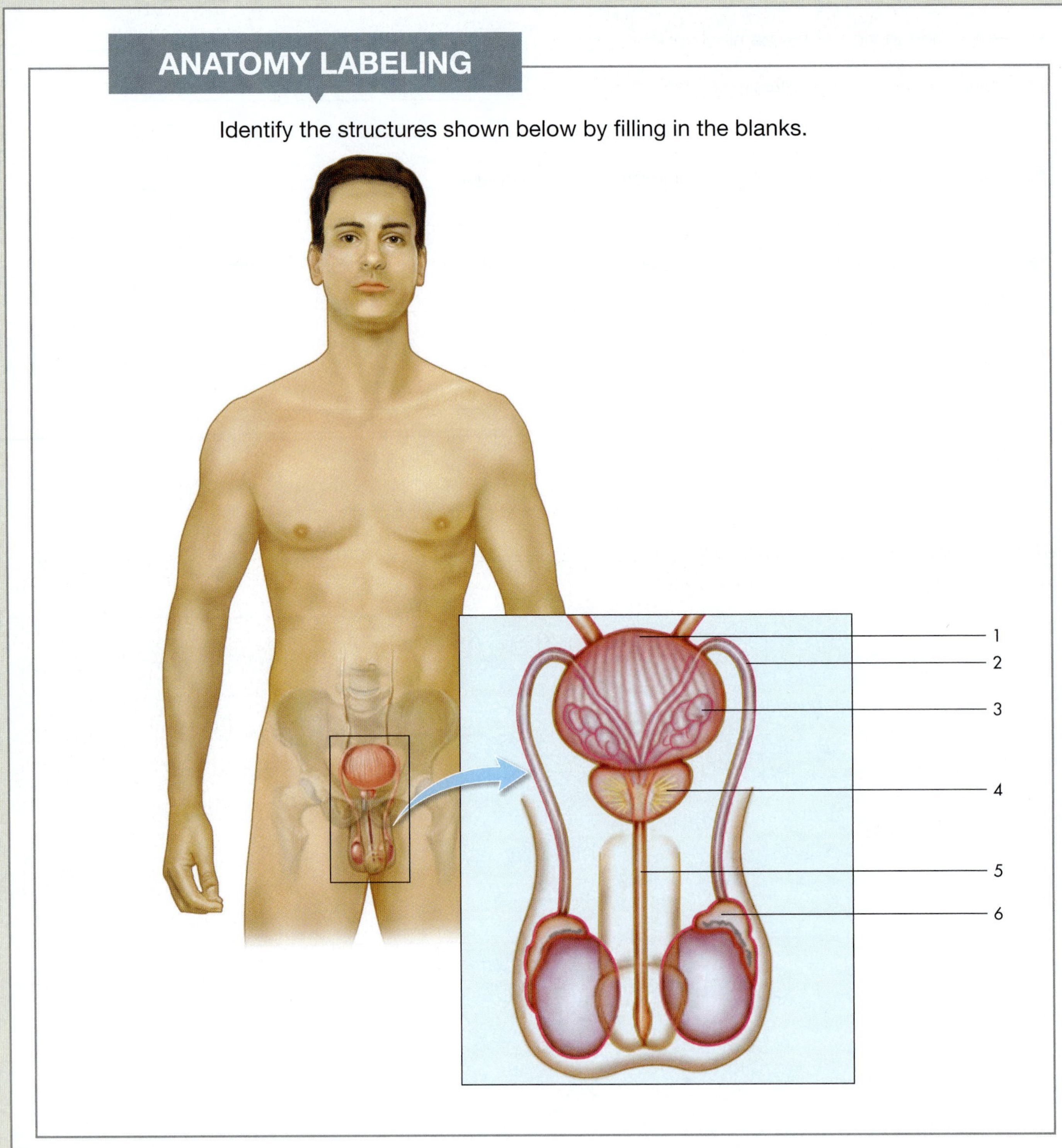

Building Your Medical Vocabulary

This section provides the foundation for learning medical terminology. Review the following alphabetized word list. Note how common prefixes and suffixes are repeatedly applied to word roots and combining forms to create different meanings. The word parts are color-coded: prefixes are yellow, suffixes are blue, roots/combining forms are red. A combining form is a word root plus a vowel. The chart below lists the combining forms for the word roots in this chapter and can help to strengthen your understanding of how medical words are built and spelled.

Remember These Guidelines

1. If the suffix begins with a vowel, drop the combining vowel from the combining form and add the suffix. For example, balan/o (*glans penis*) + -itis (*inflammation*) becomes balanitis.
2. If the suffix begins with a consonant, keep the combining vowel and add the suffix to the combining form. For example, gon/o (*genitals*) + -rrhea (*flow*) becomes gonorrhea.

You will find that some terms have not been divided into word parts. These are common words or specialized terms that are included to enhance your medical vocabulary.

Combining Forms of the Male Reproductive System			
balan/o	glans penis	**orchid/o**	testicle
cis/o	to cut	**prostat/o**	prostate
crypt/o	hidden	**sperm/o, sperm/i**	seed, sperm
didym/o	testis	**spermat/o**	seed, sperm
ejaculat/o	to throw out	**testicul/o**	testicle
gon/o	genitals	**varic/o**	twisted vein
gynec/o	female	**vas/o**	vessel
mast/o	breast	**vesicul/o**	seminal vesicle
mit/o	thread	**zo/o**	animal
orch/o	testicle		

Medical Word	Word Parts: Part	Word Parts: Meaning	Definition
anorchism (ăn-ōr´ kĭzm)	an- orch -ism	lack of testicle condition	Condition in which there is a lack of one or both testes
artificial insemination (ăr″ tĭ-fĭsh´ ăl ĭn-sĕm″ ĭn-ā´ shŭn)			Process of artificially placing semen into the vagina so that conception can take place. *Artificial insemination homologous (AIH)* means using the husband's or mate's semen and *artificial insemination heterologous* refers to using sperm from a donor other than the husband or mate.
aspermia (ă-spĕr´ mē-ă)	a- sperm -ia	lack of seed condition	Condition involving lack of sperm or failure to ejaculate sperm
azoospermia (ă-zō″ ō-spĕr´ mē-ă)	a- zo/o sperm -ia	lack of animal seed condition	Condition in which the semen lacks spermatozoa
balanitis (băl″ ă-nī´ tĭs)	balan -itis	glans penis inflammation	Inflammation of the glans penis

RULE REMINDER

The ***o*** has been removed from the combining form because the suffix begins with a vowel.

insights In ICD-10-CM, the code for Diseases of the Male Genital Organs is N40–N53. Some of these codes will have an instruction to also use an additional code from B95–B97 to identify the specific infectious agent.

Medical Word	Word Parts: Part	Word Parts: Meaning	Definition
benign prostatic hyperplasia (BPH) (bē-nīn´ prŏs-tăt´ ĭk hī″ pĕr-plā´zē-ă)			Enlargement of the prostate gland. As the prostate enlarges, it compresses the urethra, thereby restricting the normal flow of urine. See Figure 18.8. This restriction generally causes a number of symptoms and can be referred to as *prostatism*. **Prostatism** is any condition of the prostate gland that interferes with the flow of urine from the bladder. Symptoms usually include weak or difficult-to-start urine stream; feeling that the bladder is not empty; need to urinate often, especially at night (nocturia); feeling of *urgency* (a sudden need to urinate); abdominal straining; decrease in size and force of the urinary stream; and interruption of the stream.

(*continued*)

Medical Word	Word Parts		Definition
	Part	Meaning	

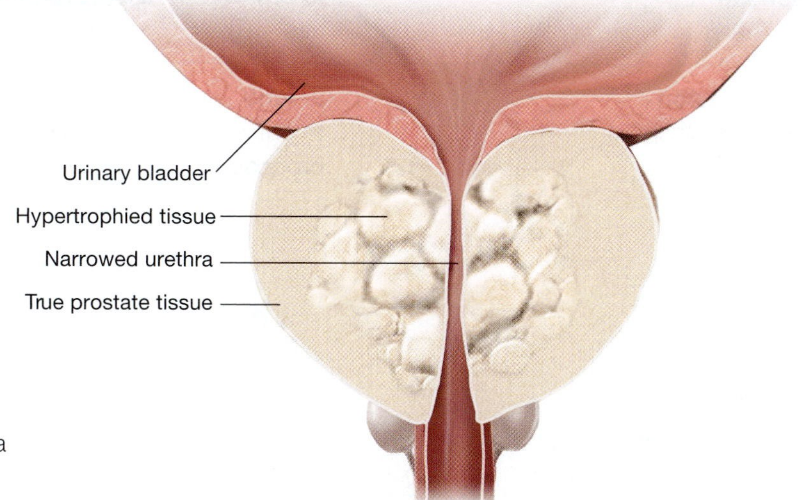

Figure 18.8 Benign prostatic hyperplasia (BPH) showing an enlarged prostate compressing the urethra.

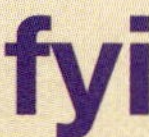

By age 60, four out of five men have an enlarged prostate. A normal prostate is about 4 cm and weighs about 20 grams (about the size of a whole walnut). To determine the size of the prostate gland, the physician will perform a digital rectal exam (DRE). See Figure 18.15. In checking for abnormalities, the physician uses a gloved, lubricated finger to examine the lower rectum. Treatment for benign prostatic hyperplasia includes drug therapy (see *Drug Highlights*), nonsurgical procedures, and/or surgery.

Nonsurgical treatments for benign prostatic hyperplasia include:

1. **Transurethral microwave thermotherapy (TUMT)**. A treatment that employs microwaves to heat and destroy excess prostate tissue, sending computer-regulated microwaves through an antenna to heat selected portions of the prostate to at least 111°F. A cooling system protects the urinary tract during the procedure.
2. **Transurethral needle ablation (TUNA)**. A minimally invasive treatment that delivers low-level radiofrequency energy through twin needles to burn away a well-defined region of the enlarged prostate. Shields protect the urethra from heat damage. Improves urine flow and relieves symptoms with fewer side effects when compared with transurethral resection of the prostate (TURP).

Types of surgery used for benign prostatic hyperplasia include:

1. **Transurethral resection of the prostate (TURP or TUR)**. During this procedure, the most common form of surgery used for this condition, an endoscopic instrument that has ocular and surgical capabilities is introduced directly through the urethra to the prostate and small pieces of the prostate gland are removed by using an electrical cutting loop.
2. **Transurethral incision of the prostate (TUIP)**. Used to widen the urethra by making a few small cuts in the bladder neck where the urethra joins the bladder and in the prostate gland itself.
3. **Open surgery**. Used when a transurethral procedure cannot be done: when the gland is greatly enlarged, when there are complicating factors, or when the bladder has been damaged and needs to be repaired.
4. **Laser surgery**. Employs side-firing laser fibers and Nd:YAG (neodymium:yttrium–aluminum–garnet) lasers to vaporize obstructing prostate tissue.

Medical Word	Word Parts		Definition
	Part	**Meaning**	
castrate (kăs´ trāt)	castr -ate	to prune use	Removal of the testicles in a man or ovaries in a woman
circumcision (sĕr″ kŭm-sĭ′ shŭn)	circum- cis -ion	around to cut process	Surgical procedure of removing the foreskin of the penis. See Figure 18.9.

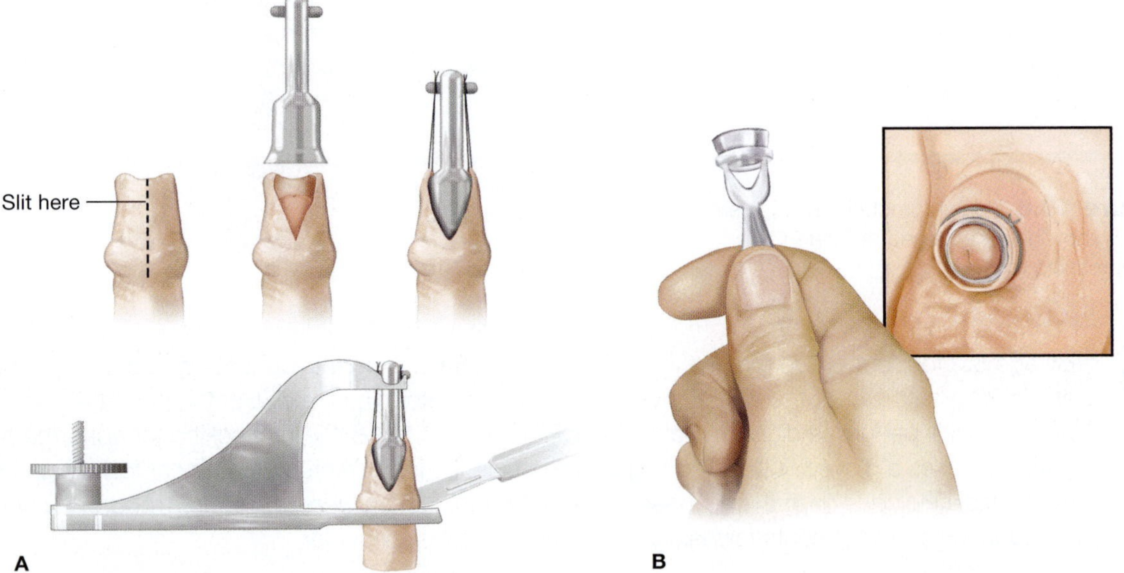

Figure 18.9 Circumcision using the Plastibell. (A) The bell is fitted over the glans. A suture is tied around the bell's rim, and then the excess prepuce is cut away. (B) The plastic rim remains in place for 3 to 4 days until healing occurs. The bell may be allowed to fall off; it is removed if still in place after 8 days.

Medical Word	Part	Meaning	Definition
coitus (kō´ ĭ-tŭs)			Sexual intercourse between a man and a woman; *copulation*
condom (kŏn´ dŭm)			Thin, flexible protective sheath, usually rubber (latex), worn over the penis during copulation to help prevent impregnation (block the passage of sperm) or sexually transmitted infections (STIs).

Medical Word	Word Parts		Definition
	Part	Meaning	
condyloma (kŏn″ dĭ-lō′ mă)			Wartlike growth on the skin, most often seen on the external genitalia; either viral or syphilitic in origin. See Figure 18.10.

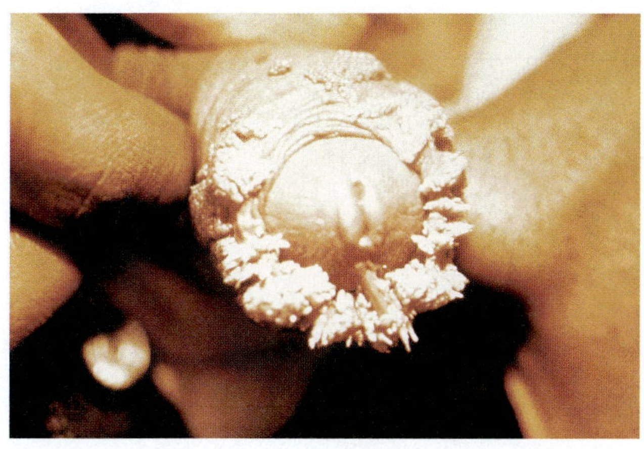

Figure 18.10 Genital warts.
(Centers for Disease Control and Prevention)

Medical Word	Part	Meaning	Definition
cryptorchidism (krĭpt-ōr′ kĭd-ĭzm)	crypt orchid -ism	hidden testicle condition	Condition in which one or both testes fail to descend into the scrotum. See Figure 18.11.

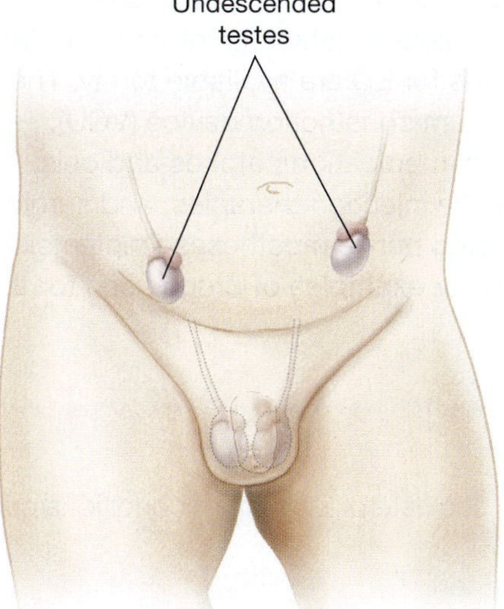

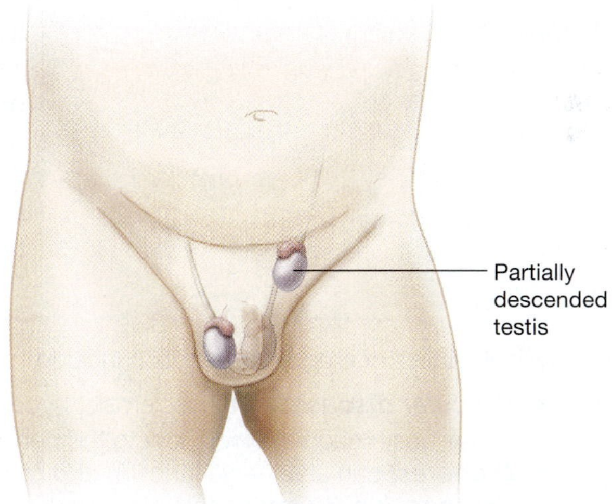

Figure 18.11 Cryptorchidism showing (A) undescended testes and (B) a partially descended testis.

Medical Word	Part	Meaning	Definition
ejaculation (ē-jăk″ ū-lā′ shŭn)	ejaculat -ion	to throw out process	Process of expulsion of seminal fluid and sperm from the male urethra
epididymitis (ĕp″ ĭ-dĭd″ ĭ-mī′ tĭs)	epi- didym -itis	upon testis inflammation	Inflammation of the epididymis

Medical Word	Word Parts: Part	Word Parts: Meaning	Definition
epispadias (ĕp″ ĭ-spā´ dĭ-ăs)	epi- spadias	upon a rent, an opening	Congenital defect in which the urethra opens on the dorsum of the penis. See Figure 18.12A.

Figure 18.12 Epispadias and hypospadias. (A) In epispadias the canal is open on the dorsal surface. (B) In hypospadias the urethral canal is open on the ventral surface of the penis.

Medical Word	Word Parts: Part	Word Parts: Meaning	Definition
erectile dysfunction (ED) (ĕ-rĕk´ tīl dĭs-fŭnk´ shŭn)			Inability to achieve and maintain penile erection sufficient to complete satisfactory intercourse. Many treatment options for ED are available today. These include the vacuum constriction device (VCD); oral medications; medication patches and gels; urethral and penile injection therapies; and surgical therapies including penile prostheses (implants). See *Drug Highlights* for examples of drugs used for this condition.

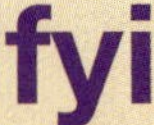

Physical causes of erectile dysfunction include:

- ***Vascular diseases:*** arteriosclerosis, hypertension, high cholesterol, and other conditions can cause obstruction of blood flow to the penis
- ***Diabetes:*** can alter nerve function and blood flow to the penis
- ***Prescription drugs:*** certain antihypertensive and cardiac medications, antihistamines, psychiatric medications, and other prescription drugs can cause ED
- ***Substance abuse:*** excessive smoking, alcohol consumption, and illegal drugs constrict blood vessels, limiting blood flow to the penis
- ***Neurological diseases:*** multiple sclerosis, Parkinson disease, and other diseases can interrupt nerve impulses to the penis
- ***Surgery:*** prostate, colon, bladder, and other types of pelvic surgery can damage nerves and blood vessels
- ***Spinal injury:*** interruptions of nerve impulses from the spinal cord to the penis can cause ED
- ***Other:*** hormonal imbalance, kidney failure, dialysis, and reduced testosterone levels can contribute to ED

Medical Word	Word Parts		Definition
	Part	**Meaning**	
gamete (găm´ ēt)			Mature reproductive cell of the male or female; a *spermatozoon* or *ovum*
gonorrhea (GC) (gŏn″ ŏ-rē´ă)	gon/o -rrhea	genitals flow	Highly contagious sexually transmitted infection of the genital mucous membrane of either sex; the infection is transmitted by the gonococcus *Neisseria gonorrhoeae*.

RULE REMINDER

This term keeps the combining vowel ***o*** because the suffix begins with a consonant.

Medical Word	Part	Meaning	Definition
gynecomastia (gī″ nĕ-kō-măs´ tĭ-ă)	gynec/o mast -ia	female breast condition	Pathological condition of excessive development of the mammary glands in the male
heterosexual (hĕt″ ĕr-ō-sĕk´ shū-ăl)	hetero- sexu -al	different sex pertaining to	Pertaining to the opposite sex; refers to an individual who has a sexual preference and relationship with the opposite sex
homosexual (hō″ mō-sĕks´ ū-ăl)	homo- sexu -al	similar, same sex pertaining to	Pertaining to the same sex; refers to an individual who has a sexual preference and relationship with the same sex
hydrocele (hī´ drō-sēl)	hydro- -cele	water hernia, swelling, tumor	Accumulation of fluid in a saclike cavity. One that occurs during prenatal development is caused by a failure of the closure of the canal between the peritoneal cavity and the scrotum. See Figure 18.13A.

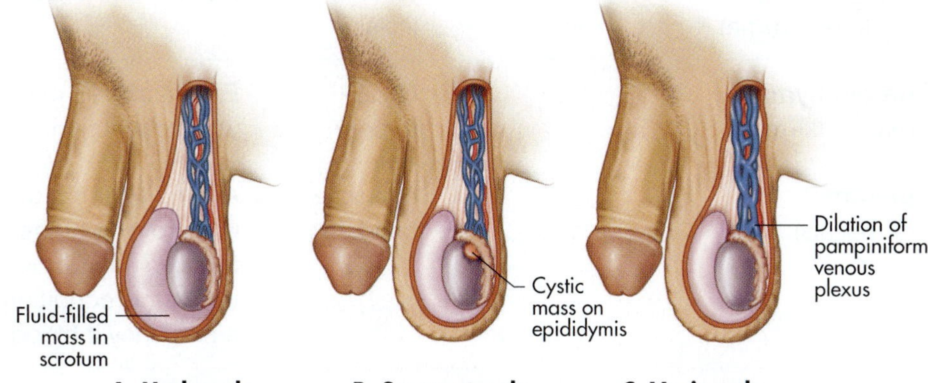

Figure 18.13 Common disorders of the scrotum. (A) and (B) Hydroceles and spermatoceles do not usually require treatment unless they become large and cause pain. (C) Varicoceles are usually treated to prevent infertility.

Medical Word	Word Parts		Definition
	Part	**Meaning**	
hypospadias (hī″ pō-spā′ dĭ-ăs)	hypo- spadias	under a rent, an opening	Congenital defect in which the urethra opens on the underside of the penis. Symptoms depend on the severity of the defect. An abnormal direction of urine spray is common. Circumcision is not recommended, as the foreskin should be kept for use in a surgical repair. Urologists usually recommend repair before the child is 18 months old. During the surgery, the penis is straightened and the opening is corrected using tissue grafts from the foreskin. The repair may require multiple surgeries. See Figure 18.12B.
infertility (ĭn″ fĕr-tĭl′ ĭ-tē)			Inability of a heterosexual couple to produce a viable offspring
mitosis (mī-tō′ sĭs)	mit -osis	thread condition	Ordinary condition of cell division
oligospermia (ŏl″ ĭ-gō-spĕr′ mĭ-ă)	oligo- sperm -ia	scanty seed condition	Condition in which there is insufficient (scanty) amount of spermatozoa in the semen
orchidectomy (or″ kĭ-dĕk′ tō-mē)	orchid -ectomy	testicle surgical excision	Surgical excision of a testicle; also called *orchiectomy*

RULE REMINDER

The ***o*** has been removed from the combining form because the suffix begins with a vowel.

Medical Word	Part	Meaning	Definition
orchiditis (or″ kĭ-dī′ tĭs)	orchid -itis	testicle inflammation	Inflammation of a testicle; also called *orchitis*
orchidotomy (or″ kĭd-ŏt′ ō-mē)	orchid/o -tomy	testicle incision	Incision into a testicle
parenchyma (păr-ĕn′ kĭ-mă)	par- enchyma	beside to pour	Essential cells of a gland or organ that are involved with its function
phimosis (fī-mō′ sĭs)	phim -osis	a muzzle condition	A condition that can be present at birth in which there is narrowing of the opening of the prepuce and the foreskin cannot be drawn back over the glans penis. When this condition occurs later in life, it can be an emergency if blood flow is blocked to the penis.

Medical Word	Word Parts		Definition
	Part	Meaning	
prostate cancer (prŏs´ tāt)			Malignant tumor of the prostate gland. See Figure 18.14. Diagnosis of prostate cancer can be confirmed with a medical history; physical examination, including a digital rectal exam (DRE) to assess the size and condition (firm, soft, hard) of the prostate gland (Figure 18.15); and results of a PSA blood test.

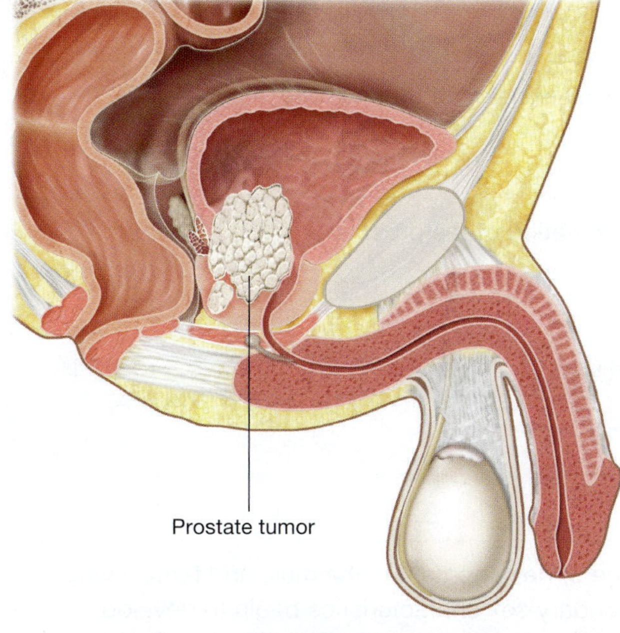

Figure 18.14 Prostate cancer showing metastasis to the urinary bladder. Note the large tumor mass.

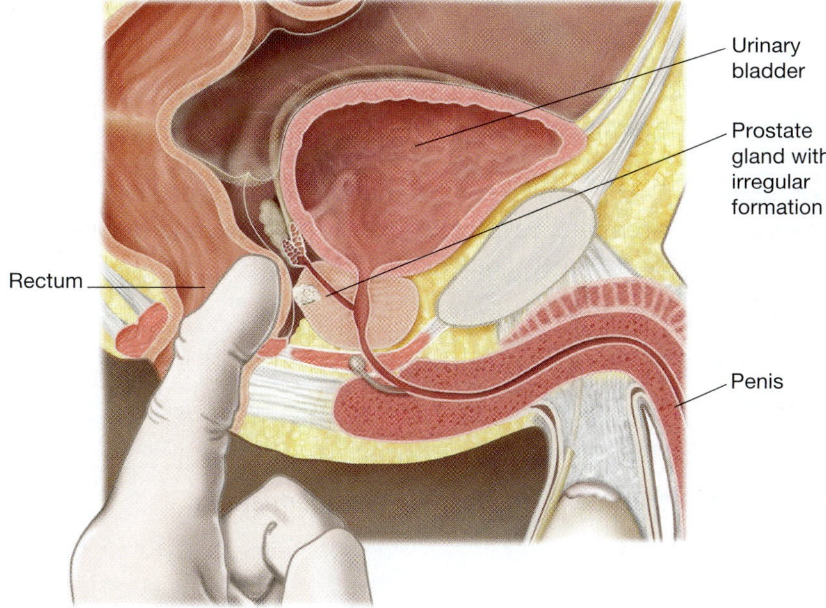

Figure 18.15 Digital rectal exam (DRE) showing palpitation of the prostate gland.

(continued)

Medical Word	Word Parts		Definition
	Part	Meaning	

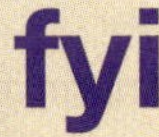

Prostate cancer is the most common type of cancer found in American men, and by age 50, up to one in four men have some cancerous cells in the prostate gland. It is the second leading cause of cancer death in men, exceeded only by lung cancer. While one man in seven will have prostate cancer during his lifetime, only one man in 39 will die of this disease. A man is more likely to die *with* prostate cancer than to die *from* prostate cancer.

Medical Word	Part	Meaning	Definition
prostatectomy (prŏs″ tă-tĕk′ tō-mē)	prostat -ectomy	prostate surgical excision	Surgical excision of the prostate
prostatitis (prŏs″ tă-tī′ tĭs)	prostat -itis	prostate inflammation	Inflammation of the prostate

insights In ICD-10-CM, the code for Inflammatory Diseases of the Prostate is N41.0–N41.9. Prostatitis is classified as *acute*, *chronic*, *abscess*, *prostatocystitis* (inflammation of bladder and prostate), *granulomatous prostatitis*, *other*, and *unspecified*.

Medical Word	Part	Meaning	Definition
puberty (pū′ ber-tē)			Stage of development in the male and female when secondary sex characteristics begin to develop and the individual becomes functionally capable of reproduction
spermatid (spĕr′ mă-tĭd)			Sperm germ cell; also called *spermatoblast*, *spermoblast*
spermatocele (spĕr-măt′ ō-sēl)	spermat/o -cele	seed, sperm hernia, swelling, tumor	Cystic swelling of the epididymis that contains spermatozoa; mobile, usually painless, and requires no treatment. See Figure 18.13B.
spermatogenesis (spĕr″ măt-ō-jĕn′ ĕ-sĭs)	spermat/o -genesis	seed, sperm formation, produce	Formation of spermatozoa
spermatozoon (spĕr″ măt-ō-zō′ ŏn)	spermat/o zoon	seed, sperm life	Male sex cell; plural form is *spermatozoa*

ALERT!

How many words can you build using the combining form ***spermat/o***?

Medical Word	Word Parts		Definition
	Part	**Meaning**	
spermicide (spĕr´ mĭ-sīd)	sperm/i -cide	seed, sperm to kill	Agent that kills sperm
testicular (tĕs-tĭk´ ū-lar)	testicul -ar	testicle pertaining to	Pertaining to a testicle
varicocele (văr´ ĭ-kō-sēl)	varic/o -cele	twisted vein hernia, swelling, tumor	Enlargement and twisting of the veins of the spermatic cord. See Figure 18.13C.
vasectomy (văs-ĕk´ tō-mē)	vas -ectomy	vessel surgical excision	Surgical procedure in which the vas deferens are cut, then tied or sealed to prevent the transport of sperm out of the testes. See Figure 18.16.

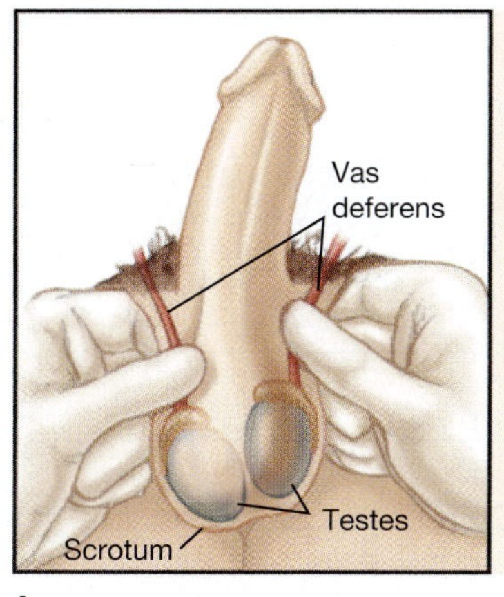

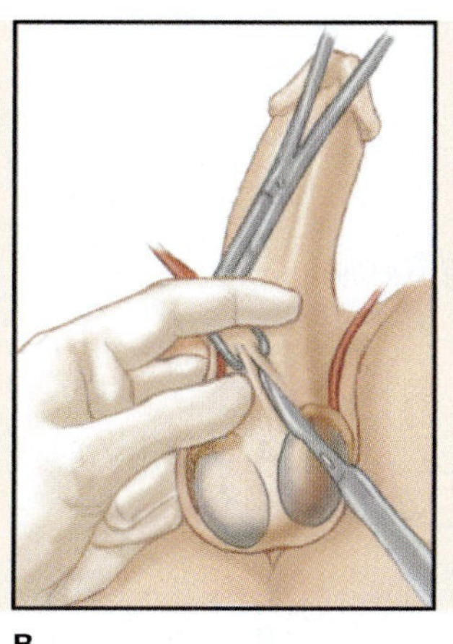

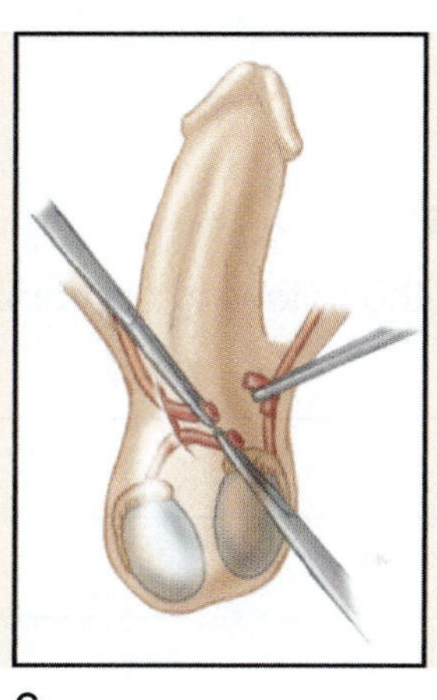

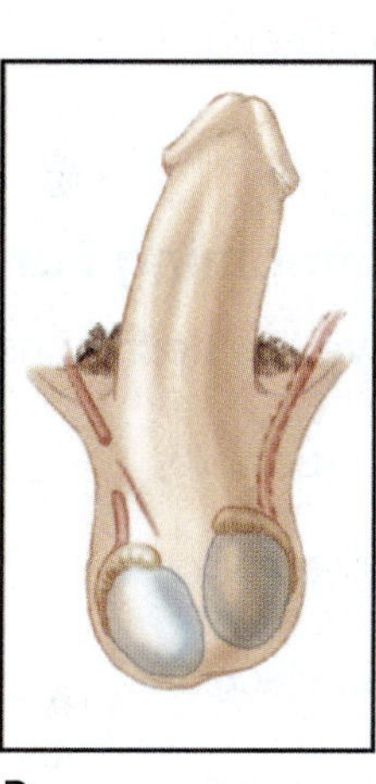

Figure 18.16 Vasectomy. (A) The spermatic cords are located as they ascend from the scrotum. (B) The vas deferens are severed. (C) A 1 cm section is removed. (D) The cut ends cannot reconnect thereby preventing the passage of sperm cells and providing surgical sterilization.

fyi A vasectomy does not affect a man's ability to achieve orgasm, ejaculate, or achieve erections. After 4–6 weeks, sperm are no longer present in the semen. A semen specimen must be examined and found to be totally free of sperm a month or more after vasectomy before the patient can rely on the vasectomy for birth control.

vesiculitis (vĕ-sĭk˝ ū-lī´ tĭs)	vesicul -itis	seminal vesicle inflammation	Inflammation of a seminal vesicle

Study and Review II

Word Parts

Prefixes

Give the definitions of the following prefixes.

1. a- ______________________
2. an- ______________________
3. circum- ______________________
4. epi- ______________________
5. hydro- ______________________
6. hypo- ______________________
7. oligo- ______________________
8. par- ______________________
9. in- ______________________
10. hetero- ______________________
11. homo- ______________________

Combining Forms

Give the definitions of the following combining forms.

1. balan/o ______________________
2. cis/o ______________________
3. crypt/o ______________________
4. didym/o ______________________
5. ejaculat/o ______________________
6. gon/o ______________________
7. gynec/o ______________________
8. mast/o ______________________
9. mit/o ______________________
10. orch/o ______________________
11. orchid/o ______________________
12. prostat/o ______________________
13. sperm/o ______________________
14. spermat/o ______________________
15. testicul/o ______________________
16. varic/o ______________________
17. vas/o ______________________
18. vesicul/o ______________________
19. zo/o ______________________

Suffixes

Give the definitions of the following suffixes.

1. -al ______________________
2. -ar ______________________
3. -cele ______________________
4. -cide ______________________
5. -ectomy ______________________
6. -genesis ______________________
7. -ia ______________________
8. -ion ______________________
9. -ism ______________________
10. -itis ______________________
11. -ate ______________________
12. -osis ______________________
13. -rrhea ______________________
14. -tomy ______________________

Identifying Medical Terms

In the spaces provided, write the medical terms for the following meanings.

1. ______________________ Inflammation of the glans penis
2. ______________________ Surgical excision of the epididymis
3. ______________________ Surgical excision of a testicle
4. ______________________ Foreskin over the glans penis
5. ______________________ Accumulation of fluid in a saclike cavity
6. ______________________ Wartlike growth on the skin
7. ______________________ Sperm germ cell
8. ______________________ Male sex cell
9. ______________________ Agent that kills sperm
10. ______________________ Pertaining to a testicle

Matching

Select the appropriate lettered meaning for each of the following words.

__________ **1.** circumcision
__________ **2.** coitus
__________ **3.** condom
__________ **4.** gamete
__________ **5.** orchiditis
__________ **6.** gonorrhea
__________ **7.** infertility
__________ **8.** prepuce
__________ **9.** spermicide
__________ **10.** parenchyma

a. Agent that kills sperm
b. Mature reproductive cell of the male or female
c. Sexual intercourse between a man and a woman
d. Essential cells of a gland or organ that are involved with its function
e. Surgical procedure of removing the foreskin of the penis
f. Thin, flexible protective sheath worn over the penis during copulation to help prevent impregnation or sexually transmitted infection
g. Inflammation of a testicle
h. Inability to produce a viable offspring
i. Causes purulent urethral discharge in the male and purulent vaginal discharge in the female
j. Caused by the bacterium *Chlamydia trachomatis*
k. The foreskin over the glans penis in the male

Medical Case Snapshots

This learning activity provides an opportunity to relate the medical terminology you are learning to a precise patient case presentation. In the spaces provided, write in your answers.

Case 1

A 45-year-old male presents with an inability to achieve and maintain penile erection sufficient to complete satisfactory intercourse. This condition is known as __________ __________. There are many treatment options for ED, with the most popular being drug therapy (see *Drug Highlights*).

Case 2

During the assessment of the newborn male it was noted that the urethra opened on the underside of the penis. This condition is referred to as __________ and an abnormal direction of urine spray is common. In this case, __________ is not recommended for the baby as the foreskin should be kept for use in a surgical repair. Urologists usually recommend repair before the child is __________ months of age.

Case 3

A 60-year-old male complains of difficulty with urinating, "I tend to urinate more frequently, especially at night." This is called ____________. "I feel this sudden need to urinate." This is known as ____________. "Then I have trouble starting my stream." After a complete physical and a digital rectal exam (DRE), the diagnosis was confirmed to be BPH also known as benign ____________ ____________. BPH can also be referred to as having ____________, (which is any condition of the prostate gland that interferes with the flow of urine from the bladder).

Drug Highlights

Type of Drug	Description and Examples
testosterone (male hormone)	Responsible for growth, development, and maintenance of the male reproductive system and secondary sex characteristics.
therapeutic use	As replacement therapy in primary hypogonadism and to stimulate puberty in carefully selected males. It can be used to relieve symptoms of the male climacteric due to androgen deficiency and to help stimulate sperm production in oligospermia and impotence due to androgen deficiency. It can also be used with advanced inoperable metastatic breast cancer in women who are 1–5 years postmenopausal. In 2015, the FDA required labeling changes for testosterone products that clarifies the approved uses of these medications and includes information about a possible increased risk of heart attacks and strokes in aging patients taking testosterone. EXAMPLES: AndroGel (testosterone), Depo-Testosterone (testosterone cypionate [in oil]), Delatestryl (testosterone enanthate in oil), and Androderm (testosterone transdermal systems)
patient teaching	Educate the patient to be aware of possible adverse reactions and report any of the following to the physician. *All patients:* nausea, vomiting, jaundice, edema. *Males:* frequent or persistent erection of the penis. *Females:* hoarseness, acne, changes in menstrual periods, growth of hair on face and/or body.
special considerations	Testosterone can decrease blood glucose and insulin requirements in diabetic patients. It also can decrease the anticoagulant requirements of patients receiving oral anticoagulants. These patients require close monitoring when testosterone therapy is begun and then when it is stopped. Individuals who seek to increase muscle mass, strength, and overall athletic ability can abuse anabolic steroids (testosterone). This form is illegal; signs of abuse include flulike symptoms; headaches; muscle aches; dizziness; bruises; needle marks; increased bleeding (nosebleeds, petechiae, gums, conjunctiva); enlarged spleen, liver, and/or prostate; edema; and in the female increased facial hair, menstrual irregularities, and enlarged clitoris.

(*continued*)

Definition	Medical Term
7. Male sex cell	__________zoon
8. Agent that kills sperm	spermi________
9. Pertaining to a testicle	____________ar
10. Enlargement and twisting of the veins of the spermatic cord	varico________

Combining Form Challenge

Using the combining forms provided, write the medical term correctly.

balan/o	orchid/o	prostat/o
gon/o	mit/o	vesicul/o

1. Inflammation of the glans penis: __________itis
2. Highly contagious sexually transmitted infection of the genital mucous membrane: __________rrhea
3. Incision into a testicle: __________tomy
4. Ordinary condition of cell division: __________osis
5. Surgical excision of the prostate: __________ectomy
6. Inflammation of a seminal vesicle: __________itis

Select the Right Term

Select the correct answer, and write it on the line provided.

1. Condition in which there is a lack of one or both testes is __________.

   aspermia **anorchism** **azoospermia** **testicular**

2. Surgical procedure of removing the foreskin of the penis is __________.

   condyloma **coitus** **circumcision** **castrate**

3. Condition in which one or both testes fail to descend into the scrotum is __________.

   cryptorchidism **epispadias** **hydrocele** **cryptochidism**

4. Pertains to the same sex is __________.

   eugenics **gamete** **homosexual** **phimosis**

5. Surgical procedure in which the vas deferens are cut, then tied or sealed to prevent the transport of sperm out of the testes, is __________.

   vasectomy **vasotomy** **vesiculitis** **orchidectomy**

6. Sexually transmitted infection caused by *treponema pallidum* is __________.

   herpes **chlamydia** **gonorrhea** **syphilis**

Diagnostic and Laboratory Tests

Select the best answer to each multiple-choice question. Circle the letter of your choice.

1. Test performed on blood serum to detect syphilis.

a. paternity
b. semen
c. FTA-ABS
d. HSV-2

2. Test to determine whether a certain man is the father of a specific child.

a. paternity
b. semen
c. FTA-ABS
d. HSV-2

3. Increased level indicates prostate disease or possibly prostate cancer.

a. fluorescent treponemal antibody
b. prostate-specific antigen
c. semen
d. VDRL

4. Used to determine infertility in men.

a. paternity
b. prostate-specific antigen
c. semen
d. VDRL

5. Increased level can indicate benign prostatic hyperplasia.

a. fluorescent treponemal antibody
b. prostate-specific antigen
c. VDRL
d. venereal disease research laboratory

Abbreviations

Place the correct word, phrase, or abbreviation in the space provided.

1. benign prostatic hyperplasia ______________________

2. GC ______________________

3. human papillomavirus ______________________

4. HSV-2______________________

5. STIs ______________________

6. erectile dysfunction ______________________

7. TURP ______________________

8. NGU ______________________

9. venereal disease research laboratory ______________________

10. prostate-specific antigen ______________________

Practical Application

CDC Study

Read the adapted CDC study and then answer the questions that follow.

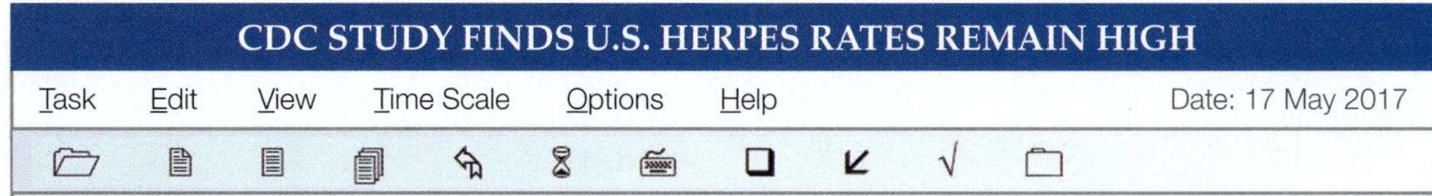

1 in 6 Americans Infected; Highest Prevalence among Women and African Americans

About 1 in 6 Americans (16.2%) between the ages of 14 and 49 is infected with herpes simplex virus type 2 (HSV-2), according to the Centers for Disease Control and Prevention. HSV-2 is a lifelong and incurable infection that can cause recurrent and painful genital sores. It remains one of the most common sexually transmitted infections (STIs) in the United States. Research shows that people with herpes are two to three times more likely to acquire HIV, and that herpes can also make HIV-infected individuals more likely to transmit HIV to others. The CDC estimates that over 80% of those with HSV-2 are unaware of their infection. Symptoms may be absent, mild, or mistaken for another condition. And people with HSV-2 can transmit the virus even when they have no visible sores or other symptoms.

"Many individuals are transmitting herpes to others without even knowing it," said John M. Douglas, Jr., M.D., director of CDC's Division of STD Prevention. "We can't afford to be complacent about this disease. It is important that persons with symptoms suggestive of herpes—especially recurrent sores in the genital area—seek clinical care to determine if these symptoms may be due to herpes and might benefit from treatment."

Combination of Prevention Approaches Needed to Reduce National Herpes Rates

Although HSV-2 infection is not curable, there are effective medications available to treat symptoms and prevent outbreaks. Those with known herpes infection should avoid sex when herpes symptoms or sores are present and understand that HSV-2 can still be transmitted when sores are not present. Effective strategies to reduce the risk of HSV-2 infection include abstaining from sexual contact, using condoms consistently and correctly, and limiting the number of sex partners.

CDC Study Questions

Place the correct answer in the space provided.

1. ______________________________ remains one of the most common sexually transmitted infections (STIs) in the United States.

2. About one in six Americans (16.2%) between the ages of __________ and __________ is infected with herpes simplex virus type 2 (HSV-2).

3. Is herpes a lifelong and incurable infection that can cause recurrent and painful genital sores?

   ____

4. The CDC estimates that over ______________________________ percent of those with HSV-2 are unaware of their infection.

5. People with HSV-2 can transmit the virus even when they have no ______________ sores or other symptoms.

Chapter

19 Oncology

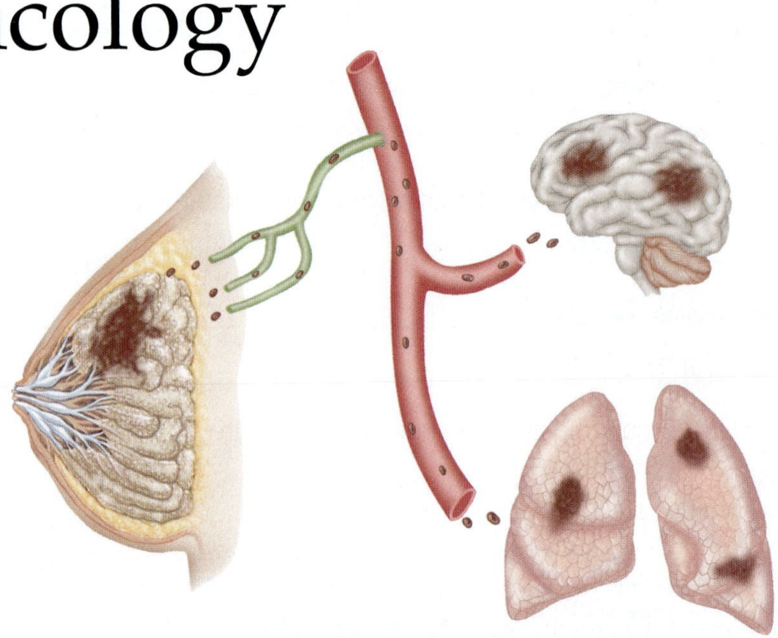

Learning Outcomes

On completion of this chapter, you will be able to:

1. Define cancer.
2. Describe cell differentiation.
3. Identify the staging system that evaluates the spread of a tumor.
4. Contrast the characteristics of benign and malignant tumors.
5. List the seven warning signals of cancer.
6. Describe the methods that can be used in diagnosing cancer.
7. List the various forms of treatment for cancer.
8. Define radiation therapy.
9. Describe important factors that must be considered when determining the use of radiotherapy for the cancer patient.
10. Recognize terminology included in the ICD-10-CM.
11. Analyze, build, spell, and pronounce medical words.
12. Identify and define selected abbreviations.
13. Apply your acquired knowledge of medical terms by successfully completing the *Practical Application* exercise.

Overview of Cancer

Cancer (CA), a Latin word meaning *crab*, was first identified around 400 B.C. during the time of Hippocrates. Early reports on cancer compared the disease to a crab because of its tendency to stretch out and spread like the crab's four pairs of legs. Today, cancer refers to any malignant tumor.

The incidence of cancer is now five times higher than it was 100 years ago. Cancer will strike one of every three Americans, according to recent statistics from the American Cancer Society (ACS). However, there is hope for those afflicted. Cancer has become one of the more treatable of the major diseases in the United States. Highly advanced surgical techniques are being used to remove cancerous tissue, and it is usually possible to excise all the cancer cells when the malignancy is discovered in its earliest stages (St). Chemotherapy (chemo) and radiation therapy are the other two principal means of treatment for patients with cancer. These treatments employ agents to kill cancerous cells that remain after surgery or in malignancies deemed inoperable.

Immunotherapy and photodynamic therapy are two newer methods employed in the treatment of cancer. These forms of therapy utilize unique treatment plans that are customized for each patient. Oncologists can now focus on the nature of the cancer and what seems to "turn on" the cancer cells.

Research has shown that some cancers can be prevented, especially those associated with environmental factors. Oncologists searching for the causes of cancer have identified numerous factors that play a role in the development of cancer. See Figure 19.1.These factors are generally grouped under three main classifications: environmental, hereditary, and biological.

The American Cancer Society recommends various safeguards against cancer, which encourages individuals to take specific steps to safeguard their health and aid in the early detection of cancer. For additional information, go to *www.cancer.org*.

fyi More than 60% of cancers in the United States occur in people over the age of 65. It is estimated that by the year 2050, 79 million people will be older than 65. Cancers of the skin, breast, bladder, colon, rectum, lung, pancreas, prostate, and stomach are the most common cancers in people over age 65.

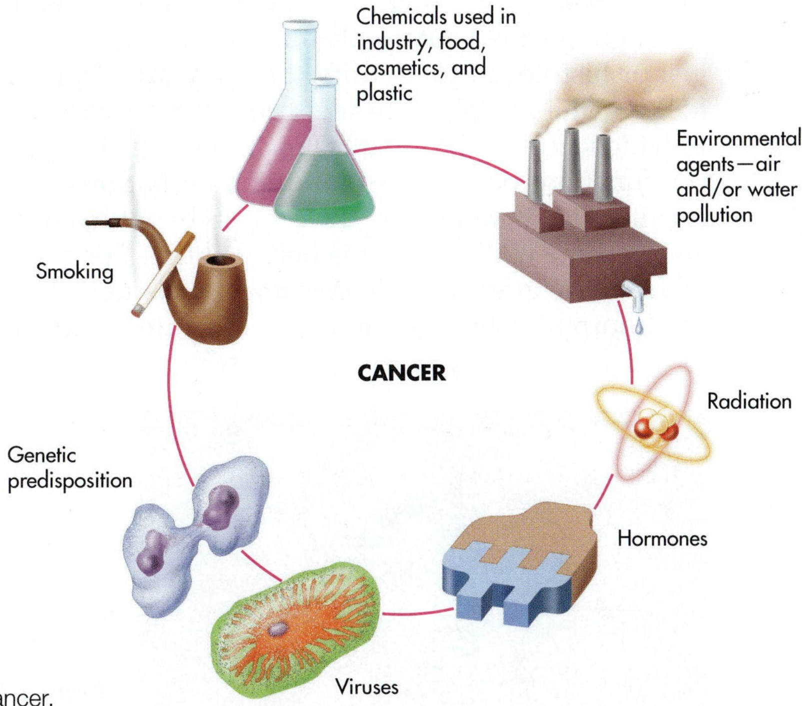

Figure 19.1 Possible causes of cancer.

Classification of Cancer

Classification of cancer helps determine appropriate treatment and prognosis. Tumors are classified according to their anatomical site of origin, grading, and staging. Cell differentiation and the invasive process are also elements of the classification process.

Anatomical Site

The anatomical site indicates where the cancer originated in the body. **Carcinomas** make up the great majority of all cancers and are malignant tumors of epithelial tissues. Epithelial tissue lines body surfaces including those of glands and organs; therefore, carcinomas make up the majority of the glandular cancers and are generally found in the breast, stomach, uterus, tongue, and skin. They are named according to the type of epithelial cell in which the malignancy occurs or the primary site of the tumor. For instance, a cancer of squamous epithelium is called a **squamous carcinoma** (see Figure 19.2 and refer to Figure 5.40), and a type of skin cancer is called a **basal cell carcinoma (BCC)** (see Figure 19.7 and refer to Figure 5.9). Likewise, a cancer originating in the bronchus of the respiratory tract is a **bronchogenic carcinoma**.

Sarcomas originate in connective or supportive tissues of the body such as the muscles, tendons, fat, joints, and bone. They are named by adding the suffix *-oma* (*tumor*) with the root *sarc* (*flesh*) to the word part that identifies the tissue of origin. A cancer of the bone, for example, is an **osteosarcoma**: oste/o (*bone*); sarc (*flesh*); -oma (*tumor*).

Leukemias are cancers of the blood-forming tissues. **Lymphomas** are cancerous tumors of the lymph nodes, and **myelomas** are cancerous tumors arising in the hematopoietic portion of the bone marrow.

Cell Differentiation and Grading

Normal cells reproduce themselves through **mitosis**, an orderly process that ensures growth, tissue repair, and cell reproduction. In normal cell development, immature cells undergo normal changes as they mature and assume their specialized functions. This process, by which normal cells have a distinct appearance and specialized function, is called **differentiation**. Knowledge of cell differentiation allows a pathologist or histologist to identify the body area from which the tissue was removed by looking at a sample of tissue through a microscope. In cancer, an abnormal process in which a cell or group of cells undergoes changes and no longer carries on normal cell functions occurs. This failure of immature cells to develop specialized functions is called **dedifferentiation**, the process by which normal cells lose their specialization and become malignant. It is believed that this process involves a disturbance in the DNA of the affected cells. **Malignant cells** usually multiply rapidly, forming a mass of abnormal cells that enlarges, ulcerates, and sheds malignant cells that invade

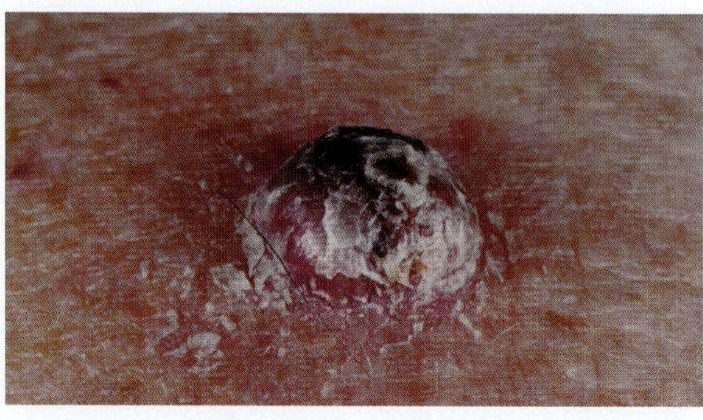

Figure 19.2 Squamous cell carcinoma.
(Courtesy of Jason L. Smith, MD)

surrounding tissues. This process destroys the normal cells, and malignant cells take their places. Microscopic analysis of a malignant cell reveals a loss of differentiation, anaplasia, nuclei of various sizes that are hyperchromatic, and cells in the process of rapid and disorderly division.

Based on microscopic analysis, malignant tumors are further classified as grades 1, 2, 3, or 4. The following describes each of the four grades of tumors in this system:

Grade 1. The most differentiated and the least malignant tumors. Only a few cells are undergoing mitosis; however, some abnormality does exist.

Grade 2. Moderately undifferentiated. More cells are undergoing mitosis, and the pattern is fairly irregular.

Grade 3. Many undifferentiated cells. Tissue origin can be difficult to recognize. Many cells are undergoing mitosis.

Grade 4. The least differentiated and high degree of malignancy.

This system of grading tumors is used to report the prognosis of the disease and to determine whether the tumor is likely to respond to radiation therapy or chemotherapy, as well as the prognosis for surgery.

Invasive Process

Two ways in which malignant cells spread to body parts are by invasive growth and metastasis.

INVASIVE GROWTH

Invasive growth is the spreading process of a malignant tumor into adjacent normal tissue. See Figure 19.3. Young malignant cells divide at the periphery of the tumor and spread by active migration or direct extension. In **active migration**, the malignant cells break away from the neoplasm (new growth), invade surrounding tissue, divide, form secondary tumors (neoplasms), and then reunite with the primary tumor as growth continues. In **direct extension**, multiplication of malignant cells is rapid, and they

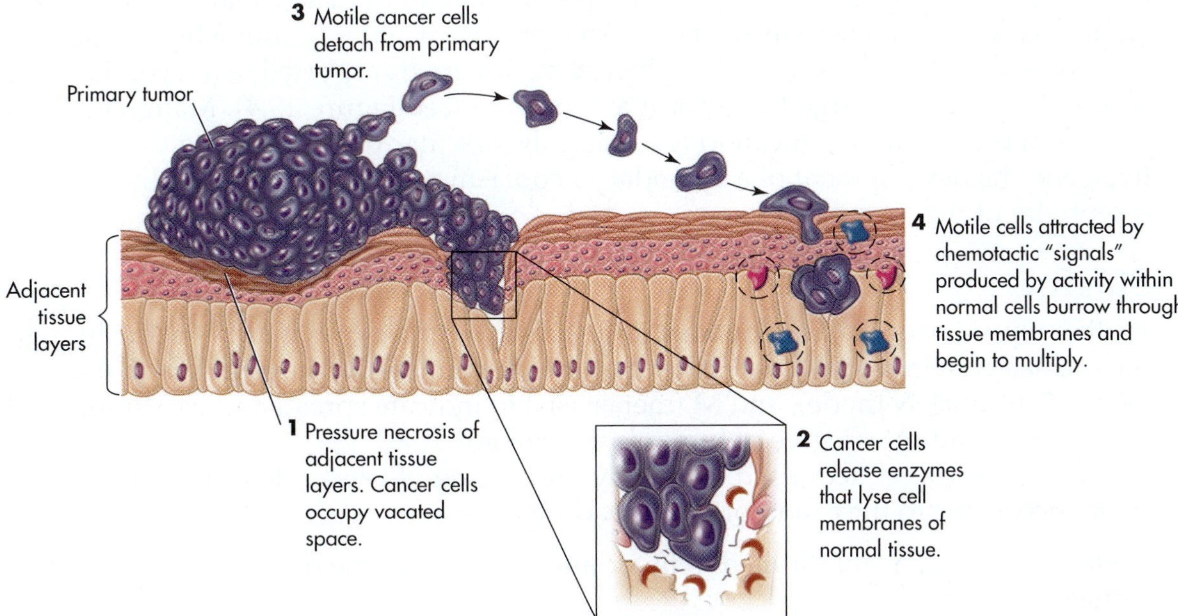
3 Motile cancer cells detach from primary tumor.
Primary tumor
Adjacent tissue layers
4 Motile cells attracted by chemotactic "signals" produced by activity within normal cells burrow through tissue membranes and begin to multiply.
1 Pressure necrosis of adjacent tissue layers. Cancer cells occupy vacated space.
2 Cancer cells release enzymes that lyse cell membranes of normal tissue.

Figure 19.3 How cancer cells invade normal tissue.

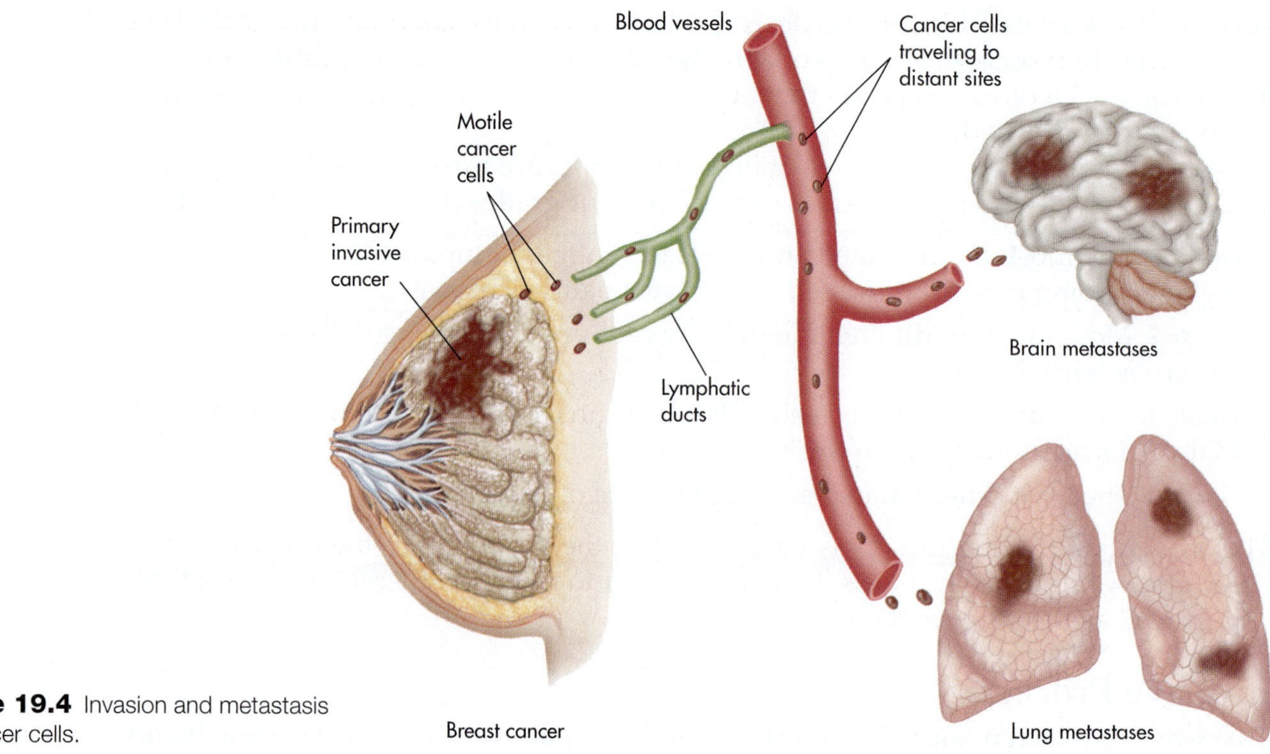

Figure 19.4 Invasion and metastasis by cancer cells.

subsequently spread into surrounding tissues via the interstitial (situated between the cells of a structure) spaces accompanied by engulfment and destruction of normal cells. As a tumor's mass enlarges, its weight is supported by connective fibers that attach to surrounding structures. These fibers invade adjacent veins and lymph vessels and become pathways for the spread of malignant cells to distant locations, such as breast cancer spreading to the bone, lung, or liver.

METASTASIS

Metastasis is the process whereby cancer cells are spread from a primary site to distant secondary sites elsewhere in the body. This process usually occurs when malignant cells invade the bloodstream or lymph system and are transported to a secondary site where they become lodged and form a neoplasm (see Figure 19.4). Malignant cells carried in the bloodstream can lodge in highly vascular organs such as the lungs or liver, and the development of a secondary neoplasm depends on the viability and the receptivity of the organ.

Staging

Further reporting of the development and spread of cancer cells may be made through the use of a system that evaluates the spread of the tumor. The staging system uses the letters **T** (tumor), **N** (node), and **M** (metastasis) to indicate spread and uses numerical subscripts to indicate degree of tumor involvement.

The numerical system used to classify the staging of cancer describes the various stages according to the extent of the spreading process.

Stage 0. Cancer in situ (limited to inner lining surface of the organ and not invading the organ)

Stage I. Cancer limited to the tissue of origin and has not spread past the tissue or organ where it started

Stage II. Limited local spread of cancerous cells, sometimes to lymph nodes

Stage III. Extensive local and regional spread of cancer, usually to draining lymph nodes

Stage IV. Distant metastasis, has spread beyond the regional lymph nodes to distant parts of the body

For example, $T_2N_1M_0$ indicates a primary tumor at stage II, abnormality of regional lymph nodes at stage I, and no evidence of distant metastasis.

Characteristics of Tumors

Tumors or *neoplasms* may be **benign** or **malignant**. See Table 19.1 for characteristics that distinguish the differences between benign and malignant tumors.

As malignant cells proliferate and begin the invasive process, the patient is unaware of the development of the cancer. In its early stages, cancer is said to be silent; however, *cytological* (at the cellular level) changes are occurring that could be detected if a tissue sample were taken and analyzed by a pathologist. With the proliferation of malignant cells and the continuation of the invasive process, tissues, organs, and surrounding structures become compressed, and ischemia can occur, causing necrosis, inflammation, ulceration, and bleeding. This bleeding is usually **occult** (hidden). Because of the silent development of cancer, the patient does not usually become aware of its symptoms until its systemic effects are evident. These systemic effects depend on the site and type of cancer but usually result in an imbalance in the patient's physiology, leading to subtle but noticeable changes that can warn of the disease.

Table 19.1 Characteristics of Benign and Malignant Tumors

Benign Tumors	Malignant Tumors
Grow slowly	Grow rapidly
Encapsulated	Not encapsulated
Have cells that resemble the normal cells from which they arose	Have cells that undergo permanent change, abnormal rapid proliferation
Grow by expansion and cause pressure on surrounding tissue	Have invasive growth and metastasis
Remain localized	Spread via the bloodstream
Do not recur when surgically removed	Can recur when surgically removed if invasive growth has occurred
Have minimal tissue destruction	Have extensive tissue destruction if invasive growth has occurred
Have no cachexia	Have cachexia (extreme weakness, fatigue, wasting, and malnutrition)
Usually not a threat to life	A threat to life unless detected early and properly treated

The American Cancer Society lists seven warning signals of cancer. The first letters of each warning signal combine to spell the word **CAUTION**, and persons who develop any of the following symptoms should bring it to the attention of a physician immediately:

- **C**hange in bowel or bladder habits
- **A** sore that does not heal
- **U**nusual bleeding or discharge
- **T**hickening or lump in breast or elsewhere
- **I**ndigestion or difficulty in swallowing
- **O**bvious change in a wart or mole
- **N**agging cough or hoarseness

Diagnosis

A variety of diagnostic tools and procedures is used to detect the possible presence of cancer. Principal among these are examination, visualization by endoscopy, laboratory analysis, biopsy (Bx), and diagnostic radiology.

Examination

An *annual physical examination* could be the best means to protect a person's state of health. The American Cancer Society publishes a cancer detection examination that recommends certain tests be included in an annual physical examination in addition to the medical history and usual tests. For more specific information, visit the American Cancer Society's website at *www.cancer.org*.

Visualization by Endoscopy

Endoscopy provides the physician a direct view of certain portions of the body. The following is a list of endoscopic procedures used to assess specific locations within the body:

Sigmoidoscopy. Use of a sigmoidoscope to examine the lower 10 inches of the large intestines

Laryngoscopy. Use of a laryngoscope to examine the interior of the larynx

Bronchoscopy. Use of a bronchoscope to examine the bronchi

Gastroscopy. Use of a gastroscope to examine the interior of the stomach

Cystoscopy. Use of a cystoscope to examine the bladder

Colposcopy. Use of a colposcope to examine the cervix and vagina

Proctoscopy. Use of a proctoscope to examine the anus and rectum

Colonoscopy. Use of a colonoscope to examine the colon

Laparoscopy. Use of a laparoscope to examine the abdomen

Laboratory Analysis

Laboratory analysis plays a key role in detecting specific types of cancer. The following are some of the laboratory tests that may be helpful in diagnosing cancer:

Pap smear/test. Cytological screening test developed by Dr. George Papanicolaou and used to detect the presence of abnormal or cancerous cells from the cervix and vagina.

Fecal occult blood test. Test to detect occult (hidden) blood in the stool (feces); if present, further testing would be needed to check for possible cancer of the colon.

Sputum cytology test. Microscopic examination of sputum to detect abnormal or cancerous cells of the bronchi and lungs.

Tumor marker tests. Tumor markers are chemicals made by tumor cells that can be detected in the blood. Examples of tumor markers include prostate-specific antigen (PSA) for prostate cancer; cancer antigen 125 (CA-125) for ovarian cancer; calcitonin for medullary thyroid cancer; alpha-fetoprotein (AFP) for liver cancer; and human chorionic gonadotropin (hCG) for germ cell tumors, such as testicular cancer (TC) and ovarian cancer.

Blood protein test. Test to examine various proteins in the blood (electrophoresis), which can aid in detecting certain abnormal immune system proteins (immunoglobulins) that are sometimes elevated in people with multiple myeloma.

Bone marrow study. A test to detect abnormal bone marrow cells, which can indicate leukemia or multiple myeloma.

Urine assay test. Test providing useful information about catecholamines, which can indicate pheochromocytoma of the adrenal medulla.

Carcinoembryonic antigen (CEA). Test that measures the amount of a protein that can appear in the blood of some people who have certain kinds of cancers, especially large intestine (colon and rectal) cancer; also can be present in people with cancer of the pancreas, breast, ovary, or lung.

Human epidermal growth factor receptor–2 (HER-2/neu). Tests can be performed on breast cancer cells to determine the presence of HER-2/neu protein, a genetic protein that is in part responsible for how certain cancer cells grow, divide, and repair themselves. This information is useful when making treatment decisions.

Circulating tumor cell tests. Experimental blood tests are being developed to find cells that have broken away from an original cancer site and are floating in the bloodstream. More research is needed to understand how these tests can help doctors diagnose advanced cancers.

Biopsy

The surgical removal of a small piece of tissue for microscopic examination is known as **biopsy (Bx)**. It is the method of providing the proof of cancer in the diagnosis of the disease. The following different types of biopsy can be used for tissue removal:

Excisional biopsy. Surgical removal of a piece of tissue from the suspected body site.

Incisional biopsy. Surgical incision to remove a section or wedge of tissue from the suspected body site.

Needle biopsy. Puncture of a tumor for the removal of a core of tissue through the lumen of a needle.

Fine needle aspiration (FNA). Form of breast biopsy in which a small needle is used to withdraw a sample of cells from the breast lump. If the lump is a cyst, removal of the fluid will cause the cyst to collapse. If the lump is solid, cells can be smeared onto slides for examination.

Stereotactic biopsy. Alternative to traditional surgical biopsy; the procedure, which uses a mammogram-guided needle, is performed by a radiologist and assisted by mammography technologists. It is most helpful when mammography shows a mass, a cluster of microcalcifications (tiny calcium deposits that are closely grouped together), or an area of abnormal tissue change but no lump can be felt on careful breast examination.

Core biopsy. Large-bore needle removal of a generous sample of breast tissue and a vacuum-assisted needle biopsy device (VAD), which uses vacuum suction to obtain a tissue sample.

Cone biopsy. Removal of a cone of tissue from the uterine cervix.

Sternal biopsy. Removal of a piece of bone marrow from the sternum.

Endoscopic biopsy. Removal of a piece of tissue through an endoscope.

Punch biopsy. Removal of a plug of tissue (epidermis, dermis, and subcutaneous tissue) from the skin.

Sentinel node biopsy. Process by which a physician pinpoints the first lymph node into which a tumor drains (the sentinel node) and removes only the nodes most likely to contain cancer cells. To locate the sentinel node, the physician injects a radioactive tracer in the area around the tumor. The tracer travels the same path to the lymph nodes that cancer cells would take, making it possible for the surgeon to determine the one or two nodes most likely to test positive. The surgeon then removes the nodes most likely to be cancerous for evaluation and staging.

Diagnostic Radiology

Encompassing a wide range of tests and procedures, **diagnostic radiology** can reveal tumors that were not detected by other diagnostic procedures. See Chapter 20, *Radiology and Nuclear Medicine*, for a discussion of diagnostic radiology.

Treatment

The treatment of cancer can employ one or a combination of the following methods: surgery, chemotherapy, radiation therapy, immunotherapy, or photodynamic therapy (PDT). The treatment of choice depends on the type of cancer, its location, its invasive process, and the patient's state of health. The ultimate goal of treatment is to kill every cancer cell. Therefore, the need to treat tumors at an early stage is critical. For example, a 1 cm breast tumor can contain 1 billion cancer cells before it is detected. A drug killing 99% of these cells would be considered an excellent drug, but 10 million cancer cells would still remain in the body. The relationship between cell kill and chemotherapy is shown in Figure 19.5.

Surgery

Surgery can be the treatment of choice when the tumor is small and localized and the surrounding tissue is accessible for removal. The aim of surgery is to remove all cancerous tissue plus some of the surrounding normal tissue. Surgery is also used to alleviate some of the complications of cancer, such as the obstruction of an area caused by the enlargement of a tumor.

A type of microscopically controlled surgery, Mohs, created by a general surgeon, Dr. Frederic E. Mohs, can be used to remove the two most common forms of skin cancer, basal cell carcinoma and squamous cell carcinoma. The Mohs procedure is essentially a pathology sectioning method that allows for the complete examination of the surgical margin, while the patient is still present in the office. It is different from the standard technique of sectioning in which random samples of the surgical margin are examined, sent to a laboratory for analysis, and then the patient is notified of the

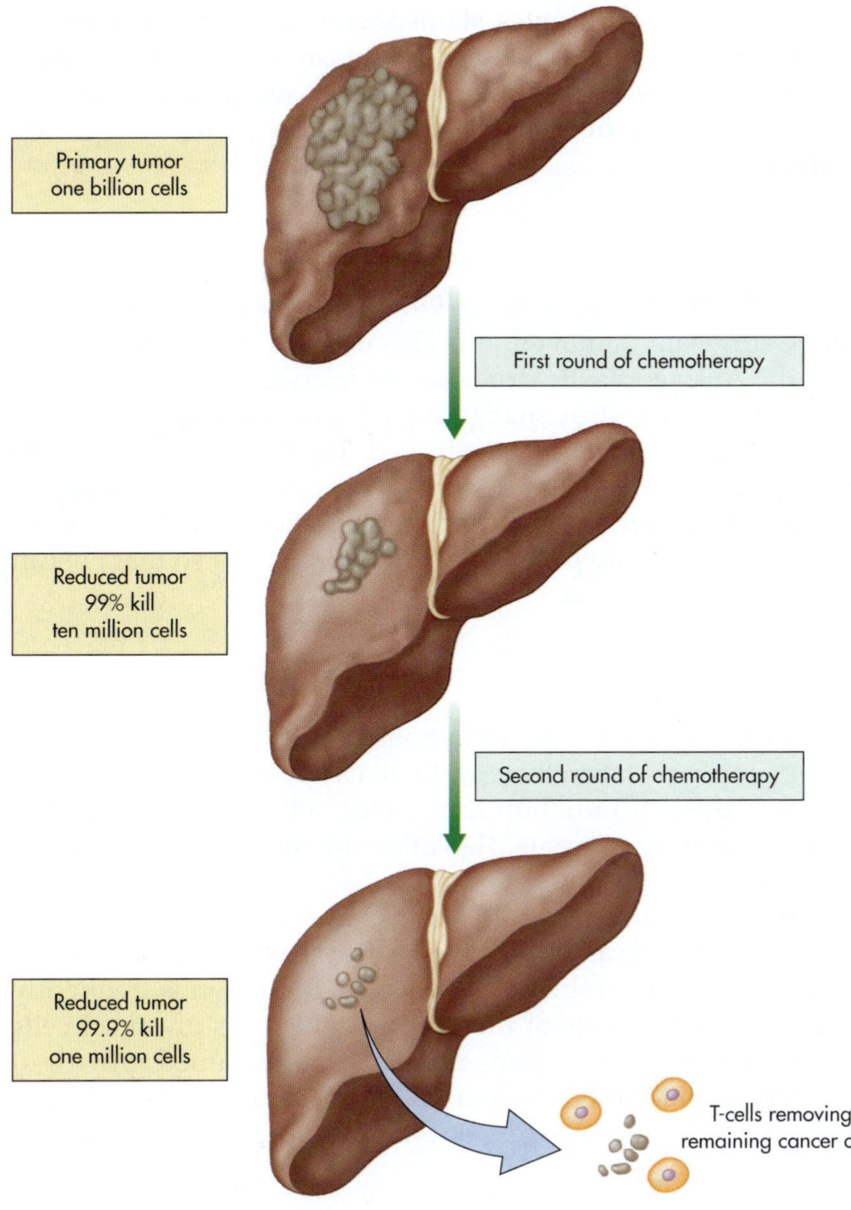

Figure 19.5 Cell kill and chemotherapy.

results and, if indicated, must schedule another visit for further treatment. The Mohs surgery is performed in four steps during one visit:

1. Surgical removal of tissue
2. Mapping the piece of tissue, freezing and cutting the tissue between 5 and 10 micrometers using a cryostat (device for maintaining very low [cold] temperatures), and staining with hematoxylin and eosin (H&E), a popular stain used in medical diagnosis
3. Interpretation of microscope slides for the presence of cancerous cells
4. Reconstruction of the surgical site as needed

The procedure is usually performed in a physician's office using a local anesthetic. A small scalpel is utilized to cut around the visible tumor. A very small surgical margin is utilized, usually with 1 to 1.5 mm of *free margin* or uninvolved skin. The amount of free margin removed is much less than the usual 4 to 6 mm required for the standard excision of skin cancers. After each surgical removal of tissue, the specimen is processed, cut on the cryostat and placed on slides, stained with H&E, and then read by the Mohs surgeon/pathologist who examines the sections for cancerous cells. If cancer is found, its location is marked on the map (drawing of the tissue) and the surgeon removes the indicated cancerous tissue from the patient. This procedure is repeated until no further cancer is found.

Chemotherapy

Chemotherapy (chemo) can be the treatment of choice when the cancer is disseminated (widespread) and cannot be surgically removed. It is also used when a tumor fails to respond to radiation therapy. Antineoplastic drugs injure individual cells, interfere with their vital functions, and kill or destroy malignant cells. In rendering cancerous cells harmless, certain normal cells could also be destroyed. The normal cells with the greatest sensitivity to destruction are the hematopoietic cells, epithelial cells, and the hair follicles. The plan of treatment for patients undergoing chemotherapy is individualized. The aim of chemotherapy is to put the patient in remission so that life can continue without exacerbation of symptoms.

Radiation Therapy

The treatment of disease by the use of ionizing radiation is called **radiotherapy**, **x-ray therapy**, **cobalt treatment**, or simply **radiation therapy**. In all cases, this treatment seeks to deliver a precise, calculated dose of radiation to a tumor, while causing the least possible damage to surrounding normal tissue. **Radiation therapy** can be defined as the process whereby energy is beamed from its source to a selected target tissue. See Figure 19.6. Substances that emit radiation are said to be *radioactive*.

Malignant cells are more sensitive to radiation because these cells divide frequently, making the DNA replication more vulnerable to destruction. Radiation is frequently used as either a *curative* or a *palliative* mode of therapy. Certain types of cancer cells can be destroyed by radiation therapy, thus preventing the unrestrained growth of such tumors. In other cancers, radiation has only a palliative effect, preventing cell growth and reducing pain, pressure, and bleeding but not providing complete tumor

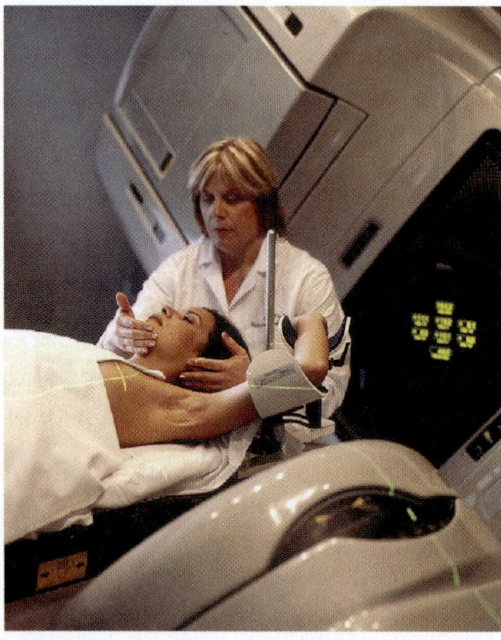

Figure 19.6 Radiation therapy.
(National Cancer Institute/Photographer: Rhoda Baer)

destruction. Important factors that must be considered when determining the use of radiotherapy for the cancer patient include the following:

- The tumor must be surrounded by normal tissue that can tolerate the radiation and then repair itself.
- The tumor must not be widespread. If the tumor has metastasized, radiation can be used as a palliative form of treatment.
- The tumor must be moderately sensitive to radiation (a radiosensitive tumor).

Radiotherapy is often the treatment of choice for cancers of the skin, uterus, cervix, or larynx or those located within the oral cavity. With other types of cancer, radiotherapy is frequently used in combination with other forms of treatment, including surgery and chemotherapy.

TECHNIQUES OF RADIATION THERAPY

The two methods for the administration of radiation are **external radiation therapy (ERT)** and **internal radiation therapy (IRT)**. The following is an overview of these two methods.

External Radiation Therapy. A type of radiation therapy that uses a machine to aim high-energy rays at the cancer from outside of the body, ERT is also called *external-beam radiation therapy*. Many types of external-beam radiation therapy are delivered using a machine called a linear accelerator (LINAC). A LINAC uses electricity to form a stream of fast-moving subatomic particles. This creates high-energy radiation that may be used to treat cancer. Patients usually receive external-beam radiation therapy in daily treatment sessions over the course of several weeks. The number of treatment sessions depends on many factors, including the total radiation dose that will be given.

One of the most common types of external-beam radiation therapy is called *three-dimensional conformal radiation therapy (3D-CRT)*. 3D-CRT uses sophisticated computer software and advanced treatment machines to deliver radiation to precisely delineated target areas. Many other methods of external-beam radiation therapy are currently being tested and used in cancer treatment.

In undergoing ERT, the patient is carefully prepared for treatment by a radiation therapist, sometimes assisted by the **dosimetrist** or a radiation physicist. The precise size and location of the tumor are determined, and the **port**, or point of entry for the radiation, is marked using dye or a tattoo. In formulating the treatment plan, a computer is used to calculate the radiation dosage needed to effect maximal destruction of malignant cells and minimal damage to surrounding normal tissue. Special lead blockers or shields can be constructed by a radiation physicist to protect surrounding normal tissue from the harmful effects of radiation.

Internal Radiation Therapy. IRT is also called *brachytherapy*, *implant radiation therapy*, and *radiation brachytherapy*. It is a type of radiation therapy in which radioactive material sealed in tiny pellets called "seeds" is placed directly into or near a tumor in the body using delivery devices such as needles, catheters, or some other type of carrier. As the isotopes decay naturally, they give off radiation that damages nearby cancer cells. Left in place, after a few weeks or months, the isotopes decay completely and no longer give off radiation; they will not cause harm if they are left in the body.

Several brachytherapy techniques are used in cancer treatment. *Interstitial brachytherapy* uses a radiation source placed within tumor tissue, such as within a prostate tumor. *Intracavitary brachytherapy* uses a source placed within a body cavity, such as the chest cavity, near a tumor. *Episcleral brachytherapy*, which is used to treat melanoma inside the eye, uses a source that is attached to the eye.

Administered as a low-dose-rate or a high-dose-rate treatment, brachytherapy may be able to deliver higher doses of radiation to some cancers than external-beam radiation therapy while causing less damage to normal tissue.

SIDE EFFECTS OF RADIATION

Because radiotherapy unavoidably affects normal tissue while destroying malignant cells, patients usually experience some unpleasant **side effects**. The degree of severity associated with the side effects depends on the individual, the cancer, its location, and the amount of radiation. Some side effects that can occur as a result of radiation therapy are anorexia, nausea, vomiting, diarrhea, malaise, mild erythema, edema, ulcers, alopecia, taste blindness, stomatitis, mucositis, and xerostomia.

TomoTherapy® Highly Integrated Adaptive Radiotherapy

The TomoTherapy® Highly Integrated Adaptive Radiotherapy (HI-ART) system combines an advanced form of intensity-modulated radiation therapy (IMRT) with the accuracy of CT scanning technology, all in one machine. This approach treats hard-to-reach tumors that often sit close to healthy tissues and organs, while minimizing damage to these surrounding tissues.

TomoTherapy offers several advantages:

- Before every treatment, advanced scanning technology provides a 3D image of the body, so the radiation beams can be targeted according to the size, shape, and location of the tumor(s) on that specific day.
- During treatment, the doctor can adjust the intensity and direction of the radiation beams in real time. The revolutionary "slice therapy" approach treats tumors one layer at a time.
- After treatment, side effects are minimized because less radiation reaches healthy tissues and organs.

Each TomoTherapy treatment takes about 20 minutes, including roughly 5 minutes for the CT scan, 5 minutes for the radiation treatment itself, and time for setup. Many cancer patients who have reached their maximum tolerance dose of traditional radiation may be candidates for TomoTherapy.

CyberKnife® Robotic Radiosurgery System

The CyberKnife® Robotic Radiosurgery System is a noninvasive option for patients who have inoperable or surgically complex tumors, or who may be looking for an alternative to surgery. This system's continual image guidance software enables radiation oncologists to deliver high doses of radiation with pinpoint accuracy to a broad range of tumors throughout the body while automatically correcting for tumor movement due to the patient's breathing cycle.

Prior to the procedure, a high-resolution CT scan determines the size, shape, and location of the tumor. This data is then digitally transferred to the CyberKnife System's workstation, where the oncologist precisely plans treatment to match the desired radiation dose to the exact tumor location. Once treatment planning is complete, the patient is positioned on a table and the system's computer-controlled robot slowly moves around the table, targeting radiation to the tumor from various angles while sparing surrounding healthy tissue. Unlike traditional radiation therapy, which can be ongoing for several weeks, each treatment session lasts 30–90 minutes for 1–5 days, depending on the location and type of tumor being treated. Potential benefits of the CyberKnife system include:

- No incision
- No pain
- No anesthesia or hospitalization
- Greater comfort (patient can breathe normally during treatment)
- Little or no recovery time
- Immediate return to normal activities

Immunotherapy

Immunotherapy is the treatment of disease by stimulation of the body's immune system, its natural defense system. The immune system (see Chapter 10) is a collection of organs, cells, and special molecules that helps protect an individual from infections, cancer, and other diseases. When a foreign substance/organism enters the body, the immune system recognizes the invader and attacks it, preventing it from causing harm. This process is called the *immune response*. Cancer cells, however, often find ways to disguise themselves as normal cells so that the immune system does not always recognize them as dangerous. In addition, cancer cells can *mutate* (change over time) and escape the immune response or the immune response is just not strong enough to fight them off and they multiply. Immunotherapies activate the immune system, making it better able to recognize cancer cells and destroy them. These therapies represent a breakthrough in cancer therapy that has the potential to revolutionize the way cancer is treated.

There are three types of immunotherapy: **active specific** (the use of various agents [medications] to produce a specific host–immune response), **passive** (the use of serum or other products from an immunocompetent individual that are given to an immunodeficient individual to produce an immune response), and **adoptive** (the process of transferring a form of specific immune response from a donor to a recipient).

New immunotherapy options include precision medications, which generally work by stimulating a patient's own immune system. Examples of these prescription medicines are Yervoy, Opdivo, and Keytruda, which are approved by the FDA for metastatic melanoma, lung cancer, or kidney cancer. These drugs are administered intravenously, usually in a cancer treatment center or physician's office.

Photodynamic Therapy

Photodynamic therapy (PDT), a type of laser therapy, involves the use of a special chemical that is injected into the bloodstream and absorbed by cells all over the body. The chemical rapidly leaves normal cells but remains in cancer cells for a longer time. A *laser* light aimed at the cancer activates the chemical, which then kills the cancer cells that have absorbed it. Photodynamic therapy can be used to reduce symptoms of non–small cell **lung cancer**, for example, to control bleeding or to relieve breathing problems due to blocked airways when the cancer cannot be removed through surgery. Photodynamic therapy can also be used to treat very small tumors in patients for whom the usual treatments for lung cancer are not appropriate and in patients with esophageal cancer.

Medical Word	Word Parts		Definition
	Part	**Meaning**	
adenocarcinoma (ACA) (ăd″ ĕ-nō-kăr″ sĭn-ō′ mă)	aden/o carcin -oma	gland cancer tumor	Malignant neoplasm (tumor) arising in a glandular organ

ALERT!

How many words can you find in this table that end with the suffix ***-oma***?

insights In ICD-10-CM, Chapter 2, *Neoplasms*, contains the codes (C00–D49) for most benign and all malignant neoplasms (tumors). To properly code a neoplasm, it is necessary to determine from the record if the neoplasm is *benign*, *in situ*, *malignant*, or *of uncertain histologic behavior*. If malignant, any secondary (metastatic) sites should also be determined.

Medical Word	Part	Meaning	Definition
adjuvant therapy (ăd′ jū-vănt)			Adjuvant therapy is any treatment given after primary therapy to increase the chance of long-term survival. Neoadjuvant therapy is treatment given before primary therapy. Adjuvant therapy for breast cancer, for example, can include chemotherapy, hormonal therapy, the targeted drug Herceptin® (trastuzumab), radiation therapy, or a combination of treatments.
anaplasia (ăn″ ă-plā′ zĭ-ă)	ana- -plasia	up, apart, backward formation	Characteristic of most cancerous cells in which there is a loss of differentiation and an irreversible alteration in adult cells toward more embryonic cell types
astrocytoma (ăs″ trō-sī-tō′ mă)	astro- cyt -oma	star-shaped cell tumor	Tumor composed of star-shaped neuroglial cells
brachytherapy (brăk″ ĭ-thĕr′ ă-pē)	brachy- -therapy	short treatment	Radiation therapy in which the radioactive substance is inserted into a body cavity or organ. The source of radiation is located a short distance from the body area being treated.
Burkitt lymphoma (bŭrk′ ĭt lĭm-fō′ mă)			Malignant tumor, most commonly found in Africa, that affects children; the characteristic symptom is a massive, swollen jaw
carcinogen (kăr″ sĭn′ ō-jĕn)	carcin/o -gen	cancer formation, produce	Agent or substance that incites or produces cancer

Medical Word	Word Parts: Part	Word Parts: Meaning	Definition
carcinoid (kăr´ sĭ-noid)	carcin -oid	cancer resemble	Tumor derived from the argentaffin cells in the intestinal tract, bile duct, pancreas, bronchus, or ovary

RULE REMINDER

The ***o*** has been removed from the combining form because the suffix begins with a vowel.

Medical Word	Word Parts: Part	Word Parts: Meaning	Definition
carcinoma (kăr˝ sĭ-nō´ mă)	carcin -oma	cancer tumor	Malignant tumor arising in epithelial tissue. See Figure 19.7.

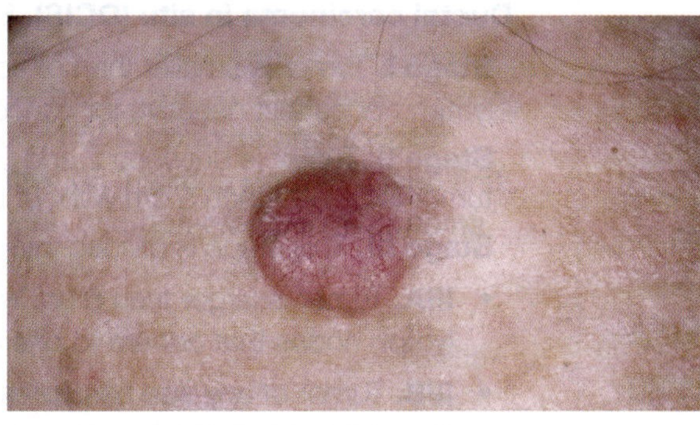

Figure 19.7 Basal cell carcinoma.
(Courtesy of Jason L. Smith, MD)

Medical Word	Word Parts: Part	Word Parts: Meaning	Definition
chondrosarcoma (kŏn˝ drō-săr-kō´ mă)	chondr/o sarc -oma	cartilage flesh tumor	Cancerous tumor derived from cartilage cells
choriocarcinoma (kō˝ rĭ-ō-kăr˝ sĭ-nō´ mă)	chori/o carcin -oma	chorion cancer tumor	Cancerous tumor of the uterus or at the site of an ectopic pregnancy
deoxyribonucleic acid (DNA) (dē-ŏk˝ sĭ-rī˝ bō-nū-klē´ ĭk)			Complex protein of high molecular weight found in the nucleus of every cell; controls all of the cell's activities and the genetic material necessary for the organism's heredity

Medical Word	Word Parts: Part	Word Parts: Meaning	Definition
nephroblastoma (nĕf″ rō-blăs-tō′ mă)	nephr/o -blast -oma	kidney immature cell tumor	Cancerous tumor of the kidney; also called *Wilms tumor*; most often found in children 2–3 years of age
neuroblastoma (nū″ rō-blăs-tō′ mă)	neur/o -blast -oma	nerve immature cell tumor	Cancerous tumor composed chiefly of neuroblasts; can appear anywhere but usually in the abdomen as a swelling; most often diagnosed during the first year of life
oligodendroglioma (ŏl″ ĭ-gō-dĕn″ drō-glī-ō′ mă)	oligo- dendr/o gli -oma	little tree glue tumor	Cancerous tumor composed chiefly of neuroglial cells and located in the cerebrum
oncogenes (ŏng′ kō-jēnz)	onc/o -genes	tumor produce	Cancer-causing genes; genes in a virus that can induce tumor formation

RULE REMINDER

This term keeps the combining vowel ***o*** because the suffix begins with a consonant.

Medical Word	Word Parts: Part	Word Parts: Meaning	Definition
oncogenic (ŏng″ kō-jĕn′ ĭk)	onc/o -genic	tumor formation, produce	Pertaining to the potential formation of tumors, especially cancerous ones
oncologist (ŏng-kŏl′ ō-jĭst)	onc/o log -ist	tumor study of one who specializes	A physician who specializes in the study and treatment of tumors
oncology (ŏng-kŏl′ ō-jē)	onc/o -logy	tumor study of	The study of tumors
osteogenic sarcoma (ŏs″ tē-ō-jĕn′ ĭk săr-kō′ mă)	oste/o -genic sarc -oma	bone formation, produce flesh tumor	Cancerous tumor composed of osseous (bone) tissue

Medical Word	Word Parts		Definition
	Part	**Meaning**	
Paget disease of the breast (păj´ ĕt)			Paget disease of the breast (also called *mammary Paget disease [MPD]*) is a rare form of breast cancer. The condition was originally reported in 1874 by Sir James Paget, an English surgeon, who also described an unrelated skeletal condition known as Paget disease of the bone. These disorders are distinct disease entities that are medically unrelated. Paget disease of the breast is characterized by inflammatory, "eczema-like" changes of the nipple that may extend to involve the areola. See Figure 19.12.

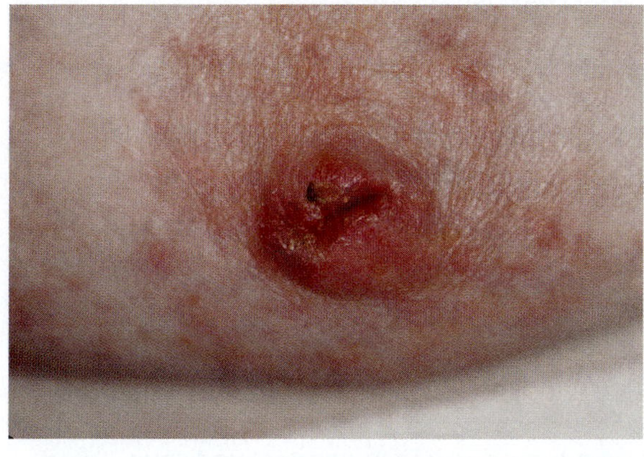

Figure 19.12 Paget disease of the breast.
(Courtesy of Jason L. Smith, MD)

Medical Word	Part	Meaning	Definition
palliative (păl´ ĭ-ā-tĭv)	palliat -ive	cloaked nature of	Pertaining to a form of treatment to relieve or alleviate symptoms without curing
port			In radiation therapy, refers to the skin area of entry for the radiation
precancerous (prē-kăn´ sĕr-ŭs)	pre- cancer -ous	before crab, cancer pertaining to	Pertaining to changes or conditions before the onset of cancer
primary site			Original, initial, or principal site; the tissue of origin of a metastatic tumor
proliferation (prō-lĭf″ ĕr-ā´ shŭn)			Process of rapid production; growth by multiplying
remission (rē-mĭsh´ ŭn)	remiss -ion	remit process	Process of lessening the severity of symptoms; time when symptoms of a disease are controlled
reticulosarcoma (rĕ-tĭk″ ū-lō-săr-kō´ mă)	reticul/o sarc -oma	net flesh tumor	Cancerous tumor of the lymphatic system
retinoblastoma (rĕt″ ĭ-nō-blăs-tō´ mă)	retin/o -blast -oma	retina immature cell tumor	Cancerous tumor of the retina. Although relatively rare, it accounts for 5% of childhood blindness.

Medical Word	Word Parts		Definition
	Part	**Meaning**	
rhabdomyosarcoma (răb″ dō-mī″ ō-săr-kō′ mă)	rhabd/o my/o sarc -oma	rod muscle flesh tumor	Cancerous tumor originating from the same embryonic cells that develop into striated muscles. It is the most common soft tissue sarcoma in children.

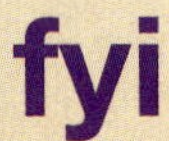

Atypical teratoid rhabdoid tumor (AT/RT) is a rare tumor generally diagnosed in childhood. Although usually a brain tumor, AT/RT can occur anywhere in the central nervous system including the spinal cord. In the United States, three children per 1,000,000 or around 30 new AT/RT cases are diagnosed each year. Because it is highly malignant, AT/RT has a high mortality rate. Current research is focusing on using chemotherapy protocols that are effective against rhabdomyosarcoma in combination with surgery and radiation therapy. The initial diagnosis of a tumor is made with a radiographic study, an MRI, or a CT scan.

Medical Word	Part	Meaning	Definition
ribonucleic acid (RNA) (rī″ bō-nū-klē′ ĭk)			Nucleic acid found in all living cells; responsible for protein synthesis
sarcoma (săr-kō′ mă)	sarc -oma	flesh tumor	Cancerous tumor arising in connective tissue
secondary site			Second site usually derived from the primary site; refers to any additional sites where a cancer has spread
seminoma (sĕm″ ĭ-nō′ mă)	semin -oma	seed tumor	Cancerous tumor of the testis generally diagnosed by biopsy; testicular cancer

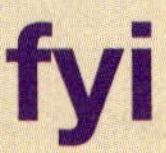

Testicular cancer (TC) is a disease in which malignant cells form in the tissues of one or both testicles. It is the most common cancer in men age 20–35. Most testicular tumors are discovered by patients themselves, either by accident or while performing a *testicular self-examination (TSE)*.

Medical Word	Part	Meaning	Definition
tamponade (cardiac) (tam″ pŏn-ād′ [kăr′ dē-ăk])			Excessive fluid in the pericardial sac surrounding the heart; can be caused by advanced cancer of the lung or a tumor that has metastasized to the pericardium
teratoma (tĕr″ ă-tō′ mă)	terat -oma	monster tumor	Malignant teratoma is a type of cancer made of cysts that contain one or more of the three layers of cells found in a developing embryo; it can contain embryonic tissues of hair, teeth, bone, or muscle; teratomas occur most often in the ovaries or testicles; may also be a benign tumor
thymoma (thī-mō′ mă)	thym -oma	thymus tumor	Tumor of the thymus gland
trismus (trĭz′ mŭs)	trism -us	grating pertaining to	Pertaining to the inability to open the mouth fully; occurs in patients with oral cancer who undergo a combination of surgery and radiation therapy

Medical Word	Word Parts		Definition
	Part	**Meaning**	
tumor (tū´ mor)			Abnormal growth, swelling, or enlargement
viral (vī´ răl)	vir -al	virus (poison) pertaining to	Pertaining to a virus, which means *poison* in Latin
Wilms tumor (vĭlmz tū´ mor)			Cancerous tumor of the kidney occurring mainly in children
xerostomia (zē″ rō-stō´ mē-ă)	xer/o stom -ia	dry mouth condition	Condition of dryness of the mouth; oral change caused by radiation therapy or chemotherapy

Study and Review II

Word Parts

Prefixes

Give the definitions of the following prefixes.

1. ana- ______________________
2. astro- ______________________
3. hyper- ______________________
4. neo- ______________________
5. oligo- ______________________
6. pre- ______________________
7. en- ______________________
8. in- ______________________
9. meta- ______________________
10. brachy- ______________________

Combining Forms

Give the definitions of the following combining forms.

1. cancer/o ______________________
2. capsul/o ______________________
3. carcin/o ______________________
4. chori/o ______________________
5. dendr/o ______________________
6. filtrat/o ______________________
7. gli/o ______________________
8. immun/o ______________________
9. lei/o ______________________
10. malign/o ______________________
11. melan/o ______________________
12. mucos/o ______________________
13. mutat/o ______________________
14. myc/o ______________________
15. myel/o ______________________
16. onc/o ______________________
17. palliat/o ______________________
18. remiss/o ______________________
19. reticul/o ______________________
20. rhabd/o ______________________
21. suppress/o ______________________
22. terat/o ______________________
23. tox/o ______________________
24. vir/o ______________________

Suffixes

Give the definitions of the following suffixes.

1. -blast ______________________
2. -emia ______________________
3. -gen ______________________
4. -genes ______________________
5. -genic ______________________
6. -ia ______________________
7. -in ______________________
8. -itis ______________________
9. -oma ______________________
10. -ous ______________________
11. -plakia ______________________
12. -plasia ______________________
13. -plasm ______________________
14. -ate(d) ______________________
15. -therapy ______________________
16. -us ______________________
17. -al ______________________
18. -ar ______________________
19. -ion ______________________
20. -ive ______________________
21. -ant ______________________
22. -stasis ______________________
23. -oid ______________________

Identifying Medical Terms

In the spaces provided, write the medical terms for the following meanings.

1. ______________________ Agent or substance that incites or produces cancer
2. ______________________ Cancerous tumor derived from cartilage cells
3. ______________________ Cancerous tumor of the brain
4. ______________________ Cancerous tumor of smooth muscle tissue
5. ______________________ Cancer of the blood characterized by overproduction of leukocytes
6. ______________________ Cancerous tumor of lymphoid tissue
7. ______________________ Literally means *a black tumor*
8. ______________________ Cancerous tumor of muscle tissue
9. ______________________ Cancerous tumor of the kidney occurring mainly in children
10. ______________________ Cancerous tumor arising in connective tissue

Matching

Select the appropriate lettered meaning for each of the following words.

_______________ **1.** Hodgkin disease

_______________ **2.** exacerbation

_______________ **3.** differentiation

_______________ **4.** in situ

_______________ **5.** encapsulated

_______________ **6.** photodynamic therapy

_______________ **7.** fungating

_______________ **8.** hyperplasia

_______________ **9.** Kaposi sarcoma

_______________ **10.** metastasis

a. Spreading process of cancer from a primary site to a secondary site

b. Excessive formation and growth of normal cells

c. Enclosed within a sheath

d. Process by which normal cells have a distinct appearance and specialized function

e. Form of lymphoma that occurs in young adults

f. Type of laser therapy that involves the use of a special chemical that is injected into the bloodstream and absorbed by cells all over the body

g. Enclosed within a site, sheath, or capsule

h. Malignant neoplasm that causes violaceous (purplish discoloration), vascular lesions, and general lymphadenopathy

i. Process of increasing the severity of symptoms

j. Process of growing rapidly

k. Agent that causes a change in the genetic structure of an organism

Medical Case Snapshots

This learning activity provides an opportunity to relate the medical terminology you are learning to a precise patient case presentation. In the spaces provided, write in your answers.

Case 1

A 45-year-old female is diagnosed with ductal carcinoma in situ (abbreviated as _______________) of the right breast. This type of cancer is confined to the _______________ or milk-producing glands or ducts and has not invaded nearby breast tissue. The patient is in stage I. The _______________ is smaller than or equal to 2 centimeters in diameter and the _______________ lymph nodes test _______________ for cancer.

Case 2

A 29-year-old male presents stating, "I was taking a shower and washing my genitals when I found a lump in my right testicle." Upon examination it was noted that the right testicle was firm with a nontender, oval, pea-sized mass that did not reduce with patient lying down. The patient was suspected of having _______________ _______________, which is a disease in which malignant cells form in the tissues of one or both testicles. To confirm the diagnosis several procedures and tests were ordered. The biopsy was positive for a ___________, a cancerous tumor of the testis.

Case 3

A 70-year-old female presents with a cough that has not gone away. She states that in the last 3 months the cough has gotten worse. She is a smoker, with a history of a pack-a-day for over 35 years. A ___________ cytology (the microscopic examination of cells obtained from a deep-cough sample of mucus in the lungs) is ordered. To confirm the presence of lung cancer, the doctor must perform a ___________ in order to examine tissue from the lung.

Abbreviations

Abbreviation	Meaning
ACA	adenocarcinoma
ACS	American Cancer Society
AFP	alpha-fetoprotein
AIDS	acquired immunodeficiency syndrome
AT/RT	atypical teratoid rhabdoid tumor
BCC	basal cell carcinoma
Bx	biopsy
CA	cancer
CA-125	cancer antigen 125
CEA	carcinoembryonic antigen
chemo	chemotherapy
cm	centimeter
DCIS	ductal carcinoma in situ
DNA	deoxyribonucleic acid
ERT	external radiation therapy
ETS	environmental tobacco smoke
FNA	fine needle aspiration
hCG	human chorionic gonadotropin
HD	Hodgkin disease
H&E	hematoxylin and eosin
HER-2/neu	human epidermal growth factor receptor–2
HI-ART	highly integrated adaptive radiotherapy
HTLV	human T-cell leukemia-lymphoma virus
IMRT	intensity-modulated radiation therapy
IRT	internal radiation therapy
KS	Kaposi sarcoma
LCIS	lobular carcinoma in situ
mL	milliliter
mm	millimeter
MPD	mammary Paget disease
MRI	magnetic resonance imaging
NHL	non-Hodgkin lymphoma
PDT	photodynamic therapy
PSA	prostate-specific antigen
RNA	ribonucleic acid
St	stage (of disease)
TC	testicular cancer
TSE	testicular self-examination
VAD	vacuum-assisted needle biopsy device

Study and Review III

Building Medical Terms

Using the following word parts, fill in the blanks to build the correct medical terms.

lymph	terat	-oma
melan	-plasia	-us
onc/o	-plasm	
remiss	-ive	

Definition	Medical Term
1. Excessive formation and growth of normal cells	hyper_________
2. Cancerous tumor of lymphoid tissue	_________oma
3. Literally means *a cancerous black mole or tumor*	_________oma
4. New tissue formed, such as an abnormal growth or tumor	neo_________
5. Cancer-causing genes	_________genes
6. A form of treatment to relieve symptoms without curing	palliat_________
7. Process of lessening the severity of symptoms	_________ion
8. Cancerous tumor of the testes	semin_________
9. Cancerous tumor of the ovary or testicles	_________oma
10. Pertaining to the inability to open the mouth fully	trism_________

Combining Form Challenge

Using the combining forms provided, write the medical term correctly.

carcin/o	leuk/o	myel/o
immun/o	malign/o	sarc/o

1. Agent or substance that incites or produces cancer: __________ gen

2. Treatment of disease by active, passive, or adoptive immunity: __________ therapy

3. Cancer of the blood characterized by overproduction of leukocytes: __________ emia

4. Pertaining to a bad wandering: __________ ant

5. Tumor arising in the hematopoietic portion of the bone marrow: __________ oma

6. Cancerous tumor arising in connective tissue: __________ oma

Select the Right Term

Select the correct answer, and write it on the line provided.

1. Process by which normal cells lose their specialization and become malignant is ________.

carcinoid **dedifferentiation** **differentiation** **exacerbation**

2. Spreading process of cancer from a primary site to a secondary site is ________.

invasive **in situ** **metastasis** **mutation**

3. In radiation therapy, refers to the skin area of entry for the radiation is ________.

primary site **port** **secondary site** **derma-entry**

4. Process of rapid production; growth by multiplying is ________.

proliferation **exacerbation** **remission** **invasive**

5. Cancerous tumor of the kidney occurring mainly in children is ________.

Hodgkin disease **Kaposi sarcoma** **neuroblastoma** **Wilms tumor**

6. Condition of dryness of the mouth is ________.

trismus **stomatitis** **xerostomia** **mucositis**

Abbreviations

Place the correct word, phrase, or abbreviation in the space provided.

1. adenocarcinoma ________

2. biopsy ________

3. CA ________

4. chemo ________

5. deoxyribonucleic acid ________

6. IRT ________

7. human epidermal growth factor receptor–2/neu ________

8. ductal carcinoma in situ ________

9. BCC ________

10. testicular cancer ________

Practical Application

Medical Record Analysis

This exercise contains information, abbreviations, and medical terminology from an actual medical record or case study that has been adapted for this text. The names and any personal information have been created by the author. Read and study each form or case study and then answer the questions that follow. You may refer to Appendix III, *Abbreviations and Symbols*.

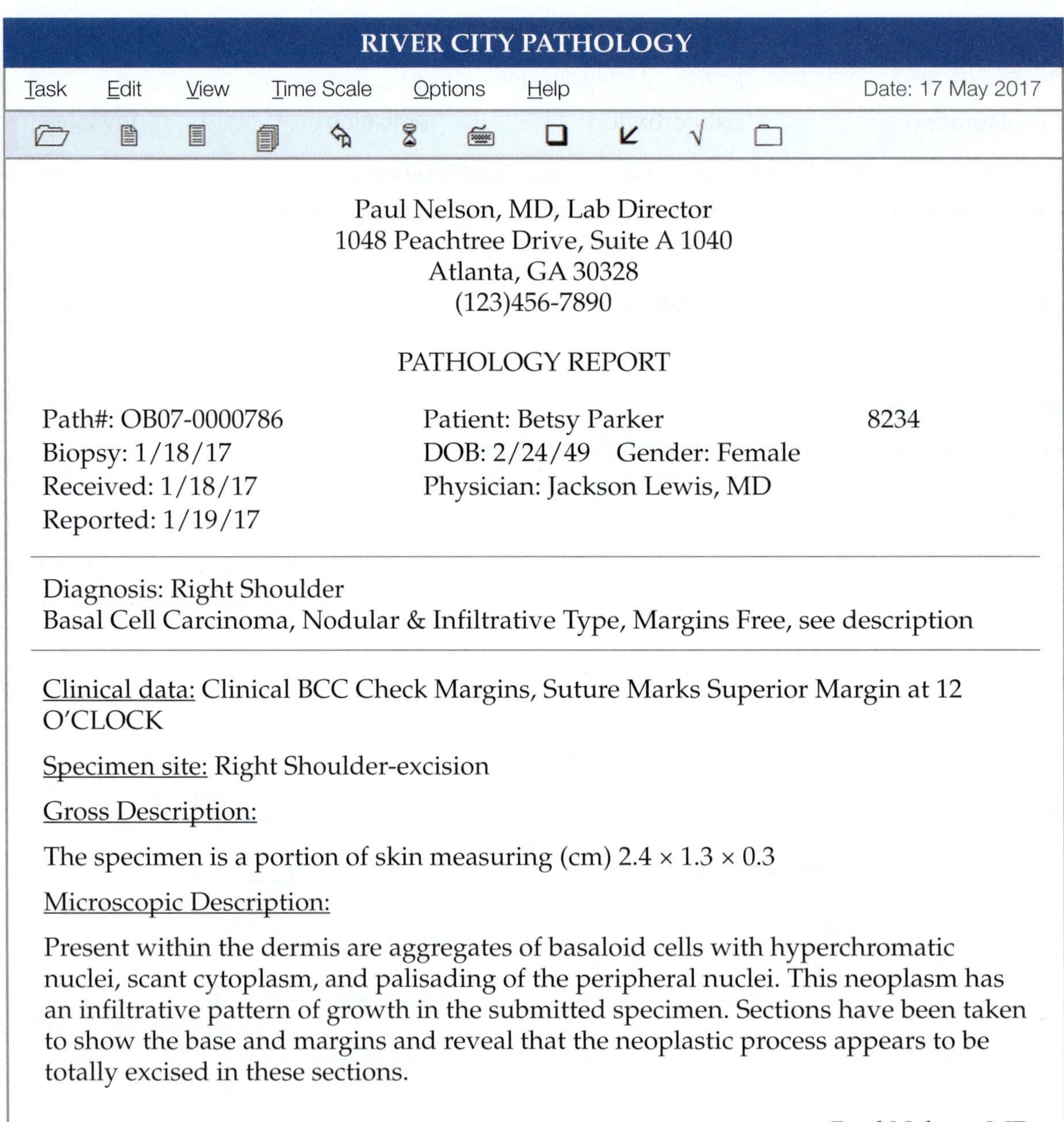

RIVER CITY PATHOLOGY

Task Edit View Time Scale Options Help Date: 17 May 2017

Paul Nelson, MD, Lab Director
1048 Peachtree Drive, Suite A 1040
Atlanta, GA 30328
(123)456-7890

PATHOLOGY REPORT

Path#: OB07-0000786	Patient: Betsy Parker	8234
Biopsy: 1/18/17	DOB: 2/24/49 Gender: Female	
Received: 1/18/17	Physician: Jackson Lewis, MD	
Reported: 1/19/17		

Diagnosis: Right Shoulder
Basal Cell Carcinoma, Nodular & Infiltrative Type, Margins Free, see description

Clinical data: Clinical BCC Check Margins, Suture Marks Superior Margin at 12 O'CLOCK

Specimen site: Right Shoulder-excision

Gross Description:

The specimen is a portion of skin measuring (cm) 2.4 × 1.3 × 0.3

Microscopic Description:

Present within the dermis are aggregates of basaloid cells with hyperchromatic nuclei, scant cytoplasm, and palisading of the peripheral nuclei. This neoplasm has an infiltrative pattern of growth in the submitted specimen. Sections have been taken to show the base and margins and reveal that the neoplastic process appears to be totally excised in these sections.

Paul Nelson, MD

Medical Record Questions

Place the correct answer in the space provided.

1. What is a neoplasm? ______________________
2. What is the meaning of BCC? ______________________
3. Why is it important to indicate "margins free" in the diagnosis? ______________________
4. What was the location of this specimen? ______________________
5. What is the meaning of cm? ______________________

Chapter

20 Radiology and Nuclear Medicine

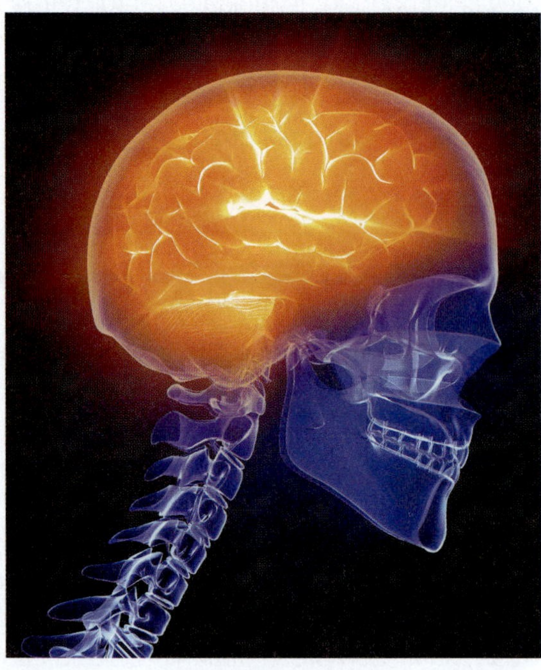

Learning Outcomes

On completion of this chapter, you will be able to:

1. Define radiology.
2. Explain the dangers and safety precautions associated with x-rays.
3. Identify the positions used in radiography.
4. Discuss diagnostic imaging as used by the radiologist and the computer-assisted x-ray machines that are described in this chapter.
5. Describe nuclear medicine and some of the general uses of this specialty.
6. Define interventional radiology and state some interventional procedures described in this chapter.
7. Analyze, build, spell, and pronounce medical words.
8. Identify and define selected abbreviations.
9. Apply your acquired knowledge of medical terms by successfully completing the *Practical Application* exercise.

Radiology

Radiology is the scientific discipline of medical imaging using radionuclides, ionizing radiation, nuclear magnetic resonance, and ultrasound. This medical specialty was developed after the discovery of an unknown ray in 1895 by Wilhelm Konrad-Roentgen, a German physicist, who called his discovery *x-ray*. An **x-ray** is produced by the collision of a stream of electrons against a target (usually an anode of one of the heavy metals) contained within a vacuum tube. This collision produces electromagnetic rays of short wavelengths and high energy. The physician who specializes in radiology, roentgen diagnosis, and roentgen therapy is called a **radiologist**.

Characteristics of X-Rays

The following are the characteristics of x-rays applicable to its medical use.

1. X-rays are an invisible form of radiant energy with short wavelengths traveling at 186,000 miles per second. They are able to penetrate different substances to varying degrees.
2. X-rays cause **ionization** of the substances through which they pass. Ionization is a process resulting in the gain or loss of one or more electrons in neutral atoms. The gain of an electron creates a negative electrical charge, whereas the loss of an electron results in a positively charged particle. These negatively or positively charged particles are called *ions*.
3. X-rays cause fluorescence of certain substances, thus allowing for the process known as **fluoroscopy** (Figure 20.1), the examination of the tissues and deep structures of the body by x-ray, using a **fluoroscope**, a device that shows a continuous x-ray image on a monitor, much like an x-ray movie. This process allows the physician to visualize internal structures that are in motion and to make permanent records of the examination for future study.
4. X-rays allow the x-ray beam to be directed at a specific site during radiotherapy or to produce high-quality shadow images on **film** (radiographs). Today much

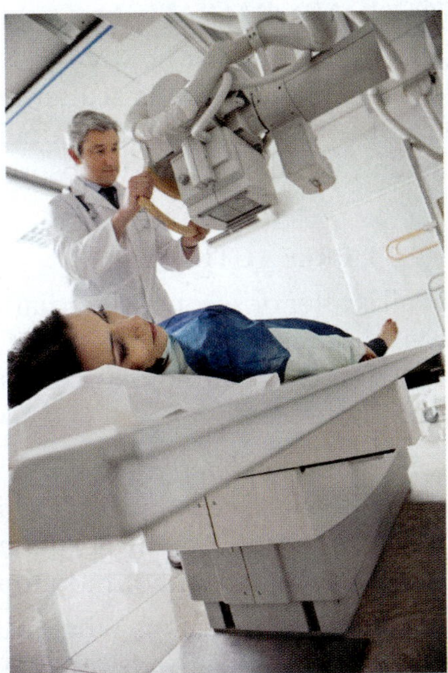

Figure 20.1 The patient is positioned for a fluoroscopy.
(Tyler Olson/Fotolia)

of medical image processing is by digital means and transmitted electronically. These images can be viewed and shared on computer screens and on other types of electronic devices.

5. X-rays are able to penetrate substances of different densities. In the body, x-rays pass through air in the lungs, fluids such as blood and lymph, and fat around muscles. Such substances are said to be **radiolucent**. Substances that obstruct the passage of radiant energy—in other words, absorb radiant energy—such as calcium in bones, lead, or barium (Ba), are called **radiopaque**. Control of the voltage and amperage applied to the x-ray tube plus the duration of the exposure allows images of body structures of varying densities. A contrast medium can be introduced into the body to enhance certain x-ray images. This characteristic allows x-rays to be used as a diagnostic tool.
6. X-rays can destroy body cells. Radiation can be used to destroy malignant tumors. In these cases, the x-ray voltage is administered by a radiotherapist using radiotherapy machines such as a linear accelerator or betatron. Care must be exercised in administering radiotherapy because x-rays can destroy healthy as well as abnormal tissue.

Dangers and Safety Precautions

Because x-rays are invisible and produce no sound or smell, those working around and with them need to take certain precautions to avoid unnecessary exposure. Following are some of the dangers known to be associated with x-rays and the safety precautions designed to prevent unnecessary exposure.

PROLONGED EXPOSURE

Prolonged and continued exposure to x-rays can cause damage to the gonads (testes or ovaries) and/or depress the hematopoietic system, which can cause leukopenia and/or leukemia. Personnel involved with radiation therapy should spend the minimal amount of time necessary when caring for patients receiving internal radiation therapy. The farther away an individual is from the source of radiation, the less the degree of exposure.

SECONDARY RADIATION

X-rays can scatter or be diverted from their normal straight paths when they strike radiopaque objects. This scatter or secondary radiation tends to add unwanted density to the image; therefore, a device known as a **grid** is positioned between the x-ray machine and the patient to absorb scatter before it reaches the x-ray film.

SAFETY PRECAUTIONS

Not all scatter or secondary radiation is absorbed by a grid; therefore, those working in areas adjacent to x-ray equipment risk unintentional exposure from this source unless proper safety precautions are observed. Generally, these safety precautions include the five described below.

1. ***Personal dosimeter.*** A device, usually attached to a medical worker's clothing, that is sensitive to ionizing radiation and monitors exposure to beta and gamma rays. A periodic analysis (generally quarterly or monthly) of the dosimeter reveals the amount of radiation the individual has received. See Figure 20.2.
2. ***Lead barrier.*** Persons who operate x-ray machines do so from behind barriers equipped with a lead-treated window for viewing the patient.

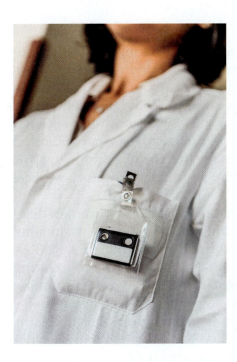

Figure 20.2 Personal dosimeters must be worn by all staff around x-ray equipment.
(Dario Lo Presti/Fotolia)

3. ***Lead-lined room.*** X-ray equipment should be housed in an area featuring lead-lined walls, floors, and doors to prevent the escape of radiation from the room.
4. ***Protective clothing.*** People who hold or position patients for x-ray examination should wear lead-lined gloves and aprons, especially if they hold a patient, such as a child, while an x-ray is being taken.
5. ***Gonad shield.*** The reproductive organs are radiosensitive and must be protected by a lead shield while x-rays are being taken. X-rays can cause damage to the genetic material within the reproductive organs, which could lead to birth defects or cancer.

Positions Used in Radiography

- **Anteroposterior (AP) position.** The patient is placed with the anterior (front) part of the body facing the x-ray tube and the posterior (back) of the body facing the film. X-rays pass through the body from the front to the back in reaching the film.
- **Posteroanterior (PA) position.** The patient is placed with the posterior (back) portion of the body facing the x-ray tube and the anterior (front) of the body facing the film. The x-rays pass through the body from the back to the front to reach the film.
- **Lateral (lat) position.** The x-ray beam passes from one side of the patient's body to the opposite side to reach the film. Placing the patient's right side next to the film and passing x-rays through the body from left to right is known as the *right lateral position*. Placing the patient's left side next to the film and passing x-rays through the body from right to left is known as the *left lateral position*.
- **Supine position.** The patient rests on the back, face upward, allowing the x-rays to pass through the body from the front to the back.
- **Prone position.** The patient is placed lying face down with the head turned to one side. The x-rays pass from the back to the front side of the body.
- **Oblique position.** The patient is placed so that the body or body part to be imaged is at an angle to the x-ray beam.

Diagnostic Imaging

Diagnostic imaging involves the use of x-rays, ultrasound, radiopharmaceuticals, radiopaque media, and computers to provide the radiologist images of internal body organs and processes. These images are used to identify and locate tumors, fractures, hematomas, disease processes, and other abnormalities within the body. In recent years, advances in the field of electronics have produced a variety of computer-assisted x-ray machines to enhance the images obtained by the radiologist. These sophisticated machines now make possible noninvasive procedures for the visualization of organs and processes that were previously not accessible or that required exploratory surgical procedures for examination.

Pregnant healthcare practitioners are permitted to work in and around certain diagnostic imaging machines. Acceptable activities include, but are not limited to, positioning patients, scanning, archiving, injecting contrast, and entering the scan room in response to an emergency. Pregnant practitioners are requested not to remain in the room during the actual data acquisition or scanning. Pregnant patients may undergo certain scanning if, in the determination of a designated attending radiologist, the risk–benefit ratio for the patient warrants that the study be performed. The radiologist should confer with the referring physician and document that the data is needed and the physician does not believe that it is prudent to wait until the patient is no longer pregnant.

COMPUTED TOMOGRAPHY

Computed tomography (CT) is sometimes referred to as a **CAT scan** (computerized axial tomography). It combines an advanced x-ray scanning system with a powerful minicomputer and has vastly improved imaging quality while making it possible to view parts of the body and abnormalities not previously open to radiography. The CT scanner combines tomography, the process of imaging structures by focusing on a specific body plane and blurring all details from other planes, with a microprocessor that provides high-speed analysis of the tissue variances scanned (Figure 20.3).

CT scans reveal both bone and soft tissues, including organs, muscles, and tumors (Figure 20.4). Image tones can be adjusted to highlight tissues of similar density and, through graphics software, the data from multiple cross-sections can be assembled into three-dimensional images. CT aids diagnosis, surgery, and treatment, including radiation therapy, in which effective dosage depends highly on the precise density, size, and location of a tumor.

A person having a CT scan is asked to refrain from eating or drinking for 4 hours before the scan. All jewelry and metal objects that could interfere with the exam need

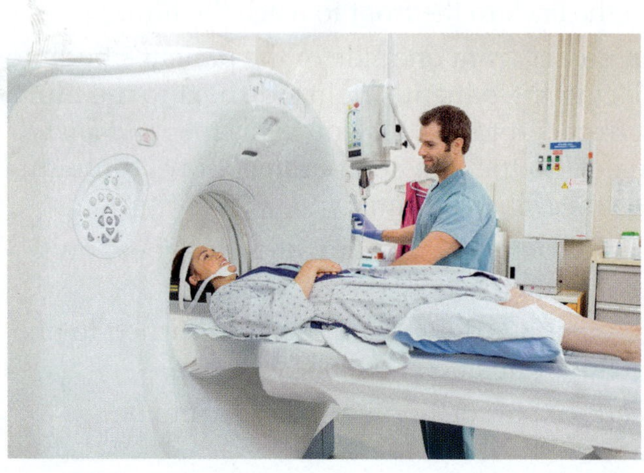

Figure 20.3 Technician preparing patient for CT scan in hospital.
(Tyler Olson/Fotolia)

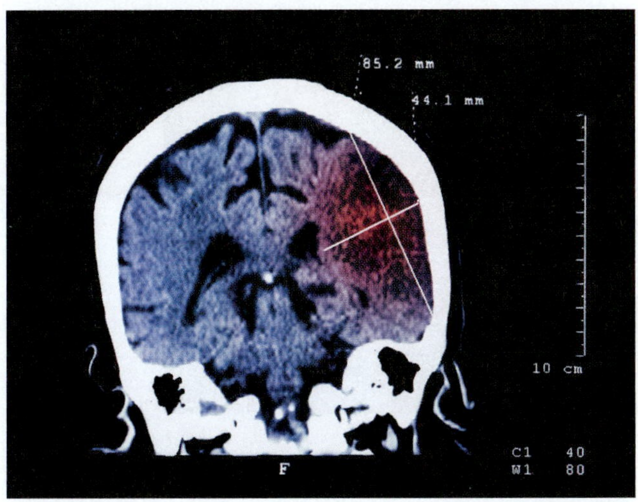

Figure 20.4 CT scan of the brain showing cerebral infarction (ischemic stroke). (stockdevil/Fotolia)

to be removed beforehand. Women are asked if they are pregnant. A person having a CT scan needs to undress and put on an exam gown.

Next, the person lies on a narrow table that slides through the opening in a machine that is shaped like a doughnut with a hole in its center. The opening is called the *gantry*. While in the gantry, an x-ray tube travels around the individual, creating computer-generated x-ray images. Some types of exams require the patient to receive an intravenous injection of iodinated contrast, which is a dye that makes some tissues show up better. Scans of the intestines sometimes call for the person to drink diluted iodinated contrast solution prior to the exam. After the exam, the technologist views the pictures. If they are adequate, the person is free to leave.

MAGNETIC RESONANCE IMAGING

Magnetic resonance imaging (MRI) is a noninvasive imaging technique. The MRI machine is used to view organs, bone, and other internal body structures. The imaged body part is exposed to radio waves while in a magnetic field. The picture is produced by energy emitted from hydrogen atoms in the human body. The patient is not exposed to radiation during this test.

MRI can be used for a variety of purposes. A physician can order an MRI of the brain, known as a *cranial MRI*, to evaluate a person's tumor, seizure disorder, or headache symptoms. An MRI of the spine examines a disk or other problem in a person's spine. See Figure 20.5. If an individual has sustained injury to the shoulder or knee, an MRI is frequently used to study these large joints. Diseases of the heart, chest, abdomen, and pelvis are also commonly evaluated with MRI.

Before the test, the physician assesses the patient for any drug or food allergies (especially shellfish or foods with added iodine such as table salt) and whether the person has experienced claustrophobia or anxiety in enclosed spaces. If this is a problem, mild sedating medication may be given. A woman is asked if she is pregnant.

The person is asked to remove all metal objects such as belts, jewelry, and any pieces of removable dental work. Internal metal objects that cannot be removed can distort the final images so the person should inform the MRI technologist about any previous surgery that required placement of metal in the body, such as a hip pinning. Because the magnetic field can damage watches and credit cards, these objects are not taken into the MRI scanner.

Typically, the person having the test does not need to restrict food or fluids before an MRI scan. Certain tests, such as an MRI-guided biopsy, do require certain food and

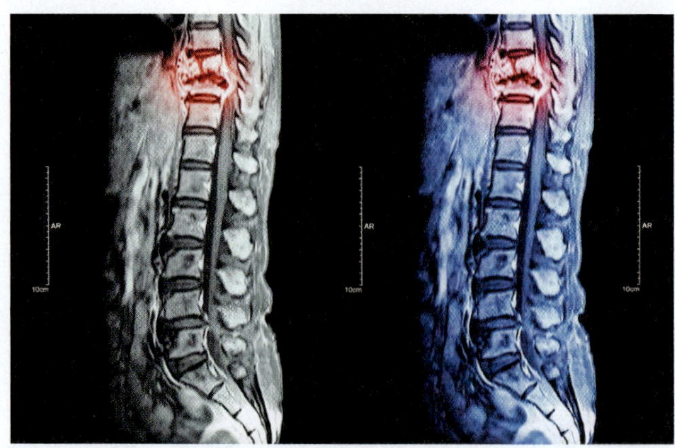

Figure 20.5 Spinal metastasis. MRI of the thoracic and lumbar spine showing cancer in the thoracic region with spinal compression. (stockdevil/Fotolia)

fluid restrictions. The person should consult the healthcare provider for instructions prior to the MRI.

As the test begins, the person lying on his or her back slides into the **bore** (horizontal tube running through the magnet from front to back) on a special table. To prevent image distortion on the final images, the person must lie very still for the duration of the test. Commonly, a special substance called a *contrast agent* is administered prior to or during the test. The contrast agent is used to enhance internal structures and improve image quality. Typically, this material is injected into a vein in the arm.

The scanning process is painless. However, the part of the body being imaged can feel a bit warm. This sensation is harmless and normal. The person hears loud banging and knocking noises during many stages of the exam. Earplugs are provided for people who find the noises disturbing.

A radiologist analyzes the MRI images. Frequently, the MRI helps to better evaluate a disease or disorder affecting organs and blood vessels. MRI is particularly useful in evaluating the size and location of tumors as well as bleeding at various clotting stages. The healthcare provider and the radiologist use this information to help guide the next course of action for the individual's condition.

ULTRASOUND

Ultrasound literally means *beyond sound.* It is sound whose frequency is beyond the range of human hearing. Ultrasound is widely used in diagnostic imaging to evaluate a patient's internal organs. Its energy is transmitted into the patient and, because various internal organs and structures reflect and scatter sound differently, returning echoes can be used to form an image of a particular structure. These ultrasonic echoes are then recorded as a composite picture of the internal organ and/or structure. See Figure 20.11.

Ultrasonography is the process of using ultrasound to produce a record of ultrasonic echoes as they strike tissues of different densities. The record produced by this process is called a **sonogram** or **echogram**. An adaptation of ultrasound technology is **Doppler echocardiography**. It is a noninvasive technique for determining the blood flow velocity in different locations in the heart. This same technique can be used to determine the uterine artery blood flow velocity during pregnancy as well as the fetal heart rate.

The test is done in the ultrasound or radiology department. The patient lies down for the procedure. A clear, water-based conducting gel is applied to the skin over the area being examined to help with the transmission of the sound waves. A handheld probe called a *transducer* is then moved over the area being examined. The patient can be asked to change position so that other areas can be examined.

Preparation for the procedure depends on the body region being examined. Ultrasound procedures generally cause little discomfort, although the conducting gel can feel slightly cold and wet.

Results are considered normal if the organs and structures in the area being examined are normal in appearance. The significance of abnormal results depends on the body region being examined and the nature of the symptom.

OTHER IMAGING TECHNIQUES

Other diagnostic imaging techniques being used include **thermography**, in which detailed images of body parts are developed from data showing the degree of heat and cold present in areas being studied, and **scintigraphy**, which involves the production of two-dimensional images of tissue areas from the scintillations emitted by an internally administered radiopharmaceutical device that concentrates on a targeted site.

Nuclear Medicine

Nuclear medicine is a subspecialty within the field of radiology that uses radioactive substances to produce images of body anatomy and function. The images are developed based on the detection of energy emitted from the radioactive substance given to the patient either intravenously (IV) or by mouth (PO). These images are used to diagnose disease processes and evaluate organ functioning. Some of the general uses of nuclear medicine are:

- Image blood flow and heart function
- Scan lungs
- Evaluate kidney function
- Identify blockage of the gallbladder
- Evaluate bones for fracture, infection, arthritis, and tumors
- Identify bleeding into the colon
- Locate an infection site
- Measure thyroid function for hyperactivity or hypoactivity

Certain imaging procedures, including PET scanning, employ radionuclides to provide real-time visuals of biochemical processes. One device, a nuclear imaging machine, employs a scintillation camera that can rotate around the body to pick up radiation emitted by an injected substance, such as radioactive iodine, which localizes in the thyroid, or radioactive thallium, which localizes in the heart. Through computerization, a digitized image of a particular organ is produced.

Positron Emission Tomography

Positron emission tomography (PET), commonly called a **PET scan**, is a nuclear medicine imaging technique that helps physicians see how the organs and tissues inside the body are actually functioning. The test involves injecting a very small dose of a radioactive chemical, called a radiotracer, into the vein of the patient's arm. The tracer travels through the body and is absorbed by the organs and tissues being studied. The

PET scan detects and records the energy given off by the tracer substance and, with the use of a computer, this energy is converted into three-dimensional pictures. A physician can then look at cross-sectional images of the body organ from any angle in order to detect functional problems.

A PET scan can measure such vital functions as blood flow, oxygen use, and glucose metabolism, which helps doctors identify abnormal from normal-functioning organs and tissues. The scan can also be used to evaluate the effectiveness of a patient's treatment plan, allowing the course of care to be adjusted if necessary.

PET scans are most commonly used to detect cancer, heart problems (such as coronary artery disease and damage to the heart following a heart attack), brain disorders (including brain tumors, memory disorders, seizures) and other central nervous system disorders.

Interventional Radiology

Interventional radiology (IR) is a medical subspecialty of **radiology** utilizing minimally invasive image-guided procedures to diagnose and treat diseases in nearly every organ system. An **interventional radiologist** is a physician who has had special training in imaging and who specializes in treating diseases percutaneously. An interventional radiologist uses radiological imaging to guide catheters, balloons, stents, filters, and other tiny instruments through the body's vascular system and/or other systems.

The procedures and/or surgeries are performed in an interventional suite, generally on an outpatient basis. General anesthesia is usually unnecessary, and conscious sedation and/or local anesthesia is more commonly used. These procedures are cost-effective and are increasingly replacing traditional surgery for certain conditions and procedures as described in Table 20.1.

Radiation Therapy

The treatment of disease by ionizing radiation is called **radiotherapy**, **x-ray therapy**, **cobalt treatment**, or simply **radiation therapy**. In all cases, this treatment seeks to deliver a precise, calculated dose of radiation to diseased tissue, such as a tumor, while causing the least possible damage to surrounding normal tissue. See Chapter 19, *Oncology*, for more information about radiation therapy.

Table 20.1 Selected Interventional Procedures

Procedure	Description
Balloon angioplasty	Opens blocked or narrowed blood vessels
Chemoembolization	Delivers cancer-fighting agents directly to the tumor site
Embolization	Delivers clotting agents directly to an area that is bleeding or to block blood flow to a problem area, such as a fibroid tumor
Fallopian tube catheterization	Opens blocked fallopian tubes, a cause of infertility in women
Needle biopsy	Diagnostic test for breast or other cancers; an alternative to surgical biopsy
Stent-graft placement	Reinforces a ruptured or ballooning section of an artery with a fabric-wrapped stent, a small cagelike tube that serves to patch the vessel
Thrombolysis	Dissolves blood clots
Transjugular intrahepatic portosystemic shunt (TIPS)	Improves blood flow for patients with severe liver dysfunction
Varicocele occlusion	Treats varicose veins in the testicles, a cause of infertility in men
Vena cava filters	Prevents blood clots from reaching the heart

Study and Review I

Overview of Radiology and Nuclear Medicine

Write your answers to the following questions.

1. Define radiology. ________________________________

2. Name three characteristics of x-rays.

   a. ____________________ **b.** ____________________

   c. ____________________

3. Name two dangers of x-rays.

   a. ____________________ **b.** ____________________

4. List five safety precautions designed to prevent unnecessary exposure to x-rays.

   a. ____________________ **b.** ____________________

   c. ____________________ **d.** ____________________

   e. ____________________

5. Name five techniques used in diagnostic imaging.

   a. ____________________ **b.** ____________________

   c. ____________________ **d.** ____________________

   e. ____________________

Building Your Medical Vocabulary

This section provides the foundation for learning medical terminology. Review the following alphabetized word list. Note how common prefixes and suffixes are repeatedly applied to word roots and combining forms to create different meanings. The word parts are color-coded: prefixes are yellow, suffixes are blue, roots/combining forms are red. A combining form is a word root plus a vowel. The chart below lists the combining forms for the word roots in this chapter and can help to strengthen your understanding of how medical words are built and spelled.

Remember These Guidelines

1. If the suffix begins with a vowel, drop the combining vowel from the combining form and add the suffix. For example, physic/o (*nature*) + -ist (*one who specializes*) becomes physicist.
2. If the suffix begins with a consonant, keep the combining vowel and add the suffix to the combining form. For example, bronch/o (*bronchus*) + -gram (*record*) becomes bronchogram.

You will find that some terms have not been divided into word parts. These are common words or specialized terms that are included to enhance your medical vocabulary.

Combining Forms of Radiology and Nuclear Medicine			
act/o	acting	**lymph/o**	lymph
angi/o	vessel	**mamm/o**	breast
arteri/o	artery	**myel/o**	spinal cord
arthr/o	joint	**oscill/o**	to swing
bronch/o	bronchus	**physic/o**	nature
chol/e	gall, bile	**pyel/o**	renal pelvis
cinemat/o	motion	**radi/o**	ray, x-ray
cyst/o	bladder	**salping/o**	fallopian tube
dermat/o	skin	**sial/o**	salivary
digit/o	finger or toe	**son/o**	sound
ech/o	echo	**therm/o**	hot, heat
encephal/o	brain	**tom/o**	to cut
fluor/o	fluorescence, luminous	**tract/o**	to draw
gen/o	kind	**ven/o**	vein
hyster/o	womb, uterus		

Medical Word	Word Parts		Definition
	Part	**Meaning**	
angiocardiogram (ăn″ jĭ-ō-kăr′ dĭ-ō-grăm)	angi/o cardi/o -gram	vessel heart record	X-ray record of the heart and great vessels made visible through the use of a radiopaque contrast medium
angiography (ăn″ jĭ-ŏg′ ră-fē)	angi/o -graphy	vessel recording	A medical imaging technique used to visualize the inside, or lumen, of blood vessels and organs of the body, with particular interest in the arteries, veins, and the heart chambers
arteriography (ăr″ tē-rĭ-ŏg′ ră-fē)	arteri/o -graphy	artery recording	Process of making an x-ray record of the arteries
arthrography (ăr-thrŏg′ ră-fē)	arthr/o -graphy	joint recording	Process of making an x-ray record of a joint

RULE REMINDER

This term keeps the combining vowel ***o*** because the suffix begins with a consonant.

Medical Word	Part	Meaning	Definition
barium (Ba) sulfate (bă′ rĭ-ŭm sŭl′ fāt)			Radiopaque barium compound used as a contrast medium in x-ray examination of the digestive tract; may be administered orally or via a barium enema (BE)
beam			Ray of light; in radiology and nuclear medicine, radiant energy emitted by a group of atomic particles traveling a parallel course
bronchogram (brŏng′ kō-grăm)	bronch/o -gram	bronchus record	X-ray record of the bronchial tree made visible through the use of a radiopaque contrast medium
cassette			Light-proof case or holder for x-ray film
cathode (kăth′ ōd)			Negative pole of an electrical current
cholangiogram (kō-lăn′ jĭ-ō-grăm)	chol angi/o -gram	gall, bile vessel record	X-ray record of the bile ducts made visible through the use of a radiopaque contrast medium
cholecystogram (kō″ lē-sĭs′ tō-grăm)	chole cyst/o -gram	gall bladder record	X-ray record of the gallbladder made visible through the use of a radiopaque contrast medium
cinematoradiography (sĭn″ ĭ-măt″ ō-ră″ dĭ-ŏg′ ră-fē)	cinemat/o radi/o -graphy	motion x-ray recording	Process of making an x-ray record of an organ in motion

Medical Word	Word Parts		Definition
	Part	**Meaning**	
cineradiography (sĭn″ ĭ-rā″ dē-ŏg′ ră-fē)	cine radi/o -graphy	motion x-ray recording	Process of making a motion picture record of successive x-ray images appearing on a fluoroscopic screen
cobalt-60 (kō′ balt)			Radionuclide that serves as the radioactive substance in teletherapy machines; also used for implantation (interstitial) in the treatment of some malignancies
contrast medium			Radiopaque substance used in certain x-ray procedures to permit visualization of organs or structures
curie (Ci) (kūr′ ē)			Unit of radioactivity
digital subtraction angiography (dĭj′ ĭ-tăl sŭb-trăk′ shŭn ăn″ jĭ-ŏg′ ră-fē)	digit -al sub- tract -ion angi/o -graphy	finger or toe pertaining to below to draw process vessel recording	Method by which a computer performs instantaneous subtraction of x-ray images, giving high-quality x-ray images of blood vessels with less x-ray dye. *Note:* In this instance, digital refers to an Arabic number from 0 to 9, so named from counting on the fingers.
dose			Amount of medication or radiation to be administered
echoencephalography (ĕk″ ō-ĕn-sĕf″ ă-lŏg′ ră-fē)	ech/o encephal/o -graphy	echo brain recording	Process of using ultrasound to study intracranial structures of the brain. Useful for diagnosing conditions that cause a shift in the midline structures of the brain.
echography (ĕk-ŏg′ ră-fē)	ech/o -graphy	echo recording	Process of using ultrasound as a diagnostic tool by making a record of the echo produced when sound waves are reflected back through tissues of different density
film			Thin, cellulose-coated, light-sensitive sheet or slip of material used in taking images
fluorescence (floo″ ō-rĕs′ ĕnts)			Property of certain substances to emit light as a result of exposure to and absorption of radiant energy
fluoroscopy (floo-or″ ŏs′ kō-pē)	fluor/o -scopy	fluorescence, luminous visual examination, to view, examine	Process of examining internal structures by viewing the shadows cast on a fluorescent screen after the x-ray has passed through the body (refer to Figure 20.1)

Medical Word	Word Parts		Definition
	Part	**Meaning**	
hysterosalpingogram (hĭs″ tĕr-ō-săl-pĭn′ gō-grăm)	hyster/o salping/o -gram	uterus fallopian tube record	X-ray record of the uterus and fallopian tubes that is made visible through the use of a radiopaque contrast medium
intravenous pyelogram (ĭn″ tră-vē′ nŭs pī′ ĕ-lō-grăm)	intra- ven -ous pyel/o -gram	within vein pertaining to renal pelvis record	X-ray record of the kidney, renal pelvis, ureters, and bladder made visible through the use of an injected radiopaque contrast medium
ion (ī′ ŏn)			Atomic particle consisting of an atom or a group of atoms that carry an electrical charge, either negative or positive
ionization (ī″ ŏn-ĭ-zā′ shŭn)			Process of breaking up molecules into their component parts
ionizing radiation (ī′ ŏn-ī-zĭng rā″ dĭ-ā′ shŭn)			Powerful invisible energy capable of producing ions
irradiation (ĭ-rā″ dē-ā′ shŭn)	ir- radiat -ion	in radiant process	Process of using x-rays, radium rays, ultraviolet rays, gamma rays, or infrared rays in the diagnosis or therapeutic treatment of a patient
isotope (ī′ sō-tōp)			One of a series of nuclides that are chemically identical yet differ in atomic weight and electrical charge. Radioactive isotopes are composed of unstable atoms, and most are artificially produced. For example, cobalt-60 is a radioactive isotope artificially produced from naturally occurring cobalt-59.
lead (Pb) (lĕd)			Metallic chemical element; soft, heavy, inelastic, malleable, ductile, bluish-gray metallic element used in its metallic form as a protective shielding against x-rays. See Figure 20.6.

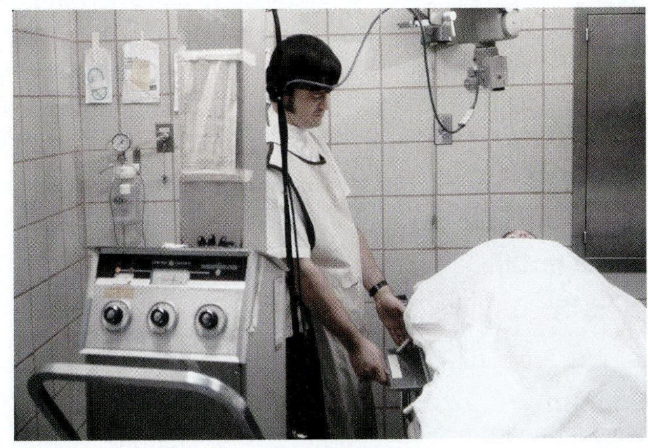

Figure 20.6 X-ray technician in a lead apron prepares to take an x-ray of a patient. This apron is a protective shield of lead and rubber worn by a patient or those taking x-rays to protect the genitals and other vital organs from excessive exposure to x-rays.

Source: Pearson Education, Inc.

Medical Word	Word Parts		Definition
	Part	**Meaning**	
lymphangiogram (lĭm-făn″ jē-ō-grăm)	lymph angi/o -gram	lymph vessel record	X-ray record of the lymph vessels made visible with radiopaque contrast medium
lymphangiography (lĭm-făn″ jē-ŏg′ ră-fē)	lymph angi/o -graphy	lymph vessel recording	Process of making an x-ray record of the lymph vessels
mammography (măm-ŏg′ ră-fē)	mamm/o -graphy	breast recording	Process of obtaining x-ray pictures of the breast using a low-dose x-ray system. The *mammogram* is the actual x-ray record (picture) of the breast. See Figure 20.7. The two types of mammograms are *screening*, which is generally used to detect breast cancer or other changes in the breast tissue in women who do not have symptoms, and *diagnostic*, which can be ordered when a screening mammogram shows something abnormal in the breast. A diagnostic mammogram can also be ordered if the woman has symptoms that suggest breast cancer.

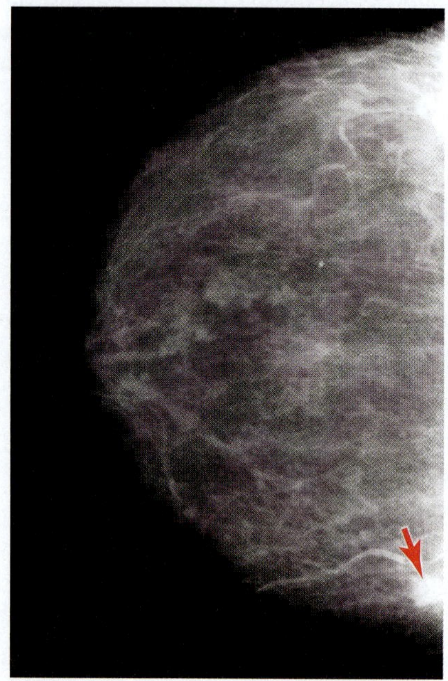

Figure 20.7 Mammogram with cancer indicated by arrow.
(Dr. Dwight Kaufman/National Cancer Institute)

fyi Mammogram screenings have reduced deaths from breast cancer; however, it remains the second leading cause of cancer death among women overall. A mammogram can detect changes in the breast, such as cancer, often before a lump can be felt. It can also show calcifications, or mineral deposits, cysts or fluid-filled masses, leaking breast implants, and noncancerous tumors or growths.

Approximately 2,600 men a year are diagnosed with breast cancer. A male who is scheduled for a mammogram may be embarrassed because he believes that breast cancer is strictly a female disease. The male breast generally does not contain as much adipose tissue as the female breast, so it can be difficult to place the man's breast onto the film holder and obtain the proper amount of compression.

Medical Word	Part	Meaning	Definition
millicurie (mCi) (mĭl″ ĭ-kū′ rē)	milli- curie	one-thousandth curie	0.001 Ci
myelogram (mī″ ĕ-lō-grăm)	myel/o -gram	spinal cord record	X-ray record of the spinal cord made visible with a radiopaque contrast medium

Medical Word	Word Parts		Definition
	Part	**Meaning**	
oscilloscope (ŏ-sĭl´ ō-skōp)	oscill/o -scope	to swing instrument for examining	Instrument used to record an electrical wave visually on a fluorescent screen of a cathode-ray tube
physicist (fĭz´ ĭ-sĭst)	physic -ist	nature one who specializes	Literally means *one who specializes in nature*; person who studies the energy, mass, and laws of nature

RULE REMINDER

The ***o*** has been removed from the combining form because the suffix begins with a vowel.

Medical Word	Part	Meaning	Definition
rad (răd)			Amount of radiation absorbed; the letters stand for **r**adiation **a**bsorbed **d**ose
radiation (rā-dĭ-ā´ shŭn)	radiat -ion	radiant process	Process by which radiant energy is propagated through space or matter
radioactive (rā˝ dĭ-ō-ăk´ tĭv)	radi/o act -ive	ray, x-ray acting nature of	Characterized by emitting radiant energy

ALERT!

The combining form ***radi/o*** means *ray, x-ray*. How many words in this chapter begin with ***radi/o***?

Medical Word	Part	Meaning	Definition
radiodermatitis (rā´ dĭ-ō-der-mă-tī´ tĭs)	radi/o dermat -itis	ray, x-ray skin inflammation	Inflammation of the skin caused by exposure to x-rays or radioactive substances
radiograph (rā´ dĭ-ō-grăf)	radi/o -graph	ray, x-ray instrument for recording	Picture produced on a sensitized film or plate by rays; an *x-ray record*
radiographer (rā˝ dĭ-ŏg´ ră-fĕr)	radi/o -graph -er	ray, x-ray instrument for recording one who	Person skilled in making x-ray records

Medical Word	Word Parts		Definition
	Part	**Meaning**	
radiography (rā″ dĭ-ŏg′ ră-fē)	radi/o -graphy	ray, x-ray recording	Process of making an x-ray record

RULE REMINDER

This term keeps the combining vowel ***o*** because the suffix begins with a consonant.

Medical Word	Part	Meaning	Definition
radiologist (rā″ dĭ-ŏl′ ō-jĭst)	radi/o log -ist	ray, x-ray study of one who specializes	Literally means *one who specializes in radiology*; a physician who specializes in the production and interpretation of medical images. See Figure 20.8.

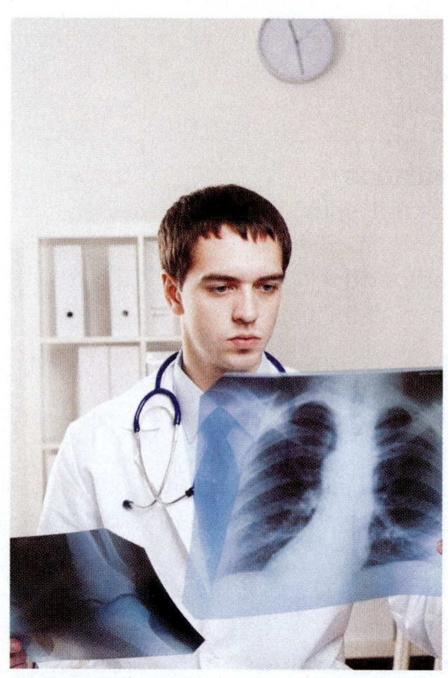

Figure 20.8 Radiologist examines an x-ray of the chest.
(adam121/Fotolia)

Medical Word	Part	Meaning	Definition
radiology (rā″ dĭ-ŏl′ ō-jē)	radi/o -logy	ray, x-ray study of	Scientific discipline of medical imaging using radionuclides, ionizing radiation, nuclear magnetic resonance, and ultrasound
radiolucent (rā″ dĭ-ō-lū′ sĕnt)	radi/o -lucent	ray, x-ray to shine	Pertaining to property of permitting the passage of radiant energy
radionuclide (rā″ dĭ-ō-nū′ klīd)	radi/o nucl -ide	ray, x-ray nucleus having a particular quality	An atom that disintegrates by emitting electromagnetic rays

Medical Word	Word Parts: Part	Word Parts: Meaning	Definition
radiopaque (rā″ dĭ-ō-pāk′)	radi -opaque	ray, x-ray dark, non-transparent	Pertaining to property of obstructing the passage of radiant energy
radioscopy (rā″ dĭ-ŏs′ kō-pē)	radi/o -scopy	ray, x-ray visual examination, to view, examine	Process of viewing and examining the inner structures of the body through the process of x-rays
radiotherapy (rā″ dĭ-ō-thĕr′ ă-pē)	radi/o -therapy	ray, x-ray treatment	Treatment of disease by the use of x-rays, radium, and other radioactive substances
radium (Ra) (rā′ dĭ-ŭm)			Radioactive isotope used to treat certain malignant diseases
roentgen (R) (rĕnt′ gĕn)			International unit for describing the exposure dose of x-rays or gamma rays
roentgenology (rĕnt″ gĕn-ŏl′ ō-jē)	roent gen/o -logy	roentgen kind study of	Study of roentgen rays for diagnostic and therapeutic purposes
scan			Process of using a moving device or a sweeping beam of radiation to produce images of organs or structures of the body. Figure 20.9 shows a PET scan and Figure 20.10 shows a CAT scan.

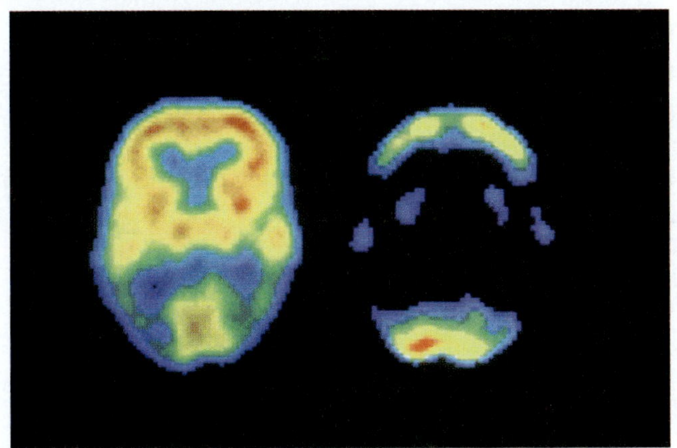

Figure 20.9 PET scans of normal (left) and Alzheimer disease–afflicted (right) human brains. Yellow color indicates normal brain activity.
(Science Source)

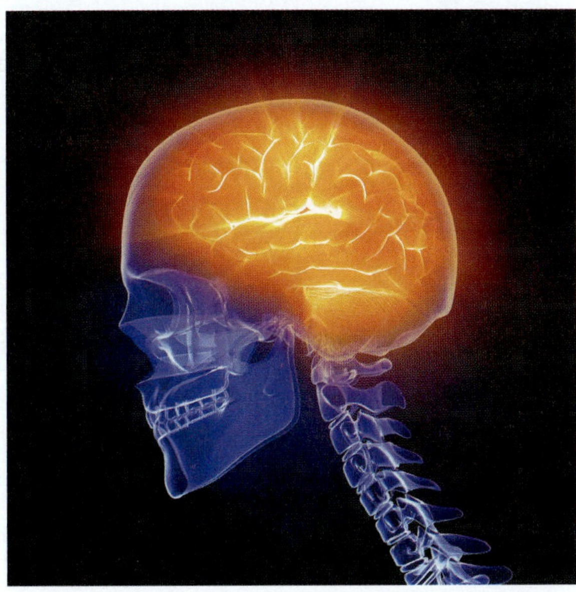

Figure 20.10 CAT scan of a human head in profile.
(cliparea.com/Fotolia)

(*continued*)

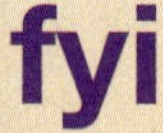

A **bone scan** is a test used to find cancer, infection, fractures, or other injuries in the bone and to check a person's response to treatment for certain bone conditions, such as Paget disease. A radioactive substance is injected into a vein in the arm of the person having the scan. The test usually begins after a wait of 2–3 hours.

A bone scan can:

- Show specific areas of irregular bone metabolism, which can suggest certain diseases based on the pattern of abnormality.
- Detect abnormal blood flow to a particular bony region.
- Help evaluate metabolic diseases that affect bones, such as certain thyroid conditions.
- Detect the spread of cancer to the bones and help the physician evaluate results of cancer treatment.
- Provide information for the physician to diagnose bone changes from a condition called *reflex sympathetic dystrophy*, a disorder of nerves that causes pain, usually in the hands or feet.

Medical Word	Word Parts: Part	Word Parts: Meaning	Definition
shield			Protective structure used to prevent or reduce the passage of particles or radiation
sialography (sī″ ă-lŏg′ ră-fē)	sial/o -graphy	salivary recording	Process of making an x-ray record of the salivary ducts and glands
sonogram (sŏn′ ō-grăm)	son/o -gram	sound record	Record produced by ultrasonography
tagging			Process of tracing a radioactive isotope that has become involved in metabolic or chemical actions
thermography (thĕr-mŏg′ ră-fē)	therm/o -graphy	hot, heat recording	Process of recording heat patterns of the body's surface; useful in the detection of breast cancer
tomography (tō-mŏg′ ră-fē)	tom/o -graphy	to cut recording	Process of cutting across and producing images of single tissue planes that help place into focus a very particular object within a larger field
ultrasonic (ŭl″ tră-sŏn′ ĭk)	ultra- son -ic	beyond sound pertaining to	Pertaining to sounds of frequencies beyond 20,000 cycles/sec

Medical Word	Word Parts		Definition
	Part	Meaning	
ultrasonography (ŭl″ tră-sŏn-ŏg′ ră-fē)	ultra- son/o -graphy	beyond sound recording	Process of using ultrasound to produce a record of ultrasonic echoes as they strike tissues of different densities. See Figure 20.11.

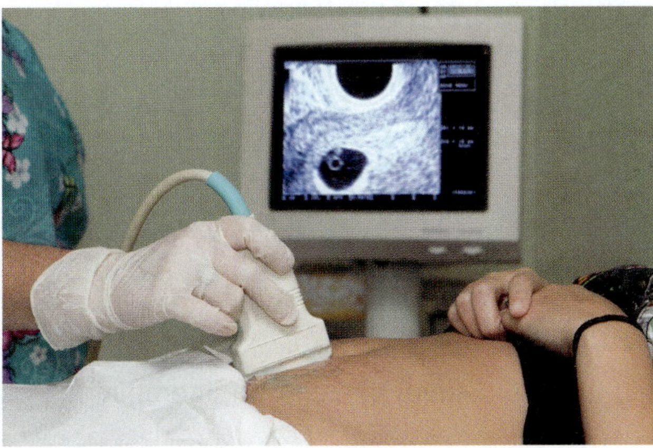

Figure 20.11 Ultrasound scanning permits visualization of the fetus in utero.

Source: Steven Frame/Shutterstock

Medical Word	Part	Meaning	Definition
venography (vē-nŏg′ ră-fē)	ven/o -graphy	vein recording	Process of making an x-ray record of veins
x-ray			Electromagnetic wave of high energy produced by the collision of a beam of electrons with a target in a vacuum tube (x-ray tube). See Figure 20.12.

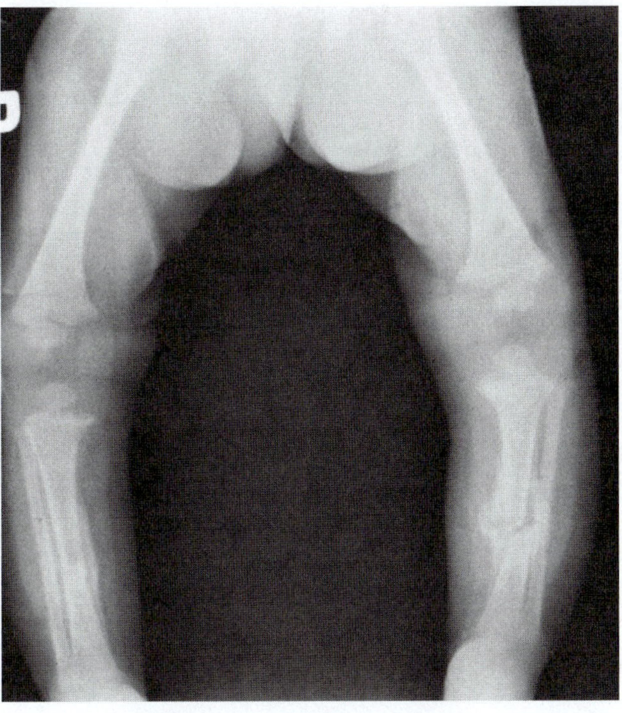

Figure 20.12 X-ray of a child's legs showing fractures in the right tibia and right fibula.

Source: Pearson Education, Inc.

Study and Review II

Word Parts

Prefixes

Give the definitions of the following prefixes.

1. sub- ______________________
2. intra- ______________________
3. milli- ______________________
4. ultra- ______________________
5. ir- ______________________

Combining Forms

Give the definitions of the following combining forms.

1. act/o ______________________
2. angi/o ______________________
3. arteri/o ______________________
4. arthr/o ______________________
5. bronch/o ______________________
6. cinemat/o ______________________
7. digit/o ______________________
8. ech/o ______________________
9. fluor/o ______________________
10. gen/o ______________________
11. mamm/o ______________________
12. oscill/o ______________________
13. physic/o ______________________
14. pyel/o ______________________
15. radi/o ______________________
16. salping/o ______________________
17. sial/o ______________________
18. son/o ______________________
19. therm/o ______________________
20. tom/o ______________________
21. tract/o ______________________

Suffixes

Give the definitions of the following suffixes.

1. -er ______________________
2. -genic ______________________
3. -al ______________________
4. -gram ______________________
5. -graph ______________________
6. -graphy ______________________
7. -ic ______________________
8. -ion ______________________

9. -ist ______________________

10. -itis ______________________

11. -ive ______________________

12. -logy ______________________

13. -ous ______________________

14. -scope ______________________

15. -scopy ______________________

16. -therapy ______________________

17. -ide ______________________

Identifying Medical Terms

In the spaces provided, write the medical terms for the following meanings.

1. ______________________ A medical imaging technique used to visualize the inside, or lumen, of blood vessels and organs of the body
2. ______________________ Process of making an x-ray record of a joint
3. ______________________ X-ray record of the gallbladder made visible through the use of a radiopaque contrast medium
4. ______________________ A process resulting in the gain or loss of one or more electrons in neutral atoms
5. ______________________ Process of obtaining x-ray pictures of the breast
6. ______________________ 0.001 Ci
7. ______________________ Literally means *one who specializes in nature*
8. ______________________ Process whereby radiant energy is propagated through space or matter
9. ______________________ Characterized by emitting radiant energy
10. ______________________ Person skilled in making x-ray records
11. ______________________ Pertaining to property of permitting the passage of radiant energy
12. ______________________ Pertaining to property of obstructing the passage of radiant energy
13. ______________________ Record produced by ultrasonography

Chapter

21 Mental Health

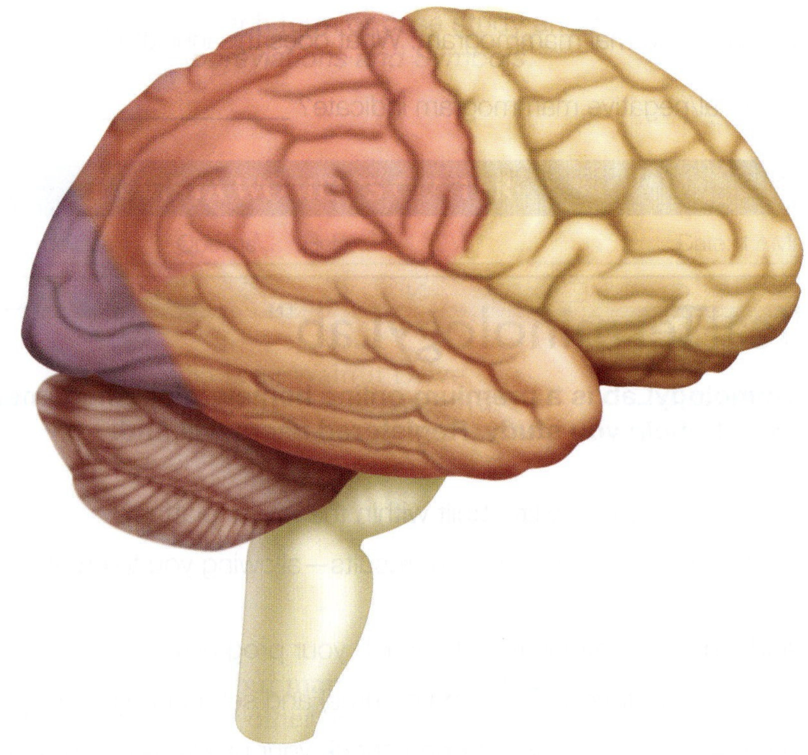

Learning Outcomes

On completion of this chapter, you will be able to:

1. Define mental health.
2. Describe mental disorders and several possible contributing factors.
3. Identify general symptoms (according to age group) that can suggest a mental disorder.
4. Explain how the diagnosis of mental disorders may be obtained.
5. Describe three basic forms of treatment that can be employed.
6. Recognize terminology included in the ICD-10-CM.
7. Analyze, build, spell, and pronounce medical words.
8. Comprehend the drugs highlighted in this chapter.
9. Identify and define selected abbreviations.
10. Apply your acquired knowledge of medical terms by successfully completing the *Practical Application* exercise.

Mental Health and Mental Disorders

Please note that much of the information on mental disorders has been adapted from the National Institute of Mental Health (NIMH), which is a component of the National Institutes of Health (NIH), a part of the U.S. Department of Health and Human Services (HHS), and the Diagnostic and Statistical Manual of Mental Disorders, *Fifth Edition (DSM-5).*

The World Health Organization (WHO) defines **health** as a state of complete physical, mental, and social well-being, not merely the absence of disease or infirmity. It defines **mental health** as a state of well-being in which an individual realizes his or her own abilities, can cope with the normal stresses of life, can work productively and fruitfully, and is able to make a contribution to his or her community.

A **mental disorder** is an abnormal condition of the brain or mind. It affects the way a person thinks, feels, behaves, and relates to others and to his or her surroundings. In most cases, the exact cause of a mental disorder is not known. Possible contributing factors include genetics, the environment, chemical changes occurring in the brain, use of certain drugs, and psychological, social, and cultural conditions. See Figure 21.1.

Many different conditions are classified as mental disorders. Examples include bipolar disorders, depressive disorders, anxiety disorders, attention-deficit/hyperactivity disorder, trauma- and stressor-related disorders, feeding and eating disorders, schizophrenia, obsessive–compulsive disorders, and autism spectrum disorder. Other types of mental disorders are adjustment disorder, dissociative disorders, factitious disorders,

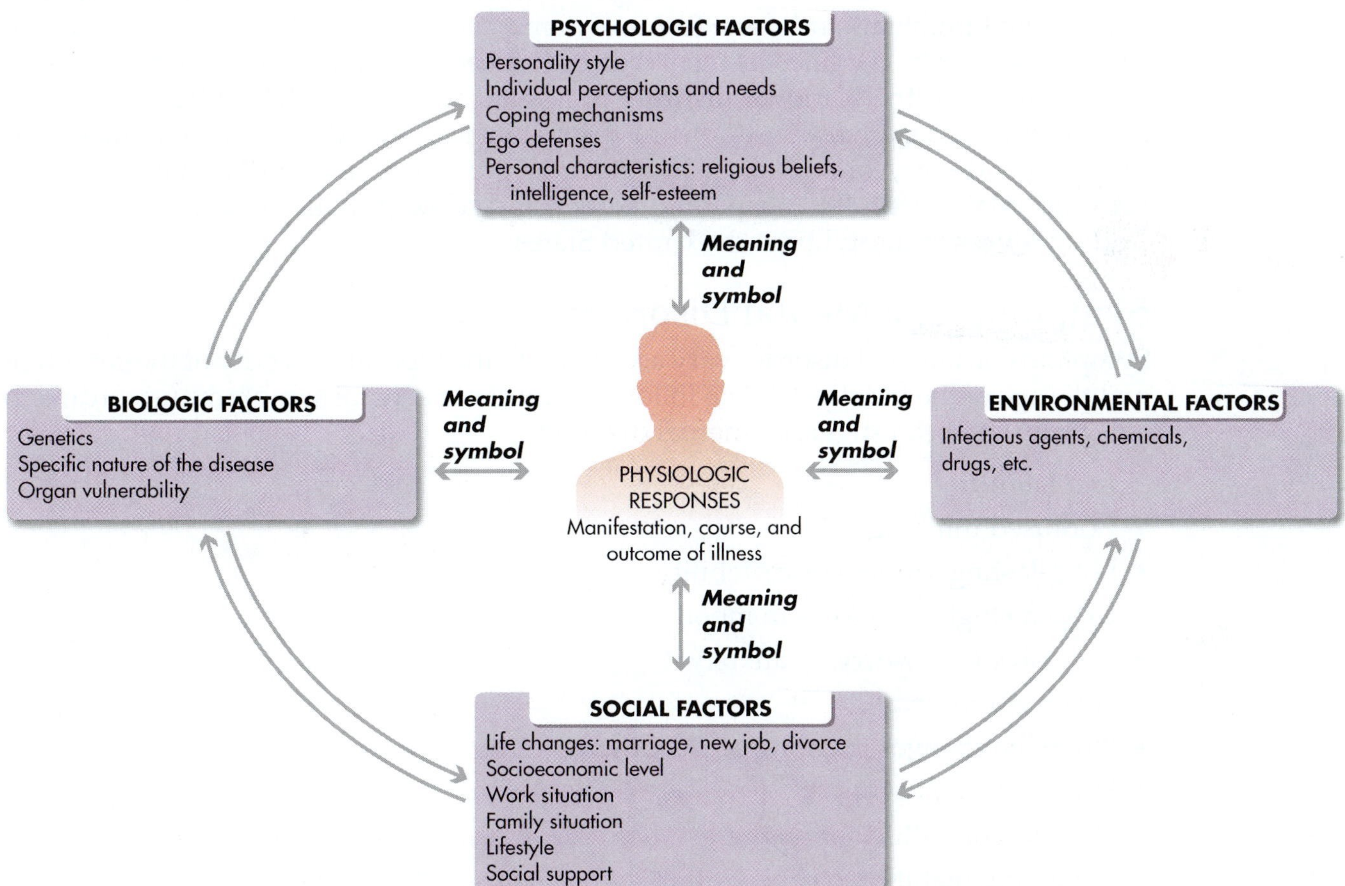

Figure 21.1 Multicausational concept of the illness process. The phrase *meaning and symbol* refers to the fact that a patient interprets all experiences in a highly individual manner according to his or her specific meaning and the broader meaning in the patient's culture.

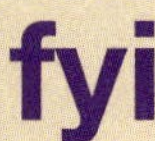

Science has identified six ingredients that can boost one's mood. These ingredients are contained in what is being called "superfoods." Some examples are described below.

- *Tomatoes* contain carotenoids, antioxidants that counteract the damage caused by free radicals, which can destroy mood-protecting fats in the brain.
- *Whole grains* promote the release of insulin, a hormone produced by the pancreas, which can stimulate serotonin, a neurotransmitter, vasoconstrictor, and smooth muscle stimulant. Serotonin plays an important role in the regulation of learning, mood, sleep, and vasoconstriction. It also might have a role in anxiety, migraine, vomiting, and appetite. Changes in serotonin levels in the brain may affect mood. Some antidepressant medications affect the action of serotonin and can be used to treat depression.
- *Fatty fish* such as salmon and mackerel contain omega-3 fats DHA and EPA. These fats are necessary for brain health and seem to be crucial to mood.
- *Dark chocolate* is believed to increase the brain's serotonin levels. This may increase mental alertness.
- *Spinach* contains folate, a B vitamin used by the brain to make mood-regulating chemicals: serotonin, dopamine, and norepinephrine. Folate may be effective in treating depression.
- *Red meat* is a good source of iron, which the brain uses to make mood-regulating dopamine. People who are iron deficient may become more depressed than those who have higher levels of iron.

sexual and gender disorders, somatic symptom disorders, and tic disorders. Various sleep-related problems and some forms of dementia, including Alzheimer disease (see Chapter 14), can be classified as mental disorders because they involve the brain.

According to the National Institute of Mental Health (NIMH) (2015), 10 million American adults experience serious functional impairment due to mental illness and in children 13–18 years of age, 1 in 5 have or previously had a debilitating mental disorder. Major depression, bipolar disorder, and schizophrenia are among the top 10 leading causes of disability in the United States.

Symptoms of a Mental Disorder

Symptoms of a mental disorder vary according to the type and severity of the condition and the age of the individual. The following are some general symptoms (according to age group) that can suggest a mental disorder:

In an adult:

- Confused thinking
- Long-lasting sadness or irritability
- Extreme highs and lows in mood
- Excessive fear, worry, or anxiety
- Social withdrawal
- Dramatic changes in eating or sleeping patterns
- Strong feelings of anger
- Delusion or hallucinations
- Increasing inability to cope with daily problems and activities
- Thoughts of suicide

- Denial of obvious problems
- Many unexplained physical problems
- Abuse of drugs and/or alcohol

In an adolescent:

- Abuse of drugs and/or alcohol
- Inability to cope with daily problems and activities
- Changes in eating or sleeping patterns
- Excessive complaints of physical problems
- Defying authority, skipping school, stealing, or damaging property
- Intense fear of gaining weight
- Long-lasting negative mood
- Thoughts of death
- Frequent outbursts of anger

In younger children:

- Changes in school performance
- Poor grades despite strong efforts
- Excessive worry or anxiety
- Hyperactivity
- Persistent nightmares
- Continual disobedience and/or aggressive behavior
- Frequent temper tantrums

Diagnosis of Mental Disorders

The standard manual used by experts for the diagnosis of recognized mental disorders in the United States is the *Diagnostic and Statistical Manual of Mental Disorders*, Fifth Edition (DSM-5).

This official manual of mental health disorders is compiled by the American Psychiatric Association (APA) and identifies categories of mental disorders. Psychiatrists, psychologists, social workers, and other healthcare providers use it to understand and diagnose mental health disorders. Insurance companies and healthcare providers also use it to classify and then code mental health disorders, as per ICD-10-CM, for reimbursement of services rendered.

Psychiatry is the branch of medicine that deals with the study, diagnosis, and treatment of mental disorders. A person who specializes in this field of medicine is a **psychiatrist**, who is a medical doctor (MD) with specialized training in **psychotherapy** and drug therapy. Psychiatrists can further specialize in the treatment of children (child psychiatry) or in the legal aspects of psychiatry, such as the determination of mental competence in criminal cases (forensic psychiatry). **Psychoanalysts** are psychiatrists with specialized training in **psychoanalysis**, a method of obtaining a detailed account of past and present mental and emotional experiences and repressions.

Psychology is the study of the mind. A **psychologist** is a person who is not a medical doctor but has a master's degree or doctor of philosophy (PhD) degree in a specific field of psychology, such as clinical, experimental, or social.

Clinical psychologists are patient-oriented and can use various methods of psychotherapy to treat patients but cannot prescribe medications or electroconvulsive therapy (ECT). They are trained in the use of tests to evaluate various aspects of a patient's mental health and intelligence. Examples are **intelligence quotient (IQ)** tests such as the **Stanford–Binet Intelligence Scale** and the **Wechsler Adult Intelligence Scale–R (WAIS-R)**. Other tests used are the **Rorschach Inkblot Test** and the **Thematic Apperception Test (TAT)**, in which pictures are used as stimuli for the patient to create stories. The **Minnesota Multiphasic Personality Inventory–2 (MMPI-2)** consists of true–false questions that can reveal aspects of personality, such as dominance, sense of duty or responsibility, and ability to relate to others; it is used as an objective measure of psychological disorders in adolescents and adults. A patient's responses to the questions can be compared with responses made by individuals with diagnoses of schizophrenia, depression, and many other mental disorders.

Psychiatrists and psychologists also use specially designed interview and assessment tools to evaluate a person for a mental disorder. The therapist bases the diagnosis on the person's report of symptoms, including any social or functional problems caused by the symptoms. The therapist then determines whether the person's symptoms and degree of disability indicate a diagnosis of a specific disorder.

Treatments for Mental Disorders

The three basic forms of treatment for mental disorders are **drug therapy**, **psychotherapy**, and **electroconvulsive therapy**.

DRUG THERAPY

Drugs that are generally used to treat mental disorders include antianxiety agents, antidepressant agents, antimanic agents, and antipsychotic agents. Drugs used for attention-deficit/hyperactivity disorder (ADHD) include stimulants. See *Drug Highlights* for more information on drug therapy for mental disorders.

PSYCHOTHERAPY

Psychotherapy is a method of treating mental disorders using psychological techniques instead of physical methods. It involves talking, interpreting, listening, rewarding, and role-playing. Psychotherapy should be performed by a trained mental health professional, such as a psychiatrist, psychologist, social worker, or counselor. See Figure 21.2.

Types of psychotherapy include cognitive-behavioral therapy, family therapy, group therapy, play therapy, art therapy, hypnosis, and psychoanalysis.

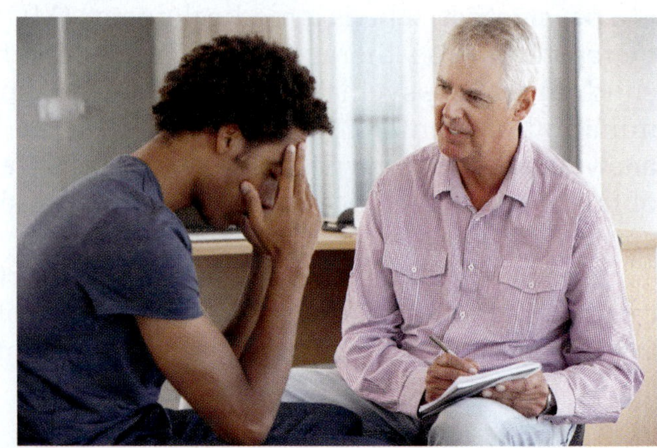

Figure 21.2 Young man having counseling session with his psychologist.
(Monkey Business/Fotolia)

- **Cognitive-behavioral therapy (CBT)** has two components. The cognitive component helps people change thinking patterns that keep them from overcoming their fears. The behavioral component seeks to change people's reactions to anxiety-provoking situations. A key element of this component is exposure, in which people confront the things they fear. Research has shown that CBT is an effective form of psychotherapy for several anxiety disorders, particularly panic disorder and social phobia.
- **Family therapy** involves an entire family. The focus is on resolving and understanding conflicts and problems as a *family* situation, not just as an individual member's problem.
- **Group therapy** involves small groups of people with similar problems attending meetings together. There are discussions and interactions between group participants; a therapist helps to focus and guide the therapy sessions. See Figure 21.3.
- **Play therapy** involves a child using toys, such as dolls and puppets, to express thoughts, feelings, fantasies, and conflicts. Because most emotionally disturbed children will not talk about their problems, play therapy provides an alternative method to encourage children to open up about what is troubling them. Children reveal themselves when they play with toys provided by the therapist and often act out their problems. See Figure 21.4.
- **Art therapy** can be used to encourage a child to portray his or her feelings in drawings. When asked to draw the family or a picture of him- or herself, information about the child, the family, and their interactions can be revealed.
- **Hypnosis** is a state of altered consciousness, usually artificially induced, used in treating mental disorders by lessening the mind's unconscious defenses and allowing some patients to be able to recall and even re-experience important childhood events that have long been forgotten or repressed. Historically, Dr. Sigmund Freud, a noted Austrian neurologist and psychoanalyst, developed the theory of the unconscious as a result of his experiments with a hypnotized patient.

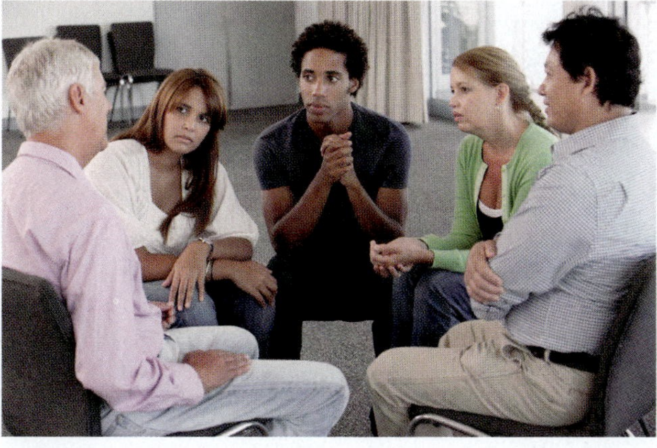

Figure 21.3 Members of a support group listening to the therapist guiding the session.
(Monkey Business/Fotolia)

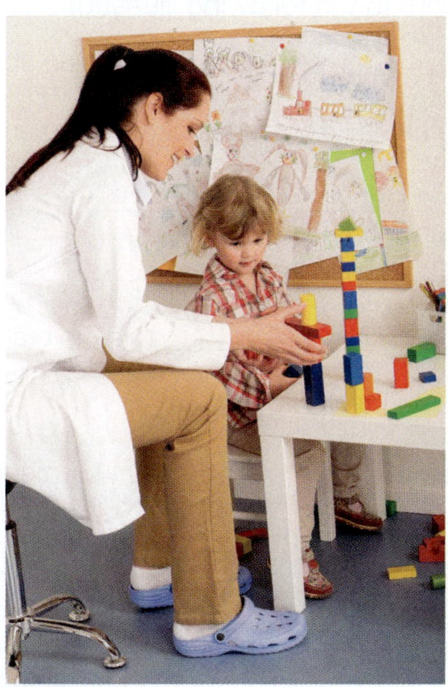

Figure 21.4 The therapist is using toys to encourage Kelly to talk about what is troubling her.
(CandyBox Images/Fotolia)

- **Psychoanalysis** is a method of obtaining a detailed account of past and present mental and emotional experiences and repressions. It was also developed by Dr. Freud. Psychoanalysis attempts, through free association and dream interpretation, to reveal and resolve the unconscious conflicts that are considered to be at the root of some mental disorders. It is believed that these conflicts have been repressed since childhood and after being brought to the conscious level can be resolved.

ELECTROCONVULSIVE THERAPY

Electroconvulsive therapy (ECT) is the use of an electric shock to produce convulsions. It is useful for individuals whose depression is severe or life threatening, particularly for those who cannot take antidepressant medication. In recent years, ECT has been much improved. A muscle relaxant is given to the patient before treatment, which is performed under brief anesthesia. Electrodes are placed at precise locations on the head to deliver electrical impulses. The stimulation causes a brief (about 30 seconds) seizure within the brain. The person receiving ECT does not consciously experience the electrical stimulus. For full therapeutic benefit, at least several sessions of ECT, typically given at the rate of three per week, are required.

Study and Review I

Overview: Mental Health and Mental Disorders

Write your answers to the following questions.

1. A ______________________________ is an abnormal condition of the brain or mind.

2. List the three mental disorders that are listed among the top 10 causes of disability in the United States.

a. ______________________________ **b.** ______________________________

c. ______________________________

3. ______________________________ is the branch of medicine that deals with the study, diagnosis, and treatment of mental disorders.

4. Give the three basic forms of treatment for mental disorders.

a. ______________________________ **b.** ______________________________

c. ______________________________

5. ______________________________ is a method of obtaining a detailed account of past and present mental and emotional experiences and repressions.

Building Your Medical Vocabulary

This section provides the foundation for learning medical terminology. Review the following alphabetized word list. Note how common prefixes and suffixes are repeatedly applied to word roots and combining forms to create different meanings. The word parts are color-coded: prefixes are yellow, suffixes are blue, roots/combining forms are red. A combining form is a word root plus a vowel. The chart below lists the combining forms for the word roots in this chapter and can help to strengthen your understanding of how medical words are built and spelled.

Remember These Guidelines

1. If the suffix begins with a vowel, drop the combining vowel from the combining form and add the suffix. For example, aut/o (*self*) + -ism (*condition*) becomes autism.
2. If the suffix begins with a consonant, keep the combining vowel and add the suffix to the combining form. For example, agor/a (*marketplace*) + -phobia (*fear*) becomes agoraphobia.

You will find that some terms have not been divided into word parts. These are common words or specialized terms that are included to enhance your medical vocabulary.

Combining Forms of Mental Health			
agor/a	marketplace	**path/o**	disease
aut/o	self	**phren/o**	mind
centr/o	center	**psych/o**	mind
compuls/o	compel, drive	**schiz/o**	to divide
cycl/o	circle, cycle	**somat/o**	body
delus/o	to cheat	**thym/o**	mind, emotion
neur/o	nerve	**trop/o**	turning

Medical Word	Word Parts		Definition
	Part	Meaning	
affect (ăf´ fĕkt)			In psychology, observable evidence of an individual's emotional reaction associated with an experience
affective disorder (ăf-fĕk´ tĭv)			Characterized by a disturbance of mood accompanied by a manic or depressive syndrome; this syndrome is not caused by any other physical or mental disorder
agoraphobia (ăg″ ō-ră-fō´ bē-ă)	agor/a -phobia	marketplace fear	An anxiety disorder; agoraphobia involves intense fear and anxiety in any place or situation where escape might be difficult, leading to avoidance of being alone outside of the home; traveling in a car, bus, or airplane; or being in a crowded area.

RULE REMINDER

This term keeps the combining vowel ***a*** because the suffix begins with a consonant.

Medical Word	Part	Meaning	Definition
anorexia nervosa (ăn-ō-rĕk´ sē-ă nĕr-vō´ să)	an- -orexia	lack of, without appetite	Complex psychological disorder in which the individual refuses to eat or has an abnormally limited eating pattern. People with eating disorders may engage in self-induced vomiting and abuse of laxatives, diuretics, or prolonged exercise to control their weight. The condition could lead them to become excessively thin or even emaciated. In severe cases, this condition can be life threatening.

insights In ICD-10-CM, the code for *Behavioral syndromes associated with physiological disturbances and physical factors* is F50–F59. *Eating disorders* is coded F50 with subcategories of *anorexia nervosa*, *bulimia*, *other eating disorders*, and *unspecified*, with their own codes.

Medical Word	Part	Meaning	Definition
anxiety (ăng-zī´ ĕ-tē)			Feeling of uneasiness, apprehension, worry, or dread; involuntary or reflex reaction of the body to stress. Anxiety can be a normal reaction to stress and can help us deal with a tense situation, study harder for an exam, or keep focused on an important speech. In general, it can help us cope.

Medical Word	Word Parts		Definition
	Part	**Meaning**	
anxiety disorders			Mental disorders that can affect adults and children and are chronic, growing progressively worse if not treated. These disorders appear to be caused by an interaction of biopsychosocial factors, including genetic vulnerability, which interact with situations, stress, or trauma to produce clinically significant syndromes. Symptoms, which may begin in childhood or adolescence, include excessive, irrational fear or dread. Examples include obsessive–compulsive disorder, posttraumatic stress disorder, social phobia, specific phobia, and generalized anxiety disorder. See Figure 21.5 for physiological responses in anxiety disorders.

Central Nervous System
Voluntary
Involuntary
Sympathetic
Parasympathetic
Mobilizes
Excites
Maintains normal smooth muscle function
• Adrenal stimulation
• Racing heart
• Rapid, shallow respirations
• Inhibited flow of saliva
• Excessive sweating
• Shaking, trembling
• Cold hands and feet
• Muscle contractions (cause smothering sensation)
• Excess gastric acid
• Slowed digestion
• More glucose in bloodstream
• Increased metabolism
• Dilated pupils

Figure 21.5 Physiological responses in anxiety disorders.

insights In ICD-10-CM, the code for *Anxiety, dissociative, stress-related, somatoform and other non-psychotic mental disorders* is F40–F48. Included in this classification are categories and subcategories for various types of affective disorders, with their own code.

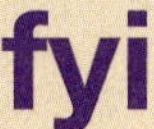

fyi A form of anxiety disorder, **panic disorder** (often called *panic attacks)* causes feelings of terror that strike suddenly and repeatedly with no warning. People with this disorder cannot predict when an attack will occur, and many develop intense anxiety between episodes, worrying about when and where the next one will strike.

When having a panic attack, a person feels sweaty, flushed or chilled, weak, faint, or dizzy. The hands can tingle or feel numb. There can be nausea, chest pain or a smothering sensation, a sense of unreality, or fear of impending doom or loss of control. The individual can genuinely believe that he or she is having a heart attack, losing his or her mind, or on the verge of death.

Medical Word	Part	Meaning	Definition
apathy (ăp´ ă-thē)	a- -pathy	without, lack of emotion	Condition in which a person lacks feelings and emotions and is indifferent

Medical Word	Word Parts		Definition
	Part	Meaning	
apperception (ăp″ ĕr-sĕp′ shŭn)			Comprehension or assimilation of the meaning and significance of a particular sensory stimulus as modified by an individual's own experiences, knowledge, thoughts, and emotions
attention-deficit/ hyperactivity disorder (ADHD)			One of the most common childhood disorders, ADHD can continue through adolescence and adulthood. Symptoms include difficulty staying focused and paying attention, difficulty controlling behavior, and hyperactivity.

fyi ADHD has three subtypes:

- *Predominantly hyperactive-impulsive*: Child can't sit still; walks, runs, or climbs when others are seated; talks when others are talking.
- *Predominantly inattentive*: Child daydreams or seems to be in another world; is sidetracked by what is going on around him or her.
- *Combined hyperactive-impulsive and inattentive*: Six or more symptoms of inattention and six or more symptoms of hyperactivity-impulsivity are present in the child.

Most children have the combined type of ADHD.

Medical Word	Part	Meaning	Definition
autism spectrum disorder (ASD) (aw′ tĭzm)	aut -ism	self condition	A DSM-5 term that reflects a scientific consensus that four previously separate disorders are actually a single condition with different levels of symptom severity. Some children are mildly impaired by their symptoms, but others are severely disabled. DSM-5 currently defines four disorders: • Autistic disorder (autism) • Asperger disorder (Asperger syndrome) • Childhood disintegrative disorder (CDD) • Pervasive developmental disorder not otherwise specified (PDD-NOS) See Figure 21.6.

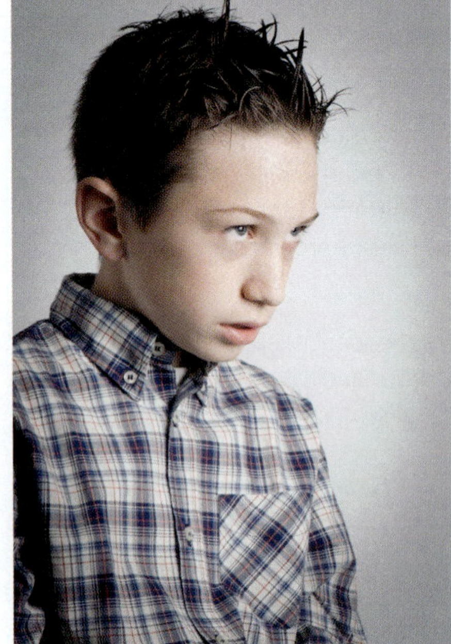

Figure 21.6 The child with autism may be self-absorbed, inaccessible, and unable to relate to others.
(umbertoleporini/Fotolia)

(continued)

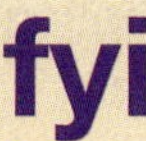

fyi According to the National Institute of Neurological Disorders and Stroke (NINDS), autism spectrum disorders (ASD) are a range of complex neurodevelopment disorders, characterized by social impairments, communication difficulties, and restricted, repetitive, and stereotyped patterns of behavior. Although ASD varies significantly in character and severity, it occurs in all ethnic and socioeconomic groups and affects every age group. About 1 in 68 children has been identified with ASD, according to estimates from the CDC's Autism and Developmental Disabilities Monitoring (ADDM) Network. Males are four times more likely to have ASD than females. The hallmark feature of ASD is impaired social interaction.

Children with **Rett syndrome** often exhibit *autistic-like* behaviors in the early stages. This neurodevelopmental disorder affects girls almost exclusively. It is characterized by normal early growth and development followed by a slowing of development, loss of purposeful use of the hands, distinctive hand movements, slowed brain and head growth, problems with walking, seizures, and intellectual disability. **Apraxia**, the inability to perform motor functions, is perhaps the most severely disabling feature, interfering with every body movement, including eye gaze and speech.

insights In ICD-10-CM, the code for *Pervasive Developmental Disorders* is F84–F89. Included in this classification are categories and subcategories including *Autistic disorder*, *Rett syndrome*, *Other childhood disintegrative disorder*, *Asperger syndrome*, and others, with their own codes.

Medical Word	Word Parts		Definition
	Part	Meaning	
bipolar disorder (bī-pōl′ ăr)			Brain disorder also known as *manic-depressive illness* that causes unusual shifts in a person's mood, energy, and ability to carry out day-to-day tasks. Bipolar disorder is characterized by cycling mood changes: mania or hypomania (a less severe form of mania) and severe lows (depression). In the DSM-5, a specifier, *with mixed features*, can be applied to episodes of mania/hypomania and depression that occur simultaneously.
compulsion (kŏm-pŭl′ shŭn)	compuls -ion	compel, drive process	Uncontrollable, recurrent, and distressing urge to perform an act in order to relieve fear connected with obsession. Common compulsions involve excessive handwashing, touching objects, and continual counting and checking.
cyclothymic disorder (sī-klō-thī′ mĭk)	cycl/o thym -ic	circle, cycle mind, emotion pertaining to	Mood disorder characterized by alternating moods of elation and depression, similar to bipolar disorder but of milder intensity
delirium (dē-lĭr′ ĭ-ŭm)			State of mental confusion marked by illusions, hallucinations, excitement, restlessness, delusions, and speech incoherence

Medical Word	Word Parts		Definition
	Part	**Meaning**	
delusion (dē-loo´ zhŭn)	delus -ion	to cheat process	Characterized by bizarre thoughts that have no basis in reality; a fixed, false belief or abnormal perception held by a person despite evidence to the contrary

RULE REMINDER

The ***o*** has been removed from the combining form because the suffix begins with a vowel.

Medical Word	Part	Meaning	Definition
dementia (dē-mĕn´ shē-ă)			Problem in the brain that makes it difficult for a person to remember, learn, and communicate and eventually to take care of him- or herself; can also affect a person's mood and personality. Dementia of the Alzheimer type is the most common form.
depression (dē-prĕsh´ ŭn)			Mental disorder marked by altered mood and loss of interest in things that are usually pleasurable such as food, sex, work, friends, hobbies, or entertainment. See Figure 21.7. A less severe type of depression, *dysthymia*, involves long-term, chronic symptoms that do not disable but keep an individual from functioning well or feeling good. Many people with dysthymia also experience major depressive episodes at some time in their lives.

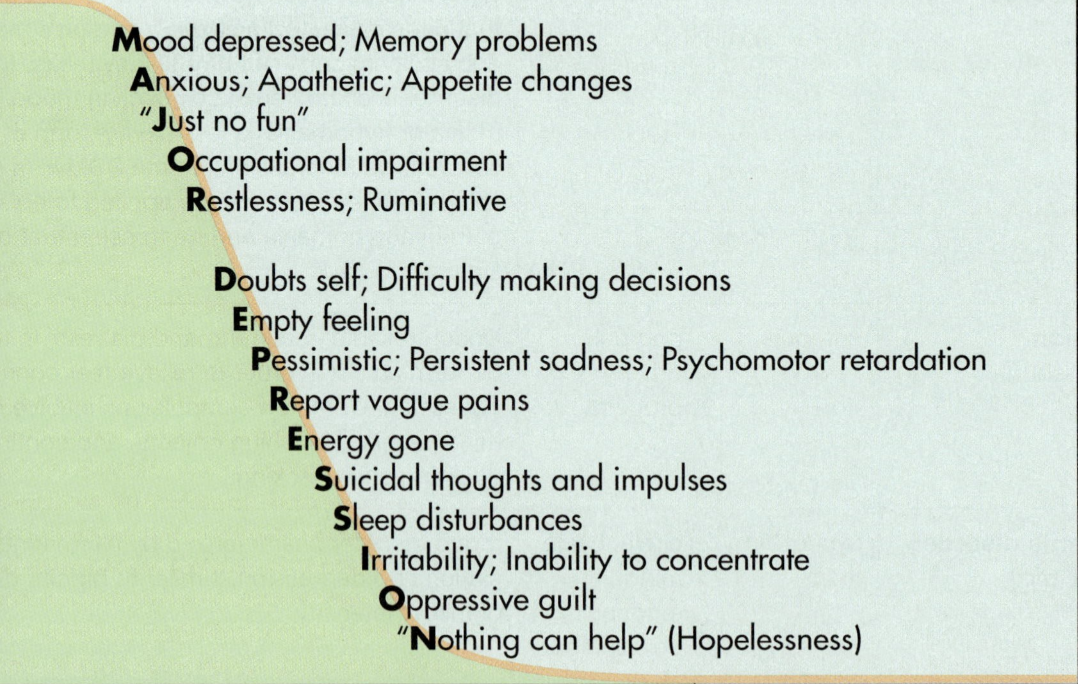

Mood depressed; Memory problems
Anxious; Apathetic; Appetite changes
"Just no fun"
Occupational impairment
Restlessness; Ruminative
Doubts self; Difficulty making decisions
Empty feeling
Pessimistic; Persistent sadness; Psychomotor retardation
Report vague pains
Energy gone
Suicidal thoughts and impulses
Sleep disturbances
Irritability; Inability to concentrate
Oppressive guilt
"Nothing can help" (Hopelessness)

Figure 21.7 Characteristics of major depression.

(continued)

Medical Word	Word Parts		Definition
	Part	Meaning	

insights In ICD-10-CM, the code for *Major depressive disorder, single episode* is F32.0–F32.9. For *Major depressive disorder, recurrent*, the code is F33.0–F33.3. For *Major depressive disorder, recurrent, in remission*, the code is F33.4–F33.42.

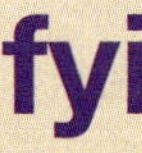

The depressed child can pretend to be sick, refuse to go to school, cling to a parent, or worry that the parent could die. Older children sulk; get into trouble at school; and are negative, grouchy, and feel misunderstood. Because normal behaviors vary from one childhood stage to another, it can be difficult to tell whether a child is just going through a temporary phase or suffering from depression. Symptoms of depression in the child:

Toddlers. Sadness, inactivity, complaints of stomachaches, and, in rare cases, self-destructive behavior.
Elementary school–age children. Unhappiness, poor school performance, irritability, refusal to take part in activities he or she used to enjoy, and occasional thoughts of suicide.
Adolescents. Sadness, withdrawal, feelings of hopelessness or guilt, changes in sleeping or eating habits, and frequent thoughts of suicide.

A child does not understand feelings of stress, anxiety, or depression and does not know how to ask for help, so when a child exhibits dramatic mood or behavior shifts, a physician should be consulted immediately. The physician could recommend psychotherapy or prescribe an antidepressant for children who are at least 5 years of age or older.

Medical Word	Part	Meaning	Definition
dissociation (dĭs-sō″ sē-ā′ shŭn)			Defense mechanism in which a group of mental processes become separated from normal consciousness and, thus separated, function as a unitary whole. In *dissociative disorder* there is a severe disturbance or trauma that causes changes in memory, consciousness, identity, and general awareness of oneself and one's environment. There are four primary types of dissociative disorders: *psychogenic amnesia*, *psychogenic fugue*, *dissociative identity disorder (DID)*, and *depersonalization disorder*.
eating disorders			Disorders that cause serious disturbances to an individual's everyday diet, such as eating extremely small amounts of food or severely overeating; *anorexia nervosa*, *bulimia nervosa*, and *binge-eating disorder* are the most common types.

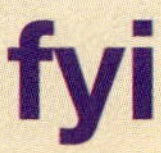

Bulimia nervosa is a potentially life-threatening eating disorder. Preoccupied with weight and body shape, people with bulimia may judge themselves severely and secretly binge—eating excessive amounts of food—and then purge, trying to get rid of the extra calories in an unhealthy way, such as forcing vomiting, taking laxatives, or exercising excessively. Effective treatment can help a person with bulimia feel better about his or her self-image, adopt healthier eating patterns, and reverse serious complications.

Binge-eating disorder is a serious eating disorder characterized by uncontrollable, excessive eating, followed by feelings of shame and guilt. Unlike those with bulimia, the person with binge-eating disorder does not purge. However, a person with bulimia may also binge-eat.

Medical Word	Word Parts		Definition
	Part	Meaning	
egocentric (ē″ gō-sĕn′ trĭk)	ego centr -ic	I, self center pertaining to	Pertaining to being self-centered
factitious disorder (făk-tĭsh′ ŭs)			Disorder that is not real, genuine, or natural. The physical and psychological symptoms are produced by the person to place him- or herself or another in the role of a patient or someone in need of help. These patients have a severe personality disturbance. *Munchausen syndrome* is a chronic factitious disorder in which a healthy person habitually seeks medical treatment; in the rare *Munchausen-by-proxy syndrome (MBPS)*, a parent (usually the mother) or other caregiver is the deliberate cause of a child's illness (by poisoning, for instance) to gain sympathy or attention.
fugue (fūg)			Dissociative disorder in which amnesia is accompanied by physical flight from customary surroundings. In psychogenic fugue, there is sudden, unexpected travel away from an individual's home or place of work with inability to recall the past. The individual can assume a partial or completely new identity. This condition is usually of short duration but can last for months. Following recovery, the person does not recall anything that happened during the fugue.
generalized anxiety disorder (GAD)			Characterized by much higher levels of anxiety than people normally experience day to day. It is chronic and fills a person's day with exaggerated worry and tension. Having this disorder means always anticipating disaster, often worrying excessively about health, money, family, or work.
hallucination (hă-loo-sĭ-nā′ shŭn)	hallucinat -ion	to wander in mind process	Process of experiencing sensations that have no source. Some examples of hallucinations include hearing nonexistent voices, seeing nonexistent things, and experiencing burning or pain sensations with no physical cause.
hypomania (hī″ pō-mā′ nē-ă)	hypo- -mania	deficient, below madness	Abnormal mood of mild mania characterized by hyperactivity, inflated self-esteem, talkativeness, heightened sexual interest, quickness to anger, irritability, and a decreased need for sleep
impulse control disorder			Mental condition in which the person is unable to resist urges or impulses to perform acts that could be harmful to him- or herself or others. *Pyromania* (starting fires), *kleptomania* (stealing), and compulsive gambling are examples of impulse control disorders.

Medical Word	Word Parts		Definition
	Part	**Meaning**	
mania (mā´ nē-ă)			Mental disorder characterized by excessive excitement; literally means *madness*
mood			Pervasive and sustained emotion that plays a key role in an individual's perception of the world. Examples include depression, joy, elation, anger, and anxiety.
neurotic (nū-rŏt´ ĭk)	neur/o -tic	nerve pertaining to	Pertaining to one who has an abnormal emotional or mental disorder
norepinephrine (nor-ĕp˝ ĭ-nĕf´ rĭn)			Hormone produced by the adrenal medulla that acts as a neurotransmitter. It is believed that disturbances in its metabolism at important brain sites can be implicated in affective disorders.
obsession	obsess -ion	besieged by thoughts process	Neurotic state in which an individual has a recurrent, persistent thought, image, or impulse that is unwanted and distressing and comes involuntarily to mind despite attempts to resist

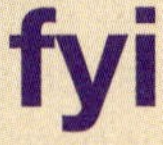

Obsessive–compulsive disorder (OCD) involves persistent, unwelcome thoughts or images or the urgent need to engage in certain rituals that the person cannot control. For example, individuals can exhibit the following:

- Obsession with germs or dirt, thus they repeatedly wash their hands
- Doubt and the need to check things repeatedly
- Frequent thoughts of violence and the fear that they will harm someone close to them
- Long periods of touching or counting things or being preoccupied with order or symmetry
- Persistent thoughts of performing repulsive sexual acts
- Thoughts against their religious beliefs

The disturbing thoughts or images are called *obsessions*, and the rituals performed to try to prevent or get rid of them are called *compulsions*. The person experiences only temporary relief, not pleasure, in carrying out the rituals, caused by the anxiety that increases when they are not performed. DSM-5 includes four new obsessive–compulsive disorders: (1) excoriation (skin-picking) disorder, (2) hoarding disorder, (3) substance- or medication-induced obsessive–compulsive and related disorder, and (4) obsessive–compulsive and related disorder due to another medical condition. Other specified obsessive–compulsive and related disorders can include body-focused repetitive behavior disorder, such as nail biting, lip biting, and cheek chewing.

Medical Word	Part	Meaning	Definition
paranoia (păr˝ ă-noy´ ă)	para- -noia	beside, abnormal mind	Mental disorder characterized by highly exaggerated or unwarranted mistrust or suspiciousness; generally classified into three categories: *paranoid personality disorder*, *delusional (paranoid) disorder*, and *paranoid schizophrenia*. Delusional (paranoid) disorder is characterized by persistent delusions of persecution or grandeur, or a combination of the two.

Medical Word	Word Parts: Part	Word Parts: Meaning	Definition
personality disorder			Mental disorder characterized by inflexible and maladaptive personality traits that are exhibited across many contexts and deviate markedly from those accepted by the individual's culture; often causes problems in work, school, or social relationships
phobia (fō´ bē-ă)	phob -ia	fear condition	Morbid and persistent fear of a specific object, activity, or situation that results in a compelling desire to avoid the feared stimulus. Examples include *claustrophobia* (fear of enclosed places), *acrophobia* (fear of heights), *photophobia* (fear of light), *arachnophobia* (fear of spiders), *nyctophobia* (fear of darkness/night), and *hematophobia* or *hemophobia* (fear of blood/bleeding).
posttraumatic stress disorder (PTSD)			Debilitating anxiety disorder that can develop following a terrifying event. It was brought to public attention by war veterans. In the DSM-5, the diagnostic thresholds have been lowered for children and adolescents and separate criteria have been added for children age 6 years or younger. PTSD can result from any number of traumatic incidents, such as a mugging, rape, or torture; being kidnapped or held captive; child abuse; serious accidents; and natural disasters.
psychiatrist (sī-kī´ ă-trĭst)	psych iatr -ist	mind treatment one who specializes	Physician who specializes in the study and treatment of mental disorders
psychopath (sī´ kō-păth)	psych/o path	mind disease	Mentally ill individual with an antisocial personality disorder; also called *sociopath*. *Note:* Path is the root for the combining form path/o.
psychosis (sī-kō´ sĭs)	psych -osis	mind condition	Serious, abnormal mental condition in which the individual's mental capacity to recognize reality and communicate with and relate to others is impaired; the person can experience delusions and hallucinations
psychosomatic (sī´ kō-sō-măt´ ĭk)	psych/o somat -ic	mind body pertaining to	Pertaining to the interrelationship of the mind and the body; a manifestation of physical disease that has a mental origin

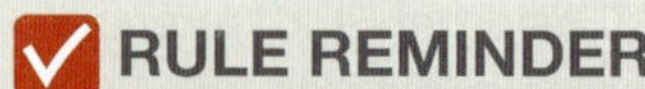

The *o* has been removed from the second combining form because the suffix begins with a vowel.

Medical Word	Word Parts: Part	Word Parts: Meaning	Definition
psychotropic (sī″ kō-trō′ pik)	psych/o trop -ic	mind turning pertaining to	Drug that affects psychic function, behavior, or experience
pyromania (pī″ rō-mā′ nē-ă)	pyro- -mania	fire madness	Impulsive disorder consisting of a compulsion to set fires or to watch fires; literally means *a madness for fire*; person suffering from this disorder (pyromaniac) receives pleasure and emotional relief from these activities
schizophrenia (skĭz″ ō -frĕn′ ē-ă)	schiz/o phren -ia	to divide mind condition	Mental disorder characterized by *positive* and *negative* symptoms. Positive (psychotic) symptoms include delusions, hallucinations, and disorganized speech. Negative symptoms include social withdrawal, extreme apathy, diminished motivation, and blunted emotional expression.

insights In ICD-10-CM, the code for *Schizophrenia, schizotypal, delusional, and other non-mood psychotic disorders* is F20–F29. Included in this classification are categories and subcategories for various types of schizophrenia, with their own codes.

Medical Word	Word Parts: Part	Word Parts: Meaning	Definition
seasonal affective disorder (SAD)			Form of depression that appears related to fluctuations in a person's exposure to natural light; usually strikes during autumn and often continues through the winter when natural light is reduced. Researchers have found that people who have SAD can be helped if they spend blocks of time bathed in light from a special full-spectrum light source called a *light therapy box*. See Figure 21.8.

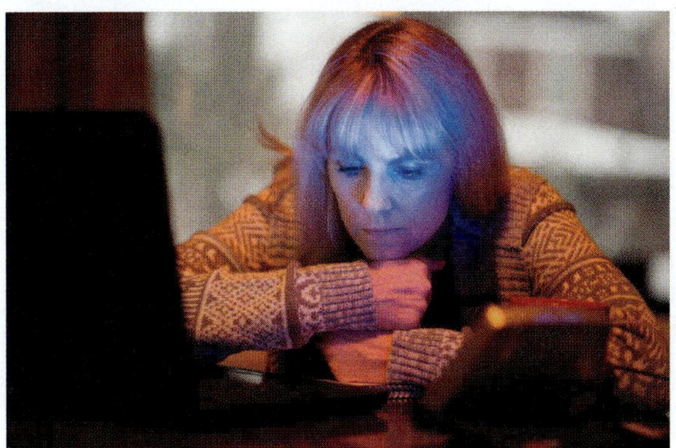

Figure 21.8 Woman using seasonal affective disorder (SAD) light therapy box.
(jrwasserman/Fotolia)

Medical Word	Word Parts: Part	Word Parts: Meaning	Definition
serotonin (sĕr″ ō-tōn′ ĭn)			Chemical present in gastrointestinal mucosa, platelets, mast cells, and carcinoid tumors; a vasoconstrictor and a neurotransmitter in the central nervous system (CNS); affects sleep and sensory perception

Medical Word	Word Parts		Definition
	Part	Meaning	
sexual disorders			Disorders that affect sexual desire, performance, and behavior. *Sexual dysfunction*, *gender dysphoria* (characterized by a persistent discomfort concerning one's anatomical sexual makeup and the desire to live as a member of the opposite sex), and *paraphilias* are examples. In paraphilia, sexual arousal requires unusual or bizarre fantasies or acts involving nonhuman objects, sexual activity with humans in which real or simulated suffering or humiliation occurs, or sexual activity with nonconsenting partners. Included in this disorder are *bestiality*, *fetishism*, *transvestism*, *zoophilia*, *pedophilia*, *exhibitionism*, *voyeurism*, *sexual masochism*, and *sexual sadism*.
somatic symptom disorder (SSD) (sō-măt´ ĭk)	somat -ic	body pertaining to	Mental disorder in which the person experiences the physical symptoms of an illness that are not explained by a medical condition or a medication. SSD is characterized by somatic symptoms that are either very distressing or result in significant disruption of functioning, as well as excessive and disproportionate thoughts, feelings, and behaviors regarding those symptoms. To be diagnosed with SSD, the individual must be persistently symptomatic (typically at least for 6 months).
substance abuse			Misuse of medications, alcohol, or illegal substances
suicide			Willfully ending one's own life. In the United States, suicide is the seventh leading cause of death for males, the fourteenth for females, and the third for young people 15–24 years of age. Research shows that the risk for suicide is associated with changes in brain chemicals, *neurotransmitters*, including serotonin. Decreased levels of serotonin have been found in people with depression, impulsive disorders, and a history of suicide attempts, and in the brains of suicide victims.

insights In ICD-10-CM, the code for *Suicide attempt* is T14.91, and is found in Chapter 19, *Injury, Poisoning, and Certain Other Consequences of External Causes*.

(*continued*)

Medical Word	Word Parts		Definition
	Part	Meaning	

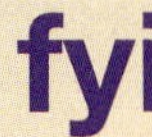

According to the National Institute of Mental Health (NIMH), older Americans are disproportionately likely to die by suicide.

Depression, which can lead to suicide, is a serious problem in the older adult. Depressive symptoms are *not* a normal part of aging. Persistent sadness or grief or loss of interest in food, sex, work, family, friends, and hobbies should be noted in an older person. See Figure 21.9.

Depression often co-occurs with other serious conditions such as heart disease, stroke, diabetes, cancer, and Parkinson disease. Because many older adults face these conditions as well as various social and economic difficulties, healthcare professionals often mistakenly conclude that depression is a normal consequence of these problems—an attitude often shared by patients themselves. These factors together contribute to the underdiagnosis and undertreatment of depressive disorders in older people. See Figure 21.10.

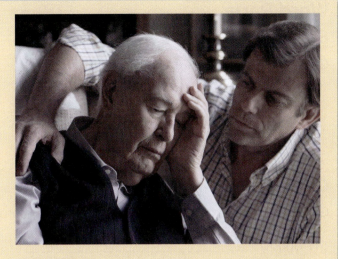

Figure 21.9 An elderly man suffering from depression being comforted by a family member.
(fresnel6/Fotolia)

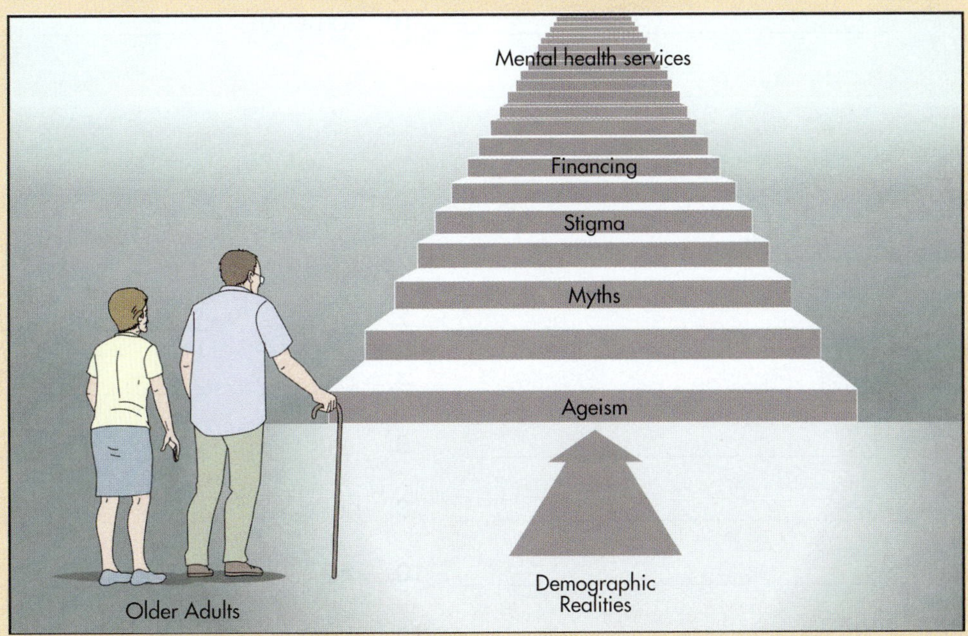

Figure 21.10 Roadblocks to mental health services for older adults.

tic disorder			Characterized by spasmodic muscular contractions most commonly involving the face, mouth, eyes, head, neck, or shoulder muscles. People with tic disorders make sounds or display body movements that are repeated, quick, sudden, and/or uncontrollable. In general, tics are of psychological origin.

Study and Review II

Word Parts

Prefixes

Give the definitions of the following prefixes.

1. an- ____________________
2. hypo- ____________________
3. para- ____________________
4. pyro- ____________________

Combining Forms

Give the definitions of the following combining forms.

1. agor/a ____________________
2. centr/o ____________________
3. cycl/o ____________________
4. delus/o ____________________
5. neur/o ____________________
6. path/o ____________________
7. phren/o ____________________
8. psych/o ____________________
9. schiz/o ____________________
10. somat/o ____________________
11. thym/o ____________________

Suffixes

Give the definitions of the following suffixes.

1. -form ____________________
2. -ia ____________________
3. -ic ____________________
4. -ion ____________________
5. -ism ____________________
6. -ist ____________________
7. -mania ____________________
8. -noia ____________________
9. -orexia ____________________
10. -osis ____________________
11. -phobia ____________________
12. -therapy ____________________
13. -tic ____________________

Identifying Medical Terms

In the spaces provided, write the medical terms for the following meanings.

1. ______________________________ Intense fear and anxiety of any place or situation where escape might be difficult, leading to avoidance of such situations
2. ______________________________ Condition in which a person lacks feelings and emotions
3. ______________________________ Fixed, false belief or abnormal perception
4. ______________________________ Mental disorder marked by altered mood and loss of interest in things that are usually pleasurable
5. ______________________________ Pertaining to being self-centered
6. ______________________________ Mental disorder characterized by excessive excitement; literally means *madness*
7. ______________________________ Morbid and persistent fear of a specific object, activity, or situation that results in a compelling desire to avoid the feared stimulus
8. ______________________________ Physician who specializes in the study and treatment of mental disorders
9. ______________________________ Method of treating mental disorders by using psychological techniques instead of physical methods
10. ______________________________ Literally means *a madness for fire*

Matching

Select the appropriate lettered meaning for each of the following words.

_____________ **1.** dysthymia

_____________ **2.** seasonal affective disorder

_____________ **3.** bipolar disorder

_____________ **4.** schizophrenia

_____________ **5.** delusion

_____________ **6.** hallucination

_____________ **7.** obsessive–compulsive disorder

_____________ **8.** posttraumatic stress disorder

_____________ **9.** generalized anxiety disorder

_____________ **10.** attention-deficit/hyperactivity disorder

a. Mental disorder characterized by positive, negative, and cognitive symptoms

b. Process of experiencing sensations that have no source

c. Brain disorder also known as *manic-depressive illness* that causes unusual shifts in a person's mood, energy, and ability to function

d. Less severe type of depression involving long-term, chronic symptoms that do not disable but keep the person from functioning well or from feeling good

e. Debilitating anxiety disorder that can develop following a terrifying event

f. Characterized by bizarre thoughts that have no basis in reality

g. Form of depression that appears related to fluctuations in a person's exposure to natural light

h. Characterized by much higher levels of anxiety than people normally experience day to day

i. Involves persistent, unwelcome thoughts or images or the urgent need to engage in certain rituals that the person cannot control

j. One of the most common childhood disorders and can continue through adolescence and adulthood

k. Anxiety syndrome and panic disorder

Medical Case Snapshot

This learning activity provides an opportunity to relate the medical terminology you are learning to a precise patient case presentation. In the spaces provided, write in your answers.

A 67-year-old female complains of sadness. She describes loss of interest in eating and social activities.

After careful evaluation and examination, it was determined that this patient was experiencing depression.

This is a ___________ ___________ marked by altered ___________ and loss of interest in things that are usually pleasurable. A less severe type of this condition known as ___________ involves long-term, chronic symptoms.

Drug Highlights

Type of Drug	Description and Examples
antianxiety agents	Chemical substances that relieve anxiety and muscle tension are indicated when anxiety interferes with a person's ability to function properly.
benzodiazepines	The *benzodiazepines* are a group of drugs with similar chemical structures and pharmaceutical activities. They are the most widely prescribed drugs for the treatment of anxiety. EXAMPLES: Xanax (alprazolam), Klonopin (clonazepam), Tranxene (clorazepate), Librium (chlordiazepoxide HCl), Valium (diazepam), and Ativan (lorazepam).
antidepressant agents	Chemical substances that relieve the symptoms of depression are indicated when depression interferes with a person's ability to function properly. Antidepressant agents can be grouped as SSRIs, SNRIs, TCAs, or MAOIs.
selective serotonin reuptake inhibitors (SSRIs)	Drugs in this group specifically block reabsorption of serotonin. EXAMPLES: Prozac (fluoxetine), Zoloft (sertraline), Paxil (paroxetine), and Luvox (fluvoxamine)
tricyclic antidepressants (TCAs)	Drugs in this group raise the level of norepinephrine and serotonin in the brain by slowing the rate at which they are reabsorbed by nerve cells. EXAMPLES: Tofranil (imipramine HC1), Pamelor (nortriptyline HC1), and amoxapine
monoamine oxidase inhibitors (MAOIs)	Drugs in this group work by blocking the breakdown of two potent neurotransmitters—norepinephrine and serotonin—and by allowing them to bathe the nerve endings for an extended length of time. EXAMPLES: Nardil (phenelzine sulfate) and Parnate (tranylcypromine sulfate)
lithium carbonate	Although not a group of drugs, various lithium medications control mood disorders by directly affecting internal nerve cell processes in all of the neurotransmitter systems. Lithium is best known as an antimanic drug used in the treatment of bipolar disorder. EXAMPLE: lithium carbonate
miscellaneous drugs	There are many miscellaneous drugs used to treat depression. Some of these drugs are used for other conditions and are being tested for treating depression; others do not fit into any of the described groups. EXAMPLES: Mirapex (pramipexole dihydrochloride), nefazodone HC1, Wellbutrin (bupropion HC1), and Remeron (mirtazapine)
antipsychotic agents	Also called *neuroleptics*, these agents modify psychotic behavior. Many antipsychotic agents are derivatives of phenothiazine (an organic compound used in the manufacture of certain of these drugs). These agents are used in the treatment of acute and chronic schizophrenia, organic psychoses, the manic phase of bipolar disorder, and psychotic disorders. EXAMPLE: chlorpromazine HCl Some antipsychotic agents are not actually phenothiazines but resemble them in action. Others resemble tricyclic antidepressants, while some are miscellaneous compounds. EXAMPLES: Clozaril (clozapine), Zyprexa (olanzapine), Orap (pimozide), and loxapine

(*continued*)

Type of Drug	Description and Examples
atypical antipsychotics	Drugs in this group affect serotonin and dopamine. EXAMPLES: Risperdal (risperidone), Clozaril (clozapine), and Zyprexa (olanzapine)
stimulants	These drugs stimulate the central nervous system (CNS) and are generally prescribed for attention-deficit/hyperactivity disorder. Patients using these drugs must take care to avoid abuse and excessive CNS stimulation by overdose. Many of these drugs are Schedule II agents with a very high potential for abuse. EXAMPLES: Dexedrine (dextroamphetamine sulfate), Ritalin (methylphenidate HCl), and Adderall, which is a combination of amphetamine salts

Abbreviations

Abbreviation	Meaning
ADHD	attention-deficit/hyperactivity disorder
APA	American Psychiatric Association
ASD	autism spectrum disorder
BDD	body dysmorphic disorder
CBT	cognitive-behavioral therapy
CNS	central nervous system
DSM-5	*Diagnostic and Statistical Manual of Mental Disorders*, Fifth Edition
ECT	electroconvulsive therapy
GAD	generalized anxiety disorder
HHS	Department of Health and Human Services
IQ	intelligence quotient
MAOIs	monoamine oxidase inhibitors
MBPS	Munchausen-by-proxy syndrome
MD	medical doctor
MMPI-2	Minnesota Multiphasic Personality Inventory-2
NIH	National Institutes of Health
NIMH	National Institute of Mental Health
NINDS	National Institute of Neurological Disorders and Stroke
OCD	obsessive–compulsive disorder
PDD-NOS	pervasive developmental disorder not otherwise specified
PTSD	posttraumatic stress disorder
SAD	seasonal affective disorder
SNRI	serotonin-norepinephrine reuptake inhibitor
SSD	somatic symptom disorder
SSRIs	selective serotonin reuptake inhibitors
TAT	Thematic Apperception Test
TCAs	tricyclic antidepressants
WAIS-R	Wechsler Adult Intelligence Scale–Revised
WHO	World Health Organization

Study and Review III

Abbreviations

Place the correct word, phrase, or abbreviation in the space provided.

1. cognitive-behavioral therapy ______________________________

2. *Diagnostic and Statistical Manual of Mental Disorders*, Fifth Edition ______________________________

3. ECT ______________________________

4. MMPI-2 ______________________________

5. National Institute of Mental Health ______________________________

6. OCD ______________________________

7. posttraumatic stress disorder ______________________________

8. SAD ______________________________

9. TAT ______________________________

10. World Health Organization ______________________________

Practical Application

Medical Record Analysis

This exercise contains information, abbreviations, and medical terminology from an actual medical record or case study that has been adapted for this text. The names and any personal information have been created by the author. Read and study each form or case study and then answer the questions that follow. You may refer to Appendix III, *Abbreviations and Symbols*.

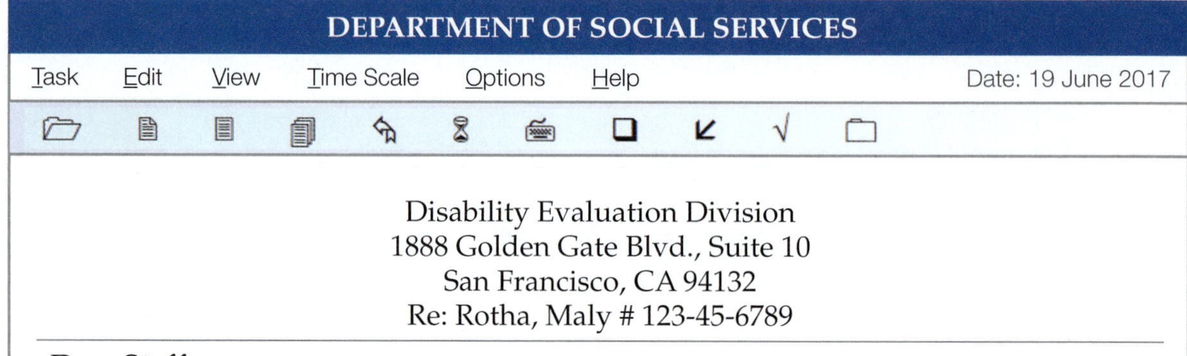

DEPARTMENT OF SOCIAL SERVICES

Task Edit View Time Scale Options Help Date: 19 June 2017

Disability Evaluation Division
1888 Golden Gate Blvd., Suite 10
San Francisco, CA 94132
Re: Rotha, Maly # 123-45-6789

Dear Staff:

Thank you for referring to me the case of Ms. Rotha for psychiatric evaluation. She was examined in psychiatric consultation on June 17, 2017. No physical exam was performed. No psychological testing was given. Medical records provided were reviewed. The patient was a clean, neatly dressed, well-groomed Asian female. She understood English and responded to questions. There was no evidence of any ambulation difficulties or speech impediments. Energy level was described as poor, with description of fatigue with minimal exertion.

History of Present Illness

Ms. Rotha is a 42-year-old Cambodian female. She lives in an apartment with her husband and three children. She describes feeling sick all the time and too weak and tired, dizzy and depressed to do anything except "rest." Currently, she is taking a combination of five different medications under the care of two different physicians. She takes Proventil inhaler for relief of asthmatic symptoms, analgesics, decongestants, and two different forms of tricyclic antidepressants. She feels that the medications are helping her. She is not receiving any formal psychiatric treatment with or without medication.

Mental Examination

There is no evidence or history of alcoholism or illicit drug use. She is oriented to time, place, persons, and events. There is no evidence of delusion or hallucinations at the present time and no history of such in the past. There is no evidence of paranoia such as feelings of being persecuted or plotted against. Thought content is generally well organized, coherent, and relevant without flight of ideas or loose associations.

Depression is manifested by occasional crying, usually occurring every other day. There is fitful sleep. There are occasional nightmares. There is no suicidal ideation or history of any suicide attempts.

(*continued*)

Memory for recent and remote events, she feels, is impaired. She cannot recall her Social Security number. She can recall her address and phone number. She can do simple arithmetic.

Medical Opinion

It is my medical opinion that at Ms. Rotha's current level of daily functioning, she has minimal difficulty in relating to others. In appearance she seems to have the ability to care for her personal needs. How much her interest, habits, and daily activities are constricted as a result of mental impairments is difficult to assess because it is my medical opinion that this represents a factitious disorder, although posttraumatic stress disorder should not be ruled out.

Very truly yours,

Hana Eun Kim, MD

Medical Record Questions

Place the correct answer in the space provided.

1. State the symptoms Ms. Rotha described. ______________________________
2. What medications does this patient take? ______________________________
3. What is a delusion? ______________________________
4. Define hallucination. ______________________________
5. Define factitious disorder. ______________________________

APPENDIX I Answer Key

CHAPTER 1

Study and Review

Word Parts

Prefixes

1. without
2. away from
3. against
4. bad
5. one hundred, one-hundredth
6. through
7. different
8. bad
9. small
10. one-thousandth
11. many, much
12. beside
13. before
14. together
15. apart
16. upon
17. out
18. in, into

Roots and Combining Forms

1. stuck to
2. armpit
3. center
4. chemical
5. a shaping
6. formation, produce
7. a thousand
8. large
9. death
10. rule
11. tumor
12. organ
13. fever
14. heat, fire
15. ray, x-ray
16. to examine
17. putrefaction
18. hot, heat
19. cough
20. to infect
21. people
22. cause
23. to cut
24. bad kind
25. greatest
26. least
27. palm
28. guarding

Suffixes

1. pertaining to
2. pertaining to
3. surgical puncture
4. that which runs together
5. shape
6. formation, produce
7. knowledge
8. a step
9. a weight
10. condition
11. pertaining to
12. process
13. condition
14. nature of, quality of
15. liter
16. study of
17. instrument to measure
18. condition
19. pertaining to
20. to carry
21. instrument for examining
22. decay
23. treatment
24. pertaining to

Identifying Medical Terms

1. adhesion
2. asepsis
3. axillary
4. chemotherapy
5. heterogeneous
6. malformation
7. microscope
8. multiform
9. oncology

Matching

1. f	2. d
3. j	4. g
5. a	6. k
7. b	8. i
9. c	10. e

Abbreviations

1. chief complaint
2. axillary
3. Bx
4. Wt
5. neurology
6. ENT
7. Derm
8. g
9. gynecology
10. orthopedics

Practical Application

1. alphanumeric
2. Diagnosis
3. medical terminology
4. Centers for Medicare & Medicaid Services
5. Current Procedural Terminology

Matching

1. c
2. e
3. a
4. b
5. i
6. d
7. j
8. f
9. h
10. g

CHAPTER 2

Study and Review

Identifying Suffixes

1. cardiac
2. cephalad
3. enuresis
4. obstetrician
5. bronchiole
6. pustule
7. dentalgia
8. diabetes
9. hyperemesis
10. hemoptysis

Defining Suffixes

1. weakness
2. process
3. inflammation
4. softening
5. enlargement, large
6. disease
7. deficiency
8. to digest
9. fear
10. rupture
11. pertaining to
12. pertaining to
13. use, action
14. condition
15. to make
16. resemble
17. one who
18. pertaining to
19. pertaining to
20. tissue, structure

Using Suffixes to Build Medical Words

1. hyperhidrosis
2. muscular
3. macula
4. alopecia
5. ventricle
6. decubitus
7. integumentary
8. penile
9. congenital
10. anterior

Identifying Medical Terms

1. abrasion
2. anesthetize
3. arousal
4. asymmetrical
5. infection
6. comatose
7. turgor
8. grandiose
9. gynecoid
10. palpate

Practical Application

1. arthropods
2. phylum
3. helminthiases
4. prion
5. protozal
6. vector
7. sanguineous
8. mycoses
9. spirochetal
10. nonsuppurative

CHAPTER 3

Study and Review

Identifying Prefixes

1. apnea
2. bradypnea
3. dyspnea
4. eupnea
5. hyperpnea
6. hypopnea
7. tachypnea

8. binary
9. concentration
10. extraocular

Defining Prefixes

1. against
2. short
3. through
4. different
5. similar, same
6. water
7. micro, small
8. scanty, little
9. all
10. false
11. without
12. without
13. two
14. twice
15. with, together
16. down, away from
17. outside
18. excessive
19. under
20. not
21. between
22. many
23. beside
24. around
25. many
26. before
27. again, backward
28. below
29. upper, above
30. not

Using Prefixes to Build Medical Words

1. anicteric
2. hyperactive
3. multifocal
4. decompensation
5. intercellular
6. bifurcation
7. polydactyly
8. hypoplasia
9. subacute
10. unconscious

Identifying Medical Terms

1. afebrile
2. extraocular
3. insomnia
4. arrest
5. enucleate
6. lumen
7. patent
8. react
9. sign
10. symptom

CHAPTER 4

Study and Review I

Anatomy and Physiology

1. body . . . cells . . . sustain
2. cell membrane
3. cell membrane . . . cytoplasm . . . nucleus
4. metabolism . . . growth . . . reproduction
5. embryonic cell
6. a. protection
   b. absorption
   c. secretion
   d. excretion
   e. sensation
   f. diffusion
7. Connective
8. a. striated (voluntary)
   b. cardiac
   c. smooth (involuntary)
9. excitability . . . conductivity
10. tissue serving a common purpose
11. group of organs functioning together for a common purpose
12. a. integumentary
    b. skeletal
    c. muscular
    d. digestive
    e. cardiovascular
    f. blood and lymphatic
    g. respiratory
    h. urinary
    i. endocrine
    j. nervous
    k. reproductive
13. a. above, in an upward direction
    b. in front of, before
    c. toward the back
    d. pertaining to the head
    e. nearest the midline or middle
    f. to the side, away from the middle
    g. nearest the point of attachment
    h. away from the point of attachment
14. midsagittal plane
15. transverse or horizontal
16. coronal or frontal
17. a. thoracic
    b. abdominal
    c. pelvic
18. a. cranial
    b. spinal

Anatomy Labeling

1. posterior
2. anterior
3. cranial cavity
4. spinal cavity

5. thoracic cavity
6. diaphragm
7. abdominal cavity
8. pelvic cavity
9. pericardial membranes
10. heart

Study and Review II

Word Parts

Prefixes

1. both
2. up, apart
3. two
4. color
5. down, away from
6. apart
7. outside
8. within
9. similar, same
10. middle
11. through
12. first
13. one

Combining Forms

1. fat
2. man
3. toward the front
4. life
5. tail
6. cell
7. away from the point of origin
8. backward
9. tissue
10. water
11. below
12. groin
13. cell's nucleus
14. side
15. toward the middle
16. organ
17. disease
18. to show
19. nature
20. behind, toward the back, back
21. near the point of origin
22. body
23. near or on the belly side of the body
24. body organs

Suffixes

1. pertaining to
2. use, action
3. formation, produce
4. pertaining to
5. process
6. study of
7. form, shape
8. resemble
9. pertaining to
10. a thing formed, plasma
11. body
12. control, stop, stand still
13. incision
14. type

Identifying Medical Terms

1. android
2. bilateral
3. cytology
4. ectomorph
5. karyogenesis
6. somatotrophic
7. unilateral

Matching

1. c
2. d
3. e
4. f
5. a
6. i
7. g
8. h
9. j
10. b

Study and Review III

Building Medical Terms

1. bilateral
2. biology
3. distal
4. inguinal
5. lateral
6. pathology
7. physiology
8. systemic
9. unilateral
10. visceral

Combining Form Challenge

1. adipose
2. android
3. histology
4. karyogenesis
5. phenotype
6. somatotrophic

Select the Right Term

1. anatomy
2. anterior
3. mesomorph
4. base
5. proximal
6. horizontal

Abbreviations

1. abdomen
2. anatomy and physiology
3. deoxyribonucleic acid
4. BMI
5. GI
6. water
7. left lower quadrant
8. O_2
9. OTC
10. right upper quadrant

Practical Application

1. calories
2. overweight
3. Laterality
4. medicaments
5. underdosing

CHAPTER 5

Study and Review I

Anatomy and Physiology

1. skin
2. a. hair
   b. nails
   c. sebaceous glands
   d. sweat glands
3. a. protection
   b. regulation
   c. sensory reception
   d. secretion
4. epidermis . . . dermis
5. a. stratum germinativum
   b. stratum spinosum
   c. stratum granulosum
   d. stratum lucidum
   e. stratum corneum
6. Keratin
7. Melanin
8. dermis
9. a. papillary layer
   b. reticular layer
10. lunula

Anatomy Labeling

1. epidermis
2. dermis
3. subcutaneous layer
4. sweat gland
5. sebaceous gland
6. hair
7. nerve
8. artery
9. vein

Study and Review II

Word Parts

Prefixes

1. without, lack of
2. self
3. out
4. down
5. out
6. excessive
7. under
8. within
9. around
10. below

Combining Forms

1. white
2. burn, burning
3. skin
4. skin
5. red
6. sweat
7. jaundice
8. tumor
9. horn
10. white
11. black
12. nail
13. thick
14. a louse
15. plate
16. itching
17. wrinkle
18. hard, hardening
19. oil
20. hot, heat
21. hair
22. to pull
23. yellow
24. dry

Suffixes

1. pertaining to
2. pain
3. pertaining to
4. pertaining to
5. skin
6. pertaining to
7. sensation
8. pencil, grafting knife
9. condition
10. pertaining to
11. process
12. condition
13. one who specializes
14. inflammation
15. study of
16. dilatation
17. resemble
18. tumor
19. condition
20. pertaining to
21. surgical repair
22. flow, discharge
23. instrument to cut

Identifying Medical Terms

1. actinic dermatitis
2. cutaneous
3. dermatitis
4. dermatology
5. pruritus
6. hyperhidrosis
7. hypodermic
8. icteric
9. onychitis
10. pachyderma
11. thermanesthesia
12. xanthoderma

Matching

1. d
2. f
3. e
4. h
5. j
6. i
7. b
8. g
9. a
10. c

Medical Case Snapshot

Case 1: alopecia

Case 2: dermabrasion, rhytidoplasty

Case 3: a lying down

Study and Review III

Building Medical Terms

1. decubitus
2. dermatology
3. icteric
4. melanoma
5. onychitis
6. pachyderma
7. seborrhea
8. xanthoderma
9. xanthoma
10. xerosis

Combining Form Challenge

1. albinism
2. causalgia
3. cutaneous
4. dermatitis
5. erythroderma
6. integumentary

Select the Right Term

1. acne
2. alopecia
3. cicatrix
4. eschar
5. lentigo
6. roseola

Diagnostic and Laboratory Tests

1. c
2. d
3. a
4. b
5. a

Abbreviations

1. BCC
2. biopsy
3. decubitus
4. intradermal
5. squamous cell carcinoma
6. purified protein derivative
7. SG
8. staphylococcus
9. streptococcus
10. TIMs

Practical Application

1. Dx
2. basal cell carcinoma
3. a solid, circumscribed, elevated area of the skin
4. telangiectasia
5. solar elastosis

CHAPTER 6

Study and Review I

Anatomy and Physiology

1. 206
2. **a.** axial
   b. appendicular
3. **a.** flat . . . ribs, scapula, parts of the pelvic girdle, bones of the skull
   b. long . . . tibia, femur, humerus, radius
   c. short . . . carpal, tarsal
   d. irregular . . . vertebrae, ossicles of the ear
   e. sesamoid . . . patella

*Optional answer to question 3:

   f. sutural or wormian . . . between the flat bones of the skull
4. **a.** Provide shape, support, and the framework of the body
   b. Provide protection for internal organs
   c. Serve as a storage place for mineral salts, calcium, and phosphorus
   d. Play an important role in the formation of blood cells (hematopoiesis)
   e. Provide areas for the attachment of skeletal muscles
   f. Help make movement possible through articulation
5. **a.** ends of a developing bone
   b. shaft of a long bone
   c. membrane that forms the covering of bones except at their articular surfaces
   d. dense, hard layer of bone tissue
   e. narrow space or cavity throughout the length of the diaphysis
   f. tough connective tissue membrane lining the medullary canal and containing the bone marrow
   g. reticular tissue that makes up most of the volume of bone

6. Matching

1. f	2. k
3. d	4. m
5. h	6. j
7. i	8. n
9. a	10. l
11. b	12. c
13. g	14. e

7. a. synarthrosis
   b. amphiarthrosis
   c. diarthrosis
8. Abduction
9. moving a body part toward the midline
10. Circumduction
11. bending a body part backward
12. Eversion
13. straightening a flexed limb
14. Flexion
15. turning inward
16. Pronation
17. moving a body part forward
18. Retraction
19. moving a body part around a central axis
20. Supination

Anatomy Labeling

1. cranium
2. mandible
3. clavicle
4. scapula
5. sternum
6. humerus
7. ulna
8. radius
9. femur
10. tibia

Study and Review II

Word Parts

Prefixes

1. without
2. apart
3. water
4. between
5. beyond
6. around
7. many, much
8. under, beneath
9. together
10. back

Combining Forms

1. extremity
2. stiffening, crooked
3. joint
4. a pouch
5. heel bone
6. wrist
7. cartilage
8. coccyx, tailbone
9. rib
10. skull
11. finger or toe
12. ischium, hip
13. a hump
14. bending, curve, swayback
15. loin, lower back
16. bone
17. kneecap
18. foot
19. sacrum
20. curvature
21. spine
22. sternum, breastbone
23. ulna, elbow
24. sword

Suffixes

1. pertaining to
2. pertaining to
3. pain
4. pertaining to
5. pertaining to
6. immature cell, germ cell
7. surgical puncture
8. related to
9. process
10. pain
11. excision
12. swelling
13. formation, produce
14. formation, produce
15. mark, record
16. instrument for recording
17. pertaining to
18. inflammation
19. nature of
20. instrument for examining
21. softening
22. structure
23. resemble
24. tumor
25. condition
26. deficiency
27. growth
28. formation, produce
29. surgical repair
30. formation
31. instrument to cut
32. incision
33. structure, tissue

Identifying Medical Terms

1. acroarthritis
2. ankylosis
3. arthritis
4. calcaneal
5. chondral
6. coccygodynia
7. chondrocostal

8. craniectomy
9. dactylic
10. osteotome
11. intercostal
12. ischialgia
13. lumbar
14. myeloma
15. osteoarthritis
16. osteomyelitis or myelitis
17. osteopenia
18. pedal
19. xiphoid

Matching

1. i
2. j
3. e
4. c
5. b
6. h
7. g
8. a
9. d
10. f

Medical Case Snapshot

Case 1: osteopenia, osteoporosis

Case 2: scoliosis, asymmetry, scapula

Case 3: rheumatoid arthritis

Study and Review III

Building Medical Terms

1. coccygodynia
2. dactylic
3. lordosis
4. metacarpals
5. myelopoiesis
6. osteomalacia
7. patellar
8. phalangeal
9. scoliosis
10. xiphoid

Combining Form Challenge

1. arthroplasty
2. bursitis
3. carpal
4. chondral
5. chondrocostal
6. dactylogram

Select the Right Term

1. ankylosis
2. craniectomy
3. ischialgia
4. mandibular
5. osteosarcoma
6. spondylodesis

Diagnostic and Laboratory Tests

1. c
2. d
3. c
4. b
5. b

Abbreviations

1. ANA
2. Fx
3. long leg cast
4. osteoarthritis
5. P
6. rheumatoid arthritis
7. ROM
8. thoracic vertebra, first
9. tumor necrosis factor
10. Tx

Practical Application

1. dual-energy X-ray -absorptiometry scan
2. bone mineral density (test)
3. lumbar vertebra, first
4. osteopenia
5. XRDXA/76075

CHAPTER 7

Study and Review I

Anatomy and Physiology

1. a. skeletal
   b. smooth
   c. cardiac
2. 42
3. a. nutrition
   b. oxygen
4. a. origin
   b. insertion
5. voluntary or striated
6. aponeurosis
7. a. body
   b. origin
   c. insertion
8. a. muscle that counteracts the action of another muscle; when one contracts the other relaxes
   b. muscle that is primary in a given movement produced by its contraction
   c. muscle that acts with another muscle to produce movement
9. involuntary, visceral, or unstriated
10. a. digestive tract
    b. respiratory tract
    c. urinary tract
    d. eye
    e. skin
11. Cardiac
12. a. movement
    b. maintain posture
    c. produce heat

Anatomy Labeling

Anterior View

1. trapezius
2. deltoid

3. rectus femoris
4. pectoralis major
5. biceps brachii

Posterior View

6. gluteus maximus
7. biceps femoris
8. gastrocnemius
9. latissimus dorsi
10. triceps
11. Achilles tendon

Study and Review II

Word Parts

Prefixes

1. lack of
2. away from
3. toward
4. against
5. two
6. slow
7. with
8. through
9. difficult
10. into
11. within
12. water
13. four
14. with, together
15. three

Combining Forms

1. agony, a contest
2. to cut through
3. arm
4. clavicle
5. turmoil
6. to lead
7. a band
8. fiber
9. equal
10. to measure
11. muscle
12. muscle
13. nerve
14. disease
15. an addition
16. rod
17. to turn
18. flesh
19. synovial
20. tendon
21. tone, tension
22. twisted
23. nourishment, development
24. will
27. weakness
28. disease
29. a fence
30. surgical repair
31. stroke, paralysis
32. suture
33. pertaining to
34. tension, spasm
35. order
36. instrument to cut
37. incision
38. nourishment, development
39. condition
40. condition

Suffixes

1. pain
2. pertaining to
3. pertaining to
4. weakness
5. immature cell, germ cell
6. head
7. binding
8. pain
9. chemical
10. treatment
11. instrument for recording
12. condition
13. pertaining to
14. process
15. agent
16. inflammation
17. condition
18. motion
19. motion
20. study of
21. process
22. softening
23. resemble
24. tumor
25. a doer
26. condition

Identifying Medical Terms

1. atonic
2. bradykinesia
3. dactylospasm
4. dystrophy
5. intramuscular
6. levator
7. myasthenia gravis
8. myoparesis
9. myoplasty
10. myosarcoma
11. myotomy
12. polyplegia
13. tenodesis
14. synergetic
15. triceps

Matching

1. d
2. i
3. g
4. e
5. j
6. a
7. h
8. c
9. b
10. f

Medical Case Snapshot

Case 1: fibromyalgia, myalgia

Case 2: muscular dystrophy, Gowers

Case 3: body erect, forward, palms

Study and Review III

Building Medical Terms

1. amputation
2. ataxia
3. biceps
4. levator
5. myograph
6. polyplegia
7. rhabdomyoma
8. sarcolemma
9. tenodynia
10. voluntary

Combining Form Challenge

1. brachialgia
2. dactylospasm
3. fasciitis
4. isometric
5. myoparesis
6. sarcolemma

Select the Right Term

1. antagonist
2. clonic
3. flaccid
4. myoplasty
5. synergetic
6. torticollis

Diagnostic and Laboratory Tests

1. b **2.** d

3. b **4.** c

5. a

Abbreviations

1. above elbow
2. aspartate aminotransferase
3. Ca
4. EMG
5. full range of motion
6. musculoskeletal
7. ROM
8. myasthenia gravis
9. muscular dystrophy
10. fibromyalgia syndrome

Practical Application

1. waddling
2. electromyography
3. **a.** minimize deformities
   b. preserve mobility
4. Test to measure electrical activity across muscle membranes by means of electrodes attached to a needle that is inserted into the muscle.
5. Surgical removal of a small piece of muscle tissue for examination.

CHAPTER 8

Study and Review I

Anatomy and Physiology

1. **a.** mouth
   b. pharynx
   c. esophagus
   d. stomach
   e. small intestine
   f. large intestine
2. **a.** salivary glands
   b. liver
   c. gallbladder
   d. pancreas
3. **a.** digestion
   b. absorption
   c. elimination
4. soft mass of chewed food ready to be swallowed
5. series of wavelike muscular contractions that are involuntary
6. hydrochloric acid and gastric juices
7. duodenum
8. chyme
9. circulatory system
10. cecum, colon, rectum, and anal canal
11. liver
12. stores and concentrates bile
13. produces digestive enzymes
14. **a.** plays an important role in metabolism
    b. manufactures bile
    c. stores iron and vitamins B_{12}, A, D, E, and K
15. small intestine
16. parotid, sublingual, submandibular
17. **a.** insulin
    b. glucagon

Anatomy Labeling

1. right lobe of liver
2. gallbladder
3. appendix
4. parotid gland
5. pharynx
6. esophagus
7. spleen
8. body of stomach
9. pancreas
10. small intestine

Study and Review II

Word Parts

Prefixes

1. lack of
2. difficult
3. above
4. excessive, above
5. deficient, below
6. bad
7. around
8. after
9. through
10. below

Combining Forms

1. starch
2. appendix
3. gall, bile
4. cheek
5. abdomen, belly
6. gall, bile
7. orange-yellow
8. colon
9. tooth
10. intestine
11. esophagus
12. stomach
13. gums
14. tongue
15. liver
16. ileum
17. lip
18. abdomen
19. tongue
20. tooth
21. meal
22. anus and rectum
23. rectum
24. mouth

Suffixes

1. pertaining to
2. pertaining to
3. pain, ache
4. pertaining to
5. enzyme
6. hernia
7. resemble
8. condition
9. surgical excision
10. vomiting
11. shape
12. formation, produce
13. pertaining to
14. pertaining to
15. process
16. condition
17. one who specializes
18. inflammation
19. nature of, quality of
20. study of
21. destruction, to separate
22. enlargement, large
23. tumor
24. appetite
25. condition
26. flow
27. to digest
28. pertaining to
29. to eat, to swallow
30. instrument for examining
31. visual examination, to view, examine
32. contraction
33. new opening
34. incision
35. pertaining to
36. suture

Identifying Medical Terms

1. amylase
2. anabolism
3. anorexia
4. appendectomy
5. appendicitis
6. biliary
7. celiac
8. dysphagia
9. hepatitis
10. herniorrhaphy
11. postprandial
12. splenomegaly
13. sigmoidoscope

Matching

1. e
2. f
3. d
4. b
5. i
6. h
7. j
8. a
9. g
10. c

Medical Case Snapshot

Case 1: colonoscopy, colostomy

Case 2: constipation, hemorrhoid

Case 3: *Helicobacter pylori*, antibiotics

Study and Review III

Building Medical Terms

1. appendectomy
2. buccal
3. cirrhosis
4. colostomy
5. diverticulitis
6. dyspepsia
7. gingivitis
8. laparotomy
9. lingual
10. rectocele

Combining Form Challenge

1. absorption
2. appendectomy
3. biliary

4. esophageal
5. glossectomy
6. hepatitis

Select the Right Term

1. cholecystitis
2. ascites
3. colostomy
4. gastroesophageal
5. gavage
6. mastication

Diagnostic and Laboratory Tests

1. a
2. c
3. d
4. c
5. c

Abbreviations

1. Ba
2. carbohydrate
3. hepatitis C virus
4. HCl
5. GB
6. HAV
7. nasogastric
8. IBS
9. PP
10. PPIs

Practical Application

1. Appointment Date: October 17, 2017 Time: 8:45 A.M.
2. Referred to: Seymour Butts, MD
   Endoscopy Center
   14 Maddox Drive
   Rome, GA 30165
3. For:
   _______X___ Diagnostic Procedure Screening Colonoscopy
   _______ Consultation
   _______ Evaluate and treat, initiating appropriate diagnostic and/or therapeutic services
   _______ Report test results to: Angel De'Crohn, MD Fax (706) 235-6676
4. Patient Instructions: Bring a driver, all current medications, driver's license, and proof of insurance
5. Referring Physician's Name: Angel De'Crohn, MD
   Date: 09/28/17
   Phone #: (706) 235-7765
   Fax #: (706) 235-6676

CHAPTER 9

Study and Review I

Anatomy and Physiology

1. **a.** heart
   b. arteries
   c. veins
   d. capillaries
2. **a.** endocardium
   b. myocardium
   c. pericardium
3. 300
4. atria . . . interatrial
5. ventricles . . . interventricular
6. electrocardiogram
7. autonomic nervous system
8. sinoatrial node
9. Purkinje network
10. **a.** radial . . . on the radial side of the wrist
    b. brachial . . . in the antecubital space of the elbow
    c. carotid . . . in the neck
11. **a.** pressure exerted by the blood on the walls of the vessels
    b. difference between the systolic and diastolic readings
12. person's fist . . . 60–90 and 80–89
13. 120 and 139, 80 to 89
14. transport blood from the right and left ventricles of the heart to all body parts; transports blood away from the heart
15. transport blood from peripheral tissues back to the heart

Anatomy Labeling

1. superior vena cava
2. aorta
3. right atrium
4. tricuspid valve
5. right ventricle
6. inferior vena cava
7. mitral valve
8. endocardium
9. myocardium
10. pericardium

Study and Review II

Word Parts

Prefixes

1. lack of
2. two
3. slow
4. together
5. within
6. within
7. outside
8. excessive, above
9. deficient, below
10. around
11. difficult, abnormal
12. half
13. rapid
14. three

Combining Forms

1. vessel
2. artery
3. fatty substance, porridge
4. heart
5. dark blue
6. to widen
7. reflected sound
8. a throwing in
9. blood
10. to hold back
11. fat
12. moon
13. thin
14. mitral valve
15. to close up
16. sour, sharp, acid
17. throbbing
18. vein
19. hardening
20. a curve
21. chest
22. clot of blood
23. vessel
24. vein

Suffixes

1. pertaining to
2. pertaining to
3. pertaining to
4. surgical puncture
5. measurement
6. dilatation
7. surgical excision
8. blood condition
9. relating to
10. formation, produce
11. recording
12. condition
13. pertaining to
14. having a particular quality
15. process
16. condition
17. one who specializes
18. inflammation
19. nature of, quality of
20. study of
21. softening
22. enlargement, large
23. instrument to measure
24. tumor
25. one who
26. condition
27. disease
28. surgical repair
29. instrument for examining
30. contraction, spasm
31. incision
32. tissue

Identifying Medical Terms

1. angioma
2. angioplasty
3. angiostenosis
4. arrhythmia
5. arteritis
6. bicuspid
7. cardiologist
8. cardiomegaly
9. cardiopulmonary
10. constriction
11. embolism
12. phlebitis
13. tachycardia
14. vasodilator

Matching

1. d	2. e
3. f	4. g
5. b	6. c
7. a	8. i
9. j	10. h

Medical Case Snapshot

Case 1: angina pectoris, neck, jaw

Case 2: auscultation, arteriosclerosis, atherosclerosis

Case 3: angina pectoris, coronary artery

Study and Review III

Building Medical Terms

1. bicuspid
2. claudication
3. occlusion
4. oxygen
5. palpitation
6. septum
7. stethoscope
8. tricuspid
9. valvuloplasty
10. venipuncture

Combining Form Challenge

1. angioplasty
2. arterial
3. atheroma
4. cardiomegaly
5. cyanosis
6. phlebitis

Select the Right Term

1. bradycardia
2. hyperlipidemia
3. pericardial
4. semilunar
5. triglyceride
6. ischemia

Diagnostic and Laboratory Tests

1. c
2. a
3. b
4. c
5. b

Abbreviations

1. AMI
2. AV
3. blood pressure
4. coronary artery disease
5. CC
6. electrocardiogram
7. high-density lipoprotein
8. H & L
9. myocardial infarction
10. tissue plasminogen activator

Practical Application

1. dyspnea
2. blood enzyme
3. oxygenated
4. electrocardiogram
5. coronary vasodilator

CHAPTER 10

Study and Review I

Anatomy and Physiology

1. **a.** erythrocytes
   b. thrombocytes
   c. leukocytes
2. transport oxygen and carbon dioxide
3. 5
4. 80–120 days
5. body's main defense against the invasion of pathogens
6. 8
7. **a.** neutrophils
   b. eosinophils
   c. basophils
   d. lymphocytes
   e. monocytes
8. play an important role in the clotting process
9. 150,000–400,000
10. **a.** A
    b. B
    c. AB
    d. O
11. **a.** transports proteins and fluids
    b. protects the body against pathogens
    c. serves as a pathway for the absorption of fats
12. **a.** spleen
    b. tonsils
    c. thymus

Anatomy Labeling

1. tonsil
2. lymphatic vessel
3. thymus gland
4. thoracic duct
5. spleen
6. lymph nodes

Study and Review II

Word Parts

Prefixes

1. lack of
2. against
3. self
4. up
5. beyond
6. excessive
7. deficient
8. one
9. all
10. many
11. before
12. across
13. deficient

Combining Forms

1. clumping
2. vessel
3. unequal
4. base
5. color
6. clots, to clot
7. cell
8. rose-colored
9. red
10. sweet, sugar
11. blood
12. blood
13. immunity
14. white
15. lymph
16. large
17. neither
18. plasma
19. putrefying
20. whey, serum
21. iron
22. spleen
23. thymus
24. small vessel

Suffixes

1. capable
2. forming
3. removal
4. immature cell, germ cell
5. body
6. swelling
7. cultivation
8. cell
9. surgical excision

10. blood condition
11. work
12. formation, produce
13. protection
14. globe, protein
15. pertaining to
16. chemical
17. process
18. one who specializes
19. inflammation
20. study of
21. destruction
22. enlargement
23. mass, fluid collection, tumor
24. condition
25. lack of
26. attraction
27. formation
28. bursting forth
29. control, stop, stand still
30. incision
31. condition
32. oxygen

Identifying Medical Terms

1. agglutination
2. allergy
3. antibody
4. anticoagulant
5. antigen
6. autotransfusion
7. coagulable
8. creatinemia
9. embolus
10. granulocyte
11. hematologist
12. hemoglobin
13. hyperglycemia
14. hyperlipidemia
15. leukocyte
16. lymphostasis
17. mononucleosis
18. prothrombin
19. splenomegaly
20. thrombocyte

Matching

1. h
2. d
3. e
4. g
5. f
6. c
7. b
8. a
9. j
10. i

Medical Case Snapshot

Case 1: human immunodeficiency, T4
Case 2: hypoxia, SOB
Case 3: hemoglobin, hematocrit

Study and Review III

Building Medical Terms

1. erythropoiesis
2. globulin
3. hemolysis
4. reticulocyte
5. lymphoma
6. erythrocyte
7. seroculture
8. sideropenia
9. splenomegaly
10. thrombosis

Combining Form Challenge

1. hemolysis
2. coagulable
3. erythroblast
4. hematology
5. leukemia
6. lymphedema

Select the Right Term

1. allergy
2. antibody
3. hemophilia
4. thalassemia
5. embolus
6. thromboplastin

Diagnostic and Laboratory Tests

1. d
2. c
3. c
4. b
5. a

Abbreviations

1. AIDS
2. ALL
3. chronic myelogenous leukemia
4. Hb, Hgb
5. hematocrit
6. HIV
7. *Pneumocystis jiroveci* pneumonia
8. prothrombin time
9. red blood cell (count)
10. RIA

Practical Application

1. complete blood count
2. differential count
3. MCH (mean corpuscular hemoglobin)
4. WBC: 4.8–10.8 (thousand)
5. RBC: 4.6–6.13 (million)

CHAPTER 11

Study and Review I

Anatomy and Physiology

1. **a.** nose
   b. pharynx

c. larynx
d. trachea
e. bronchi
f. lungs

2. to furnish oxygen for use by individual cells and to take away their gaseous waste product, carbon dioxide
3. process in which the lungs are ventilated and oxygen and carbon dioxide are exchanged between the air in the lungs and the blood within capillaries of the alveoli
4. process in which oxygen and carbon dioxide are exchanged between the bloodstream and the cells of the body
5. a. serves as an air passageway
   b. warms and moistens inhaled air
   c. its cilia and mucous membrane trap dust, pollen, bacteria, and foreign matter
   d. contains special smell receptor cells (nerve cells), which assist in distinguishing various smells
   e. contributes to phonation and the quality of voice
6. a. serves as a passageway for air
   b. serves as a passageway for food
   c. contributes to phonation as a chamber where the sound is able to resonate
7. acts as a lid to prevent aspiration of food into the trachea
8. narrow slit at the opening between the true vocal folds
9. production of vocal sounds
10. serves as a passageway for air
11. provide a passageway for air to and from the lungs
12. conical-shaped, spongy organs of respiration lying on both sides of the heart
13. serous membrane composed of several layers
14. diaphragm
15. mediastinum
16. 3 . . . 2
17. alveoli
18. to bring air into intimate contact with blood so that oxygen and carbon dioxide can be exchanged in the alveoli
19. temperature, pulse, respiration, and blood pressure
20. a. amount of air in a single inspiration and expiration
    b. amount of air remaining in the lungs after maximal expiration
    c. volume of air that can be exhaled after maximal inspiration
21. medulla oblongata . . . pons
22. 30–60
23. 16–20

Anatomy Labeling

1. nasopharynx
2. hard palate
3. soft palate
4. oropharynx
5. laryngopharynx
6. epiglottis
7. trachea
8. thyroid cartilage
9. cricoid cartilage

Study and Review II

Word Parts

Prefixes

1. lack of
2. upon
3. difficult
4. within
5. good
6. out
7. below, deficient
8. excessive
9. in
10. rapid

Combining Forms

1. small, hollow air sac
2. coal
3. imperfect
4. bronchi
5. dust
6. breathe
7. larynx, voice box
8. nose
9. smell
10. mouth
11. straight
12. chest
13. pharynx, throat
14. pleura
15. air
16. pus
17. nose
18. snore
19. breath
20. chest
21. tonsil, almond
22. trachea
23. a little swelling

Suffixes

1. pertaining to
2. pain
3. surgical puncture

4. pain
5. dilation
6. surgical excision
7. pertaining to
8. condition
9. process
10. inflammation
11. instrument to measure
12. condition
13. tumor
14. dripping
15. surgical repair
16. a doer
17. breathing
18. to spit
19. flow, discharge
20. instrument for examining
21. new opening
22. incision
23. pertaining to

Identifying Medical Terms

1. alveolus
2. bronchiectasis
3. bronchitis
4. dysphonia
5. eupnea
6. hemoptysis
7. inhalation
8. laryngitis
9. pneumothorax
10. rhinoplasty
11. rhinorrhea
12. sinusitis

Matching

1. h
2. i
3. k
4. f
5. c
6. b
7. d
8. a
9. e
10. g

Medical Case Snapshot

Case 1: asthma, orthopnea

Case 2: dyspnea, shortness of breath, spirometer, chronic obstructive pulmonary disease

Case 3: tuberculosis, sputum

Study and Review III

Building Medical Terms

1. atelectasis
2. dyspnea
3. epistaxis
4. hyperpnea
5. pharyngitis
6. pneumonectomy
7. rhinoplasty
8. tachypnea
9. thoracotomy
10. tuberculosis

Combining Form Challenge

1. anthracosis
2. bronchoscope
3. hemoptysis
4. laryngoscope
5. olfaction
6. orthopnea

Select the Right Term

1. asthma
2. croup
3. hypoxia
4. pertussis
5. rale
6. rhinovirus

Diagnostic and Laboratory Tests

1. b
2. c
3. c
4. d
5. a

Abbreviations

1. AFB
2. cystic fibrosis
3. CXR
4. COPD
5. endotracheal
6. HMD
7. R
8. severe acute respiratory syndrome
9. SOB
10. tuberculosis

Practical Application

1. abnormal sound heard on auscultation of the chest; a crackling, rattling, or bubbling sound
2. directly observed therapy
3. pertaining to without fever
4. no
5. occasional cough, non-productive

CHAPTER 12

Study and Review I

Anatomy and Physiology

1. a. kidneys
   b. ureters
   c. bladder
   d. urethra
2. extraction of certain wastes from the bloodstream, conversion of these materials to urine, and transport of the urine from the kidney, via the ureters, to the bladder for elimination
3. a notch
4. saclike collecting portion of the kidney
5. inner

6. structural and functional unit of the kidney
7. renal corpuscle . . . tubule
8. glomerulus . . . Bowman capsule
9. filtration . . . reabsorption
10. 1000–1500
11. narrow, muscular tubes that transport urine from the kidneys to the bladder
12. muscular, membranous sac that serves as a reservoir for urine
13. urinary meatus
14. laboratory test that evaluates the physical, chemical, and microscopic properties of urine
15. a. yellow to amber
    b. clear
    c. 4.6–8.0 pH
    d. 1.003–1.030
    e. aromatic
    f. 1000–1500 mL/day
16. diabetes mellitus
17. renal disease, acute glomerulonephritis, pyelonephritis

Anatomy Labeling

1. kidney
2. ureter
3. bladder
4. urethra

Study and Review II

Word Parts

Prefixes

1. without
2. against
3. complete, through
4. difficult, painful
5. within
6. water
7. outside, beyond
8. not
9. scanty
10. through
11. beyond
12. excessive

Combining Forms

1. protein
2. bacteria
3. calcium
4. body
5. bladder
6. sifted out
7. glomerulus, little ball
8. glucose, sugar
9. blood
10. ketone
11. stone
12. passage
13. to urinate
14. kidney
15. night
16. perineum
17. peritoneum
18. renal pelvis
19. kidney
20. sound
21. urine, urinate, urination
22. ureter
23. urethra
24. urine

Suffixes

1. pertaining to
2. pertaining to
3. hernia
4. pain
5. pertaining to
6. pertaining to
7. surgical excision
8. blood condition
9. mark, record
10. pertaining to
11. chemical
12. process
13. one who specializes
14. inflammation
15. stone
16. study of
17. separation, loosening, dissolution
18. crushing
19. process
20. instrument to measure
21. tumor
22. condition
23. disease
24. surgical repair
25. instrument for examining
26. condition
27. new opening
28. incision
29. urine

Identifying Medical Terms

1. antidiuretic
2. cystectomy
3. cystitis
4. dysuria
5. glomerulitis
6. hypercalciuria
7. micturition
8. nephrolithiasis
9. periurethral
10. pyuria
11. ureteroplasty
12. urinalysis
13. urologist

Matching

1. d
2. e
3. b
4. f
5. a
6. g
7. j
8. c
9. h
10. i

Medical Case Snapshot

Case 1: dysuria, nocturia, hematuria

Case 2: urinalysis, blood, urinary tract infection, bacteriuria, cystitis

Case 3: nephrolithiasis, extracorporeal shock wave, ultrasonic

Study and Review III

Building Medical Terms

1. albuminuria
2. cystogram
3. incontinence
4. meatotomy
5. micturition
6. nephrolithiasis
7. oliguria
8. polyuria
9. renal
10. urination

Combining Form Challenge

1. cystocele
2. glycosuria
3. lithotripsy
4. nephroma
5. nocturia
6. ureteropathy

Select the Right Term

1. calciuria
2. edema
3. hematuria
4. nephrosclerosis
5. pyelonephritis
6. renal colic

Diagnostic and Laboratory Tests

1. c
2. c
3. b
4. c
5. b

Abbreviations

1. AGN
2. blood urea nitrogen
3. CKD
4. cystoscopy
5. genitourinary
6. hemodialysis
7. IVP
8. peritoneal dialysis
9. hydrogen ion concentration
10. UA

Practical Application

1. yellow to amber
2. weight of a substance compared with an equal amount of water; urine has a specific gravity of 1.003–1.030
3. higher
4. yes
5. early warning of hepatic or hemolytic disease

CHAPTER 13

Study and Review I

Anatomy and Physiology

1. **a.** pituitary
   b. pineal
   c. thyroid
   d. parathyroid
   e. islets of Langerhans
   f. adrenals
   g. ovaries (female)
   h. testes (male)
2. involves the production and regulation of chemical substances (hormones) that play an essential role in maintaining homeostasis
3. chemical transmitter that is released in small amounts and transported via the bloodstream to a targeted organ or other cells
4. synthesizes and secretes releasing hormones, releasing factors, release-inhibiting hormones, and release-inhibiting factors
5. because of its regulatory effects on the other endocrine glands
6. **a.** growth hormone (GH)
   b. adrenocorticotropin (ACTH)
   c. thyroid-stimulating hormone (TSH)
   d. follicle-stimulating hormone (FSH)
   e. luteinizing hormone (LH)
   f. prolactin (PRL)
   g. melanocyte-stimulating hormone (MSH)
7. **a.** antidiuretic hormone (ADH)
   b. oxytocin
8. melatonin . . . serotonin
9. plays a vital role in metabolism and regulates the body's metabolic processes
10. **a.** thyroxine (T_4)
    b. triiodothyronine (T_3)
    c. calcitonin
11. serum calcium . . . phosphorus

12. blood sugar
13. glucocorticoids, mineralocorticoids, and the androgens
14. a. regulates carbohydrate, protein, and fat metabolism
    b. stimulates output of glucose from the liver (gluconeogenesis)
    c. increases the blood sugar level
    d. regulates other physiological body processes

*Optional answers to question 14:
    e. promotes the transport of amino acids into extracellular tissue
    f. influences the effectiveness of catecholamines such as dopamine, epinephrine, and norepinephrine
    g. has an anti-inflammatory effect
    h. helps the body cope during times of stress
15. a. use of carbohydrates
    b. absorption of glucose
    c. gluconeogenesis
    d. potassium and sodium metabolism
16. Aldosterone
17. substance or hormone that promotes the development of male characteristics
18. a. dopamine
    b. epinephrine
    c. norepinephrine
19. a. elevates the systolic blood pressure
    b. increases the heart rate and cardiac output
    c. Increases glycogenolysis, thereby hastening release of glucose from the liver. This action elevates the blood sugar level and provides the body with a spurt of energy.

*Optional answers to question 19:
    d. dilates the bronchial tubes
    e. dilates the pupils
20. estrogen . . . progesterone
21. testosterone
22. a. thymosin
    b. thymopoietin
23. a. gastrin
    b. secretin
    c. cholecystokinin (pancreozymin)
    d. enterogastrone

Anatomy Labeling

1. pineal gland
2. pituitary gland
3. thyroid gland
4. parathyroid gland
5. thymus
6. adrenal gland
7. pancreas
8. ovary (female)
9. testis (male)

Study and Review II

Word Parts

Prefixes

1. through
2. within
3. good, normal
4. out, away from
5. out, away from
6. excessive
7. deficient, under
8. beside
9. before
10. upon

Combining Forms

1. acid
2. extremity, point
3. gland
4. adrenal gland
5. man
6. cortex
7. to secrete
8. female
9. old age
10. giant
11. sweet, sugar
12. seed
13. hairy
14. insulin
15. potassium (K)
16. mucus
17. pancreas
18. testicle
19. thymus
20. thyroid, shield
21. poison
22. masculine

Suffixes

1. pertaining to
2. formation, produce
3. pertaining to
4. to go
5. surgical excision
6. swelling
7. blood condition
8. formation, produce
9. condition
10. pertaining to

11. condition
12. one who specializes
13. inflammation
14. study of
15. hormone
16. enlargement, large
17. resemble
18. tumor
19. condition
20. disease
21. substance
22. growth
23. chemical
24. pertaining to

Identifying Medical Terms

1. adenoma
2. cretinism
3. diabetes
4. endocrinology
5. euthyroid
6. exocrine
7. gigantism
8. glucocorticoid
9. hyperkalemia
10. hypogonadism
11. lethargic
12. thymitis

Matching

1. e
2. f
3. b
4. g
5. h
6. i
7. c
8. j
9. d
10. a

Medical Case Snapshot

Case 1: Cushing, buffalo hump

Case 2: polydipsia, polyphagia, polyuria

Case 3: exophthalmic, Graves, swollen, light, blurring

Study and Review III

Building Medical Terms

1. adrenal
2. cortisone
3. dwarfism
4. gigantism
5. hirsutism
6. hypophysis
7. insulin
8. lethargic
9. myxedema
10. pineal

Combining Form Challenge

1. adenosis
2. androgen
3. estrogen
4. insulinogenic
5. thymectomy
6. thyroid

Select the Right Term

1. acromegaly
2. diabetes
3. epinephrine
4. hypothyroidism
5. progeria
6. virilism

Diagnostic and Laboratory Tests

1. a
2. c
3. c
4. b
5. c

Abbreviations

1. BMR
2. DM
3. fasting blood sugar
4. glucose tolerance tests
5. PBI
6. parathyroid hormone
7. radioimmunoassay
8. STH
9. thyroid-stimulating hormone
10. vasopressin

Practical Application

1. because his dad and grandfather both take insulin
2. Hb A1C and FBS
3. thirsty (polydipsia), hungry (polyphagia), and urinating a lot (polyuria)
4. fasting blood sugar
5. 25

CHAPTER 14

Study and Review I

Anatomy and Physiology

1. **a.** central
   b. peripheral
2. Neurons
3. long process reaching from the cell body to the area to be activated
4. resembles the branches of a tree and has short, unsheathed processes that transmit impulses to the cell body
5. sensory nerves transmit impulses to the central nervous system
6. **a.** single elongated process
   b. bundle of nerve fibers
   c. groups of nerve fibers
7. brain . . . spinal cord

8. a. dura mater
   b. arachnoid
   c. pia mater
9. a. cerebrum
   b. cerebellum
   c. diencephalon
   d. brainstem
10. frontal lobe
11. somesthetic area
12. auditory . . . language
13. vision
14. a. relay center for all sensory impulses
    b. relays motor impulses from the cerebellum to the cortex
15. a. is a regulator
    b. produces neurosecretions
    c. produces hormones
16. sensory perception and motor output
17. a. regulates and controls breathing
    b. regulates and controls swallowing
    c. regulates and controls coughing
    d. regulates and controls sneezing
    e. regulates and controls vomiting
18. a. conducts sensory impulses
    b. conducts motor impulses
    c. is a reflex center
19. 120 . . . 150
20. a. controls sweating
    b. controls the secretions of glands
    c. controls arterial blood pressure
    d. controls smooth muscle tissue
21. a. sympathetic
    b. parasympathetic

Anatomy Labeling

1. cerebrum
2. frontal lobe
3. parietal lobe
4. occipital lobe
5. cerebellum
6. spinal cord
7. medulla oblongata
8. pons
9. temporal lobe
10. lateral fissure

Study and Review II

Word Parts

Prefixes

1. lack of
2. lack of
3. star-shaped
4. slow
5. down
6. difficult
7. upon
8. half
9. water
10. excessive
11. within
12. small
13. little
14. beside
15. beside
16. many
17. four
18. below

Combining Forms

1. head
2. little brain
3. cerebrum
4. skull
5. tree
6. disk
7. dura, hard
8. electricity
9. brain
10. feeling
11. sleep
12. thin plate
13. membrane, meninges
14. bone marrow, spinal cord
15. numbness, sleep, stupor
16. nerve
17. globus pallidus
18. gray
19. sleep
20. thorn, spine
21. vertebra
22. vagus, wandering
23. ventricle

Suffixes

1. pertaining to
2. condition of pain
3. pain
4. pertaining to
5. weakness
6. germ cell
7. hernia
8. cell
9. binding
10. surgical excision
11. swelling
12. feeling
13. glue
14. mark, record
15. recording
16. condition
17. pertaining to
18. process
19. condition
20. one who specializes

21. inflammation
22. motion, movement
23. motion
24. seizure
25. diction, word, phrase
26. study of
27. nourishment, development
28. visual examination, to view, examine
29. tumor
30. condition
31. weakness
32. disease
33. to eat, swallow
34. to speak, speech
35. action
36. strength
37. order, coordination
38. incision
39. pertaining to
40. condition

Identifying Medical Terms

1. amnesia
2. analgesia
3. aphagia
4. ataxia
5. cephalalgia
6. cerebellar
7. craniectomy
8. dyslexia
9. encephalitis
10. epidural
11. hemiparesis
12. meningitis
13. neuralgia
14. neuritis
15. neurocyte
16. neurology
17. neuroma
18. palsy
19. polyneuritis
20. somnambulism
21. vagotomy
22. ventriculogram

Matching

1. g
2. d
3. c
4. b
5. e
6. h
7. j
8. f
9. a
10. i

Medical Case Snapshot

Case 1: epilepsy, idiopathic

Case 2: herpes zoster, chickenpox, shingles

Case 3: bradykinesia, akinesia, pallidotomy

Study and Review III

Building Medical Terms

1. analgesia
2. bradykinesia
3. concussion
4. encephalitis
5. laminectomy
6. neuralgia
7. papilledema
8. paresthesia
9. quadriplegia
10. vagotomy

Combining Form Challenge

1. cephalalgia
2. craniectomy
3. encephalopathy
4. hypnosis
5. meningitis
6. neuroglia

Select the Right Term

1. akathisia
2. anesthesia
3. coma
4. dementia
5. hyperkinesis
6. stroke

Diagnostic and Laboratory Tests

1. a
2. b
3. c
4. d
5. c

Abbreviations

1. AD
2. ALS
3. central nervous system
4. cerebral palsy
5. CT
6. HDS
7. intracranial pressure
8. lumbar puncture
9. multiple sclerosis
10. PET

Practical Application

1. cognition
2. tremor
3. difficult articulation of speech
4. antiparkinsonism
5. used for palliative relief from such major symptoms of Parkinson disease as bradykinesia, rigidity, tremor, and disorder of equilibrium and posture

CHAPTER 15

Study and Review I

Anatomy and Physiology

1. hearing . . . balance
2. external . . . middle . . . inner
3. auricle or pinna and the external acoustic meatus
4. auricle
5. a. to lubricate the ear
   b. to protect the ear
6. a. malleus (hammer)
   b. incus (anvil)
   c. stapes (stirrup)
7. mechanically transmit sound vibrations from the tympanic membrane to the oval window
8. a. transmits sound vibrations from the tympanic membrane to the cochlea
   b. equalizes external/internal air pressure on the tympanic membrane
9. cochlea, vestibule, and the semicircular canals
10. a. cochlear duct
    b. semicircular ducts
    c. utricle and saccule
11. organ of Corti
12. vestibule
13. acoustic or eighth cranial nerve
14. motion sickness
15. a. endolymph
    b. perilymph

Anatomy Labeling

1. external auditory canal
2. auricle
3. malleus
4. incus
5. stapes
6. cochlea
7. eustachian tube
8. round window
9. tympanic membrane

Study and Review II

Word Parts

Prefixes

1. within
2. within
3. around
4. twice
5. one

Combining Forms

1. to hear
2. ear
3. gall, bile
4. land snail
5. electricity
6. maze, inner ear
7. larynx, voice box
8. mastoid process, breast-shaped
9. eardrum, tympanic membrane
10. nerve
11. ear
12. pharynx
13. old
14. pus
15. hardening
16. stapes, stirrup
17. fat
18. eardrum, tympanic membrane

Suffixes

1. pertaining to
2. pain
3. hearing
4. surgical excision
5. mark, record
6. recording
7. pertaining to
8. one who specializes
9. inflammation
10. stone
11. study of
12. serum, clear fluid
13. instrument to measure
14. measurement
15. resemble
16. tumor
17. condition
18. surgical repair
19. flow
20. instrument for examining
21. instrument to cut
22. incision
23. pertaining to
24. small
25. process
26. condition

Identifying Medical Terms

1. audiologist
2. audiometry
3. auditory
4. endaural
5. labyrinthitis
6. myringoplasty
7. myringotome
8. otalgia
9. otolaryngology
10. otopharyngeal
11. otoscope
12. perilymph
13. stapedectomy
14. tympanectomy
15. tinnitus

Matching

1. h 2. e
3. i 4. a
5. g 6. b
7. j 8. c
9. d 10. f

Medical Case Snapshot

Case 1: otitis media

Case 2: tinnitus, organ of Corti

Case 3: audiologist, audiometer, deafness

Study and Review III

Building Medical Terms

1. acoustic
2. aural
3. endolymph
4. myringotome
5. otitis
6. otoplasty
7. perilymph
8. stapedectomy
9. tympanic
10. tympanoplasty

Combining Form Challenge

1. audiometer
2. auricle
3. labyrinthectomy
4. myringoplasty
5. otalgia
6. presbycusis

Select the Right Term

1. audiogram
2. equilibrium
3. fenestration
4. malleus
5. tinnitus
6. utricle

Diagnostic and Laboratory Tests

1. a 2. b
3. d 4. b
5. a

Abbreviations

1. AC
2. BC
3. decibel
4. ENG
5. ear, nose, throat
6. HD
7. OM

Practical Application

1. 102.2°F; pulling
2. otoscopy
3. analgesic/antipyretic; pain; fever
4. antibiotic; infection
5. acid; antibiotic

CHAPTER 16

Study and Review I

Anatomy and Physiology

1. orbit, muscles, eyelids, conjunctiva, and the lacrimal apparatus
2. fatty tissue
3. optic nerve . . . ophthalmic artery
4. **a.** support
   b. rotary movement
5. intense light, foreign particles . . . impact
6. mucous membrane that acts as a protective covering for the exposed surface of the eyeball
7. structures that produce, store, and remove the tears that cleanse and lubricate the eye
8. eyeball, its structures, and the nerve fibers
9. vision
10. optic disk
11. process of sharpening the focus of light on the retina
12. Matching

1. c 2. e
3. b 4. a
5. f 6. d
7. h 8. i
9. j 10. g

Anatomy Labeling

1. iris
2. lens
3. pupil
4. cornea
5. aqueous humor
6. retina
7. choroid
8. sclera
9. optic nerve

Study and Review II

Word Parts

Prefixes

1. lack of, without
2. two
3. in
4. in
5. inward
6. beyond
7. within
8. three
9. out

10. half
11. lack of
12. behind

Combining Forms

1. dull
2. unequal
3. eyelid
4. choroid
5. to join together, conjunctiva
6. pupil
7. cornea
8. cold
9. ciliary body
10. tear, lacrimal duct, tear duct
11. double
12. iris
13. cornea
14. tear, lacrimal duct, tear duct
15. lens
16. less, small
17. eye
18. eye
19. straight
20. lens
21. light
22. retina
23. foreign material
24. dry

Suffixes

1. pertaining to
2. pertaining to
3. pertaining to
4. germ cell
5. condition
6. surgical excision
7. mark, record
8. recording
9. condition
10. pertaining to
11. specialist
12. process
13. condition
14. one who specializes
15. inflammation
16. study of
17. destruction, to separate
18. formation
19. instrument to measure
20. tumor
21. sight, vision
22. condition
23. disease
24. fear
25. surgical repair
26. stroke, paralysis
27. prolapse, drooping
28. instrument for examining
29. pertaining to
30. incision
31. structure

Identifying Medical Terms

1. amblyopia
2. bifocal
3. blepharoptosis
4. corneal
5. dacryoma
6. diplopia
7. emmetropia
8. intraocular
9. keratitis
10. keratoplasty
11. lacrimal
12. ocular
13. photophobia

Matching

1. e	2. f
3. j	4. h
5. c	6. d
7. g	8. b
9. a	10. i

Medical Case Snapshot

Case 1: cataract, phacoemulsification

Case 2: conjunctivitis, redness, yellow, blurred

Case 3: glaucoma, 60, African, hypertension, type 2, mellitus

Study and Review III

Building Medical Terms

1. diplopia
2. iridectomy
3. lacrimal
4. miotic
5. nyctalopia
6. ophthalmology
7. photophobia
8. retinopathy
9. trichiasis
10. uveal

Combining Form Challenge

1. amblyopia
2. blepharoptosis
3. cycloplegia
4. dacryoma
5. gonioscope
6. keratitis

Select the Right Term

1. accommodation
2. cataract
3. entropion
4. glaucoma
5. hyperopia
6. sty(e)

Diagnostic and Laboratory Tests

1. c
2. b
3. c
4. d
5. d

Abbreviations

1. Acc
2. emmetropia
3. hyperopia
4. IOL
5. ET
6. myopia
7. visual acuity
8. intraocular pressure
9. RLF
10. exotropia

Practical Application

1. antibiotic to prevent/treat bacterial infection
2. antibiotic to prevent/treat bacterial infection
3. yes
4. any time before the day of surgery
5. Tylenol regular-strength (325 mg) acetaminophen

CHAPTER 17

Study and Review I

Anatomy and Physiology

1. **a.** ovaries
   b. fallopian tubes
   c. uterus
   d. vagina
   e. vulva
   f. breasts
2. anteflexion
3. rounded portion of the uterine body superior to the attachment of the fallopian tube
4. **a.** perimetrium
   b. myometrium
   c. endometrium
5. **a.** provides a place for the nourishment and development of the fetus during pregnancy
   b. contracts rhythmically and powerfully to help push out the fetus during the process of birthing
6. **a.** bent backward at an angle with the cervix usually unchanged from its normal position
   b. fundus forward toward the pubis with the cervix tilted up toward the sacrum
   c. bent backward with the cervix pointing forward toward the symphysis pubis
7. uterine tubes or oviducts
8. fertilization
9. **a.** production of ova
   b. production of hormones
10. **a.** female organ of copulation
    b. passageway for discharge of menstruation
    c. passageway for birth of the fetus
11. mammary glands
12. areola . . . nipple
13. thin yellowish secretion containing mainly serum and white blood cells; the "first milk"
14. **a.** follicular phase
    b. ovulation
    c. luteal phase

Overview of Obstetrics

1. Obstetrics
2. Fertilization
3. zygote
4. yolk sac and amniotic cavity
5. **a.** time period from conception to onset of labor
   b. last phase of pregnancy to the time of delivery
   c. act of giving birth, also known as *childbirth* or *delivery*
   d. the 6 weeks following childbirth and expulsion of the placenta
6. **a.** begins from the onset of true labor and lasts until the cervix is fully dilated to 10 cm
   b. continues after the cervix is dilated to 10 cm until the delivery of the baby
   c. delivery of the placenta

Anatomy Labeling

1. uterus
2. cervix
3. vagina
4. fallopian tube
5. ovary
6. symphysis pubis
7. labia majora
8. labia minora

Study and Review II

Word Parts

Prefixes

1. lack of
2. against
3. difficult, painful
4. out
5. within
6. within
7. scanty
8. around

9. after
10. backward
11. before

Combining Forms

1. to miscarry
2. cervix, neck
3. a coming together
4. vagina
5. cul-de-sac
6. bladder
7. fibrous tissue
8. female
9. womb, uterus
10. breast
11. breast
12. month, menses, menstruation
13. womb, uterus
14. muscle
15. ovum, egg
16. ovary
17. lying beside, sexual intercourse
18. rectum
19. fallopian tube
20. uterus
21. vagina
22. turning

Suffixes

1. pertaining to
2. beginning
3. hernia
4. surgical puncture
5. surgical excision
6. formation, produce
7. condition
8. pertaining to
9. process
10. one who specializes
11. inflammation
12. tumor
13. condition
14. surgical repair
15. to burst forth
16. flow
17. instrument for examining
18. resemble

Identifying Medical Terms

1. cervicitis
2. dysmenorrhea
3. fibroma
4. gynecology
5. hymenectomy
6. mammoplasty
7. menorrhea
8. oogenesis
9. dyspareunia
10. genitalia

Matching

1. e 2. b
3. a 4. c
5. d 6. h
7. j 8. g
9. i 10. f

Medical Case Snapshot

Case 1: uterine, cramping, cervix

Case 2: ectopic, pregnancy, obstetrician

Case 3: dyspareunia, perimenopause

Study and Review III

Building Medical Terms

1. bartholinitis
2. culdocentesis
3. hysterectomy
4. lumpectomy
5. mastectomy
6. menopause
7. menorrhea
8. oogenesis
9. salpingitis
10. postcoital

Combining Form Challenge

1. cervicitis
2. colposcope
3. cystocele
4. fibroma
5. genitalia
6. gynecology

Select the Right Term

1. adnexa
2. dysmenorrhea
3. gravida
4. lochia
5. preeclampsia
6. retroversion

Diagnostic and Laboratory Tests

1. a 2. c
3. d 4. b
5. d

Abbreviations

1. abortion
2. fetal heartbeat
3. COCs
4. IUD
5. PID
6. CIN
7. dysfunctional uterine bleeding
8. premenstrual syndrome
9. D&C
10. TSS

Practical Application

1. GYN
2. hot flashes
3. dyspareunia
4. two pregnancies
5. rule out uterine fibroid tumor

CHAPTER 18

Study and Review I

Anatomy and Physiology

1. **a.** testes
   b. various ducts
   c. urethra
   d. bulbourethral gland
   e. prostate gland
   f. seminal vesicles
2. **a.** scrotum
   b. penis
3. provide the sperm cells necessary to fertilize the ovum, thereby perpetuating the species
4. glans penis
5. loose skinfolds that cover the penis
6. lubricating fluid
7. **a.** male organ of copulation
   b. site of the orifice for the elimination of urine and semen from the body
8. seminiferous tubules
9. **a.** responsible for the development of secondary male characteristics during puberty
   b. essential for normal growth and development of the male accessory sex organs
   c. plays a vital role in the erection process of the penis
   d. affects the growth of hair on the face
   e. affects muscular development and vocal timbre
10. **a.** storage site for sperm
    b. duct for the passage of sperm
11. vas deferens or ductus deferens
12. production of a slightly alkaline fluid
13. about 4 cm wide and weighs about 20 g; composed of glandular, connective, and muscular tissues and lies behind the urinary bladder
14. enlargement of the prostate that can occur in older men
15. bulbourethral . . . Cowper
16. **a.** prostatic
    b. membranous
    c. penile
17. transmits urine and semen out of the body
18. 20

Anatomy Labeling

1. bladder
2. vas deferens
3. seminal vesicles
4. prostate
5. urethra
6. epididymis

Study and Review II

Word Parts

Prefixes

1. lack of
2. lack of
3. around
4. upon
5. water
6. under
7. scanty
8. beside
9. into
10. different
11. similar, same

Combining Forms

1. glans penis
2. to cut
3. hidden
4. testis
5. to throw out
6. genitals
7. female
8. breast
9. thread
10. testicle
11. testicle
12. prostate
13. seed, sperm
14. seed, sperm
15. testicle
16. twisted vein
17. vessel
18. seminal vesicle
19. animal

Suffixes

1. pertaining to
2. pertaining to
3. hernia, swelling, tumor
4. to kill
5. surgical excision
6. formation, produce
7. condition
8. process
9. condition
10. inflammation
11. use
12. condition
13. flow
14. incision

Identifying Medical Terms

1. balanitis
2. epididymectomy
3. orchidectomy
4. prepuce
5. hydrocele
6. condyloma
7. spermatid
8. spermatozoon
9. spermicide
10. testicular

Matching

1. e	2. c
3. f	4. b
5. g	6. i
7. h	8. k
9. a	10. d

Medical Case Snapshot

Case 1: erectile dysfunction

Case 2: hypospadias, circumcision, 18

Case 3: nocturia, urgency, prostatic hypertrophy, prostatism

Study and Review III

Building Medical Terms

1. castrate
2. hydrocele
3. orchiditis
4. parenchyma
5. prostatitis
6. spermatoblast
7. spermatozoon
8. spermicide
9. testicular
10. varicocele

Combining Form Challenge

1. balanitis
2. gonorrhea
3. orchidotomy
4. mitosis
5. prostatectomy
6. vesiculitis

Select the Right Term

1. anorchism
2. circumcision
3. cryptorchidism
4. homosexual
5. vasectomy
6. syphilis

Diagnostic and Laboratory Tests

1. c	2. a
3. b	4. c
5. b	

Abbreviations

1. BPH
2. gonorrhea
3. HPV
4. herpes simplex virus–2
5. sexually transmitted infections
6. ED
7. transurethral resection of the prostate
8. nongonococcal urethritis
9. VDRL
10. PSA

Practical Application

1. Herpes
2. 14 and 49
3. yes
4. 80
5. visible

CHAPTER 19

Study and Review I

An Overview of Cancer

1. a. carcinomas
   b. sarcomas
   c. mixed cancers
2. process in which normal cells have a distinct appearance and specialized function
3. process in which normal cells lose their specialization and become malignant
4. a. active migration
   b. direct extension
   c. metastasis
5. a. Change in bowel or bladder habits
   b. Sore that does not heal
   c. Unusual bleeding or discharge
   d. Thickening or lump in breast or elsewhere
   e. Indigestion or difficulty in swallowing
   f. Obvious change in a wart or mole
   g. Nagging cough or hoarseness
6. a. surgery
   b. chemotherapy
   c. radiation therapy
   d. immunotherapy

Study and Review II

Word Parts

Prefixes

1. up, apart, backward
2. star-shaped
3. excessive

4. new
5. little
6. before
7. in
8. in
9. beyond
10. short

Combining Forms

1. crab, cancer
2. a little box
3. cancer
4. chorion
5. tree
6. to strain through
7. glue
8. safe, immunity
9. smooth
10. bad kind
11. black
12. mucus
13. to change
14. fungus
15. bone marrow
16. tumor
17. cloaked
18. remit
19. net
20. rod
21. suppress
22. monster
23. poison
24. virus (poison)

Suffixes

1. immature cell
2. blood condition
3. formation, produce
4. formation, produce
5. formation, produce
6. condition
7. substance
8. inflammation
9. tumor
10. pertaining to
11. plaque
12. formation
13. a thing formed
14. use, action
15. treatment
16. pertaining to
17. pertaining to
18. pertaining to
19. process
20. nature of
21. forming
22. control
23. resemble

Identifying Medical Terms

1. carcinogen
2. chondrosarcoma
3. glioma
4. leiomyosarcoma
5. leukemia
6. lymphoma
7. melanoma
8. myosarcoma
9. Wilms tumor
10. sarcoma

Matching

1. e	2. i
3. d	4. g
5. c	6. f
7. j	8. b
9. h	10. a

Medical Case Snapshot

Case 1: DCIS, lobules, tumor, axillary, negative

Case 2: testicular cancer, seminoma

Case 3: sputum, biopsy

Study and Review III

Building Medical Terms

1. hyperplasia
2. lymphoma
3. melanoma
4. neoplasm
5. oncogenes
6. palliative
7. remission
8. seminoma
9. teratoma
10. trismus

Combining Form Challenge

1. carcinogen
2. immunotherapy
3. leukemia
4. malignant
5. myeloma
6. sarcoma

Select the Right Term

1. dedifferentiation
2. metastasis
3. port
4. proliferation
5. Wilms tumor
6. xerostomia

Abbreviations

1. ACA
2. Bx
3. cancer
4. chemotherapy
5. DNA
6. internal radiation therapy
7. HER-2/neu
8. DCIS
9. basal cell carcinoma
10. TC

Practical Application

1. new growth or tumor, may be benign or malignant
2. basal cell carcinoma
3. to reveal that the neoplastic process appears to be totally excised
4. right shoulder
5. centimeter

CHAPTER 20

Study and Review I

An Overview of Radiology and Nuclear Medicine

1. scientific discipline of medical imaging using radionuclides, ionizing radiation, nuclear magnetic resonance, and ultrasound
2. a. invisible
   b. cause ionization
   c. cause fluorescence

*Alternate characteristics to those listed:

   d. allow the x-ray beam to be directed at a specific site or to produce high-quality shadow images on film
   e. able to penetrate substances
   f. destroy cells
3. a. can depress the hematopoietic system, cause leukopenia, leukemia
   b. can damage the gonads
4. a. wearing a personal dosimeter
   b. lead screens
   c. lead-lined room
   d. protective clothing
   e. gonad shield
5. a. computed tomography
   b. magnetic resonance imaging
   c. ultrasound
   d. thermography
   e. scintigraphy

Study and Review II

Word Parts

Prefixes

1. below
2. within
3. one-thousandth
4. beyond
5. in

Combining Forms

1. acting
2. vessel
3. artery
4. joint
5. bronchus
6. motion
7. finger or toe
8. echo
9. fluorescence, luminous
10. kind
11. breast
12. to swing
13. nature
14. renal pelvis
15. ray, x-ray
16. fallopian tube
17. salivary
18. sound
19. hot, heat
20. to cut
21. to draw

Suffixes

1. one who
2. formation, produce
3. pertaining to
4. record
5. instrument for recording
6. recording
7. pertaining to
8. process
9. one who specializes
10. inflammation
11. nature of
12. study of
13. pertaining to
14. instrument for examining
15. visual examination, to view, examine
16. treatment
17. having a particular quality

Identifying Medical Terms

1. angiography
2. arthrography
3. cholecystogram
4. ionization
5. mammography
6. millicurie
7. physicist
8. radiation
9. radioactive
10. radiographer
11. radiolucent
12. radiopaque
13. sonogram

Matching

1. d	2. e
3. c	4. g
5. j	6. k
7. b	8. i
9. a	10. h

Medical Case Snapshot

mammogram, screening, changes

Study and Review III

Building Medical Terms

1. bronchogram
2. sialography
3. mammography
4. myelogram
5. physicist
6. radiation
7. radiolucent
8. radiopaque
9. radiotherapy
10. venography

Combining Form Challenge

1. arthrography
2. radiotherapy
3. radiograph
4. sonography
5. thermography
6. tomography

Select the Right Term

1. arteriography
2. cholecystogram
3. radioactive
4. roentgen
5. shield
6. ultrasonography

Abbreviations

1. AP
2. Ba
3. CT
4. interventional radiology
5. lateral
6. radium
7. MRI
8. posteroanterior
9. Ci
10. positron emission tomography

Practical Application

1. a specific type of imaging that uses a low-dose x-ray system for examination of the breasts
2. because if there is a finding on the mammogram it needs to be compared to previous mammograms
3. there is a finding on the mammogram that requires further tests for a more thorough evaluation
4. no evidence of cancer
5. the referring physician or other healthcare provider

CHAPTER 21

Study and Review I

An Overview: Mental Health and Mental Disorders

1. mental disorder
2. **a.** major depression
   b. bipolar disorder
   c. schizophrenia
3. Psychiatry
4. **a.** drug therapy
   b. psychotherapy
   c. electroconvulsive therapy
5. Psychoanalysis

Study and Review II

Word Parts

Prefixes

1. lack of, without
2. deficient, below
3. beside, abnormal
4. fire

Combining Forms

1. marketplace
2. center
3. circle, cycle
4. to cheat
5. nerve
6. disease
7. mind
8. mind
9. to divide
10. body
11. mind, emotion

Suffixes

1. shape
2. condition
3. pertaining to
4. process
5. condition
6. one who specializes
7. madness
8. mind
9. appetite
10. condition
11. fear
12. treatment
13. pertaining to

Identifying Medical Terms

1. agoraphobia
2. apathy
3. delusion
4. depression
5. egocentric
6. mania
7. phobia
8. psychiatrist
9. psychotherapy
10. pyromania

Matching

1. d **2.** g
3. c **4.** a
5. f **6.** b
7. i **8.** e
9. h **10.** j

Medical Case Snapshot

mental disorder, mood, dysthymia

Study and Review III

Abbreviations

1. CBT
2. DSM-5
3. electroconvulsive therapy
4. Minnesota Multiphasic Personality Inventory–2
5. NIMH
6. obsessive–compulsive disorder
7. PTSD
8. seasonal affective disorder
9. Thematic Apperception Test
10. WHO

Practical Application

1. feels sick all the time, too weak and tired, dizzy and depressed, to do anything except "rest"
2. Proventil inhaler for relief of asthmatic symptoms, analgesics, decongestants, and two different forms of tricyclic antidepressants
3. a fixed, false belief or abnormal perception held by a person despite evidence to the contrary
4. process of experiencing sensations that have no source
5. disorder that is not real, genuine, or natural; the physical and psychological symptoms are produced by the person to place him- or herself or another in the role of a patient or someone in need of help

APPENDIX II Glossary of Word Parts

PREFIXES

a-	no, not, without, lack of, apart
ab-	away from
ad-	toward, near
ambi-	both, both sides, around, about
an-	no, not, without, lack of
ana-	up, apart, backward, again, anew
ant-	against
ante-	before, forward
anti-	against
apo-	separation
astro-	star-shaped
auto-	self
bi-	two, double
bin-	twice, two
brachy-	short
brady-	slow
cac-	bad
centi-	one hundred, one hundredth
chromo-	color
circum-	around
con-	with, together
contra-	against, opposite
de-	down, away from
deca-	ten
di-	two, double
dia-, di(a)-	through, between, complete
dif-	apart, free from, separate
di(s)-	two, apart
dis-	apart
dys-	bad, difficult, painful, abnormal
ec-	out, outside, outer
ecto-	out, outside, outer
em-	in
en-	in, within
end-	within, inner
endo-	within, inner
ep-	upon, over, above
epi-	upon, over, above
eso-	inward
eu-	good, normal
ex-	out, away from
exo-	out, away from
extra-	outside, beyond
hemi-	half
heter-	different
hetero-	different
homeo-	similar, same, likeness, constant
homo-	similar, same
hydr-	water
hyp-	below, deficient
hyper-	above, beyond, excessive
hypo-	below, under, deficient
in-	in, into, not
infer-	below
inter-	between
intra-	within
ir-	in
mal-	bad
mega-	large, great
meso-	middle
meta-	beyond, over, between, change
micro-	small
milli-	one-thousandth
mon(o)-	one

mono-	one
multi-	many, much
neo-	new
nulli-	none
olig-	little, scanty
oligo-	little, scanty
pan-	all
par-	around, beside
para-	beside, alongside, abnormal
per-	through
peri-	around
poly-	many, much, excessive
post-	after, behind
pre-	before, in front of
primi-	first
pro-	before, in front of
proto-	first
pseudo-	false
pyro-	fire
quadri-	four
re-	back, backward, again
retro-	backward
semi-	half
sub-	below, under, beneath
super-	upper, above
supra-	above, beyond, superior
sym-	together, with
syn-	together, with
tachy-	rapid, fast
trans-	across
tri-	three
ultra-	beyond
un-	back, reversal, not, annulment
uni-	one

WORD ROOTS/COMBINING FORMS

abdomin	abdomen
abort, abort/o	to miscarry
absorpt, absorpt/o	to suck in
acanth	thorn
acetabul, acetabul/o	acetabulum, hip socket
acid, acid/o	acid
acoust	hearing
acr, acr/o	extremity, point
act, act/o	acting, act
actin	ray
acute	sharp
aden, aden/o	gland
adhes	stuck to
adip, adip/o	fat
adren, adren/o	adrenal gland
agglutinat	clumping
agglutin/o	clumping
agon, agon/o	agony
agor/a	marketplace
albin, albin/o	white
albumin, albumin/o	protein
aliment, aliment/o	nourishment
all, all/o	other
alveol, alveol/o	small, hollow air sac
ambly, ambly/o	dull
ambul	to walk
amni/o	amniotic fluid
ampere	ampere
amputat, amputat/o	to cut through
amyl, amyl/o	starch
an/o	anus
anabol, anabol/o	building up
anastom	opening
andr, andr/o	man
angi, angi/o	vessel

angin, angin/o	to choke
anis/o	unequal
ankyl, ankyl/o	stiffening, crooked
anter, anter/o	toward the front
anthrac, anthrac/o	coal
aort, aort/o	aorta
append, append/o	appendix
appendic, appendic/o	appendix
arachn	spider
arche	beginning
arous	alertness, to rise
arteri, arteri/o	artery
arthr, arthr/o	joint, to articulate
aspirat, aspirat/o	to draw in
atel, atel/o	imperfect
ather, ather/o	fatty substance, porridge
atri, atri/o	atrium
audi/o	to hear
auditor	hearing
aur, aur/i	ear
auscultat, auscultat/o	listen to
aut	self
axill	armpit
bacteri/o	bacteria
balan, balan/o	glans penis
bartholin	Bartholin glands
bas/o	base
bi/o	life
bil, bil/i	bile
blast/o	germ cell
blephar, blephar/o	eyelid
brach/i, brachi/o	arm
bronch, bronch/o	bronchus
bronchiol, bronchiol/o	bronchiole
bucc, bucc/o	cheek
burs, burs/o	pouch
calc, calc/i, calc/o	lime, calcium

calcan/e	heel bone
cancer, cancer/o	crab, cancer
capn	smoke
capsul, capsul/o	little box
carcin, carcin/o	cancer
cardi, cardi/o	heart
carp, carp/o	wrist, carpus
cartil	gristle
cartilagin/o	cartilage
castr	to prune
catabol, catabol/o	casting down
caud, caud/o	tail
caus, caus/o	burn, burning
cavit	cavity
celi, celi/o	abdomen, belly
cellul, cellul/o	little cell
centr, centr/i, centr/o	center
centrat	center
cephal, cephal/o	head
cept	receive
cerebell, cerebell/o	little brain
cerebr/o	cerebrum
cervic, cervic/o	cervix, neck
cheil, cheil/o	lip
chem/o	chemical
chir/o	hand
chlor/o	green
chol, chole, chol/e	gall, bile
choledoch/o	common bile duct
chondr, chondr/o	cartilage
chord	cord
chori/o	chorion
choroid, choroid/o	choroid
chromat, chromat/o	color
chrom/o	color
chym	juice

cine	motion
cinemat/o	motion
circulat, circulat/o	circular
cirrh, cirrh/o	orange-yellow
cis, cis/o	to cut
claudicat, claudicat/o	to limp
clavicul, clavicul/o	clavicle, collar bone
cleid/o	clavicle
clon/o	turmoil
coagul, coagul/o	to clot
coagulat	to clot
coccyg/e, coccyg/o	coccyx, tailbone
cochle/o	land snail
coit, coit/o	coming together
col, col/o	colon
coll/a	glue
collis	neck
colon, colon/o	colon
colp/o	vagina
comat	a deep sleep
compensat	to make good
compuls/o	compel, drive
coni/o	dust
concuss	shaken violently
condyle	knuckle
conjunctiv, conjunctiv/o	conjunctiva, to join together
connect	to bind together
consci	aware
constipat	to press together
continence	to hold
cor, cor/o	pupil
cord/o	cord
coriat	corium
corne, corne/o	cornea
corpor, corpore/o, corpor/o	body
cortic, cortic/o	cortex
cortis	cortex
cost, cost/o	rib
coxa	hip
crani, cran/i, crani/o	skull
creat	flesh
creatin	flesh, creatine
crine, crin/o	to secrete
crur	leg
cry/o	cold
crypt, crypt/o	hidden
cubit	to lie
cubit/o	elbow
culd/o	cul-de-sac
curie	curie
cutane, cutane/o	skin
cyan, cyan/o	dark blue
cycl, cycl/o	ciliary body of eye, circle, cycle
cyst, cyst/o	bladder, sac
cyt, cyt/o	cell
cyth	cell
dacry, dacry/o	tear, lacrimal duct, tear duct
dactyl, dactyl/o	finger or toe
defecat	to remove dregs
delus, delus/o	to cheat
dem	people
dendr/o	tree
dent, dent/i, dent/o	tooth
derm, derm/a, derm/o	skin
dermat, dermat/o	skin
dextr/o	to the right
didym, didym/o	testis
digit, digit/o	finger or toe
dilat, dilat/o	to widen
dipl/o	double
disk, disk/o	disk
dist, dist/o	away from the point of origin
diverticul, diverticul/o	diverticula
dors, dors/i, dors/o	backward

duct, duct/o	to lead
duoden, duoden/o	duodenum
dur, dur/o	dura, hard
dwarf	small
dynam, dynam/o	power
ech/o	echo, reflected sound
ectop	displaced
eg/o	I, self
ejaculat, ejaculat/o	to throw out
electr/o	electricity
embol, embol/o	to cast, to throw
eme	to vomit
emulsificat	disintegrate
encephal, encephal/o	brain
enchyma	to pour
enter/o	intestines (usually small intestine)
enucleat	to remove the kernel of
eosin/o	rose-colored
episi/o	vulva, pudenda
erget	work
erg/o	work
eructat	breaking out
erysi	red
erythr/o	red
esophag/o, esophage/o	esophagus
esthesi/o	feeling, sensation
esthet	feeling, sensation
estr/o	female
eti/o	cause
excret/o, excretor	sifted out
fasc	band (fascia)
fasci/o	band (fascia)
febr	fever
femor, femor/o	femur, thigh bone
fenestrat	window
fibr, fibr/o	fibrous tissue, fiber
fibrillat	fibrils (small fibers)
fibrin/o	fiber
fibul, fibul/o	fibula
filtrat, filtrat/o	to strain through
fixat, fixat/o	fastened
flex	to bend
fluor/o	fluorescence, luminous
foc, foc/o	focus
follicul, follicul/o	little bag
format	shaping
fungat	mushroom, fungus
furc	fork
fus, fus/o	to pour
ganglion	knot
gastr, gastr/o	stomach
gen, gene, genet	formation, produce
gen/o	kind
genital	belonging to birth
ger, ger/o	old age
gester	to bear
gigant, gigant/o	giant
gingiv, gingiv/o	gums
glandul	little acorn
gli, gli/o	glue
glob, globul/o	globule, globe
globin	globule
glomerul, glomerul/o	glomerulus, little ball
gloss/o	tongue
gluc/o	sweet, sugar
glyc, glyc/o, glycos, glycos/o	glucose, sweet, sugar
gnost	knowledge
gonad, gonad/o	seed
gon/o	genitals
goni/o	angle
grand/i	great
granul/o	little grain, granular
gravida, gravidar	pregnancy
gryp	curve
gurgitat	to flood
gynec/o	female
halat, halat/o	breathe

halit/o	breath
hallucinat	to wander in mind
hallux	great (big) toe
hem, hem/o, hemat, hemat/o	blood
hemorrh, hemorrh/o	vein liable to bleed
hepat, hepat/o	liver
herni/o	hernia
hidr, hidr/o	sweat
hirsut, hirsut/o	hairy
hist/o	tissue
hol/o	whole
horizont	horizon
humer, humer/o	humerus
hydr, hydr/o	water
hymen	hymen
hypn, hypn/o	sleep
hyster, hyster/o	womb, uterus
iatr	treatment
icter, icter/o	jaundice
ile, ile/o	ileum
ili, ili/o	ilium
illus	foot
immun/o	safe, immunity
infarct, infarct/o	infarct (necrosis of an area)
infect	to infect
infer, infer/o	below
inguin, inguin/o	groin
insul, insulin/o	insulin
integument, integument/o	covering
intern	within
irid, irid/o	iris
isch, isch/o	to hold back
is/o	equal
ischi	ischium
jaund	yellow
kal, kal/i	potassium
kary/o	cell's nucleus
kel, kel/o	tumor
kerat, kerat/o	horn, cornea
keton, keton/o	ketone
kil/o	one thousand
kinet	motion
kyph, kyph/o	hump
labi, labi/o	lip
labyrinth, labyrinth/o	maze
lacrim, lacrim/o	tear, lacrimal duct, tear duct
lamin, lamin/o	lamina, thin plate
lamp(s)	to shine
lapar/o	abdomen
laryng, laryng/o	larynx, voice box
later, later/o	side
laxat	to loosen
lei/o	smooth
lent, lent/o	lens
lept	seizure
letharg	drowsiness
leuk, leuk/o	white
levat	lifter
lingu, lingu/o	tongue
lip, lip/o	fat
lipid, lipid/o	fat
lith, lith/o	stone
lob, lob/o	lobe
lobul	small lobe
locat	to place
log	study
log/o	word
lopec	fox mange
lord, lord/o	bending, curve, swayback
lumb, lumb/o	loin, lower back
lump	lump
lun, lun/o	moon
lymph, lymph/o	lymph, clear fluid
macr/o	large
malign, malign/o	bad kind
mamm/o	breast
man/o	thin

mandibul, mandibul/o	lower jawbone
mast, mast/o	mastoid process, breast-shaped, breast
masticat	to chew
mat	to ripen
maxill, maxill/o	upper jawbone
maxilla	jaw
maxim	greatest
meat, meat/o	passage
med	middle
medi, medi/o	toward the middle
medull, medull/o	marrow
melan, melan/o	black
men, men/o	month, menses, menstruation
mening, meningi/o, mening/o	membrane, meninges
menisc, menisc/i, menisc/o	meniscus, crescent-shaped
menstru	to discharge the menses
ment, ment/o	mind
mes, mes/o	middle
mester	month
metr, metr/o	to measure, womb, uterus
mi/o	less, smaller
micturit, micturit/o	to urinate
miliar	millet (tiny)
minim	least
mit, mit/o	thread
mitr, mitr/o	mitral valve
mnes	memory
mucos, mucos/o, mucus	mucus
muscul, muscul/o	muscle
muta, mutat, mutat/o	to change
my, my/o	muscle
my/o, my/o(s)	muscle
myc, myc/o	fungus
mydriat	dilation, widen
myel, myel/o	bone marrow, spinal cord
myring, myring/o	eardrum, tympanic membrane
myx, myx/o	mucus
narc/o	numbness, sleep, stupor
nas/o	nose
nat, nat/o	birth
necr, necr/o	death
nephr, nephr/o	kidney
neur, neur/o	nerve
neutr/o	neither
nid	nest
noct, noct/o	night
nom	law
norm	rule
nucl	nucleus
nucle	kernel, nucleus
nyctal	night
o/o	ovum, egg
obsess, obsess/o	besieged by thoughts
occlus, occlus/o	to close up
ocul, ocul/o	eye
odont, odont/o	tooth
olecran, olecran/o	elbow
olfact/o	smell
omnion	shoulder
omphal/o	navel, umbilicus
onc/o	tumor
onych, onych/o	nail
oophor, oophor/o	ovary
ophthalm, ophthalm/o	eye
opt, opt/o	eye
or, or/o	mouth
orch, orch/o	testicle
orchid, orchid/o	testicle
organ, organ/o	organ
orth, orth/o	straight
oscill, oscill/o	to swing
oste, oste/o	bone
ot, ot/o	ear
ovar	ovary

ovul, ovulat	ovary
ox/i	oxygen
oxy	sour, sharp, acid
pachy, pachy/o	thick
palat/o	palate
palliat, palliat/o	cloaked
pallid/o	globus pallidus
palm	palm
palp	touch
palpitat, palpit/o	throbbing
pancreat, pancreat/o	pancreas
papill, papill/o	papilla
para	to bear, bring forth
paralyt	to disable, paralysis
pareun, pareun/o	lying beside, sexual intercourse
partum	labor
parturit	in labor
patell, patell/o	kneecap, patella
path, path/o	disease
pause	cessation
pector, pector/o, pector(at)	chest
ped, ped/o, ped/i	foot, child
pedicul, pedicul/o	louse
pelv/i	pelvis
penile	penis
pept, pept/o	to digest
perine, perine/o	perineum
peritone/o	peritoneum
phac, phac/o	lens
phag, phag/o	to eat, engulf
phak, phak/o	lens
phalang/e, phalang/o	phalanges, finger/toe bones
pharyng, pharynge/o, pharyng/o	pharynx, throat
phas	speech
phe/o	dusky
phen/o	to show
phim	muzzle
phleb, phleb/o	vein
phob, phob/o	fear
phon, phon/o	voice, sound
phor	carrying
phos	light
phot/o	light
phragm	partition
phras	speech
phren, phren/o	mind
physi/o	nature, function
physic/o	nature
pil/o	hair
pine	pine cone
pineal	pineal body
pituitar	pituitary gland
plak, plak/o	plate
plasma, plasm/o	plasma
plast	developing
pleur, pleur/o	pleura
plicat	to fold
pneum/o	air
pneumon, pneumon/o	lung
pod/o	foot
poiet	formation
poli/o	gray
por	passage
porphyr	purple
poster, poster/o	behind, toward the back, back
prand/i	meal
presby, presby/o	old
press	to press
proct, proct/o	anus and rectum
prophylact	guarding
prostat, prostat/o	prostate
prosth/e	an addition
proxim, proxim/o	near the point of origin
prurit, prurit/o	itching
psych, psych/o	mind
pudend	external genitals

pulm/o	lung
pulmon/o	lung
pupill, pupill/o	pupil
purpur	purple
py, py/o	pus
pyel, pyel/o	renal pelvis
pylor, pylor/o	pylorus, gatekeeper
pyr/o	heat, fire
pyret	fever
rach, rachi/o	spinal column, vertebrae
radi/o	ray, x-ray
radiat	radiant
radic/o	spinal nerve root
radicul	spinal nerve root
ras	to scrape off
rect/o	rectum
regul	rule
relaxat	to loosen
remiss, remiss/o	remit
ren, ren/o	kidney
respirat, respirat/o	breathing
reticul/o	net
retin, retin/o	retina
rhabd/o	rod
rheumat, rheumat/o	discharge
rhin/o	nose
rhonch, rhonch/o	snore
rhytid/o	wrinkle
roent	roentgen
rotat, rotat/o	to turn
rrhyth, rrhythm, rrhythm/o	rhythm
rube/o	red
sacr, sacr/o	sacrum
salping, salping/o,	tube, fallopian
salpinx	tube
sarc, sarc/o	flesh
scapul, scapul/o	shoulder blade
schiz/o	to divide
scler, scler/o	hard, hardening, sclera
scoli, scoli/o	curvature
scop	to examine
seb/o	oil
secund	second
semin, semin/o	seed, semen
seminat	seed, semen
senil, senile	old
sept	putrefaction
sept/o	a partition
septic, septic/o	putrefying
ser(a), ser/o	whey, serum
sert	to gain
sexu	sex
sial, sial/o	saliva, salivary
sider/o	iron
sigmoid, sigmoid/o	sigmoid
sin/o	curve
sinus	a hollow curve
situ	place
som, somat, somat/o	body
somn, somn/o	sleep
son, son/o	sound
spadias	rent, opening
spastic	convulsive
sperm, sperm/i, sperm/o	seed (sperm)
spermat, spermat/o	seed (sperm)
sphygm/o	pulse
spin, spin/o	spine, thorn
spir/o	breathe
splen/o	spleen
spondyl, spondyl/o	vertebra
staped, staped/o	stapes, stirrup
steat, steat/o	fat
sten, sten/o	narrowing
ster	solid
stern, stern/o	sternum, breastbone
sterol	solid (fat)

steth, steth/o	chest
stigmat, stigmat/o	point
stom, stom/o	mouth
stomat, stomat/o	mouth
strabism	squinting
strict	to tighten, contraction
suppress, suppress/o	suppress
surrog	substitute
symmetric	symmetry
sympath	sympathy
synov, synov/o	synovial membrane
systol	contraction
systole	contraction
tars/o	ankle, tarsus
tel	end, distant
tele	distant
tempor	temples
ten/o	tendon
tend/o	tendon
tendin, tendin/o	tendon
tendon, tendon/o	tendon
tenos	tendon
tens	tension
tentori	tentorium, tent
terat, terat/o	monster
test/o	testicle
testicul, testicul/o	testicle
thalass	sea
thel, thel/o	nipple
therm, therm/o	hot, heat
thorac, thorac/o	chest
thromb, thromb/o	clot
thym, thym/o	thymus, mind, emotion
thyr, thyr/o	thyroid, shield
tibi, tibi/o	tibia
toc, toc/o	labor, birth
tom/o	to cut
ton, ton/o	tone, tension

tonsill, tonsill/o	tonsil, almond
topic, top/o	place
tors, tors/o	twisted
tort/i	twisted
tox, tox/o	poison
toxic, toxic/o	poison
trache/o	trachea
tract, tract/o	to draw
trephinat	bore
trich, trich/o	hair
trism	grating
trop, trop/o	turning
troph, troph/o	nourishment, development
tuber	bulge
tubercul, tubercul/o	little swelling
turg	swelling
tuss	cough
tympan, tympan/o	eardrum, drum
uln, uln/o	ulna
umbilic	navel
ungu	nail
ur, ur/o	urinate, urination
urea	urea
uret	urine
ureter, ureter/o	ureter
urethr, urethr/o	urethra
urin, urin/o	urine
uter, uter/o	uterus
uve, uve/o	uvea
vag/o	vagus, wandering
vagin, vagin/o	vagina
valvul/o	valve
varic/o	twisted vein
vas, vas/o	vessel
vascul, vascul/o	small vessel
vector	carrier
ven/o	vein
venere, venere/o	sexual intercourse
ventilat, ventilat/o	to air

ventr, ventr/o	near or on the belly side of the body
ventricul, ventricul/o	ventricle, little belly
vermin, verm/i	worm
vers, vers/o	turning
vertebr, vertebr/o	vertebra
vesic	bladder
vesicul, vesicul/o	seminal vesicle
vir, vir/o	virus (poison)
viril, viril/o	masculine
viscer, viscer/o	body organs
volt	volt
volunt, volunt/o	will
volvul	to roll
vuls, vuls/o	to pull
watt	watt
xanth/o	yellow
xen, xen/o	foreign material
xer, xer/o	dry
xiph, xiph/o	sword
zo/o	animal
zoon	life

SUFFIXES

-able	capable
-ac	pertaining to
-act	to act
-ad	pertaining to
-age	related to
-al	pertaining to
-algesia	condition of pain
-algia	pain, ache
-ant	forming
-apheresis	removal, remove
-ar, -ary	pertaining to
-arche	beginning
-ase	enzyme
-asthenia	weakness
-ate, -ate(d)	use, action, having the form of, possessing
-betes	to go
-blast	immature cell, germ cell, embryonic cell
-body	body
-cele	hernia, tumor, swelling
-centesis	surgical puncture
-ceps	head
-cide	to kill
-clasia	a breaking
-clasis	crushing, breaking up
-clysis	injection
-cope	strike
-crine	to secrete
-crit	to separate
-culture	cultivation
-cusis	hearing
-cuspid	point
-cyesis	pregnancy
-cyst	bladder, sac
-cyte	cell
-derma	skin
-dermis	skin
-desis	binding
-dipsia	thirst
-drome	course
-dynia	pain, ache
-eal	pertaining to
-ectasia	dilatation
-ectasis	dilatation, dilation, stretching, expansion
-ectasy	dilation
-ectomy	surgical excision, surgical removal, resection
-edema	swelling
-emesis	vomiting
-emia	blood condition
-er	relating to, one who
-ergy	work

-esis	condition
-esthesia	feeling
-form	shape
-fuge	to flee
-gen	formation, produce
-genes	produce
-genesis	formation, produce
-genic	formation, produce
-glia	glue
-globin	protein
-gnosis	knowledge
-grade	step
-graft	pencil, grafting knife
-gram	weight, mark, record
-graph	to write, record, instrument for recording
-graphy	recording
-hexia	condition
-ia	condition
-iasis	condition
-iatrics	treatment
-iatry	treatment
-ic	pertaining to
-ician	specialist, physician
-icle	small, minute
-ide	having a particular quality
-ile	pertaining to
-in	substance
-ine	pertaining to, substance
-ing	quality of
-ion	process
-ior	pertaining to
-is	pertaining to
-ism	condition
-ist	one who specializes, agent
-itis	inflammation
-ity	condition
-ive	nature of, quality of
-ize	to make, to treat or combine with
-kinesia	motion, movement
-kinesis	motion, movement
-lalia	to talk
-lemma	sheath, rind
-lepsy	seizure
-lexia	diction, word, phrase
-liter	liter
-lith	stone
-logy	study of
-lucent	to shine
-lymph	clear fluid, serum, pale fluid
-lysis	destruction, separation, breakdown, loosening, dissolution
-malacia	softening
-mania	madness
-megaly	enlargement, large
-meter	instrument to measure
-metry	measurement
-mnesia	memory
-morph	form, shape
-noia	mind
-oid	resemble, like, similar
-ole	opening, small
-oma	tumor, mass, fluid collection
-on	pertaining to
-one	hormone
-opaque	dark, nontransparent
-opia	sight, vision
-opsia	sight, vision
-opsy	to view
-or	one who, doer
-orexia	appetite
-ose	pertaining to
-osis	condition
-ous	pertaining to
-oxia	oxygen
-paresis	weakness
-pathy	disease, emotion
-penia	lack of, deficiency, abnormal reduction
-pepsia	to digest, digestion
-pexy	surgical fixation
-phagia	to eat, to swallow

ASO	antistreptolysin O
ASPD	advanced sleep phase disorder
AST	aspartate aminotransferase
AT/RT	atypical teratoid rhabdoid tumor
AV	atrioventricular
ax	axillary

B

Ba	barium
BAC	blood alcohol concentration
baso	basophil
BC	bone conduction
BCC	basal cell carcinoma
BDD	body dysmorphic disorder
BE	Barrett esophagus; below elbow; barium enema
BG	blood glucose
BK	below knee
BM	bowel movement
BMD	bone mineral density (test)
BMI	body mass index
BMR	basal metabolic rate
BP	blood pressure
BPH	benign prostatic hyperplasia (hypertrophy)
BUN	blood urea nitrogen
Bx	biopsy

C

C	centigrade; Celsius
C1, C2, etc.	first cervical vertebra; second cervical vertebra
CA	cancer
CA-125	cancer antigen 125
Ca	calcium
CABG	coronary artery bypass graft
CAD	coronary artery disease
CAPD	continuous ambulatory peritoneal dialysis
CAT	computerized axial tomography
CBC	complete blood count
CBT	cognitive-behavioral therapy
CC	cardiac catheterization; chief complaint; clean catch (urine)
CD	Crohn disease
CDC	Centers for Disease Control and Prevention
CEA	carcinoembryonic antigen
CF	cystic fibrosis
CGN	chronic glomerulonephritis
CHD	coronary heart disease
chemo	chemotherapy
CHF	congestive heart failure
CHO	carbohydrate
chol	cholesterol
Ci	curie
CIN	cervical intraepithelial neoplasia
CK	creatine kinase
CKD	chronic kidney disease
CLI	critical limb ischemia
CLIA	clinical laboratory improvement amendments
CLL	chronic lymphocytic leukemia
cm	centimeter
CMP	cardiomyopathy; comprehensive metabolic panel
CMV	cytomegalovirus
CMS	Centers for Medicare & Medicaid Services
CNS	central nervous system
c/o	complains of
CO	cardiac output
CO_2	carbon dioxide
COCs	combined oral contraceptives

COPD	chronic obstructive pulmonary disease
CP	cerebral palsy
CRF	corticotropin-releasing factor
CRP	C-reactive protein blood test
CS, C-section	cesarean section
CSF	cerebrospinal fluid
CT	computed tomography
CTA	clear to auscultation
CTE	chronic traumatic encephalopathy
CV	cardiovascular
CVA	cerebrovascular accident (stroke)
CVS	chorionic villus sampling; computer vision syndrome
CXR	chest x-ray
cysto	cystoscopic examination; cystoscopy

D

D&C	dilation (dilatation) and curettage
db, Db	decibel
DBS	deep brain stimulation
DCIS	ductal carcinoma in situ
decub	decubitus
Derm	dermatology
DHT	dihydrotestosterone
DI	diabetes insipidus
diff	differential count (white blood cells)
DM	diabetes mellitus
DMARDs	disease-modifying antirheumatic drugs
DMD	Duchenne muscular dystrophy
DNA	deoxyribonucleic acid; does not apply
DOB	date of birth
DOT	directly observed therapy
Dr.	doctor
DRE	digital rectal examination
DSM-5	*Diagnostic and Statistical Manual of Mental Disorders*, Fifth Edition
DSPS	delayed sleep phase syndrome
DUB	dysfunctional uterine bleeding
DVT	deep vein thrombosis
Dx	diagnosis
DXA	dual-energy X-ray absorptiometry scan

E

ECC	extracorporeal circulation
ECG, EKG	electrocardiogram
ECHO	echocardiogram
ECT	electroconvulsive therapy
ED	erectile dysfunction
EE	erosive esophagitis
EEG	electroencephalogram
EF	ejection fraction
EHR	electronic health record
EHT	estrogen hormone therapy
ELISA	enzyme-linked immunosorbent assay
EM	emmetropia
EMG	electromyography
ENG	electronystagmography
ENT	ear, nose, throat (otorhinolaryngology)
eos, eosin	eosinophil
EPS	electrophysiology study (intracardiac)
ER	emergency room; endoplasmic reticulum
ERCP	endoscopic retrograde cholangiopancreatography
ERT	external radiation therapy
ERV	expiratory reserve volume
ESR, sed rate	erythrocyte sedimentation rate

ESRD	end-stage renal disease
ESWL	extracorporeal shockwave lithotripsy
ET	esotropia; endotracheal
ETS	environmental tobacco smoke
Ex	examination

F

F	Fahrenheit; female
FBG	fasting blood glucose
FBS	fasting blood sugar
FDA	Food and Drug Administration
FFA	free fatty acids
FH	family history
FHB	fetal heartbeat
FIV	forced inspiratory volume
FMS	fibromyalgia syndrome
FNA	fine-needle aspiration
FP	family practice
FRC	forced residual capacity
FROM	full range of motion
FSH	follicle-stimulating hormone
FTA-ABS	fluorescent treponemal antibody absorption
F-V loop	flow volume loop
Fx	fracture

G

g	gram
GAD	generalized anxiety disorder
GB	gallbladder
GBS	group B streptococcus
GC	gonorrhea
GCS	Glasgow coma scale
GERD	gastroesophageal reflux disease
GFR	glomerular filtration rate
GGT	gamma-glutamyl transferase
GH	growth hormone
GHRF	growth hormone–releasing factor
GI	gastrointestinal
GnRF	gonadotropin-releasing factor
grav I	pregnancy one
GTT	glucose tolerance test
GU	genitourinary
GYN	gynecology

H

H_2O	water
H&E	hematoxylin and eosin
H&L	heart & lungs
HAART	highly active antiretroviral therapy
HAV	hepatitis A virus
HBIG	hepatitis B immune globulin
HBP	high blood pressure
HB_SA	hepatitis B surface antigen
HBV	hepatitis B virus
hCG	human chorionic gonadotropin
HCl	hydrochloric acid
HCO_3	bicarbonate
Hct, HCT	hematocrit
HCV	hepatitis C virus
HD	hearing distance; Hodgkin disease; hemodialysis
HDL	high-density lipoprotein
HDS	herniated disk syndrome
HDV	hepatitis D virus
HER-2/neu	human epidermal growth factor receptor–2
HEV	hepatitis E virus
HF	heart failure
Hg	mercury
Hgb, HGB, Hb	hemoglobin
HHS	Health and Human Services (Department of)
HI-ART	highly integrated adaptive radiotherapy

HIPAA	Health Insurance Portability and Accountability Act
HIV	human immunodeficiency virus
HMD	hyaline membrane disease
HNP	herniated nucleus pulposus
HPV	human papillomavirus
HSG	hysterosalpingography
HSV	herpes simplex virus
HSV-2	herpes simplex virus–2
HT	hormone therapy
Ht	height
HTLV	human T-cell leukemia-lymphoma virus
HTN	hypertension
HUD	humanitarian use device
Hx	history
Hy	hyperopia
Hz	cycles/seconds

I

IBD	inflammatory bowel disease
IBS	irritable bowel syndrome
IC	interstitial cystitis; inspiratory capacity
ICD	International Classification of Diseases
ICP	intracranial pressure
ID	intradermal
IDDM	insulin-dependent diabetes mellitus
Ig	immunoglobulin
IM	intramuscular
IMRT	intensity-modulated radiation therapy
IOL	intraocular lens
IOP	intraocular pressure
IPD	intermittent peritoneal dialysis
IQ	intelligence quotient
IR	interventional radiology
IRDS	infant respiratory distress syndrome
IRT	internal radiation therapy
IRV	inspiratory reserve volume
IUD	intrauterine device
IV	intravenous
IVP	intravenous pyelogram

J

jt	joint

K

K	potassium
kg	kilogram
KS	Kaposi sarcoma
KUB	kidney, ureter, and bladder

L

L1, L2, etc.	first lumbar vertebra, second lumbar vertebra, etc.
L	liter
LA	left atrium
LAT, lat	lateral
LCIS	lobular carcinoma in situ
LD, LDH	lactate dehydrogenase
LDL	low-density lipoprotein
LES	lower esophageal sphincter
LH	luteinizing hormone
lig	ligament
LLQ	left lower quadrant
LMP	last menstrual period
LP	lumbar puncture
LPI	laser peripheral iridotomy
LTH	lactogenic hormone
LUQ	left upper quadrant
LV	left ventricle
LVEF	left-ventricular ejection fraction
lymphs	lymphocytes

M

MALT	mucosa-associated lymphoid tissue (lymphoma)
MAOIs	monoamine oxidase inhibitors
MBPS	Munchausen-by-proxy syndrome
mcg	microgram
mCi	millicurie
MD	medical doctor; muscular dystrophy
MDR TB	multidrug-resistant tuberculosis
MG	myasthenia gravis
mg	milligram (0.001 gram)
MHI	mild head injury
MHT	minor head trauma
MI	myocardial infarction
MIF	melanocyte-stimulating hormone release-inhibiting factor
mL, ml	milliliter (0.001 liter)
mm	millimeter (0.001 meter; 0.039 inch)
MMPI-2	Minnesota Multiphasic Personality Inventory–2
MPD	mammary Paget disease
MRF	melanocyte-stimulating hormone–releasing factor
MRI	magnetic resonance imaging
MS	mitral stenosis; multiple sclerosis; musculoskeletal
MSH	melanocyte-stimulating hormone
MTBI	mild traumatic brain injury
MV	mitral valve
MVP	mitral valve prolapse
MVV	maximal voluntary ventilation
MY	myopia

N

Na	sodium
NaCl	sodium chloride
N&V	nausea and vomiting
NCI	National Cancer Institute
Neuro	neurology
NG	nasogastric (tube)
NGU	nongonococcal urethritis
NH_3	ammonia
NHL	non-Hodgkin lymphoma
NIDDM	non-insulin-dependent diabetes mellitus
NIH	National Institutes of Health
NIMH	National Institute of Mental Health
NINDS	National Institute of Neurological Disorders and Stroke
NK	natural killer (cells)
NKDA	no known drug allergies
NPO, npo	nothing by mouth
NRDS	neonatal respiratory distress syndrome
NREM	no rapid eye movement (sleep)
NSAIDs	nonsteroidal anti-inflammatory drugs
NSSC	normal size, shape, and consistency
NST	nonstress test
NSTEMI	non-ST-segment elevation myocardial infarction

O

O, O_2	oxygen
O&P	ova and parasites
OA	osteoarthritis
OB	obstetrics
OCD	obsessive–compulsive disorder
OIC	opioid-induced constipation
OM	otitis media
OP	outpatient
OPCAB	off-pump coronary artery bypass surgery
OR	operating room

Orth, ortho	orthopedics; orthopaedics
OTC	over-the-counter
OV	office visit
oz	ounce

P

P	pulse; phosphorus
PA	posteroanterior
PAD	peripheral artery disease
Pap	Papanicolaou (smear)
Path	pathology
Pb	lead
PBI	protein bound iodine
PCS	procedure coding system
PD	Parkinson disease
PDD-NOS	pervasive developmental disorder not otherwise specified
PDT	photodynamic therapy
PE	physical examination; pulmonary embolism
Peds	pediatrics
PET	positron emission tomography
pH	hydrogen ion concentration
PID	pelvic inflammatory disease
PIF	prolactin release-inhibiting factor
PIH	pregnancy-induced hypertension
PJP	*Pneumocystis jiroveci* pneumonia
PMS	premenstrual syndrome
PNS	peripheral nervous system
PO	orally, by mouth
PP	postprandial (after meals)
PPD	purified protein derivative (TB test)
PPIs	proton pump inhibitors
PrEP	pre-exposure prophylaxis
PRF	prolactin-releasing factor
PRL	prolactin hormone
PRN, prn	as necessary; as required; when necessary; as needed
PSA	prostate-specific antigen
Psych	psychiatry; psychology
PT	prothrombin time
PTCA	percutaneous transluminal coronary angioplasty
PTH	parathyroid hormone (parathormone)
PTSD	posttraumatic stress disorder
PTT	partial thromboplastin time
PUBS	percutaneous umbilical blood sampling
PUD	peptic ulcer disease
PUL	percutaneous ultrasonic lithotropsy

Q

q	every (quaque)
q2h	every 2 hours
q4h	every 4 hours
qh	every hour
qid	four times a day
qm	every morning (quaque mane)
qns	quantity not sufficient
qs	quantity sufficient
qt	quart

R

R	respiration
R, rt	right
RA	right atrium; rheumatoid arthritis
Ra	radium
rad	radiation absorbed dose
RAIU	radioactive iodine uptake
RBC(s)	red blood cell(s); red blood cell (count)
RD	respiratory disease
RDS	respiratory distress syndrome
REM	rapid eye movement (sleep)
RF	rheumatoid factor

Rh Rhesus blood factor (Rh+ or Rh–)
RIA radioimmunoassay
RLF retrolental fibroplasia
RLQ right lower quadrant
RNA ribonucleic acid
R/O rule out
ROM range of motion
RP retrograde pyelography
RSV respiratory syncytial virus
RUQ right upper quadrant
RV right ventricle; residual volume
RVEF right ventricular ejection fraction
Rx take thou; prescribe; treatment; therapy

S

SA sinoatrial (node)
SAD seasonal affective disorder
SARS severe acute respiratory syndrome
SCA sudden cardiac arrest
SCC squamous cell carcinoma
SCD sudden cardiac death
SDs standard deviations
SG skin graft
SLT selective laser trabeculoplasty
SNRI serotonin-norepinephrine reuptake inhibitor
SOAP subjective, objective, assessment, plan
SOB shortness of breath
sp. gr specific gravity
SSD somatic symptom disorder
SSRIs selective serotonin reuptake inhibitors
St stage (of disease)
staph staphylococcus
STEMI ST-segment elevation myocardial infarction
STH somatotropin hormone
STIs sexually transmitted infections
strep streptococcus

T

T1, T2, etc. thoracic vertebrae first, thoracic vertebrae second, etc.
T_3 triiodothyronine
T_3U triiodothyronine uptake
T_4 thyroxine
T temperature
TAH-BSO total abdominal hysterectomy with bilateral salpingo-oophorectomy
TAT Thematic Apperception Test
TB tuberculosis
TBSA total body surface area
TC testicular cancer
TCAs tricyclic antidepressants
TENS transcutaneous electrical nerve stimulation
TH thyroid hormone
TIA transient ischemic attacks
tid three times a day
TIMs topical immunomodulators
TIPS transjugular intrahepatic portosystemic shunt
TIS tumor in situ
TLC tender loving care; total lung capacity
TM tympanic membrane
TNF tumor necrosis factor

TOF	tetralogy of Fallot
TORCH	toxoplasmosis, rubella, cytomegalovirus, herpes simplex virus
TPA, tPA	tissue plasminogen activator
TPR	temperature, pulse, respiration
TRH	thyrotropin-releasing hormone
TSE	testicular self-exam
TSH	thyroid-stimulating hormone
TSS	toxic shock syndrome
TUIP	transurethral incision of the prostate
TUMT	transurethral microwave thermotherapy
TUNA	transurethral needle ablation
TUR	transurethral resection
TURP	transurethral resection of the prostate
TV	tidal volume
Tx	traction

U

UA	urinalysis
UC	ulcerative colitis
UE	unconjugated estriol
UG	urogenital
UGI	upper gastrointestinal
URI	upper respiratory infection
US	ultrasound
UTI	urinary tract infection
UV	ultraviolet

V

VA	visual acuity
VAD	vacuum-assisted needle biopsy device
VC	vital capacity
VCD	vacuum constriction device
VD	venereal disease
VDRL	Venereal Disease Research Laboratory (syphilis test)
VLDL	very low-density lipoprotein
VP	vasopressin
VS, V/S	vital signs
VSD	ventricular septal defect

W

WAIS-R	Wechsler Adult Intelligence Scale–Revised
WBC	white blood cell; white blood (cell) count
WHO	World Health Organization
WNL	within normal limits
Wt	weight

X

XR	x-ray
XT	exotropia

Y

y/o	year(s) old
YOB	year of birth
yr	year

E

F

G

H

S